HANDBOOK OF DIAGNOSTIC IMAGING

VOLUME 3

ADVANCED IMAGING TECHNOLOGIES AND CLINICAL APPLICATIONS

Dr. José Abraham Amaya Duarte

ALLIED HEALTH PRESS

Handbook of Diagnostic Imaging Volume 3

Advanced Imaging Technologies and Clinical Applications

Author: **Dr. José Abraham Amaya Duarte**

Allied Health Press
4164 Lakeshore Road
Burlington ON L7L 1A4
Canada
www.alliedhealthpress.com
Email: orders@arclereducation.com

ISBN: 978-1-77956-867-0

Allied Health Press publishes wide variety of books and eBooks. For more information about Allied Health Press and its products, visit our website at www.alliedhealthpress.com

ABOUT THE AUTHOR

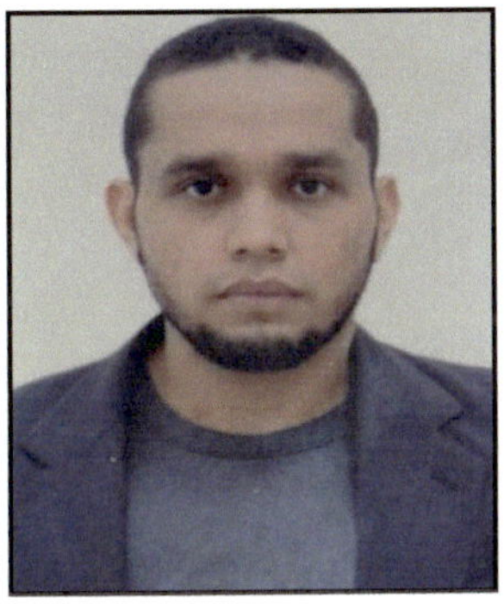

Dr. José Abraham Amaya Duarte is a radiologist with extensive clinical and academic experience in diagnostic imaging, advanced image interpretation, and image-guided procedures. His expertise includes ultrasound, computed tomography (CT), magnetic resonance imaging (MRI), and radiography across a broad range of clinical applications.

He earned his Doctor of Medicine and Surgery degree from the Universidad Nacional Autónoma de Nicaragua (UNAN-León) and completed his specialization in Diagnostic Imaging at the Universidad de Defensa de Nicaragua (UDENIC). To further enhance his expertise, Dr. Amaya pursued advanced subspecialty training in musculoskeletal, neuro, and women's imaging, and is currently completing a Master's degree in Obstetric and Gynecologic Ultrasound.

Dr. Amaya currently serves as a Radiology and Imaging Specialist at Sugar City Medical Center in Belize, where he provides comprehensive diagnostic evaluations and supports multidisciplinary clinical teams. His professional background also includes academic instruction, pediatric medicine, and international teleradiology services for hospitals and clinics worldwide.

A dedicated educator and researcher, Dr. Amaya's professional focus lies in improving diagnostic accuracy, clinical workflow, and imaging quality through continuous education and collaboration. His commitment to excellence and his contributions to clinical radiology continue to advance the field across Latin America and beyond.

Brief Table of Contents

Detailed Table of Contents

CHAPTER 5

Image-Guided Biopsy and Ablation Techniques 119

CHAPTER 6

3D Reconstruction, Printing, and Virtual Reality in Medical Imaging 147

LIST OF FIGURES

PREFACE

Medical imaging has transformed healthcare by providing noninvasive insights into the human body, enabling precise diagnosis and guiding therapeutic interventions. Over the past decades, innovations in detector technology, signal processing, and computational power have driven leaps in image resolution, contrast, and speed. Clinicians now rely on a spectrum of modalities—from X-ray and ultrasound to magnetic resonance and positron emission tomography—to characterize anatomy, physiology, and pathology with unprecedented clarity. These capabilities have not only improved disease detection but also enriched our understanding of complex conditions, from vascular anomalies to metabolic dysfunctions.

As patient populations age and the demand for personalized care grows, there is mounting pressure to further refine imaging techniques. Enhancements in spectral imaging, quantitative analysis, and data integration are enabling clinicians to distinguish subtle variations in tissue composition, track disease progression, and predict treatment response. Concurrently, the integration of real-time imaging and minimally invasive approaches has expanded the role of image guidance in procedures, reducing patient risk and shortening recovery times. The convergence of technological progress and clinical need continues to reshape diagnostic protocols, setting new standards for safety, efficiency, and patient comfort.

Handbook of Diagnostic Imaging – Volume 3 offers a comprehensive survey of the latest developments in advanced imaging technologies. This volume brings together contributions from leading experts who translate complex physics and engineering principles into practical guidance for radiologists, technologists, and researchers. Organized to facilitate both learning and reference, the book balances foundational concepts with clinical applications, helping practitioners incorporate cutting-edge tools into their daily practice.

Chapter 1 presents advanced CT techniques, focusing on dual-energy and photon-counting methodologies. It begins with a refresher on computed tomography principles and traces the evolution from conventional CT to modern spectral approaches. Detailed sections then explain how dual-energy CT distinguishes materials based on their energy-dependent attenuation profiles, followed by an exploration of photon-counting detectors that offer superior contrast resolution and dose efficiency. Technical innovations in detector design, image reconstruction software, and the integration of artificial intelligence are highlighted, along with a balanced discussion of implementation challenges, patient safety considerations, and cost factors.

Chapter 2 focuses on functional MRI and diffusion imaging, modalities that probe tissue physiology and microstructure. The text explains the mechanisms behind blood-oxygen-level-dependent contrast and diffusion tensor imaging, emphasizing their strengths and limitations in mapping neural activity and white-matter connectivity. Clinical applications include pre-surgical planning for brain tumors, assessment of neurological and psychiatric disorders, stroke diagnosis, and monitoring of neurodegenerative disease. The chapter concludes by outlining prospective directions in neuroimaging, such as combined fMRI-diffusion protocols and personalized diagnostic workflows.

Chapter 3 presents hybrid imaging systems—PET/CT and PET/MRI—that merge metabolic and anatomical information. It begins with the basics of positron emission tomography, covering radiotracer chemistry and quantitative imaging metrics. Fundamental CT and MRI principles are then reviewed before delving into the technical integration that enables simultaneous acquisition. Comparative discussions highlight the advantages of each hybrid modality in oncology staging, cardiac viability studies, and neuroimaging, supported by illustrative case studies. Practical considerations regarding system calibration, workflow optimization, and reimbursement issues are also addressed.

Chapter 4 covers molecular and cellular imaging modalities that visualize biological processes at the microscopic level. After introducing the core concepts of molecular imaging and contrast agent design, the chapter explores optical techniques such as fluorescence and bioluminescence imaging, as well as near-infrared approaches. Ultrasound methods are then examined, with emphasis on high-frequency probes and targeted microbubble agents. Clinical applications range from early cancer detection to assessment of therapeutic response, with summaries of sensitivity, spatial resolution, and safety profiles for each modality.

Chapter 5 explores image-guided biopsy and ablation techniques for diagnosing and treating lesions with precision. The text describes fine-needle aspiration, core needle biopsy, and vacuum-assisted methods, outlining indications for tumor diagnosis, lymph node evaluation, and assessment of inflammatory disease. It then reviews ablation tools—radiofrequency, microwave, and cryoablation—detailing procedure planning, energy delivery parameters, and strategies for minimizing complications. Risk management sections provide guidelines for patient selection, periprocedural care, and post-procedure monitoring.

Chapter 6 describes 3D reconstruction, printing, and virtual reality applications in medical imaging. The chapter explains algorithms for volumetric rendering and mesh generation, then surveys biocompatible materials and additive manufacturing techniques for creating anatomical models and surgical guides. Virtual reality platforms for immersive training and patient education are introduced, with evidence on their impact on surgical planning and communication. Integration workflows that connect imaging data to physical and virtual models are discussed, along with regulatory, ethical, and financial considerations.

Chapter 7 examines artificial intelligence and machine learning in diagnostic imaging, highlighting current and emerging applications. Sections cover automated image analysis, anomaly detection algorithms, and the integration of AI into radiology reporting systems. Discussions address performance metrics, challenges in obtaining high-quality training data, and strategies to mitigate algorithmic bias. Ethical topics such as accountability in AI-assisted diagnoses and informed consent are explored. Future trends include advances in deep learning and models that adapt dynamically to individual patient characteristics.

Chapter 8 covers quantitative imaging biomarkers and radiomics, a field that transforms images into high-dimensional data for decision support. The chapter outlines principles of feature extraction, model building, and validation. Oncology applications include tumor characterization, response assessment, and prognostic modeling. Neurology sections focus on biomarkers for stroke, multiple sclerosis, and neurodegenerative diseases. Challenges such as protocol standardization and data sharing frameworks are examined, followed by prospects for integrating genomic and imaging data in precision medicine.

Chapter 9 outlines teleradiology workflows and quality assurance processes that enable remote image interpretation. The chapter reviews the historical evolution of teleradiology services, then details protocols for image acquisition, secure transmission, and report delivery. Technology platforms are evaluated for interoperability, user interfaces, and cybersecurity measures. Quality assurance guidelines from accreditation bodies are summarized, with recommendations for continuous performance monitoring, peer review, and error reduction.

Chapter 10 addresses radiation protection regulations and accreditation standards governing imaging practices. The text surveys national and international guidelines on dose limits, equipment certification, and facility accreditation. It explains the accreditation process for imaging centers and the role of professional organizations in maintaining safety and quality. Discussions cover the impact of regulatory changes on training requirements, risk management strategies, and implementation challenges as imaging technology advances.

Intended for radiologists, imaging technologists, medical physicists, and trainees in these fields, this volume serves as both an educational resource and a practical reference. Readers will find guidance on selecting appropriate modalities, optimizing protocols, and interpreting advanced imaging results to support clinical decision-making and research.

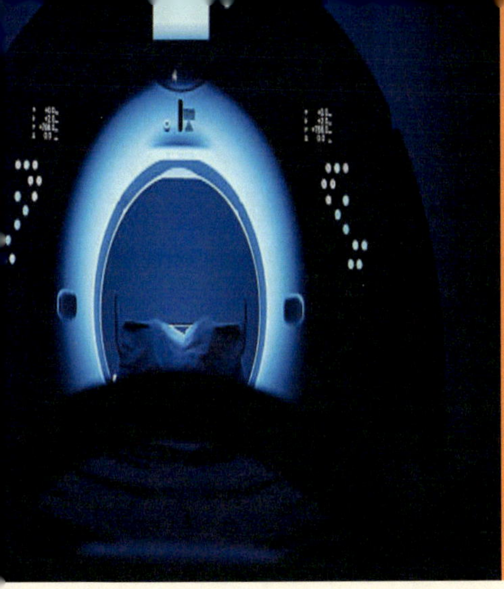

Chapter 1

ADVANCED CT TECHNIQUES: DUAL-ENERGY AND PHOTON-COUNTING

Contents

Introduction

The development of computed tomography (CT) has revolutionized diagnostic imaging with great increases in accuracy and efficiency. Older CT methods have used single-energy X-rays for years, handicapping their ability to differentiate among various materials within a scan. More recent improvements like dual-energy CT and photon-counting detectors have become a strong methodology that has the potential to break through these limitations. By applying various X-ray energies, dual-energy CT can differentiate between materials based on electron density and atomic number, enabling more comprehensive material characterization. It has the added benefit of offering new possibilities for clinicians to obtain important information about complex medical disorders and to plan treatment in the process. The introduction of photon-counting detectors represents a qualitative leap in image quality and diagnostic capability (Figure 1.1).

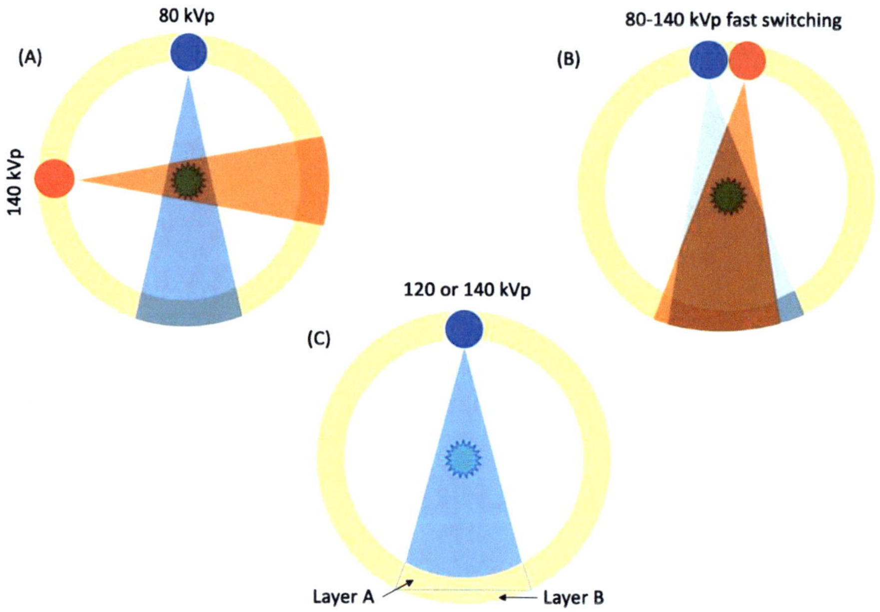

Figure 1.1. Illustrations showing the main DECT scanning techniques in clinical use. (A) Dual-source DECT, consisting of two-source X-ray tubes and the corresponding detectors; (B) Single-source DECT consisting of a single tube with rapid kVp switching; and (C) Detector-based DECT consisting of a single source and a dual-layer detector to obtain low- and high-energy spectra.

Source: https://www.mdpi.com/2313-433X/8/9/236.

In contrast to conventional energy-integrating detectors, photon-counting technology can detect and identify X-ray photons by energy level and then provide better spatial resolution with reduced image noise. This has been particularly useful for applications requiring very high-resolution imaging, such as musculoskeletal assessments and imaging of hard, mineralized structures. Besides that, the native spectral imaging capability of photon-counting detectors enables precise discrimination of specific materials and thus better visualization of disease. The technology's promise lies in its ability to merge multiple imaging capabilities into a single system with superior overall diagnostic performance. With continued advances in advanced CT technology, the clinical applications of dual-energy and photon-counting technologies are being pursued more vigorously. In musculoskeletal imaging, for instance, hybrid modalities through combining CT with other imaging modalities, such as MRI, demonstrate synergistic effects to offer complete evaluations. Dual-energy CT's ability to differentiate crystal deposits and evaluate metal hardware is a good example of its clinical usefulness. Further, ongoing research highlights the potential applications of photon-counting CT in high-resolution performance imaging processes involving the monitoring of soft tissue diseases and the assessment of intricate fractures. With more preclinical and clinical validations to emerge, the promise of these innovative CT technologies to enhance diagnostic imaging can undoubtedly lead to significant improvements in patient treatment and therapy.

1.1. Fundamentals of Computed Tomography

Computed tomography (CT) evolution has been driven by the need for better imaging techniques that can overcome the limitations of traditional techniques. One way forward in this evolution is the development of newer techniques such as dual-energy computed tomography (DECT). DECT uses two energy tiers to capture images, and from these it can differentiate between materials based on atomic content. This capability is particularly valuable in fields such as medicine and materials science, where discovering specific substances is crucial. In the microelectronics industry, for instance, DECT can effectively examine materials and detect defects in components containing elements with both high and low atomic numbers. This technology makes it possible to improve diagnostic accuracy and patient care, ultimately helping to improve clinical decision-making and treatment protocols. The integration of DECT into standard CT platforms is a milestone in the ongoing pursuit of accurate imaging. In addition to DECT, photon-counting CT is another innovative technique to enhance imaging performance. Unlike the standard CT systems that measure the overall X-ray intensity, photon-counting detectors measure individual X-ray photons and hence provide improved energy resolution and improved image quality. This resolution at the high level is especially valuable while distinguishing between various types of tissues or materials, particularly in complicated anatomical structures. This photon-counting technology provides better quantification of contrast agents, supporting improved diagnosis and treatment monitoring. Moreover, the relatively higher dose reduction ability without sacrificing quality demonstrates this as an up-and-coming technology for application in clinical settings where patient protection is of the highest priority. As the medical community continues to focus on reducing radiation exposure, photon-counting CT is an exciting solution. The limitations posed by high metal content in imaging, as typically found in electronic components, highlight the need for constant innovation in CT technology. Conventional CT methods often fail to produce clear images in the presence of metallic artifacts, leading to misdiagnosis or missed defects. As suggested in contemporary literature, integrating energy-sensitive methods into computed tomography can address most of these concerns. By leveraging energy data within projection data, novel applications can enhance image quality and enable better characterization of defects, especially in the microelectronics industry (Hasn, 2023). These innovations underscore the benefits of adopting multi-faceted measures, such as dual-energy methods and photon-counting detectors, to push the edge in medical imaging. Lastly, developing solutions to overcome such limitations will enhance diagnostic capabilities and improve patient care across numerous clinical applications (Ståhl et al., 2023).

1.1.1. Basic Principles of CT Imaging

CT imaging is based on X-ray technology, in which multiple X-rays are acquired from various angles around an object and later reconstructed to create cross-sectional images, or slices, of the body. The method relies on the differential absorption of X-rays by different tissues, which is critical in differentiating structures based on density. The reconstructed images have a high-resolution representation of anatomical features, and hence, CT is very helpful in the diagnosis of conditions with high-contrast structures such as bone. By creating accurate, three-dimensional images, CT imaging enhances diagnostic quality in challenging cases. It is a basic imaging modality that forms the foundation for advanced techniques such as dual-energy and photon-counting CT (Figure 1.2).

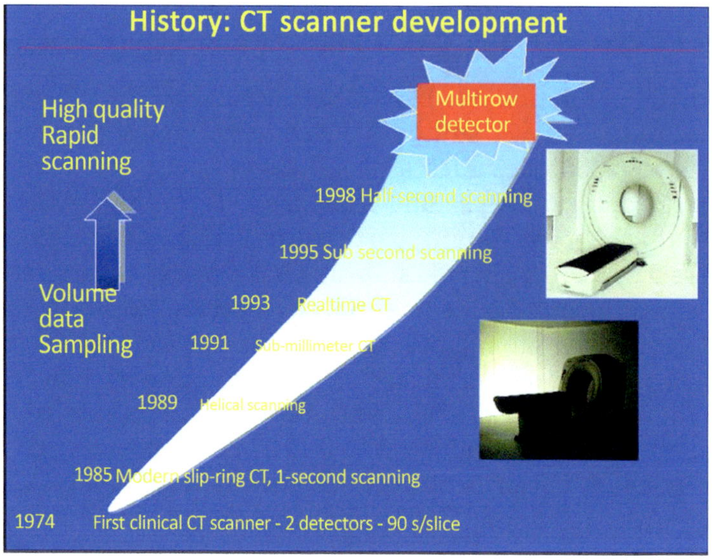

Figure 1.2. CT history.

Source: https://thecommonvein.com/wp-content/uploads/2023/03/web-CT-018.jpg.

The evolution of CT technology has greatly influenced its applications and functionality, especially with the innovation of dual-energy CT. The technology allows images to be captured at two different energy levels simultaneously, thereby enhancing the ability to differentiate between materials based on their atomic structure. Dual-energy CT exploits this idea to provide improved tissue characterization and contrast resolution, particularly in cases with overlapping materials, such as the separation of different types of kidney stones or the assessment of vascular structures. With two energy levels being employed, the technique can offer spectral information that gets beyond the majority of restrictions for usual CT imaging, thereby opening up possibilities for improved diagnostic insight and a more personalized approach to imaging disease. One of the recent developments in CT imaging is the development of photon-counting detectors (PCDs), an advancement in the imaging ability. Unlike conventional energy-integrating detectors, PCDs offer greater spatial sensitivity and resolution through individual photon counting, resulting in reduced noise and improved image quality. This PCD technology application area is particularly important in musculoskeletal imaging, where high-resolution imaging is critical for assessing fine details, such as bone health and fine crystal deposits. PCD introduction paves the way for a plethora of applications from low-dose whole-body imaging to intricate spectral imaging. With ongoing advancements in research, validation, and implementation of these innovative techniques, the potential of CT imaging can be further enhanced, which can ultimately improve patient outcomes and optimize diagnostic processes (Becce et al., 2024).

1.1.2. Historical Development of CT Technology

The history of CT technology has profoundly transformed medical diagnostic imaging ever since its introduction. From its beginnings in the early 1970s with Allan Cormack and Godfrey Hounsfield, CT has grown from rudimentary techniques to advanced methods that significantly enhance the diagnostic value. Early on, CT had only limited resolution and was primarily used in brain scanning, producing cross-sectional images that revolutionized cerebral lesion detection. The technical trajectory took a giant step in the 1980s with spiral (or helical) CT, which enabled continuous rotation of the X-ray tube and faster image acquisition. This led to the development of multi-slice CT systems that opened the prospect of simultaneous image acquisition across multiple slices and thus extended its application to thoracic and abdominal imaging, in addition to neurology. Advancements in CT technology also continued in the 21st century, the most prominent being dual-energy CT, which has continued to push diagnostic accuracy. It is a technique in which two energies are imaged simultaneously, which improves discrimination of various tissue types based on their atomic number and density. For instance, dual-energy CT is particularly useful for imaging coronary artery calcification and plaque characterization, which will benefit understanding of atherosclerosis. Examinations revealed that standard CT has low spatial resolution and blooming artifacts, which make precise characterization of coronary artery narrowing impossible. With the inclusion of the additional information obtained using dual-energy imaging, clinicians gain a more comprehensive knowledge of their patients' vascular health and can modify treatment with improved effectiveness, thus also constituting evidence for ongoing advances in CT technology within healthcare practice (Figure 1.3).

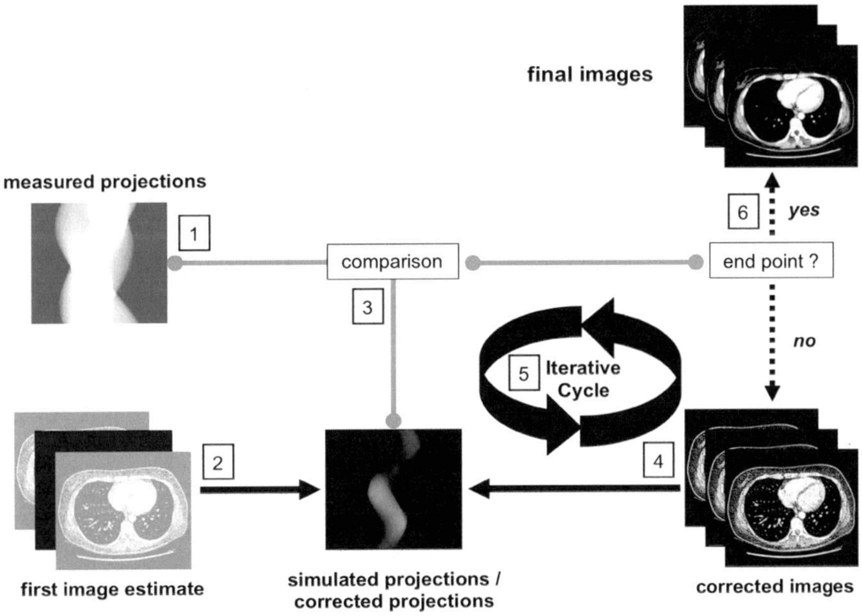

Figure 1.3. The process of iterative image reconstruction algorithms.

Source: https://www.researchgate.net/profile/Siiri-Rautio-2/publication/335757447/figure/fig7/AS:802237920051212@1568279833959/The-process-of-iterative-image-reconstruction-algorithms-28.jpg.

With the advancement in CT technology, the dawn of photon-counting CT has arrived as a new horizon of innovation in imaging. Photon-counting detectors have the potential to revolutionize image acquisition by increasing sensitivity and resolution while reducing radiation exposure.

This is particularly critical in patients requiring repeated imaging, particularly in chronic conditions where early assessment is crucial. Latest advances in computing methods, such as iterative reconstruction algorithms, also provide improved image quality alongside efficient radiation dose management. Such technologies enable a paradigm shift towards more precise diagnosis, particularly cardiovascular imaging. The growing emphasis on quantifying coronary artery disease through measures such as coronary calcium scoring and plaque severity assessment demonstrates the potential of newer CT techniques not only to improve diagnostic capability but also to provide prognostic data that guide patient management. With these ongoing innovations, CT continues to be at the forefront of diagnostic imaging, driving further clinical insights and better patient outcomes across a variety of healthcare settings (Ananthasubramaniam et al., 2017; Boi et al., 2024).

1.1.3. Comparison of Traditional and Advanced CT Techniques

The evolution of CT has significantly transformed imaging procedures, particularly through the introduction of sophisticated techniques. Standard CT methods have traditionally been based on energy-integrating detectors (EIDs), which provide full imaging via traditional X-ray attenuation. Effective as they are, they do have some limitations, mainly regarding spectral resolution and controlling noise. Specifically, EIDs face the challenge of distinguishing between materials with the same atomic numbers, leading to diagnostic uncertainties, notably in musculoskeletal imaging. Conversely, new technologies such as dual-energy CT have revolutionized the field by allowing clinicians to acquire images at two energy levels. This enables improved material differentiation, allowing accurate characterization of pathologies such as gout or infection by distinguishing calcified tissues from adjacent structures, thereby improving diagnostic accuracy in clinics (Becce et al., 2024). Another revolutionary CT technological advancement is the appearance of PCDs. While conventional EIDs detect all impinging photons and sum them into an image, the individual photons are counted separately in PCDs, yielding several remarkable advantages. One of these obvious advantages is an increased spatial resolution and lower noise in images, which is very valuable for high-contrast image applications. This kind of technological shift makes it possible for PCDs to facilitate advanced applications such as spectral imaging and characterization of complex tissues.

For instance, in musculoskeletal imaging, PCDs enhance the assessment of highly dense structures such as bones as well as the analysis of less dense materials such as soft tissues and crystal deposits. The ability to reliably image a variety of tissue types with greater resolution makes the PCDs an optimistic tool for reliable diagnosis and treatment planning, yet another indicator of their clinical relevance compared to standard techniques (Becce et al., 2024). The implications for these newer CT techniques in real-world terms extend beyond mere image enhancement; they also significantly impact patient care and safety. Traditional CT modalities often necessitate higher doses of radiation to achieve high image quality, which could be harmful to patients, particularly in a setting that requires multiple scans. With advancements such as photon-counting technology and dual-energy, low-dose functionality is a core design consideration, considerably reducing patient radiation exposure without degrading diagnostic efficacy. The dual-energy technique not only reduces the need for repeated imaging but also enables whole-body measurements that can adapt screening techniques to varying conditions. Ultimately, as scientists continue to refine the clinical usability of these newer technologies, there is a need to establish their effectiveness through further preclinical and clinical trials, providing a solid foundation for their general use in diagnostic imaging (Becce et al., 2024) (Figure 1.4).

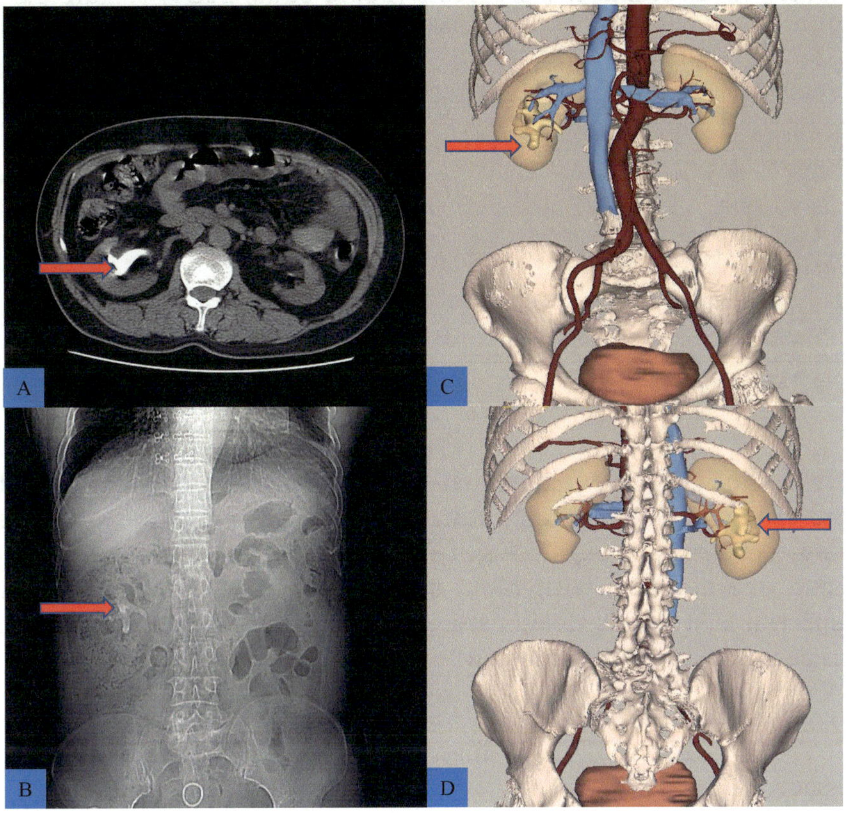

Figure 1.4. The difference between traditional CT scans and 3D reconstructive CT scans. (A,B) The CT scan showing a staghorn stone (red arrow); (C) The front view of the reconstructive urinary system, including calculi (red arrow), kidney, collective system, and blood vessels, hiding the ureter to reveal the location of the stone better; and (D) Posterior view of the puncture location, during PCNL.

Source: https://www.researchgate.net/publication/355472439/figure/fig2/AS:11431281153709847@1682525484988/The-difference-between-traditional-CT-scans-and-3D-reconstructive-CT-scans-A-B-The-CT.tif

1.2. Dual-Energy CT: Overview

The introduction of dual-energy computed tomography (DECT) has significantly transformed diagnostic imaging, particularly in areas where improved tissue characterization is required. Through this technique, two different X-ray energies are used for data acquisition to enhance material discrimination based on atomic composition. By exploiting the varying attenuation properties of tissues across energy bands, DECT images that distinguish individual tissue types, such as calcified structures and soft-tissue components, are generated. This feature is particularly advantageous in musculoskeletal imaging because demarcation between mineralized tissue and surrounding soft tissue is critical for obtaining an accurate diagnosis and treatment planning. As clinical use continues to increase for DECT, its capacity to provide extensive diagnostic information strengthens its position in modern medical imaging protocols (Becce et al., 2024) (Figure 1.5).

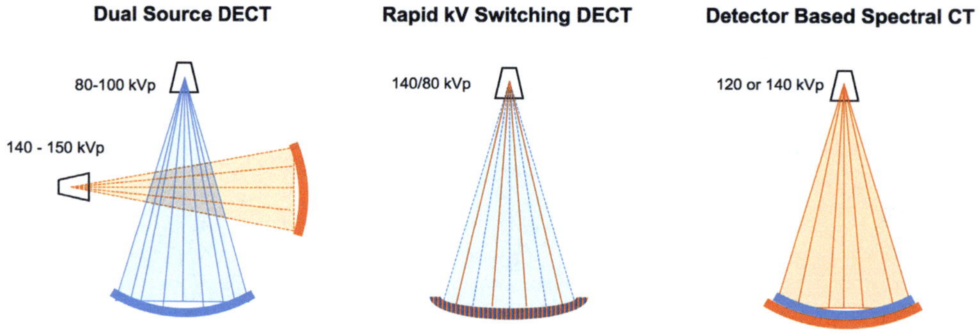

Figure 1.5. Illustration of the three major dual-energy CT (DECT) techniques. Dual-source DECT (Siemens Healthcare, Forchheim, Germany) utilizes two X-ray tubes and two detectors to generate low-and high-energy spectra. Single-source DECT (GE Healthcare, Milwaukee, Wisconsin) employs one X-ray tube and one detector, with rapid switching between low- and high-energy levels. Detector-based spectral CT (Philips Healthcare, Andover, Massachusetts) uses a single X-ray tube with a "sandwich detector" to obtain low-and high-energy spectra.

Source: https://www.researchgate.net/profile/Joseph-Grajo/publication/319993747/figure/fig1/AS:616375919861785@1523966879812/llustration-of-the-three-major-dual-energy-CT-DECT-techniques-Dual-source-DECT.png.

In medical practice, DECT has proved to be valuable for diagnosing disorders, particularly musculoskeletal disorders. It provides high-resolution imaging with minimal radiation exposure, which is indispensable for patient safety. The technique is better in identifying bone abnormalities, crystal deposition, and even metallic implantation, where single-energy CT falls short. In addition, DECT's ability to produce high-resolution spectral imaging further optimizes incident detection by enabling differentiation between closely related substances—e.g., uric acid and calcium pyrophosphate crystals in gout pathology. Such qualities demonstrate the utility of DECT in routine clinical practice, suggesting its role in enhancing the accuracy of diagnosis in complex cases, where composition knowledge is essential to an optimal treatment response (Becce et al., 2024).

The addition of PCDs further improves the strength of DECT, providing greater depth of detail and diagnostic capability. PCDs have unique strengths relative to conventional energy-integrating detectors, including improved spatial resolution and lower noise. This translates into improved image quality, allowing clinicians to better visualize subtle tissue variations. Thus, the integration of PCDs within DECT platforms holds promise for enhancing various diagnostic applications, including measurements of crystal deposits and visualization of metal hardware. However, it should be acknowledged that while the theoretical promise of PCD-CT is vast, its real-world applications must be validated through rigorous clinical trials. In the future, further research will be required to maximize and fully exploit the clinical potential of DECT and PCDs, thereby enriching the progressive arsenal of advanced imaging techniques (Becce et al., 2024) (Figure 1.6).

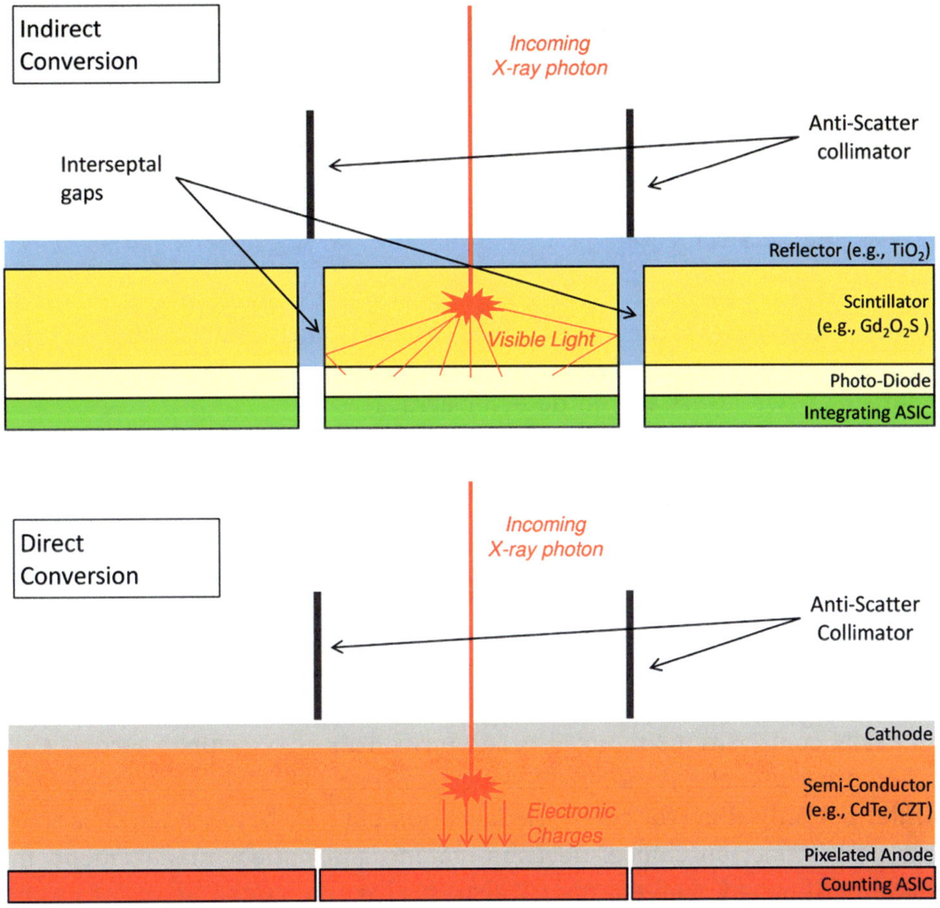

Figure 1.6. Spectral photon-counting CT technology in chest imaging.

Source: https://www.mdpi.com/jcm/jcm-10-05757/article_deploy/html/images/jcm-10-05757-g001-550.jpg.

1.2.1. Definition and Working Principle of Dual-Energy CT

Dual-energy CT is a significant advancement in imaging technology because it maximizes material discrimination by tissue using two different X-ray energy levels. As opposed to conventional single-energy CT, which responds equally to the body's tissue spectrum, dual-energy CT images at high and low photon energies, thereby making the most of attenuation differences across various substances' properties. This capability allows radiologists not just to tell tissues apart but also to identify certain materials such as calcium, iodine, and fat more precisely. By studying how different substances absorb and scatter energy, dual-energy CT enriches diagnostic data, enabling the detection of diseases such as tumors, pulmonary emboli, and cardiovascular disease (Figure 1.7).

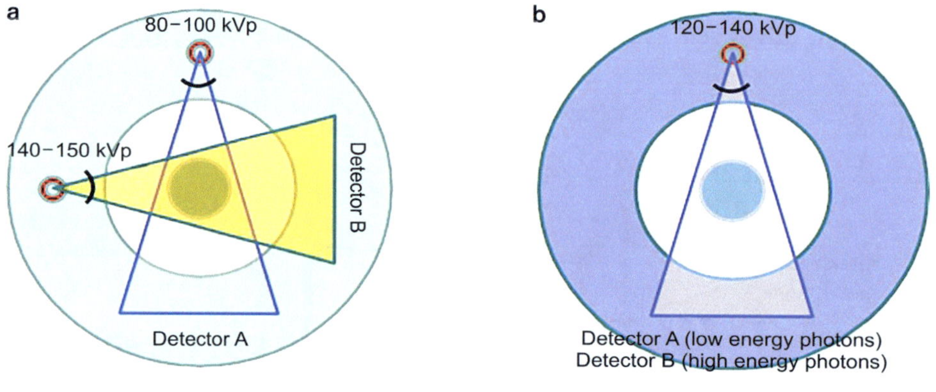

Figure 1.7. Structure and mechanism of (a) dual-energy computed tomography (CT) system (adopts two X-ray tubes and corresponding detector arrays); and (b) detector-based spectral CT system (single X-ray tube and two layers within detector arrays).

Source: https://www.researchgate.net/publication/350528455/figure/fig3/AS:1007471577530370@1617211350104/Structure-and-mechanism-of-a-dual-energy-computed-tomography-CT-system-adopt-two.png.

The mechanism of dual-energy CT is based on energy-selective detection of the X-rays after attenuation in the body. In practice, this is achieved by rapid switching between two unlike X-ray spectra or by using two separate tubes emitting X-rays at two different energies. The images obtained are then processed using advanced algorithms that analyze differential attenuation patterns to reconstruct material compositions in voxel-based form. This is typically a virtual monochromatic image generation process that allows clinicians to view images as though at a single energy level. These capabilities not only allow for better visualization but also better quantification of materials, which has a critical impact on clinical decision-making and patient management. In addition to its increased ability to image, dual-energy CT also receives the added bonus of reduced radiation exposure over traditional imaging techniques. The ability to separate material at two energy levels generally allows lower overall radiation doses to be delivered while maintaining high-quality images. This is particularly useful for sensitive patient groups, such as pediatric patients, where reduced exposure is a priority. Moreover, dual-energy CT continues to advance with technology such as photon-counting, which can further enhance material characterization accuracy and efficiency. With its potential uses extending beyond cardiovascular disease diagnosis to tissue perfusion assessment and lesion characterization, the technology has placed itself at the forefront of next-generation imaging technologies (Doria et al., 2012; Elisa et al., 2016).

1.2.2. Advantages of Dual-Energy CT Over Conventional CT

The advantages of dual-energy CT over conventional CT are significant, particularly in its improved diagnostic accuracy. Dual-energy CT operates by applying two different X-ray energy levels, allowing discrimination of varying materials based on their atomic number. This feature is particularly helpful for identifying specific tissue types and conditions, such as distinguishing between uric acid and calcium stones in urolithiasis. Patients are assisted by increased diagnostic precision because dual-energy CT provides improved images and data to clinicians, which can affect treatment decisions. With continually advancing imaging technology, the potential of dual-energy CT to revolutionize conventional diagnostic protocols is increasingly evident, offering a robust alternative to conventional methodologies (Bove et al., 2013). Another key advantage of dual-energy CT is its functional imaging potential, allowing assessment of tissue perfusion and content. This is particularly valuable in oncology, where the delineation between benign and malignant lesions can have a profound impact on patient management.

The ability to assess contrast agent distribution and enhance tissue characterization is another aspect of imaging not available with conventional CT. Besides, dual-energy CT will reduce the need for follow-up contrast studies, thereby avoiding patient exposure to contrast materials and enhancing the diagnostic workflow. As a result, healthcare professionals can use dual-energy CT to deliver more comprehensive care while simultaneously reducing patient safety risks (Ahmed et al., 2017). Lastly, the availability of dual-energy CT will improve patient outcomes by contributing to treatment planning and follow-up. The enhanced visualization of pathologies facilitated by dual-energy CT not only aids in initial diagnosis but also in ongoing assessment of treatment efficacy. For example, in kidney stones, identifying the stone's composition can influence therapeutic intervention, leading to more individualized and effective patient management strategies. Along with this, the conventional artifact reduction observed in old CT maximizes the consistency of follow-up imaging, thereby better facilitating clinical decision-making in the long run. Ongoing improvements in dual-energy CT technology make its integration into standard practice increasingly important for enhancing the level of care in medical imaging (Bove et al., 2013).

1.2.3. Clinical Applications of Dual-Energy CT

The clinical application of DECT has significantly transformed the diagnostic process, particularly in musculoskeletal imaging. Dual-energy CT enables tissue differentiation based on composition and atomic number using two different X-ray energy levels. It is particularly useful in detecting and characterizing materials such as uric acid and calcium deposits, which are central to diseases such as gout and other crystal arthropathies. Furthermore, the accuracy with which DECT can detect such deposits enhances treatment planning and therapeutic response monitoring. In this regard, DECT not only optimizes diagnostic precision but also has proved capable of reducing the number of unnecessary surgical interventions and providing better insight into pathological conditions in musculoskeletal tissue, placing it at the center of contemporary medical practice (Becce et al., 2024). Another area where dual-energy CT is very useful is the evaluation of vascular anatomy and interventions. The modality enables better imaging of blood vessels via contrast among iodine-based contrast agents and other substances in the body. The capability significantly improves the visualization of vascular pathologies, stenosis, and aneurysms, thereby helping clinicians make decisions regarding interventions. Further, DECT can reduce total contrast agent doses by producing suitable diagnostic information with reduced amounts of contrast, thereby reducing the risk of contrast media-related adverse events. Through enhanced diagnostic clarity and safety in vascular imaging, dual-energy CT not only facilitates more accurate diagnoses but also enables patient-centered medicine across a wide range of clinical applications (Becce et al., 2024). In cancer diagnosis, dual-energy CT is used for its ability to provide comprehensive information on lesion characterization and treatment response follow-up. Its ability to discriminate between tumors based on composition is useful for designing personalized treatment plans. For example, by evaluating biochemical tumor content, clinicians can estimate malignancy risk, thereby optimizing patient management protocols. Additionally, the technology enables quantitative assessment of tumor response to therapy by monitoring changes in contrast enhancement patterns over time. The two-functionality adds to the oncologist's toolkit by facilitating more personalized treatment regimens and improved prognostic evaluation. As research continues to confirm these applications, dual-energy CT may have a profound impact on oncology practice by delivering advanced imaging capabilities aligned with emerging trends in precision medicine (Becce et al., 2024).

1.3. Photon-Counting CT: Overview

The development of photon-counting computed tomography (PCCT) is a landmark in the field of diagnostic imaging technology. Unlike traditional energy-integrating detectors, PCCT uses photon counting to detect and resolve single X-ray photons (Figure 1.8).

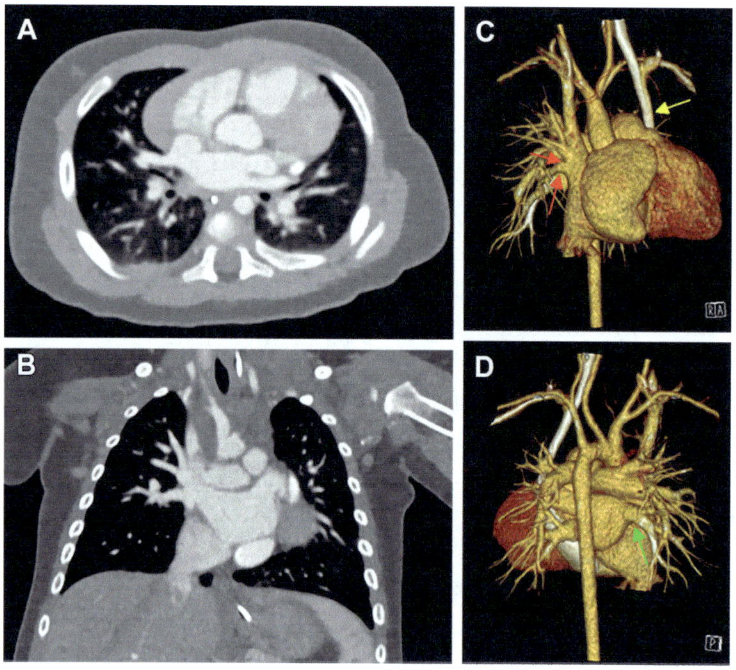

Figure 1.8. Photon-counting CT offers superior imaging in babies with heart defects.

Source: https://press.rsna.org/pressrelease/2023_resources/2437/fig_1.jpg.

This technology permits increased spatial resolution, which is significant in all but the most low-contrast applications, particularly in the examination of high-contrast material such as mineralized tissue. The ability to discriminate among the various energy levels of X-ray photons enhances material discrimination and yields a superior image of the underlying anatomy. This is particularly beneficial in musculoskeletal imaging, where accurate representation of bone and soft tissue is critical to effective diagnosis and treatment planning. The technological shift to PCCT, therefore, not only improves imaging quality but also allows for more precise clinical assessments. Additionally, the most significant advantage of PCCT is that it may enable lower radiation doses than current CT technologies. The inherent ability of photon-counting detectors to image at lower doses without sacrificing high-quality photos is a significant consideration in modern radiology, where minimizing patient risk is a top priority. This aspect aligns with broader efforts throughout the medical industry to implement dose-reduction strategies and enhance imaging capacity. Existing studies have shown that PCCT can deliver excellent image quality at suboptimal exposures, substantiating its use in a broad range of clinical scenarios, such as whole-body CT scans and settings where low-dose imaging protocols are preferable. Improvements in photon-counting technology are a significant step toward achieving safer yet efficient imaging modalities in healthcare. Apart from higher-quality images and lower doses of radiation, the integration of spectral imaging capability into PCCT systems contributes to their clinical value. Spectral imaging allows for material characterization based on its attenuation characteristics at various energy levels, which makes it easy for radiologists to discriminate between multiple tissue types or pathologies. For example, in musculoskeletal imaging, PCCT can be used to detect and characterize crystal deposits in diseases such as gout, providing valuable information to guide appropriate therapeutic interventions. Moreover, in tandem with technological advancements, there has been a growing interest in extending applications to traditional imaging challenges, such as testing advanced metallic implants. As noted in recent papers, the full potential of photon-counting detectors remains to be substantiated by clinical studies, further emphasizing the necessity for continued research in this groundbreaking area of diagnostic imaging (Becce et al., 2024).

1.3.1. Definition and Working Principle of Photon-Counting CT

Photon-counting CT represents a significant advancement over traditional imaging technology. Unlike standard CT scanners based on energy-integrating detectors, photon-counting CT employs energy-resolving detectors that can distinguish individual photons by their energies. This enables greater differentiation among materials and improved contrast resolution. The operating premise relies on single-photon detection to enable the system to acquire rich spectral information that will enable more accurate differentiation among several tissue types and densities than existing techniques. By this, photon-counting CT technology holds the potential to improve diagnosis in clinical settings (Figure 1.9).

The unique operational procedure of photon-counting CT has two major components: the photon detector and reconstruction algorithm. X-ray photons pass through the patient and are absorbed by the detector material, with each photon being detected. Interestingly, the sensors also record the energy of each incident photon, enabling spectral data acquisition. Then, sophisticated reconstruction algorithms process the data to generate high-resolution cross-sectional images. This technique not only enhances image quality by minimizing noise but also enables better quantification of materials based on their individual spectral characteristics. Therefore, photon-counting CT is at the top of diagnostic imaging, offering an efficient tool to clinicians. In addition, the advent of photon-counting CT results from the growing demand for more precise imaging technologies in medicine. By providing means to discriminate among dissimilar materials through their distinct energy signatures, this technology is used in many diagnostic challenges, such as distinguishing calcified from non-calcified lesions or discriminating among various tumor types based on metabolic characteristics. Furthermore, photon-counting CT technology will also lead to reduced radiation exposure, as increased detector sensitivity allows doses to be reduced without compromising image quality. As research continues to evolve, the integration of photon-counting technologies into clinical applications holds immense potential, addressing shortcomings of current imaging devices and improving patient care by increasing diagnostic accuracy (Will et al., 2011; Cirigliano et al., 2018).

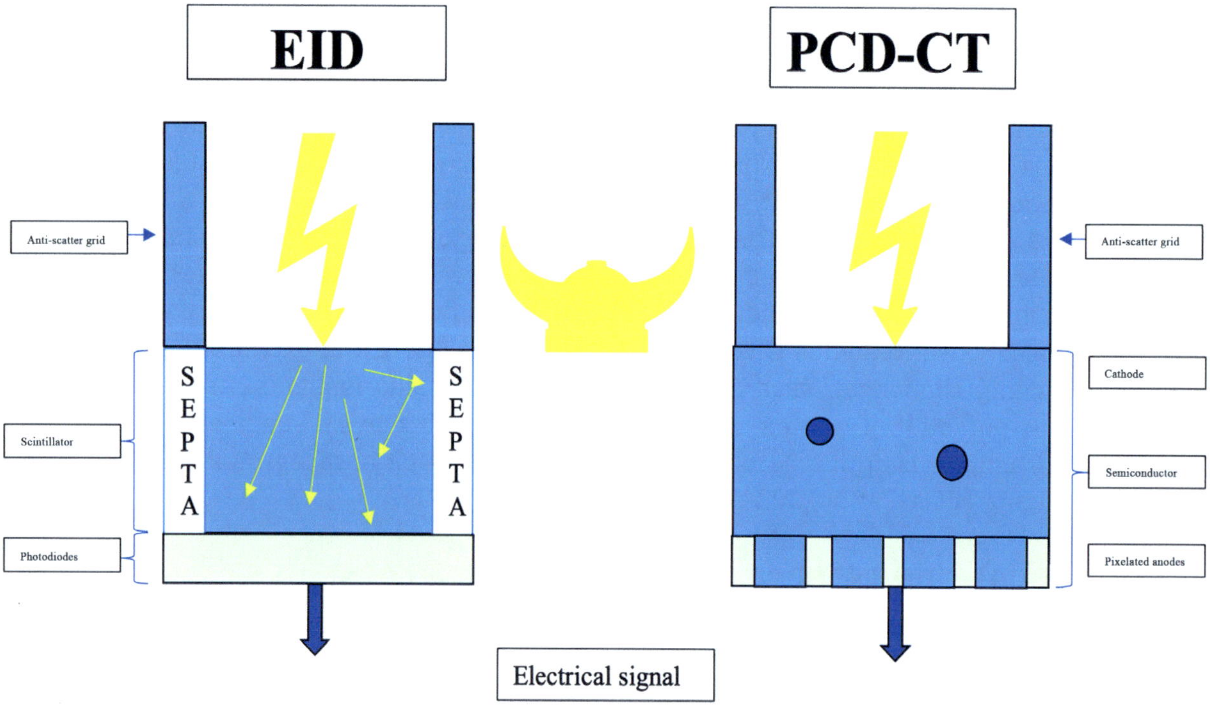

Figure 1.9. Technical principles of photon-counting detector CT (PCD-CT) compared to those of energy-integrated detector (EID)-CT. On the left side, a standard EID-CT is illustrated. The use of a scintillator and septa characterizes EID-CT. On the right side, a PCD-CT that directly converts and counts X-ray photons into electrical signals without the need for scintillator layers is shown.

Source: https://www.researchgate.net/publication/380019392/figure/fig1/AS:11431281430412205@1746736910839/Technical-principles-of-photon-counting-detector-CT-PCD-CT-compared-to-those-of.tif.

1.3.2. Benefits of Photon-Counting Technology

The use of photon-counting technology in CT represents a significant advance in imaging capability, particularly in terms of enhanced spatial resolution and noise reduction. PCDs tally individual photons, whereas conventional energy-integrating detectors (EIDs) measure cumulative energy. This precision in photon detection yields improved images that are crucial for diagnosing minute abnormalities, especially in high-contrast structures such as bones. PCDs' ability to minimize noise levels also enhances visibility of finer details within the area under scan, which is beneficial in musculoskeletal imaging where precision is critical (Figure 1.10).

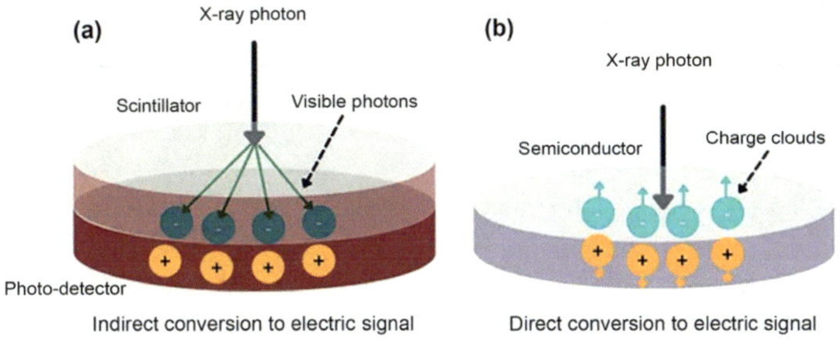

Figure 1.10. Photon-counting detectors (PCDs)

Source: https://www.azoquantum.com/images/Article_Images/ImageForArticle_273_16414751144874649.png.

Hence, the incorporation of photon-counting technology can improve the quality of patient diagnosis and treatment by enabling more accurate and earlier diagnoses of fractures or degenerative diseases, thereby reducing the need for repeated imaging tests. Photon-counting technology also helps in minimizing radiation dose, which promotes safer imaging. In a clinical setting focused on limiting patients' exposure to ionizing radiation, PCDs become essential. The inherent efficiency of photon-counting detectors enables substantial improvements in image quality at lower radiation doses. This is particularly useful in populations that have to be examined repeatedly, such as patients with chronic conditions or children, who are more sensitive to radiation. PCDs directly address one of the key issues in conventional imaging by enabling low-dose use—such as whole-body CT scans—without compromising image integrity. The ability to decrease doses without compromising the quality of diagnostically relevant images can make CT imaging universally accepted, increasingly integrating it into patient care protocols as a first-line diagnostic imaging modality. Finally, the revolutionary value of photon-counting technology lies in its potential for intrinsic spectral imaging. PCDs not only improve traditional imaging but also enable advanced applications by offering spectral data that help distinguish materials based on their energy-absorption behavior. This feature is especially beneficial in the detection of certain conditions like gout, using the identification of deposits of crystals in joints, as well as the characterization of types of metal hardware in orthopedics. The ability to access this spectral information without additional scans is a new paradigm in CT imaging. Furthermore, continued development and validation of such applications underscore the imperative to include photon-counting detectors in practice on a broad basis. Because research is continually challenging their capabilities, PCDs are being assessed to determine the future of advanced CT imaging techniques, establishing new standards of diagnostic excellence across the spectrum of healthcare practices (Becce et al., 2024).

1.3.3. Clinical Applications of Photon-Counting CT

The advent of photon-counting computed tomography (PCCT) represents a significant leap in diagnostic imaging, particularly when used in clinical settings across various areas of medicine. Although conventional computed tomography has long been the cornerstone of imaging techniques, PCCT offers a significant advantage, especially for imaging high-contrast structures such as mineralized tissues. The distinctive capabilities of the PCDs include enhanced spatial resolution and reduced noise, leading to improved visualization of anatomical structures. The additional fact that, in musculoskeletal imaging, PCDs can identify bone integrity and crystal deposits makes PCDs more useful for diagnosis (Figure 1.11).

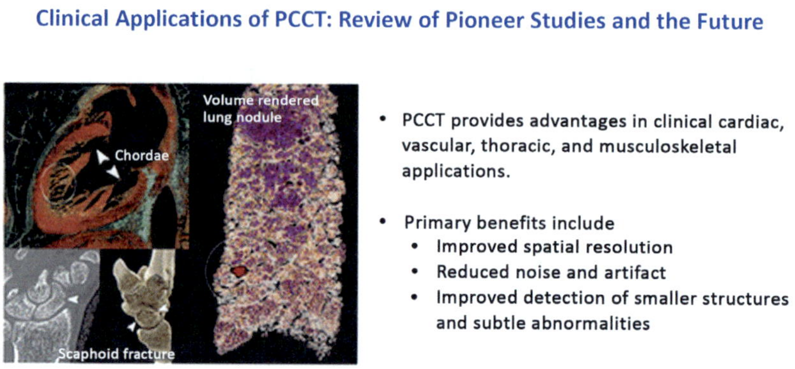

Figure 1.11. Clinical applications of photon-counting computed tomography (PCCT) demonstrate enhanced visualization in cardiac, pulmonary, and musculoskeletal imaging.

Source: https://pubs.rsna.org/cms/10.1148/radiol.222432/asset/images/medium/radiol.222432.va.gif.

The ability of PCDs to perform spectral imaging enhances their utility, enabling discrimination between various materials and disease states that are hard to distinguish using standard imaging methodologies, thereby revolutionizing patient care through more accurate diagnosis and personalized treatment regimens (Becce et al., 2024). With advances in image quality, clinical application of photon-counting CT also meets the demand for reduced radiation exposure in the imaging process. As medicine continues to seek ways to reduce risk to patients, PCCT enables low-dose whole-body imaging without compromising diagnostic performance. The precision that PCDs enable enables optimal imaging with lower radiation doses, a major issue in pediatric imaging and other at-risk patient populations. For example, studies have demonstrated that PCDs can capture high-quality images with reduced radiation doses compared to conventional energy-integrating detectors (EIDs). The latter is of concern amid growing concern about cumulative radiation exposure from multiple imaging, while retaining patient safety at the top of the diagnostic process's considerations (Becce et al., 2024). Furthermore, the evolving horizon of health technology is driving the development of emerging applications of photon-counting CT. New applications leverage the intrinsic spectral capability of PCCT for advanced analysis across various clinical applications. Such applications are metal hardware characterization, evaluation of soft tissue lesions, and multi-material imaging to identify pathological tissue alterations. The variety and precision of PCDs are unveiling new methods in musculoskeletal imaging, hinting at the prospect of holistic evaluations previously unattainable. However, the clinical community acknowledges that more preclinical and clinical proof of concept is needed to realize the potential of photon-counting CT so that these advances translate into real-world, practical, effective outcomes for disease care and patient management.

1.4. Technical Innovations in Dual-Energy CT

The emergence of DECT is a breakthrough in imaging technology that offers greater diagnostic capability than previous single-energy CT systems. DECT permits the separation of materials according to their atomic numbers by imaging at two energy levels. This capability not only improves the quality of images but is also used for advanced material characterization, which is most critical in the diagnosis of disorders with complex tissue compositions, such as tumors or calcifications. Apart from this, dual-energy techniques can significantly reduce image artifacts caused by overlapping tissue densities, thereby producing sharper and more precise images. The integration of spectral CT applications into clinical practice reflects the strength of DECT as a multi-tool, allowing radiologists to glean more clinically relevant information from scans and to reduce radiation exposure (Bousse et al., 2024). Continued enhancement of DECT technology reflects not only its diagnostic capability but also the continuously shifting paradigm of patient safety through radiation dose optimization. Where fears about radiation exposure rise among medical professionals, there is a desperate need to develop low-dose scanning technologies that do not compromise on image quality. Advances such as rapid switching of kilovolt peak (kVp), as part of DECT techniques, enable the flexibility needed to fine-tune doses without diminishing diagnostic effectiveness. These advances are complementary to the increased emphasis on patient-oriented care, ensuring that imaging technologies deliver essential information without compromising the patient's health. This has encouraged research into reducing the radiation dose for CT imaging in dual-energy contexts, which has placed DECT as an available option for future diagnostic use (Liu et al., 2018). Further, the application of machine learning techniques to DECT is transforming the technology by overcoming inherent challenges such as image and data artifacts. By leveraging data-driven approaches, researchers hope to enhance image reconstruction and the homogeneity of material decomposition in dual-energy scans. These advancements not only enable the system's ability to highlight subtle tissue composition variations but also enhance the generated image robustness. The ongoing integration of artificial intelligence into DECT will accelerate processes, reduce the time required for image interpretation, and ultimately improve patient outcomes. With such technological developments always on the move, DECT has the potential to transform diagnostic imaging, hence becoming part of modern radiology (Bousse et al., 2024).

1.4.1. Advances in Detector Technology

Recent developments in detection technology have significantly redefined the CT field, particularly with the advent of PCDs. Compared to traditional energy-integrating detectors, PCDs offer better spatial and contrast resolution, which is valuable in most imaging applications. This high performance results from their ability to accurately measure the energy of individual X-ray photons, enabling enhanced discrimination between materials based on their atomic numbers. As a result, photon-counting CT has emerged as a valuable resource in forensic medicine, enabling high-resolution virtual autopsies and advanced postmortem investigations. PCDs not only improve image quality but also reduce the dose of radiation, making them greatly useful in sensitive situations, particularly in pediatrics and trauma analysis (Gascho et al., 2024). In musculoskeletal imaging, the introduction of dual-energy CT has enabled significant improvements in diagnostic accuracy by exploiting the different X-ray absorption characteristics of tissues.

Dual-energy CT allows imaging at two energy levels simultaneously and offers a broader range of information that can lead to improved characterization of disease conditions. PCDs also enhance the performance of dual-energy imaging through intrinsic spectral imaging capabilities, enabling improved detail in the assessment of high-contrast structures such as mineralized tissues. With this integration, practitioners can obtain accurate assessments of conditions such as crystal deposits in gout or of hardware visibility in post-surgical examinations, further underscoring the need for innovative imaging technologies in modern practice (Becce et al., 2024).

The rapid development of detector technology, particularly with the emergence of PCDs, is a very promising direction in CT imaging. Improved image acquisition capabilities are driving greater diagnostic certainty across various fields of medicine. The potential for reduced noise levels and improved spatial resolution makes it feasible to provide more accurate estimates of complex anatomical objects, particularly in cases requiring meticulous detail. Moreover, the recent studies on the applications of PCDs still need to emphasize their role in pushing the frontiers of CT utilization, including low-dose protocols and high-end spectral imaging techniques. With these technologies validated by research, their use in clinical practice promises to usher in a new era of diagnostic imaging with greater precision and reduced patient risk, underscoring the significance of advances in detector technology (Gascho et al., 2024; Becce et al., 2024).

1.4.2. Software Improvements for Image Reconstruction

Advances in image reconstruction software have significantly enhanced the capabilities of CT systems, particularly when applied to advanced approaches such as dual-energy and photon-counting imaging. Higher accuracy in image reconstruction from input data is enabled by such software advancements, creating more detailed visual descriptions of anatomical structure.

With sophisticated algorithms that exploit the unique information provided by dual-energy sources, these systems can separate materials based on their energy-dependent attenuation characteristics (Figure 1.12).

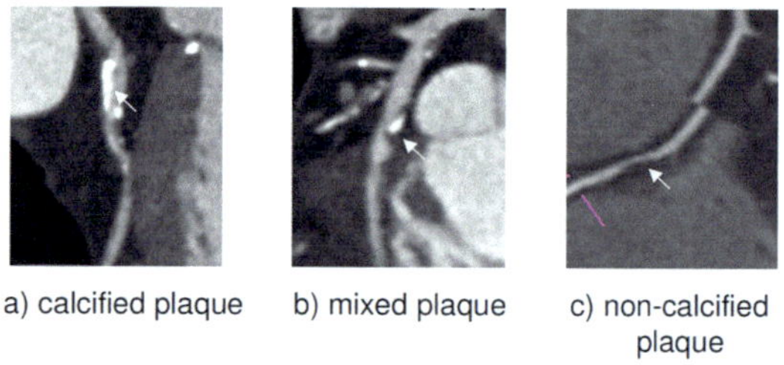

Figure 1.12. Representative images of calcified, mixed, and non-calcified plaques.

Source: https://www.researchgate.net/profile/Alexander-Becker-9/publication/26809538/figure/fig1/AS:196057599352832@1423755182511/Representative-images-of-calcified-a-mixed-b-and-non-calcified-plaques-c-as.png.

This capability is also critical for applications such as distinguishing calcified from non-calcified plaque in cardiovascular imaging. Present research has demonstrated that image-reconstruction accuracy not only enhances diagnostic confidence but also optimizes patient management, as appropriate treatments can be planned more efficiently based on accurately reconstructed data. The introduction of photon-counting CT has ushered in a new era in image quality, thanks to advanced software algorithms that further improve image reconstruction. In contrast to traditional energy-integrating detectors, photon-counting technology sums up individual photons and benefits from the energy levels (Figure 1.13).

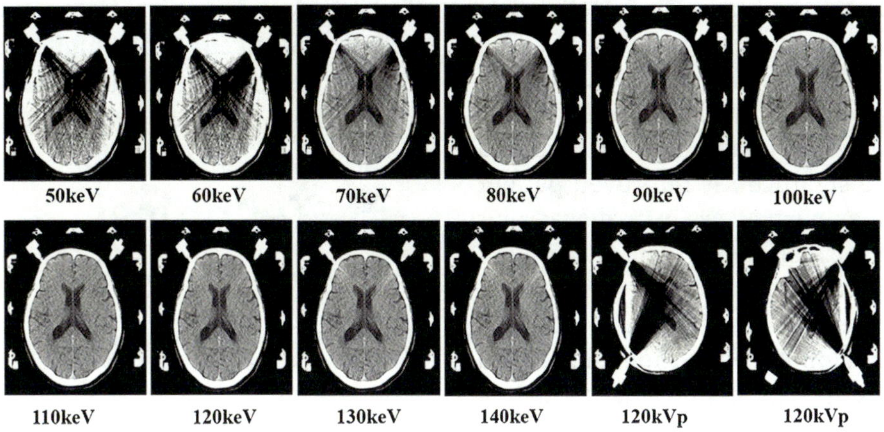

Figure 1.13. Generation of virtual monoenergetic images (VMI).

Source: https://www.researchgate.net/publication/361224193/figure/fig1/AS:1165562260520962@1654903106507/The-images-of-virtual-monoenergetic-images-VMI-and-120-kVp-images-VMI-of-a.png.

This technique enables the creation of virtual monoenergetic images (VMI), which are less sensitive to beam hardening and have a sharper definition of contrast agents. According to recent definitions, the iodine contrast-to-noise ratio (CNR) in VMIs from photon-counting CT clearly surpasses that of dual-energy methods at lower energies. This improvement, facilitated by sophisticated reconstruction algorithms, underscores the significance of software in maximizing imaging performance to deliver better diagnostic outcomes for patients undergoing assessment for cardiac conditions or oncological illnesses, thereby underscoring the importance of sustained software development in medical imaging (Booij et al., 2022). In addition, the integration of artificial intelligence (AI) within software platforms has taken hold as a fundamental element of modern image reconstruction methods. AI-powered reconstruction algorithms enable adaptive learning, allowing systems to modify their performance based on vast amounts of data. The benefit of this is not only to accelerate reconstruction but also to enhance overall image quality by minimizing artifacts and fine-tuning noise suppression routines. As hinted by research in advancements in cardiovascular imaging, this type of innovation is fundamental to enhancing not only the diagnostic accuracy but also the efficiency of patient-specific precision medicine. The intersection of emerging software platforms and imaging modalities underscores the importance of interprofessional collaboration among clinicians, software engineers, and radiologists to take full advantage of these technologies (Cabrelle et al., 2023). Through the above methods, the field of image reconstruction will be revolutionized, with improved patient care across most fields of medicine.

1.4.3. Integration with Artificial Intelligence for Enhanced Diagnostics

By integrating AI with advanced CT techniques, such as dual-energy and photon-counting imaging, diagnostic accuracy and effectiveness in radiology can be potentially revolutionized. Through machine learning algorithms, AI can analyze large volumes of data from imaging modalities, enabling clinicians to identify and characterize obscure or very subtle pathologies. Such consolidation not only improves diagnostic precision but also streamlines workflows, allowing radiologists to focus on interpretation rather than being bogged down in redundant work. As discussed in the most recent research, advances in image data capture and processing have significantly improved patient care and outcomes, particularly in cardiovascular imaging, which is experiencing explosive growth across radiological subspecialties (Cabrelle et al., 2023). Further, the integration of AI using dual-energy and photon-counting modalities introduces an additional dimension to imaging technologies. The new CT protocols provide high-quality material characterization, enabling better tissue differentiation and improved diagnostic capabilities. AI algorithms can help make these technologies more effective by providing automatic quality assurance tests and optimizing image parameters. For example, AI has the ability to dynamically modify parameters based on real-time image quality analysis, thus enhancing diagnostic yield and patient safety. New developments in medical imaging highlight the critical role of expert radiologists who possess not only technical proficiency but also a deep understanding of AI technologies in bridging the gap between advanced imaging techniques and practice (Cabrelle et al., 2023).

Additionally, the future path of AI in imaging is toward even greater integration, with algorithms that can learn from each new case and respond to evolving clinical needs. This ability to adapt ensures that AI tools remain relevant and worthwhile as diagnostic needs shift over time. The safety and precision achieved through AI-assisted imaging can lead to improved clinical decision-making and patient outcomes across various medical specialties, such as oncology and cardiology. Notably, the ongoing advancement of state-of-the-art imaging technologies, such as SPECT/CT, has demonstrated that AI can transform standard diagnostics into quantitative assessments, leading to more precise treatments. With the development of medical imaging, the synergy of AI with advanced CT techniques is a revolution that will be advantageous both to patients and healthcare professionals.

1.5. Technical Innovations in Photon-Counting CT

The development of photon-counting CT is a significant technological achievement that increases imaging capacities while addressing core clinical issues. Unlike conventional energy-integrating detectors, photon-counting detectors can detect individual X-ray photons, yielding greater spatial resolution and lower noise in the resulting images. This heightened sensitivity enables discrimination of low-contrast structures, which are essential for early detection of pathological changes, e.g., microcalcifications associated with coronary artery disease (CAD). Photon-counting technology is potentially valuable for providing more targeted diagnostic information while simultaneously decreasing radiation doses, a consideration that is increasingly occupying radiological discourse. Consequently, utilization of photon-counting CT in routine clinical practice will be anticipated to redefine diagnostic standards and improve patient outcomes by equipping clinicians with the technology to diagnose and manage cardiovascular disease more effectively. Technical advancements in photon-counting CT also align with greater efforts to reduce exposure to radiation without compromising image quality. Recent research has identified a major challenge in reconciling high-resolution imaging and low-dose protocols (Liu et al., 2018). Technologies such as automatic tube current modulation and rapid peak kilovoltage switching provide better control of the radiation delivered during scans. These technologies, when interfaced with photon-counting technology, enhance the ability to execute advanced imaging studies without compromising patient safety. The prospect of dual-energy approaches in this context also expands the capabilities of photon-counting CT for material differentiation, which is crucial for ascertaining the composition of coronary artery calcification and its impact on atherosclerosis (Liu et al., 2018). This innovation underscores technology's potential to map the future of medical imaging. In addition, the coupling of photon-counting CT and dual-energy imaging modalities will fundamentally transform cardiovascular diagnostic protocols. Using the distinct energy signatures of different tissues, photon-counting CT can elevate calcification and other structure characterization to the level necessary for individualized planning of therapy. For instance, a detailed depiction of coronary artery calcification is extremely valuable in predicting thrombogenic susceptibility. Current conventional imaging methods fall short here, making photon-counting CT a desirable alternative (Boi et al., 2024). Clinical use of photon-counting CT will ultimately offer improved prognostic assessment, improved treatment planning, and ultimately improved care of the patient in cardiovascular practice once there is ongoing research with the resolution of the technical problems with these advancements.

1.5.1. Development of Advanced Photon-Counting Detectors

The ongoing development of high-end PCDs is a crucial move for CT, especially as it is being married with dual-energy techniques. In the past, EIDs were employed in CT scanners, which integrate the energy of incoming X-ray photons, thereby compromising spatial resolution and noise. In contrast, PCDs count individual photons and measure their energy directly, which creates better spatial resolution and lower noise. This technology enables improved image quality, particularly in high-contrast applications, where precise detail is critical. Second, the ability of PCDs to discriminate among different energy levels offers promise for spectral imaging applications, thereby improving material characterization under many imaging conditions, underscoring their role-revolutionizing contribution to medical imaging technology. The combination of dual-energy CT advancements with PCDs has made CT imaging more useful, particularly for musculoskeletal imaging. As stated, while conventional imaging techniques like MRI provide softer tissue contrast, CT fares better in the case of high-contrast structures like mineralized structures. Dual-energy CT complemented the diagnostic ability of CT by enabling material distinction based on density and energy-absorption characteristics. Secondly, because of their native spectral imaging function, PCDs can give more accurate assessments of pathology and bone quality by facilitating facile measurement of mineral density. Consequently, advances in PCD technology have enabled clinicians to obtain useful information about conditions such as crystal deposits and bone lesions, ultimately improving patient outcomes during musculoskeletal exams (Becce et al., 2024). The potential of photon-counting detectors also opens avenues for novel applications in low-dose CT scans. Image quality is preserved despite reduced radiation exposure, owing to the increased detection efficiency of PCDs, a significant aspect for patient safety and public health. The promise of whole-body CT scans with PCDs holds the potential to revolutionize routine screening and follow-up scans because lower doses reduce long-term radiation risks. Moreover, PCD functionality is also well-adapted to more advanced capabilities such as characterization of crystal deposits or imaging metal hardware at unprecedented resolution (Becce et al., 2024). As the technological path is now available, there is a requirement to conduct comprehensive preclinical and clinical validations to define and optimize the clinical applications of this novel imaging modality.

1.5.2. Innovations in Data Processing Algorithms

Algorithm development for data processing has revolutionized CT, particularly in dual-energy and photon-counting technologies. One of the most prominent developments in this field is the application of machine learning methods to enhance image quality and reduce spectral CT artifacts. In this case, big data is employed to learn and predict corrections for inconsistencies in spectral data, significantly improving image reconstruction processes. Thus, integrating such high-level algorithms not only guarantees optimal performance of spectral CT but also yields superior, accurate images, ultimately leading to more efficient diagnostic outcomes in clinics. As the research continues, the possibility of further algorithm refinement guarantees a solution to existing problems, ensuring maximum trustworthiness of spectral imaging equipment (Bousse et al., 2024). Innovative data processing algorithms are particularly important in relation to low-dose CT technology. Due to growing anxiety about radiation exposure, the imperative of creating algorithms that ensure image quality without substantially reducing dose is imperative. Citizens' focus on safety and health has encouraged scientists to investigate image processing algorithms that dynamically adjust image parameters. Interestingly, techniques such as automated tube current modulation and rapid peak kilovoltage switching have gained popularity to optimize radiation delivery based on patient-specific conditions. Further, the exploration of advanced image reconstruction methods based on advanced data processing has enabled diagnostic-quality images at lower radiation doses, addressing both clinical effectiveness and patient protection (Liu et al., 2018). With evolving technologies, the challenge will be to combine them with advanced algorithms. The direction of future CT imaging is through the seamless integration of dual-energy and photon-counting CT with state-of-the-art data processing technology. By combining the advantages of these novel, complementary techniques, researchers can pursue materials characterization and diagnostic imaging at unprecedented levels. Photon-counting CT, with its high detection accuracy capability, holds out the prospect of improved quantification of most tissue types and pathologies to previously unseen levels of precision. Meanwhile, dual-energy CT enables advanced material decomposition and differential diagnosis, thereby enhancing clinical decision-making. As more sophisticated data-processing algorithms are developed, their potential to enable the integration of these technologies and to take diagnostic accuracy in CT into a new era of improved imaging resolution and patient management (Bousse et al., 2024).

1.5.3. Impact of Technology on Image Quality and Dose Reduction

The technological evolution of CT has deeply influenced both image quality and reduction of radiation doses. Of particular mention in this context is dual-energy CT, a significant imaging technology innovation that enabled more advanced tissue composition studies through energy discrimination. This enables the possibility of distinguishing between materials of the same attenuation properties, enhancing diagnostic specificity in many clinical scenarios, especially musculoskeletal imaging. With its ability to provide spectral information, dual-energy CT enables the diagnosis of disorders such as gout and more accurate characterization of rare crystal deposits. Moreover, as radiologists increasingly recognize the risks of radiation exposure, the technology benefits twice: improving image sharpness while reducing the delivered dose, a natural means of ensuring patient health and safety in imaging examinations. In addition to dual-energy methods, PCD introduction is the predominant CT technology innovation. PCDs have improved spatial resolution and lower image noise than conventionally used energy-integrating detectors, which are fundamental components of high-quality imaging. Such enhanced resolution enables more accurate visualization of intricate anatomical structures, particularly in areas where precision matters most, such as in orthopedic examinations. In addition, PCDs inherently possess spectral imaging characteristics, allowing for complex applications in a clinical setting. For instance, accurate bone density imaging or the detection of metal artifacts can be achieved with increased capability. These advancements not only enhance diagnostic accuracy but also help optimize dose by maintaining image quality at lower radiation levels, underscoring the value of developing CT techniques in modern healthcare. The impact of these emerging technologies extends beyond its direct imaging benefits, with the possible ability to fundamentally transform patient outcomes. Dual-energy CT and PCD scanners not only maximize test diagnostic quality but also the safety profile of the imaging procedure by minimizing radiation dose. With evidence-based medicine increasingly prominent in health care, the implementation of advanced CT techniques reflects an emphasis on optimizing patient care through technology. This is particularly crucial in musculoskeletal imaging, where examiners need to satisfy the need for high-quality images while limiting radiation doses. The future use of PCD technology is auspicious, hinting at an even larger array of uses that would keep on enhancing dose-reduction methods while establishing a comprehensive understanding of various pathological conditions, as documented in recent research in spectral imaging applications in relation to crystal deposits and metal hardware assessments (Becce et al., 2024).

1.6. Challenges and Limitations

The union of advanced technology CT techniques, such as dual-energy and PCDs, brings many challenges and shortcomings requiring close scrutiny. Among the challenges is the complexity of the technology itself, particularly in the case of dual-energy CT, which involves complicated algorithms and dual-source or dual-layer detectors to differentiate between tissues with similar attenuations. This complexity results in steep learning curves for technologists and radiologists to adopt new operational protocols and interpretive strategies. In addition, reliance on advanced software for image reconstruction can produce inconsistencies in image quality, particularly when the algorithms are poorly calibrated or when patients' anatomical characteristics vary. These arguments highlight the significance of proper training and standardization to guarantee valid outcomes in clinical practice (Becce et al., 2024). Additionally, although photon-counting technology has greater spatial resolution and reduced noise, its implementation comes with its set of challenges. High production costs and hardware infrastructure demands may lead to high investment, depriving most clinical settings of access to PCDs. Institutions may be hesitant to adopt such complex technologies without an unequivocal demonstration of cost-effectiveness and improved diagnostic capacity compared with conventional EIDs. Furthermore, the intrinsic spectral imaging benefits of PCDs may complicate routine imaging protocols, requiring processing time to manage spectral data. The current challenges call for extensive studies to validate the enhanced performance of PCDs in clinical applications, particularly for determining high-contrast structures such as bones and mineralized tissues (Becce et al., 2024). Finally, the limitations of dual-energy and photon-counting approaches carry over to their applications in clinics and patient safety. For instance, while dual-energy CT enables material discrimination, it can occasionally create artifacts due to patient motion or metal interference, making interpretation more challenging. In addition, the possibility of reduced doses of radiation is an appealing part of new CT technology; however, this achievement typically depends on tradeoffs in image quality. A delicate trade-off between reducing radiation exposure and yet achieving sufficient diagnostic information is a central theme in the application of these novel techniques. As the field grows, ongoing validation through rigorous clinical trials and the establishment of standard protocols will play a pivotal role in addressing problems and realizing the optimal use of dual-energy and photon-counting CT in routine clinical practice (Becce et al., 2024).

1.6.1. Technical Challenges in Implementing Advanced CT Techniques

The use of newer CT technologies, such as dual-energy CT and PCDs, is often hindered by technical challenges that could limit their clinical potential. A principal issue concerns the complex calibration and optimization of these systems, which require careful calibration to ensure accurate image reconstruction. Because these new technologies use advanced algorithms to differentiate among materials based on their energy absorption characteristics, any mis-calibration will produce gross artifacts in the final images. Furthermore, dual-energy CT involves synchronizing multiple X-ray sources and detectors, making system design more complex, increasing costs, and requiring additional training for radiologists and technologists to operate it effectively. This multi-faceted challenge underscores the importance of rigorous preclinical and clinical trials before such technologies can find their full potential in everyday clinical use, as noted in more recent literature. Another important hindrance to the use of advanced CT techniques is the need for more computational power and greater storage capacities. With increasing amounts of data generated by dual-energy and PCD technology, so do the demands placed on processing capacity and storage. Traditional image reconstruction algorithms may no longer be sufficient, and new, more complex algorithms capable of handling larger datasets in real time are needed. This shift requires not only investment in top-of-the-range computing hardware but also institutions to redesign their workflows to accommodate this. This transition from conventional methods to advanced techniques tends to disrupt existing protocols, raising concerns about the consistency and quality of patient treatment during implementation. These are major challenges to the significance of ongoing research on computational procedures that would allow seamless integration of advanced CT methodologies into clinical environments. Finally, photon-counting detector adoption is accompanied by unique challenges, most notably access and interoperability with multiple imaging platforms. While PCDs are advantageous for minimizing noise and improving spatial resolution (Becce et al., 2024), their implementation is limited by their compatibility with installed-base CT systems. Integration of new technology must be concurrent with retrofitting or replacing older machines, which can be budget- and institutional-resource-straining. In addition to economic hurdles, institutions also have to overcome regulatory challenges to bring new imaging technologies to the market. The clinical world must collaborate towards standard standardization protocols that ensure PCD systems are installed and tested consistently. Without such coordination, the potential of advanced CT methods goes to waste, preventing diagnostic imaging breakthroughs (Becce et al., 2024).

1.6.2. Limitations in Clinical Settings and Patient Safety

Introduction of new CT technologies, such as dual-energy and photon-counting computed tomography (PCCT), brings significant enhancement in imaging capability. Still, these also pose constraints that may impact the clinical setting and patient well-being. The most critical of these is the risk of increased radiation exposure associated with these novel imaging modalities. While PCCT aims to deliver enhanced image quality and diagnostic yield, the technology must be calibrated sensitively to avoid risks. Moreover, varying protocols across clinical settings may result in heterogeneous radiation doses, compromising patient safety. These variations highlight the necessity of standardizing protocol use to ensure consistency and safety across different health care settings, upholding the integrity of the diagnostic process and supporting patient well-being. Furthermore, the technical complexity of sophisticated CT technologies poses a challenge in the training of medical professionals. This limitation affects the overall efficacy and safety of these technologies in clinical settings. For instance, the advanced algorithms and computations needed for dual-energy and PCCT require radiologists to possess a strong technical background in addition to interpretation skills. Lack of training may result in misinterpretations, potentially leading to erroneous clinical deductions that significantly compromise patient outcomes. Besides this, there may be a learning process in adopting these advanced systems by healthcare centers, which may delay the benefits of improved diagnostics. Thus, ongoing education and rigorous training programs are required to bridge the knowledge gap and allow healthcare professionals to use these advanced imaging modalities optimally while ensuring patient safety. Lastly, the financial implications of incorporating dual-energy and photon-counting techniques into practice cannot be overlooked. The cost of acquiring new technology, as well as operating and maintenance expenses, can exceed healthcare budgets for small hospitals or underdeveloped regions. This financial burden may inadvertently limit the availability of advanced imaging for certain patient populations, leading to inequities in care. Additionally, with limited resources, healthcare institutions may need to invest in other services or technology aside from advanced CT imaging, which can impede progress in atherosclerotic plaque assessment and patient safety initiatives. Therefore, healthcare policymakers must consider both the clinical benefits and financial feasibility of embracing these innovative methodologies in offering equal access to high-quality diagnostic hardware that ultimately enhances patient safety and outcomes (Balestrieri et al., 2024).

1.6.3. Cost Implications and Accessibility of Advanced CT Technologies

The advent of new CT technologies, particularly dual-energy and photon-counting technologies, has very significant implications for cost containment and the affordability of imaging services. New modalities would typically require a substantial capital investment in hardware and integration into existing operational healthcare facilities. Based on several studies, their acquisition and maintenance costs are high, leading to disparities in access between facilities, particularly between urban and rural facilities. Therefore, cost-conscious hospitals may prefer conventional imaging modalities over these new modalities, to the patient's disadvantage, as improved diagnosis with these new methods can revolutionize disease detection and treatment planning. Further, the expense of maintaining high-tech CT technologies, including the training of healthcare professionals and upkeep, may play a part in healthcare disparities. Organizations may struggle to manage ongoing expenses associated with operating advanced imaging equipment, as well as higher costs for consumables and software updates. Nevertheless, the potential for dramatically increased diagnostic accuracy through methods such as dual-energy CT, with improved tissue characterization and material discrimination, is finally an investing rationale that carries powerful allure. Lastly, as healthcare environments become more and more inclined toward value-based care systems, the dilemma is in weighing high initial expenditures against long-term benefits of earlier diagnosis and reduced need for more invasive methods, which can potentially translate to overall cost savings in patient treatment. Availability of such newer CT technologies, such as dual-energy and photon-counting systems, can also be denied by insurance reimbursement and payment structures. Many healthcare providers would benefit from improved payment systems that value the additional capabilities of these new imaging technologies. As physicians and hospitals encourage advancements in diagnostic technology, strides must be made to implement insurance systems that, ideally, properly subsidize these therapies, thereby improving access for patients in resource-scarce environments. In addition, awareness and education concerning the benefits of advanced imaging must be disseminated among healthcare providers and policymakers as well. By defeating the fiscal challenges and struggling for greater insurance coverage, the healthcare community can achieve improved access to these new technologies, and ultimately promote equity in diagnostic imaging and patient outcomes (Hall et al., 2013; Moudi et al., 2014).

SUMMARY

The advancement of new CT techniques, such as dual-energy and photon-counting, has significantly enhanced diagnostic capabilities in medical imaging. Dual-energy CT differentiates materials based on their atomic structures by using two X-ray energies. This is particularly useful for diagnosing tissue properties, as it improves contrast resolution and facilitates attenuation correction, leading to better detection of disease conditions. With this new imaging technique, healthcare professionals can visualize disease processes that are not visible with conventional CT, particularly in oncology and cardiovascular imaging. Apart from dual-energy CT, PCCT is a key innovation in the field. In contrast to traditional harmonization techniques involving X-ray photon detection and summation, PCCT uses advanced detectors that count each photon and measure its energy. This development enables enhanced spatial resolution and imaging quality at lower radiation doses. As such, PCCT holds potential to be of significant value in clinical practice, particularly in the fine imaging of carotid artery atherosclerotic disease and plaque morphology. Its ability to discriminate between tissue types holds the potential to provide informative details for assessing plaque vulnerability and cerebral vascular event risk, thereby potentially impacting future clinical management (Bertacchi et al., 2024). The development of cardiac imaging with CT technology further elucidates the utility of these techniques in non-invasive diagnosis and myocardial condition monitoring. Cardiac CT has emerged as an important imaging modality that may replace or complement traditional imaging modalities such as magnetic resonance imaging (MRI) and echocardiography when they are inappropriate. The latest development enables full myocardial characterization, including quantification of conditions such as fibrosis and strain analysis. These capabilities are set to propel cardiac CT from basic anatomical assessment, possibly to a mainstay of routine clinical use for myocardial health evaluation (Alkadhi et al., 2024). This overabundance of information underscores the vast potential and necessity of integrating advanced CT imaging modalities into routine diagnostic workflows, solidifying their cornerstone role in shaping patient outcomes.

CLOSER LOOK

ADVANCED CT TECHNIQUES

The Potential Impact on Patient Care and Medical Imaging Advancements

The integration of advanced CT techniques, such as dual-energy and photon-counting technologies, has the potential to significantly enhance patient care by improving diagnostic accuracy and reducing radiation exposure. These advancements enable more precise imaging capabilities that can differentiate between various tissue types and pathologies, allowing for greater specificity in diagnoses. For instance, dual-energy CT utilizes different energy levels to characterize materials based on their attenuation properties. This ability to quantify distinct tissue characteristics can enhance the detection of cardiovascular diseases and other conditions that rely on detailed imaging, consequently facilitating timely and effective intervention. As the medical imaging field continues to evolve, these technologies will play a pivotal role in refining diagnostic processes and tailoring treatment strategies to individual patient needs, ultimately leading to better patient outcomes and reduced healthcare costs (Cabrelle et al., 2023). In addition to enhancing the sensitivity of imaging modalities, advancements in medical imaging technologies also embrace AI to optimize interpretative accuracy and efficiency. AI algorithms can analyze imaging data rapidly, identifying patterns and abnormalities that clinicians. This capability is particularly beneficial in cardiovascular imaging, where the quantitative assessment of inflammation and disease activity is critical. The automated tools developed to improve disease quantification in PET/CT scans, as exemplified by recent studies, underscore the need for AI-driven solutions in clinical practice. Such innovations promise to reduce the burden on radiologists, allowing them to focus on complex cases requiring higher-order clinical reasoning while improving diagnostic rates and treatment personalization (Van et al., 2024). Furthermore, the cumulative impact of these advanced imaging techniques extends beyond immediate diagnostic improvements to the broader spectrum of patient-centered care. Enhanced imaging capabilities facilitate better stratification of patient risk, ultimately enabling tailored therapeutic interventions. By offering high-resolution anatomical and functional data, these advancements have revolutionized the approach to managing diseases such as cancer and vascular disorders. As demonstrated through various research efforts, including those utilizing advanced imaging in oncology and cardiovascular applications, high-definition imaging can inform clinical decision-making and improve the efficacy of neoadjuvant therapies. Thus, as dual-energy and photon-counting CT techniques continue to gain traction, the field of medical imaging stands poised to deliver not only superior diagnostic tools but also a paradigmatic shift toward more individualized and effective patient care strategies (Cabrelle et al., 2023).

REFERENCES

1. Ahmed, F., & Maisano, J. (2017). *ToScA North America (6–8 June 2017, The University of Texas, Austin, TX) Program.* https://core.ac.uk/download/211334283.pdf (accessed on 5th August 2025).
2. Al Moudi, M. Z. (2014). Diagnostic value of nuclear cardiology in coronary artery disease. https://core.ac.uk/download/195631955.pdf (accessed on 5th August 2025).
3. Lisi, C., Moser, L.J., Mergen, V. *et al.* Advanced myocardial characterization and function with cardiac CT. *Int J Cardiovasc Imaging* (2024). https://doi.org/10.1007/s10554-024-03229-1Almeida, M. M., Destefani, A. C., Destefani, V. C., Mendonça, D., et al. (2024). Cutting-edge advancements in musculoskeletal radiology: A comprehensive review of innovative techniques and their impact on diagnostic capabilities. https://core.ac.uk/download/617924504.pdf (accessed on 5th August 2025).
4. AlSaadi, A., Jain, A., Al-Jabri, A., Delanerolle, G., Zabah, J., Shi, J. Q., Phiri, P., et al. (2024). Technological advances in SPECT and SPECT/CT imaging. https://core.ac.uk/download/613741130.pdf (accessed on 5th August 2025).
5. Ananthasubramaniam, K., Rudin, G., & Sareen, N. (2017). Advances in cardiac computed tomography. https://core.ac.uk/download/322431419.pdf (accessed on 5th August 2025).
6. Balestrieri, A., Bossone, E., Cademartiri, F., Cau, R., Cavaliere, C., La Grutta, L., Maffei, E., et al. (2024). Photon-counting computed tomography in atherosclerotic plaque characterization. https://core.ac.uk/download/638995753.pdf (accessed on 5th August 2025).
7. Becce, F., Booij, R., Gallego Manzano, L., Mourad, A., et al. (2024). Chances and challenges of photon-counting CT in musculoskeletal imaging. https://core.ac.uk/download/610639100.pdf (accessed on 5th August 2025).
8. Bertacchi, J., Bossone, E., Cademartiri, F., Cau, R., et al. (2024). Photon-counting computed tomography angiography of carotid arteries: A topical narrative review with case examples. https://core.ac.uk/download/621423889.pdf (accessed on 5th August 2025).
9. Boi, A., Cademartiri, F., Congiu, T., Faa, G., et al. (2024). Coronary artery calcification: Current concepts and clinical implications. https://core.ac.uk/download/614059412.pdf (accessed on 5th August 2025).
10. Booij, R., Dijkshoorn, M. L., van der Lugt, A., van der Werf, Y. D., et al. (2022). Assessment of iodine contrast-to-noise ratio in virtual monoenergetic images reconstructed from dual-source energy-integrating CT and photon-counting CT data. https://core.ac.uk/download/567462842.pdf (accessed on 5th August 2025).
11. Bousse, A., Kandarpa, V. S. S., Rit, S., Perelli, A., et al. (2024). Systematic review on learning-based spectral CT. https://core.ac.uk/download/587634376.pdf (accessed on 5th August 2025).
12. Bove, P., Finazzi Agrò, E., Kim, F. J., Miano, R., Micali, S., Rosa, M., & Usai, P. (2013). Recent findings and new technologies in nephrolithiasis: A review of the recent literature. https://core.ac.uk/download/pdf/54580708.pdf (accessed on 5th August 2025).
13. Budde, R. P. J., Hirsch, A., Lemmens, M. J. D. K., Mihl, C., et al. (2024). Photon-counting detector computed tomography in cardiac imaging. https://core.ac.uk/download/621177108.pdf (accessed on 5th August 2025).

14. Burger, M., Sawatzky, A., & Steidl, G. (2014). First order algorithms in variational image processing. https://core.ac.uk/download/34228185.pdf (accessed on 5th August 2025).
15. Cabrelle, G., Crimi, F., Gambato, S., Lupi, A., Pepe, A., Perazzolo, A., Quaia, E., et al. (2023). Medical radiology: Current progress. https://core.ac.uk/download/614221390.pdf (accessed on 5th August 2025).
16. Cirigliano, V., Dekens, W., Mereghetti, E., Walker-Loud, A., et al. (2018). Neutrinoless double beta decay in effective field theory: The light Majorana neutrino exchange mechanism. *arXiv*. http://arxiv.org/abs/1710.01729 (accessed on 5th August 2025).
17. Doria, A., Rosen, A., Pakhomov, A. G., Orlando, A. R., Born, B., Jang, B. S., Furse, C., et al. (2012). A dual-beam irradiation facility for a novel hybrid cancer therapy. *arXiv*. http://arxiv.org/abs/1206.4840 (accessed on 5th August 2025).
18. Gascho, D. (2024). Photon-counting CT for forensic death investigations—a glance into the future of virtual autopsy. https://core.ac.uk/download/621172575.pdf (accessed on 5th August 2025).
19. Hall, A., Sato, A., Schneiderman, A., Goren, A. D., Farman, A. G., Murray, A. K., Hermanson, A. S., et al. (2013). Surfing the spectrum–what is on the horizon? https://core.ac.uk/download/29032647.pdf (accessed on 5th August 2025).
20. Harris, E. D., Lin, H., & Acton, J. M. (2016). *Governance of Dual-Use Technologies: Theory and Practice*. https://core.ac.uk/download/75785647.pdf (accessed on 5th August 2025).
21. Hasn, S. (2023). Inspection of complex objects utilizing energy-sensitive X-ray imaging. https://core.ac.uk/download/643424401.pdf (accessed on 5th August 2025).
22. Liu, Y. (2018). Research status and prospect for CT imaging. https://core.ac.uk/download/322434518.pdf (accessed on 5th August 2025).
23. Schmidt, T. G. (2012). An empirical method for correcting the detector spectral response in energy-resolved CT. https://core.ac.uk/download/213084669.pdf (accessed on 5th August 2025).
24. Ståhl, F. (2023). *Dual-Energy Imaging in Stroke: Feasibility of Dual-Layer Detector Cone-Beam Computed Tomography*. https://core.ac.uk/download/588362183.pdf (accessed on 5th August 2025).
25. van Praagh, G. (2024). Towards optimal quantification in vascular PET and CT imaging. https://core.ac.uk/download/620188794.pdf (accessed on 5th August 2025).
26. Will, C. M., Nguyen, H., Overduin, J. M., Tasson, J. D., Carbone, L., Messier, M. D., et al. (2011). Matter-gravity couplings and Lorentz violation. https://core.ac.uk/download/213843423.pdf (accessed on 5th August 2025).

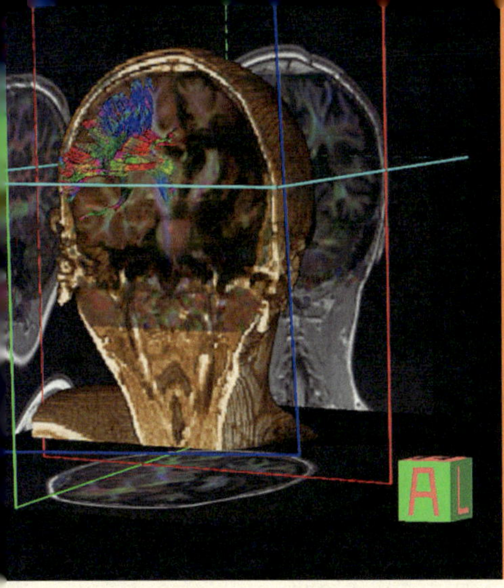

Chapter 2

FUNCTIONAL MRI AND DIFFUSION IMAGING

Contents

Introduction

The advent of functional magnetic resonance imaging (fMRI) and diffusion imaging has revolutionized medical imaging, particularly in oncology and neuroscience. fMRI enables researchers and clinicians to map brain activity by measuring changes in blood flow, thereby obtaining valuable information about cognitive processes and neural networks. Concomitantly, diffusion imaging, and above all, diffusion tensor imaging (DTI), aim at the characterization of microstructural integrity of white matter tracts of the brain. This dual approach prepares health professionals not only to diagnose disorders but also to monitor treatment outcomes and follow up, underscoring the profound impact of cutting-edge imaging technologies on patient care. The diagnosis and treatment of prostate cancer, when it is coupled with imaging modalities like mpMRI, offer superior accuracy compared to traditional procedures like transrectal ultrasound. With prostate cancer being one of the significant causes of cancer mortality in men, accurate detection, localization, and staging are currently the primary concerns. The limitations of TRUS-guided biopsy—ineffective resolution and tissue characterization—emphasize the need for improved techniques. Advances in mpMRI enable not just the identification of aggressive cancer but also play a role in active surveillance practices, which are appropriate with evolving intricacies in the management of prostate cancer. The expanding application of mpMRI calls to mind the crucial role imaging plays in enhancing cancer detection and guiding the decision to treat, practically contributing to reducing death rates due to prostate cancer (Cabarrus et al., 2017). Moreover, diffusion imaging uses extend beyond oncology, offering crucial assistance in the comprehension of neurological disorders. For instance, DTI measurements of white matter integrity have yielded important information in traumatic brain injury and multiple sclerosis. The ability to estimate internal structures and external surfaces in brain imaging is particularly relevant because it addresses broader scientific issues, such as drug delivery in critical anatomical regions. Using advanced tube-fitting algorithms, researchers can acquire meaningful information about the integrity of anatomical structures and thereby contribute to both clinical and scientific knowledge in neuroimaging (Caffo et al., 2011). Combining functional MRI with diffusion imaging provides a window into the brain's physiological processes, the development of a number of disease states, and better overall patient outcomes.

2.1. Principles of Functional MRI

Functional magnetic resonance imaging (fMRI) relies on the hemodynamic response principle, a measure of brain oxygen consumption that reflects neuronal activity. Activation of an area of the brain is followed by increases in blood flow to that area, providing oxygen and nutrients needed for enhanced function. This neural-vascular dynamic interaction underlies the blood oxygen level-dependent (BOLD) signal that fMRI uses. The BOLD signal is a measure of changes in the magnetic properties of blood, allowing researchers to observe brain activity in response to cognitive tasks or stimuli. It is crucial to understand these fundamental principles in order to properly interpret fMRI data and appreciate its applications within cognitive neuroscience, as well as in clinical practice, as they provide the brain's structure-function relationships required for the diagnosis and follow-up monitoring of neurodegenerative disorders, such as Alzheimer's disease. The addition of diffusion imaging techniques like diffusion tensor imaging (DTI) advances knowledge of the connectivity of the brain, along with fMRI. Based on the detection of water-molecule diffusion through brain tissue, DTI evaluates the microstructural integrity of white matter tracts, thereby sculpting neural pathways for communication between regions. This modality is essential for mapping the brain's architecture and for assessing how structural connectivity might correlate with functional activity, as quantified by fMRI. These modalities accurately capture the brain's complex networks and are increasingly being utilized to clarify numerous neurological diseases, including mild Alzheimer's disease. Specifically, the combination of fMRI and diffusion imaging can provide important insights into the neuroanatomical and neurophysiological substrates of cognitive deficits, making it easier to identify potential biomarkers for early intervention (Babiloni et al., 2016). Additionally, the convergence of fMRI and diffusion imaging provides a comprehensive framework for studying the functional and structural features of the brain, yielding in-depth insights into cognitive processes. For instance, integrating findings from resting-state fMRI and DTI can elucidate the intrinsic brain network pathology of mild cognitive impairment (MCI) and Alzheimer's disease. Research indicates that both structural connectivity, as measured by impaired white matter integrity, and functional connectivity, as reflected by aberrant resting-state BOLD activity, are correlated with cognitive impairment. These partnerships offer a window of opportunity to understand the trajectory of neurodegenerative disease better and to develop clinical resources geared towards improving patient outcomes. In this case, diffusion imaging's ability to highlight connectivity failures fits with fMRI's ability to chart functional alterations, thus allowing for a deeper understanding of the pathological processes underlying most cognitive disorders (Barkovich et al., 2010).

2.1.1. Mechanism of Blood-Oxygen-Level-Dependent (BOLD) Contrast

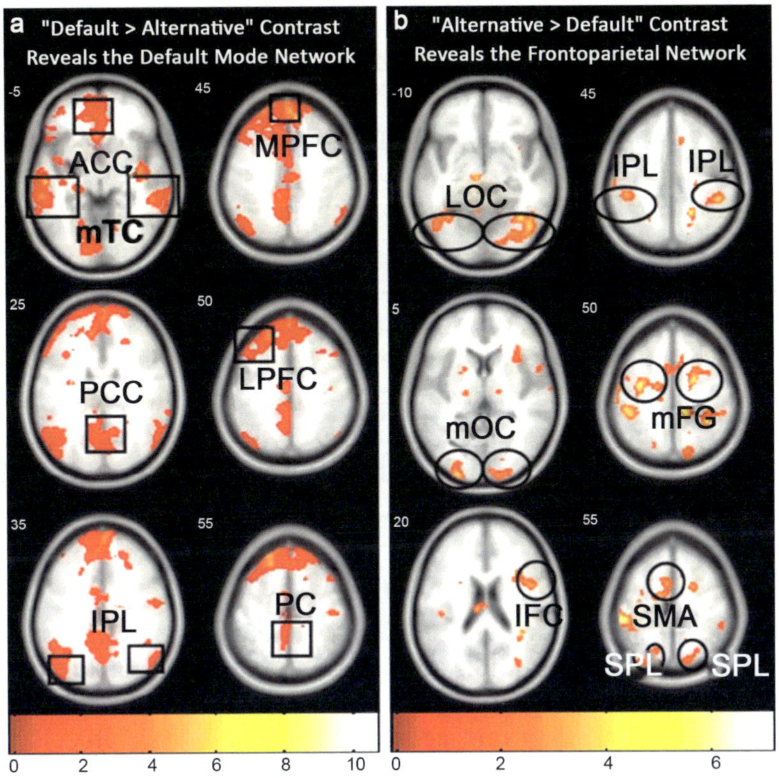

Figure 2.1. (a) Blood oxygen level-dependent (BOLD) related functional magnetic resonance imaging (fMRI) activity associated with the default percept as defined by the contrast default > alternative. The boxed clusters indicate regions previously b 4C.

Source: https://www.researchgate.net/profile/Spiro-Pantazatos/publication/236062636/figure/fig1/AS:601763811962890@1520483081669/a-Blood-oxygen-level-dependent-BOLDrelated-functional-magnetic-resonance-imaging.png.

The mechanism of BOLD contrast is fundamentally founded on the intricate relationship between neural activity and hemodynamic responses (Figure 2.1). When neurons discharge, they require more oxygen to sustain their metabolic requirements. This regional increase in neural activity triggers a cascade of physiological events, primarily of the cerebral vasculature, which leads to vasodilation. Hence, there is also an increase in blood flow to the active region, delivering oxygenated blood that is in excess of the oxygen consumption by the active neurons. This process leads to a relative decrease in the quantity of deoxyhemoglobin, which is paramagnetic and impacts T2* relaxation times, making BOLD fMRI sensitive to related signal changes. The real-time measurement of these changes enables researchers and clinicians to track brain function, which is fundamental to both basic neuroscience research and clinical diagnostics. Furthermore, understanding the intricacies of BOLD contrast is required for the effective interpretation of functional MRI data. Modulations in BOLD signals are not only produced by neuronal activity but also by alterations in systemic physiological parameters, including blood volume, blood flow, and oxygenation levels. For instance, the introduction of respiratory difficulties has proved to be a helpful experimental model and one that provided insight into the role of oxygen and carbon dioxide concentrations in the determination of cerebral hemodynamics. Such approaches help to explain the complex interactions inevitable for BOLD signals. Apart from that, the non-invasiveness inherent to BOLD imaging allows one to study clinical conditions, such as chronic kidney disease (CKD), and their impact on cerebrovascular function, thereby contributing further to the understanding of various pathophysiological states (Breidthardt et al., 2016). The study of BOLD contrast also entails knowledge regarding its limitations and variables capable of influencing findings. Although BOLD MRI is a powerful diagnostic in assessing cerebral and renal oxygenation, it can be undermined by hematocrit levels, age, and pre-existing vascular disease that impairs interpretation. The evolving state of MRI methods, as well as standard BOLD imaging, provides a rationale for extensive analysis to ensure secure clinical application. Integration of methods, such as phase contrast and diffusion-weighted imaging, provides complementary information on tissue viability and perfusion dynamics, which may aid in increased understanding of renal and cerebral physiology. Continued refinement of these imaging modalities will hold out promise for the use of BOLD contrast in the clinical setting, ushering in increased diagnostic capability (Dani et al., 2016).

2.1.2. Temporal and Spatial Resolution of fMRI

fMRI is one of the primary neuroimaging methods for visualizing brain activity via changes in blood flow. Temporal and spatial resolution are two of the most important features of fMRI that have direct effects on the accuracy of collected data. Temporal resolution is concerned with the ability to detect temporal changes in brain activity. Standard fMRI protocols typically possess a temporal resolution of two to three seconds per scan, potentially pushing the limits of detecting fast neural events. More sophisticated methods, such as multi-band imaging, can greatly surpass this resolution. This plays a critical role in capturing fast brain activity change, and therefore, temporal resolution limitation knowledge is still at the core of the fMRI's utility in cognitive neuroscience. Spatial resolution, on the other hand, is the ability to distinguish between different regions of the brain, thus the specific areas that are involved while doing tasks (Figure 2.2).

High spatial resolution allows researchers to pinpoint localized brain activity with greater accuracy, which is required for understanding sophisticated behavioral and cognitive phenomena. The old spatial resolution of fMRI ranges from 1.5 to 3 millimeters; however, ongoing hardware and imaging technology advancements, such as higher magnetic field strengths, enable higher resolution down to the millimeter or submillimeter range. Of particular interest, such advancements are best suited for studying smaller structures or functional networks of the brain. Increasing spatial resolution can lead to tremendous gains in understanding variation in neuroanatomy, as observed in studies that used fMRI to compare brain morphology across various populations. The relationship between temporal and spatial resolution in fMRI serves not only to highlight its ability to localize brain function but also to highlight the necessity of thorough quality assurance (QA) to reverse errors that have the potential to compromise data integrity. Potential sources of error, such as motion artifacts or differences in magnetic fields, can detrimentally affect both resolutions (Vogelbacher et al., 2020). Therefore, rigorous QA processes, such as the use of standardized phantom measurements in combination with human data analysis, are required to deliver secure and reproducible findings (Gozzi et al., 2013). By upholding high standards for data acquisition and interpretation, researchers can guarantee that fMRI is used to its full potential, ultimately resulting in improved comprehension of neurological diseases and improved clinical practices in brain imaging.

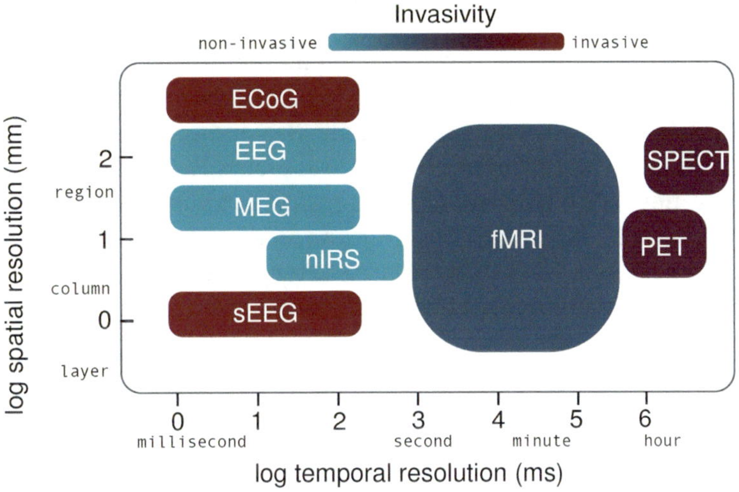

Figure 2.2. Spatial and temporal resolutions of different modalities commonly used for functional imaging. A typical fMRI acquisition (as of 2014) enjoys spatial resolution of the order of 1 – 3mm 3 and temporal resolution of the order of 1-3 seconds.

Source: https://www.researchgate.net/profile/Fabian-Pedregosa/publication/278826818/figure/fig3/AS:614336141746177@1523480558607/Spatial-and-temporal-resolutions-of-diierent-modalities-commonly-used-for-functional.png.

2.1.3. Applications of fMRI in Cognitive Neuroscience

fMRI has revolutionized our understanding of the brain's intricate functions. It allows scientists to conclude neural activity associated with specific cognitive processes by measuring changes in blood oxygen level-dependent signals. The technology's non-invasive character has played a key role in clarifying the relationship between cognitive processes and neural networks, such as memory, attention, and emotion regulation (Figure 2.3). For instance, fMRI research has identified the neural substrates that mediate episodic memory retrieval and has demonstrated the roles of the hippocampus and medial prefrontal cortex in these processes. Further, fMRI data have enabled mapping of differential brain activity patterns across varying cognitive tasks to emphasize modality-specific processing and inform the functional architecture of the brain. The recent advances in fMRI technology, particularly its integration with diffusion tensor imaging (DTI), have enabled increased understanding of brain microstructure and connectivity. DTI quantifies white matter integrity by measuring water diffusion within brain tissue, yielding critical information about the structural networks that support cognition. Integration of fMRI and DTI has enriched our understanding of many neurological disorders, such as Alzheimer's disease (AD). For example, research has identified that patients with mild cognitive impairment exhibit broken white matter integrity in significant brain areas, and this is associated with non-normal functional connectivity based on resting-state fMRI. These findings highlight the ability of a combination of DTI and fMRI to identify structural as well as functional alterations present in cognitive impairment, making early diagnosis and intervention strategy efficient in clinics, as explained by a large literature on neuroanatomical substrates of cognitive deficits of AD (Babiloni et al., 2016). In addition, new analysis techniques, such as non-negative matrix factorization, have enhanced the interpretability of fMRI data, particularly when examining complex structures like the hippocampus. Using advanced algorithms that identify patterns of microstructural change in the hippocampus, researchers can gain valuable information about cognitive ability differences between people. High-resolution imaging from resources like the Human Connectome Project, merged with multivariate analysis, enables researchers to separate specific microstructural elements linked to cognitive outcomes. The integration of fMRI with new analytical methods suggests a robust foundation for future studies to unravel the neurophysiological substrate of cognition. As depicted in more recent studies, the use of multiple indices enhances the reliability of data interpretation, opening the door to a deeper understanding of how microstructure is connected to behavioral measurements (Chakravarty et al., 2019).

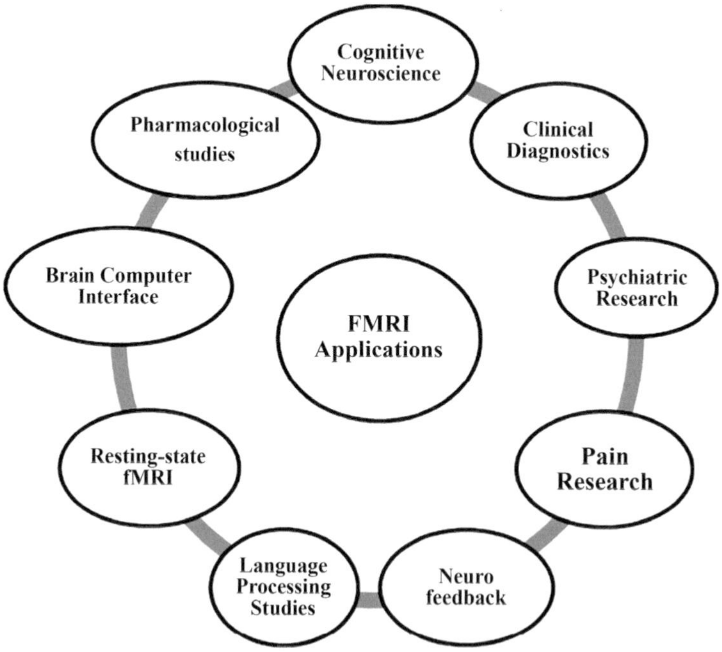

Figure 2.3. Progress and prospects in functional MRI (fMRI).

Source: https://media.springernature.com/lw685/springer-static/image/chp%3A10.1007%2F978-981-96-1124-9_13/MediaObjects/532820_1_En_13_Fig1_HTML.png.

2.2. Principles of Diffusion Imaging

Diffusion imaging, or more precisely DTI, is a cornerstone in evaluating the microstructural integrity of neural tissue. Through measuring the Brownian motion of water molecules in the brain, DTI provides essential information regarding the orientation and organization of white matter tracts. The method exploits the anisotropic diffusion of water, in which water diffuses more freely along the fiber pathway than perpendicular to it. Quantitative estimates, such as fractional anisotropy (FA), acquired as byproducts thus express brain tissue microstructural parameters. Increased FA values are more representative of normal white matter tracts, whereas low values can signal pathology, e.g., demyelination or axonal injury. Such assumptions render diffusion imaging highly valuable for clinical applications, both due to enhanced understanding of neuroanatomy and also because it facilitates the diagnosis of neurological illness and its extent. Coupling diffusion imaging with fMRI significantly improves our understanding of brain function by demystifying the relationship between structural and functional connectivity. While fMRI measures actual brain activity, as reflected in neuronal oxygen consumption, diffusion imaging provides insight into the anatomical pathways responsible for such functional interactions. For instance, both methods of investigation have indicated that disruption of white matter tracts can negatively affect functional patterns of connectivity, particularly in conditions such as epilepsy. Detailed mapping of white matter pathways using diffusion imaging allows scientists to uncover how structural disconnections may lead to functional impairments. This concordance highlights the importance given to the combination of diverse neuroimaging techniques in establishing a full understanding of brain health because alterations in either structure or function may have a profound impact on patient outcomes. Also, with further advancements in diffusion imaging techniques, our diagnostic and predictive powers are increasingly enhanced. Recent studies have identified robust relationships between FA values and clinical outcomes across numerous conditions, including cervical spondylotic myelopathy, in which preoperative FA correlates with postoperative recovery potential. Inferences from microstructural integrity allow clinicians to derive a valuable tool for individualizing interventions and monitoring therapeutic response over time. As outlined, FA values can serve as objective biomarkers of severity and recoverability, particularly in chronic neurological disease. The recoverability supports the utility of diffusion imaging in the clinic because it provides information that is vital not only to uncovering disease mechanisms but also to guiding individualized treatment plans to maximize patient quality of life.

2.2.1. Mechanism of Diffusion Tensor Imaging (DTI)

DTI was characterized as a potent instrument in the investigation of white matter microstructure of the brain. Essentially, DTI operates on the principle of water diffusion, in which the motion of water molecules is controlled by the structural integrity of the tissue beneath (Figure 2.4). DTI differs from classical diffusion imaging in that it measures diffusion in several directions, enabling the creation of tensor maps that characterize the orientation and coherence of white matter tracts. DTI's ability to estimate FA enables detection of regions with varying degrees of directional water flow. Elevated FA values are commonly found in healthy, well-organized white matter tracts, whereas decreased values can be the result of damage or degeneration. Thus, DTI has turned out to be very helpful in the study of diseases such as Alzheimer's disease, in which abnormality in the white matter is observed even at initial stages and hence becomes clinically relevant (Alves et al., 2012). The mechanism behind DTI makes us cognizant of the pathophysiology of neurodegenerative disorders by measuring the anisotropic diffusion of water. In mild cognitive impairment and Alzheimer's disease, DTI finds major alterations of FA and mean diffusivity, particularly in the important brain regions like the corpus callosum and the uncinate fasciculus. These microstructural changes indicate both primary and secondary degenerative processes, thereby providing an integrated picture of disease progression.

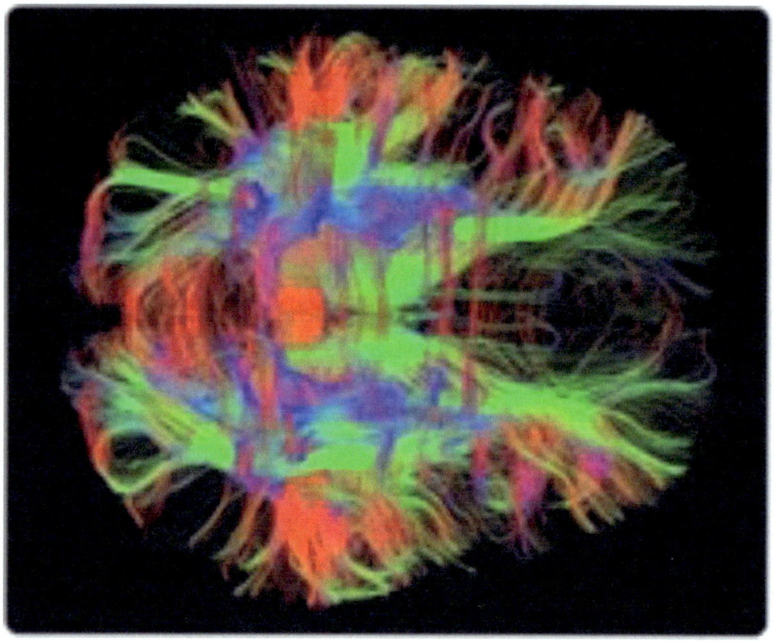

Figure 2.4. Diffusion tensor imaging (DTI).

Source: https://www.news-medical.net/image-handler/ts/20181011085702/ri/200/picture/2018/10/image7LR.jpg.

Through merging DTI estimations with brain volumetric measurements, researchers are able to chart the intricate relationship between white matter integrity and cognitive status. By this multi-modal system, not only is our understanding of disease manifestation at the microstructural level enhanced, but so is the potential for DTI as a clinical diagnostic and treatment assessment biomarker optimally served through being extremely valuable for early intervention programs for cognitive impairment (Alves et al., 2012). Ongoing research continues to uncover the intricacies of DTI, expanding its applications beyond neurodegenerative diseases. Recent research explored the dynamic nature of myelination and its impact on the integrity of white matter, particularly in the case of stress disorders. The results suggest that alterations in oligodendrocyte function, essential for myelin development, can influence white matter microstructure and, thereby, overall brain function. For instance, myelination modifications have been correlated with cholinergic stress responses, as shown in a study with veterans with PTSD. DTI measurements of myelination provide a viable mechanism for neural responses to trauma, demonstrating the flexibility of the methodology in responding to many different neurological questions. As DTI continues to mature, integration of functional imaging techniques might increasingly demonstrate how structure, function, and experience interact in the brain.

2.2.2. Measurement of Water Molecule Movement in Brain Tissue

Measurement of the movement of water molecules in the tissue of the brain is a critical component of fMRI and diffusion imaging procedures. The movement of water molecules, influenced by cellular structures and the surrounding microenvironment, provides information about various physiological and pathological conditions of the brain. Diffusion-weighted imaging (DWI) allows researchers to observe the random migration of water molecules, which is affected by the integrity of cellular membranes and the density of tissue structure. As brain function increases, alterations in blood supply and neuronal activation also affect water diffusion properties, creating variations in signal intensity. This correlation between neuronal activity and water motion enables understanding of brain function and disease and provides essential information for diagnosing neurological disorders and evaluating treatment response. Furthermore, the combination of diffusion imaging techniques with fMRI has enhanced the ability to characterize brain structure and connectivity. Recent advancements in imaging modalities, such as equipment capable of conducting PET/MRI scans simultaneously, have provided new possibilities to merge metabolic activity with structural integrity and diffusion values (Catana et al., 2008). The hybrid modalities enable a more accurate assessment of dynamic interactions within the brain's microenvironment. This is, for instance, measuring changes in the movement of water molecules to explain the mechanisms of brain disorders like multiple sclerosis and Alzheimer's disease, where altered diffusion properties can serve as indicators of disease state. The mapping function of these associations in a live brain highlights the significance of water molecule diffusion measurements in research and clinical use. Because research continues to explore the complexity of water motion in brain tissue, it is imperative to address issues related to imaging artifacts and data interpretation. Multimodal imaging, promising as it is, must be advanced in calibration and validation to ensure measurements accurately reflect biological processes (Cherry et al., 2008). Balancing different imaging modalities may produce artifacts that have to be addressed to ensure proper results. Technological advancements in imaging agents and sequences are being made to improve the accuracy of diffusion measurements in the presence of noise and motion. In these advancements, measurement of the motion of water molecules in brain tissue not only makes a better understanding of normal brain function possible but also propels us toward more effective interventions and targeted therapies for neurodegenerative disorders.

2.2.3. Applications of Diffusion Imaging in Understanding Brain Connectivity

The application of diffusion imaging, particularly DTI, plays an essential role in the comprehension of brain connectivity. By mapping the orientation and integrity of white matter tracts, DTI provides essential information about structural connectivity within the brain. The method acquires particular importance in the study of neurological disorders, where changes in brain structure may reflect underlying pathologies. Research has indicated that diffusion imaging can accurately identify disruption of white matter integrity associated with various conditions, including traumatic brain injury and neurodegenerative disorders. Clinicians and researchers can hence utilize such measurements to determine how structural disruption corresponds to functional impairment, thus improving diagnosis. The ability to visualize and quantify these tracks entirely redefines our comprehension of brain networks and their role in overall cognitive and functional capacity (Figure 2.5).

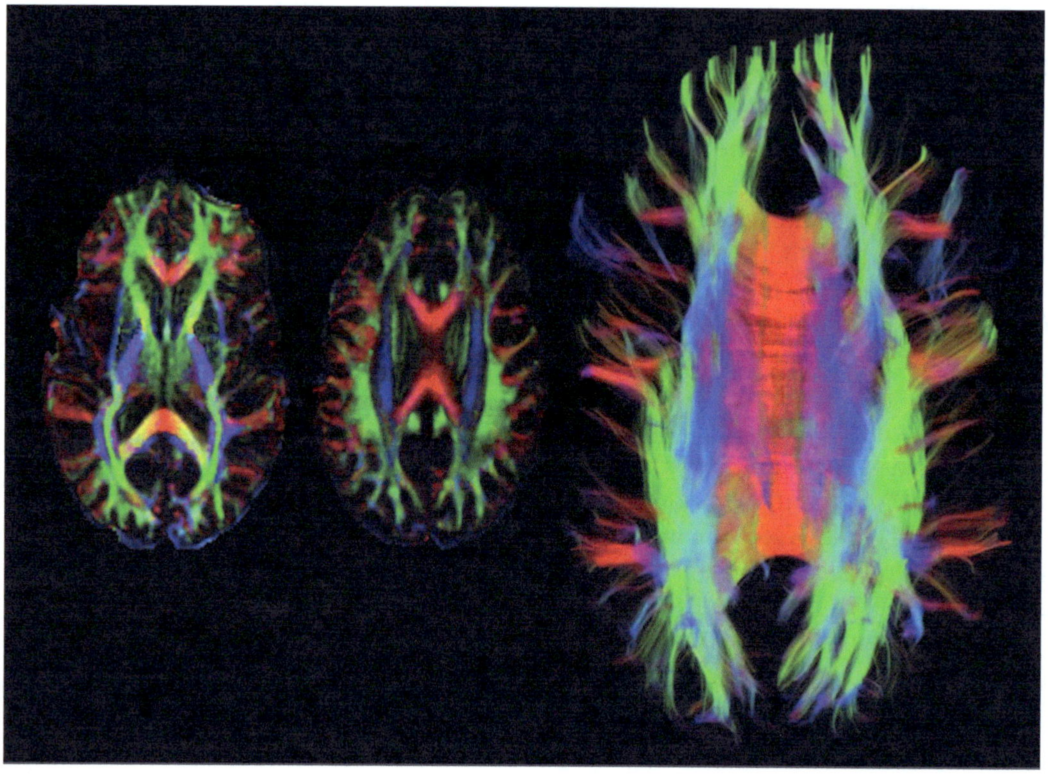

Figure 2.5. Human brain connectivity. Diffusion tensor imaging of the human brain obtained from 3-tesla MRI sequences. The technique allows visualization of the direction of tracts of white matter fibers. (Left and Middle) Panoramic views at different levels. (Right) High-magnification tractography of the corpus callosum and superior longitudinal fasciculus. The colors indicate the direction of the fibers (red, transversal; green, anteroposterior; blue, superoinferior). [Courtesy of Juan Álvarez-Linera (Fundación CIEN-Fundación Reina Sofía, Madrid)].

Source: https://www.researchgate.net/profile/Javier-Defelipe/publication/49637711/figure/fig3/AS:341713496363009@1458482254069/Human-brain-connectivity-Diffusion-tensor-imaging-of-the-human-brain-obtained-from.png.

Apart from its structural data, diffusion imaging also works alongside functional imaging techniques, such as resting-state functional MRI (rs-fMRI). Taken together, this multimodal imaging allows scientists to better understand the interactions between structural and functional brain connections. The study has found that patients with disorders such as Alzheimer's disease have significant impairments in both structural connectivity, as evidenced by diffusion imaging abnormalities, and functional connectivity, as measured by alterations in rs-fMRI metrics. Integration of the modality offers a more comprehensive understanding of how brain structure gives rise to cognition and offers potential biomarkers for the early identification and treatment of cognitive impairment. This integration of structural and functional analysis is critical to both basic neuroscience studies and clinical applications. Beyond basic neuroscience studies, diffusion imaging has practical applications in real-world clinical settings, such as neurosurgery. The use of DTI information allows neurosurgeons to visualize basic brain pathways before proceeding with an operation, minimizing the risk of damage to essential fiber tracts. Research indicates that awareness of structural connectivity from diffusion imaging can also profoundly influence the planning and results of surgery by sustaining cognitive ability and supporting the success of surgical aims. Besides surgery, diffusion imaging findings can also direct therapeutic regimens for targeted rehabilitation therapy after brain injury or neurologic illness. As highlighted by recent literature, including language mapping for epilepsy surgery, the ability to visualize and interrogate structural pathways makes significant contributions to our understanding of the brain's functional organization and its orientations in both clinical practice and research (Babiloni et al., 2016; Pur et al., 2020).

2.3. Comparison of fMRI and Diffusion Imaging

The field of neuroimaging provides a range of methods, one of which is fMRI and diffusion imaging that have become constitutive modalities to study brain activity and structure. fMRI primarily estimates changes in blood flow, indirectly mapping neural activity via the hemodynamic response. With its ability to provide temporal resolution of brain processes, fMRI is increasingly important in cognitive neuroscience and clinical research. On the other hand, Diffusion Imaging, especially through DTI, focuses on water-molecule diffusion within brain tissue. It provides insights into the integrity and organization of white matter tracts, which is crucial for understanding brain connectivity. Although the two procedures differ in function, they can complement each other when used together, providing a better understanding of brain structure and function and better supporting the overall analysis of neural processes. Comparative studies between fMRI and Diffusion Imaging reveal significant strengths and weaknesses peculiar to each method. fMRI is stronger at detecting active brain regions involved in specific tasks, with high spatial resolution, which is crucial for the localization of functions and pathologies within the brain. Its reliance on hemodynamic responses, however, can lead to indirect estimates of neural activity, which can introduce ambiguity in the interpretation of results. On the contrary, Diffusion Imaging can map white matter tracts, which are important for characterizing brain connections. It has been proven that integrating fMRI with DTI data provides better interpretative capacity, particularly in clinical diagnoses where it is important to know both functional and structural components of the brain. This two-fold approach is particularly relevant to diseases such as cancers and degenerative diseases, where activity and structure can be adversely affected, thereby offering more accurate examinations and tailored treatment protocols. The current advances point to the synergy between fMRI and Diffusion Imaging for early diagnosis and treatment of conditions such as cancer. For instance, multi-parametric MRI techniques that use DWI and DTI have been identified as holding great promise for differentiating between muscle-invasive and non-muscle-invasive bladder cancer, with high precision in staging. Methods of Neuroimaging, hence, are not only used as diagnostic agents but are also part of the treatment strategy. The growing consensus among researchers points to the fact that functional and diffusion imaging techniques can be used to improve patient outcomes, which can be achieved through early intervention (Barchetti et al., 2017). As research continues, continued exploration of functional activity and structural connectivity is vital to enhancing our understanding of complex neurological disorders and developing effective treatments (Halpern et al., 2018).

2.3.1. Differences in Imaging Techniques and Methodologies

Within neuroimaging, there are certain methodologies to match the specific requirements of investigation and principles of operation. fMRI relies primarily on the hemodynamic response to neuronal activity, yielding information about brain function using BOLD contrast. This technique is beneficial for mapping cognition to identify patterns of activation across various brain regions during tasks. On the other hand, Diffusion Imaging, specifically DTI, is interested in water molecule motion in neural tissue. Through diffusion mapping of these molecules, DTI tells us about the structure and integrity of white matter tracts and provides us with helpful information concerning structural connectivity within the brain. To value these fundamental differences, it is essential to select the appropriate imaging modality in research, diagnosis, and therapy. Though fMRI performs exceptionally well in recording real-time brain activity, it is limited (Figure 2.6).

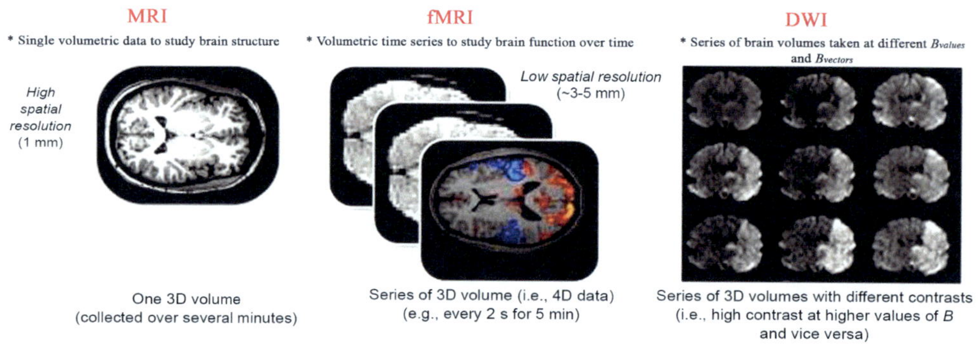

Figure 2.6. Advances and challenges in fMRI and DTI techniques.

Source: ScienceDirect.

The method's reliance on blood flow changes can lead to misinterpretations due to vascular confounds, preventing the identification of the actual neural correlates of cerebral processes. Furthermore, susceptibility to motion artifacts complicates analyses of dynamic cardiac or respiratory cycles and is frequently complicating analyses in certain populations, e.g., children or patients with neurological impairments. On the contrary, DTI, by enabling the visualization of the integrity of white matter, enables clinicians to assess developmental and degenerative disorders sufficiently. Its sensitivity to microstructural change makes it particularly useful in delineating disease course in disorders such as multiple sclerosis or traumatic brain injury. The interface between these imaging modalities underscores the need for equilibrium in interpreting neuroimaging data to address the complexities of understanding the structure and function of the brain. Advances, though, have enabled the development of improved imaging modalities that will minimize the shortcomings of fMRI and DTI, opening the door to greater consistency in their use. For instance, higher magnetic field strength in fMRI, such as 7 T systems, enhances spatial resolution, allowing brain activity to be better localized while reducing geometric distortions in images. Techniques such as B 0 field mapping or echo-planar imaging acquired with reversed phase encoding have been effective at correcting distortions typical of high-field fMRI studies, thus providing more precise interpretation of data (Michael-Schallmo et al., 2021). On top of that, advances in machine learning algorithms for image analysis can potentially bridge the gap between diffusion and functional imaging techniques by integrating structural connectivity data and functional activity measurement. Not only does this interdisciplinarity provide an extended understanding of brain networks, but it also has novel applications in research and clinical settings, which deepen the discussion on sound imaging methods in neuroscience.

2.3.2. Strengths and Limitations of Each Imaging Modality

Among neuroimaging techniques, fMRI stands out in that it can demonstrate brain function through imaging changes in blood flow, a surrogate measure for neural activity. Such inherent strength enables scientists to study resting-state networks, focusing on functional connectivity among different brain regions. A study utilizing resting state fMRI demonstrated tremendous differences in brain connectivity among subjects with migraine without aura and control volunteers, establishing fMRI's capability of discriminating subtle neuronal variation that can be employed to classify clinical status. While it has its advantages, fMRI is not without limitations, particularly in temporal resolution. The hemodynamic response observed with fMRI is not direct neuronal discharge, and this can be misleading in the interpretation of rapid cognitive processes, hence limiting its use in real-time testing of brain function. In contrast, diffusion imaging, particularly DTI, is more suited to visualize the integrity of white matter by means of measures such as fractional anisotropy and mean diffusivity (Figure 2.7).

DTI advantages	DTI disadvantages/ limitations
Short acquisition time (approximately 5 min)	
Available on most existing clinical system (acquisition, tensor reconstruction, scalar measures such as FA and ADC)	Limited in crossing and curving areas; only 1 fiber direction possible
Anisotropy measures (FA, parallel, perpendicular diffusivity) useful for clinical studies and aid for diagnosis	Scalar measures limited in non-Gaussian areas; measures must be interpreted with care

Figure 2.7. Advantages and Limitations of DTI.

Source: High Angular Resolution Diffusion Imaging (HARDI) - Scientific Figure on ResearchGate. Available from: https://www.researchgate.net/figure/Advantages-and-Limitations-of-DTI_tbl2_319558026 [accessed 8 Aug 2025]

This technique provides informative data on the microstructural properties of brain tissue to diagnose neurological disorders and injuries. DTI, for instance, can be used to assess thalamic microstructure in migraine patients, correlating structural changes with connectivity (Goel et al., 2013). Yet, even though DTI yields informative information in brain tractography, it relies on specific diffusion models that risk oversimplifying complex neurological pathways. Additionally, movement or adjacent-structure artifacts may impair image quality, rendering inferences based on such data invalid. Both fMRI and diffusion imaging have the potential to reveal novel details of brain function and structure, but each also has singular strengths and limitations that investigators must contend with. The power of fMRI to depict dynamic brain activity is strongly matched by its temporal limitations. At the same time, the strength of DTI in tracing white matter architecture is balanced against possible model limitations and vulnerability to artifacts. Together, these imaging modalities contribute strongly to the field of neuroscience; however, they need a keen understanding of their strengths and weaknesses for their optimal application. The integration of findings from both modalities can grant a deeper understanding of neurological processes, which can facilitate better diagnosis and treatment modalities in clinical environments (Goel et al., 2013).

2.3.3. Situations Where One Technique is Preferred Over the Other

In neuroimaging, the choice between fMRI and diffusion imaging is typically dependent on the final clinical purposes engaged. For instance, fMRI excels at assessing brain activity involved in cognitive functions and is hence the preferred modality in neurology research that requires the localization of functional brain areas. Areas such as language, memory, and motor function can be mapped using fMRI, which measures changes in blood flow as an indirect marker of neuronal activity. The technique is invaluable in pre-surgical planning for patients with brain tumors or epilepsy; awareness of functional cortical areas guarantees minimal risk of post-operative impairment. Diffusion imaging, however, is more appropriate for evaluating the microstructural integrity of brain tissue. This makes diffusion imaging particularly valuable in the treatment of acute stroke or traumatic brain injury, where cell viability and tracts are critical to the choice of treatment and prognosis. When applying imaging to treat prostate cancer, the imaging method employed may be adapted based on the specific clinical indication (Figure 2.8).

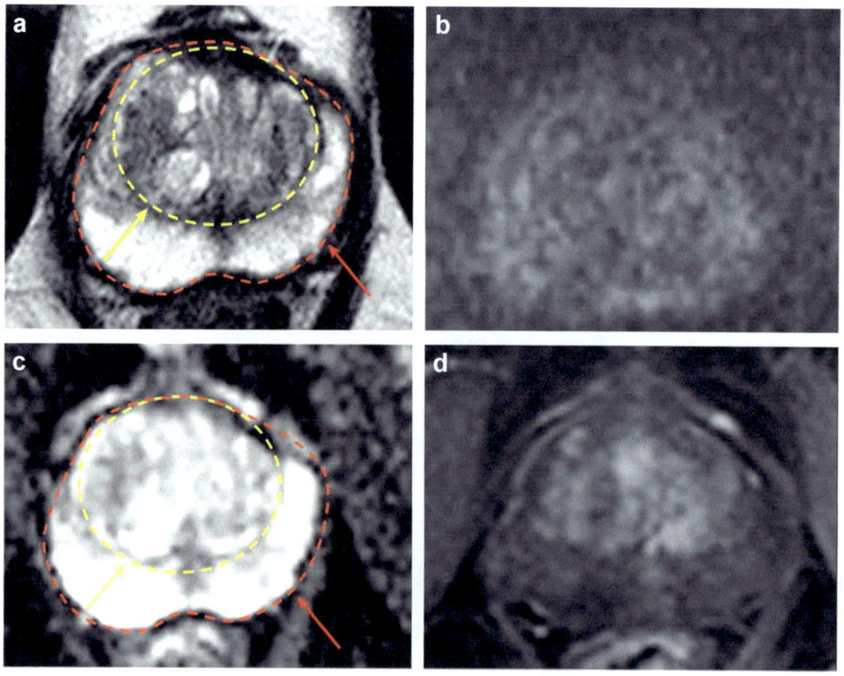

Figure 2.8. Multiparametric MRI for prostate cancer diagnosis.

Source: https://media.springernature.com/lw1200/springer-static/image/art%3A10.1038%2Fs41585-019-0212-4/MediaObjects/41585_2019_212_Fig1_HTML.png.

Multiparametric magnetic resonance imaging (mpMRI) is now the modality of choice over traditional ultrasound-guided biopsy due to its higher ability to detect and detail prostate lesions (Cabarrus et al., 2017). mpMRIs are used because their greater visual clarity of the prostate enhances diagnosis and patient outcomes. While the ultrasound is a valuable diagnostic tool, the lack of high spatial resolution and tissue characterization renders it less useful in the staging of more malignant prostate cancers. mpMRI is superior when visual separation between benign and malignant lesions is necessary, such as in active surveillance protocols, where it facilitates monitoring disease behavior. Here, inclusion of mpMRI has the ability to contribute significantly to clinical decision and ultimately enhance the treatment of patients within a complex and multidimensional setting. In the evaluation of pancreatic tumors, the use of a blend of imaging modalities with the patient's specific condition in mind is preferred. Although computed tomography (CT) remains the preferred imaging test for suspected pancreatic disease due to its ease of availability and thorough assessment of anatomical detail, multiparametric MRI is one of the central tools for characterizing complex lesions (Baccari et al., 2016). MRI, for example, can provide valuable information on the nature of solid versus cystic pancreatic tumors and demarcating tumor margins and vascular invasion. In these cases, the ability of MRI to provide contrast, emphasizing differences between healthy and pathological tissues, makes diagnostic confidence more certain. Multimodality imaging provides the clinician with the ability to join the strengths of each imaging modality, leading eventually to more accurate staging and management plans according to individual characteristics of pancreatic lesions.

2.4. Clinical Applications of Functional MRI

fMRI has rapidly emerged as an important diagnostic instrument in clinical practice, offering unparalleled access to brain functional anatomy. By detecting changes in blood flow associated with neuronal activity, fMRI allows clinicians and researchers to map brain function with unprecedented precision. This ability is of incalculable value in pre-surgical planning, particularly in neurosurgery, where critical areas dedicated to language, motor control, and sensory perception must be localized. Its use in the present context reduces the likelihood of postoperative deficits, thereby enhancing patients' overall outcome. In addition, its use is not limited to surgical applications; fMRI has also served as an unlock to the comprehension of a variety of neurological conditions, presenting valuable information guiding diagnosis and treatment pathways. Such advancements underscore the role of fMRI as a game-changer in the treatment of neurological disorders, repaving traditional models of clinical practice and research. In neurodegenerative diseases, functional MRI is likely to enable accurate diagnosis and disease monitoring. Atypical Parkinsonian disorders are challenging to diagnose since their symptoms are similar to those of idiopathic Parkinson's disease. However, advances in fMRI and other MRI techniques like DWI and DTI offer robust tools for discrimination. Research has shown that these novel imaging modalities can highlight specific patterns of brain activity and connectivity changes associated with various conditions like progressive supranuclear palsy and multiple system atrophy. These imaging modalities not only contribute to our understanding of the disease pathophysiology but also assist in establishing a baseline to measure the efficacy of therapeutic interventions. Thus, fMRI and ancillary imaging technologies hold significant potential for improving diagnostic accuracy and planning individualized treatment therapies for patients with complex neurological disorders (Brockhuis et al., 1970). Beyond diagnostics, the use of fMRI in the clinic extends to therapeutic monitoring and evaluation of intervention efficacy. For instance, in psychotherapeutic situations, fMRI has been employed to track brain activity changes as a response to different treatment modalities, for instance, cognitive-behavioral therapy for depression or anxiety disorders. By tracking neural responses over time, clinical practitioners can assess the efficacy of therapeutic interventions and adjust accordingly to optimize patient care. In addition, fMRI's non-invasiveness renders it the perfect candidate for longitudinal studies aiming to correlate brain function with treatment effect. This capacity to monitor and quantify treatment effect in real-time singles out fMRI's value as being not only that of a diagnostic, but also that of an important tool in the continuum of patient care. With continued advances in research, such clinical applications of fMRI represent a significant leap in expanding our understanding of both healthy and pathological neurological diseases (Destefani et al., 2024).

2.4.1. Role in Pre-Surgical Planning for Brain Tumors

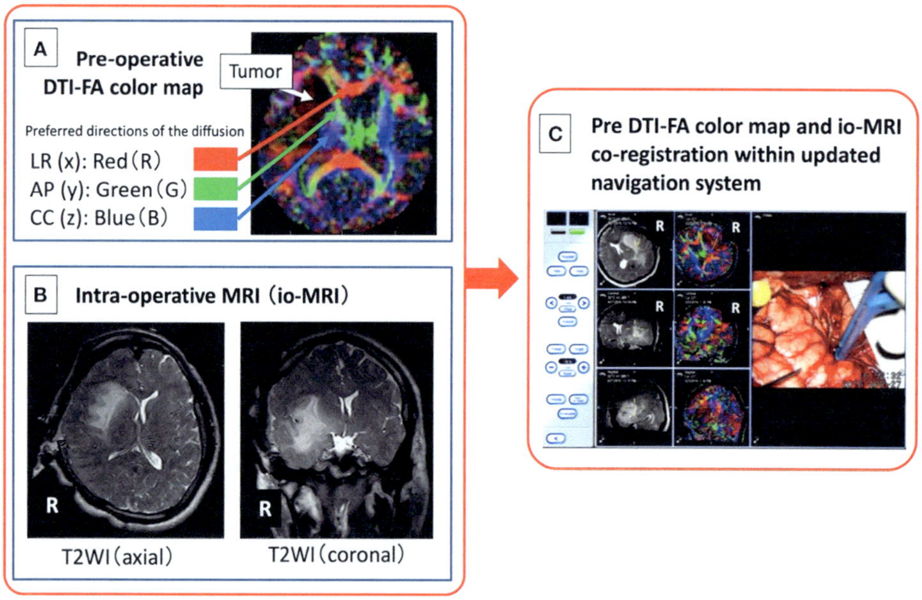

Figure 2.9. Combining pre-operative diffusion tensor images and intraoperative magnetic resonance,

Source: https://www.frontiersin.org/files/Articles/805952/fneur-12-805952-HTML/image_m/fneur-12-805952-g001.jpg.

The imaging contribution of fMRI and diffusion imaging to the pre-surgical planning of brain tumors has become a mainstay of modern neuro-oncological practice. These advanced imaging modalities provide precise measurement of tumor characteristics, including the extent of invasion into adjacent brain tissue, which is crucial for planning surgical approaches. Traditional MRI sequences, such as T1 and T2, were previously used to assess the structural integrity of the brain but lack specificity to aid surgical planning. Functional regions of the brain and tumor borders may be defined using a combination of fMRI and DTI. It results in more efficient surgical strategies that maximize functional preservation and tumor resection, thus enhancing patients' outcomes in the management of malignant brain tumors (Alexander et al., 2018) (Figure 2.9). Moreover, diffusion imaging provides useful information on the microstructural brain tumor alterations. Techniques like DTI enable white matter tract mapping, which enables the identification of eloquent brain areas to be preserved during surgery.

Data on such tracts are important since their preservation is essential to the preservation of neurological functions such as speech, motor function, and sensory perception. With the application of diffusion imaging to pre-surgical planning, neurosurgeons can produce a clearer comprehension of the tumors' relationship to such crucial pathways, allowing for targeted surgical methods with reduced risks of postoperative deficits. Such precise planning not only improves surgical precision but also directly contributes to better long-term functional outcomes for patients (N/A, 2018).

In addition to enhancing surgical methods, functional MRI also helps extensively with pre-surgical planning by providing details on the functional reorganization of the brain due to tumors. Tumors tend to induce compensatory rearrangements in brain function, leading to reorganization of neural circuits. fMRI helps detect such rearrangements so that neurosurgeons can detect areas within the brain that have compensated for diminished functions. Such information is invaluable when planning interventions because it reduces the risk of injury to the functional brain areas. Ultimately, the use of fMRI and diffusion imaging promotes a multidisciplinary approach towards planning surgery such that the intervention not only aims at the resection of the tumor but also considers the preservation of quality of life and neurological function in patients (Alexander et al., 2018).

2.4.2. Use in Assessing Brain Function in Neurological Disorders

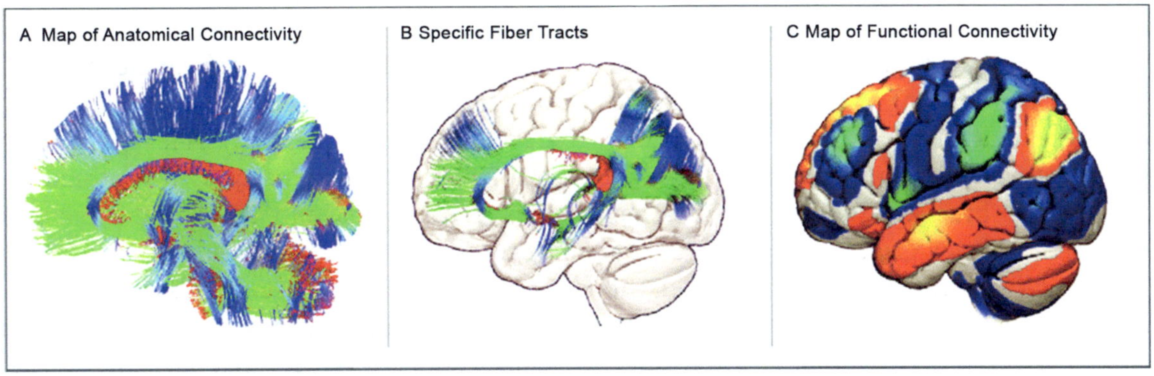

Figure 2.10. FMRI aids in diagnosing and treating mental health disorders.

Source: https://kryptonite.global/wp-content/uploads/2023/09/Introduction.png.

The assessment of brain function in neurological disorders has been greatly enhanced by employing advanced imaging techniques such as fMRI and DTI (Figure 2.10). fMRI takes advantage of the brain's hemodynamic response to quantify functional activity and allows scientists to visualize active brain regions during tasks or stimulation. This capability is also significant for the investigation of conditions such as stroke, epilepsy, and neurodegenerative disease, where the identification of alterations in brain activity can be employed to characterize disease processes and to aid therapeutic intervention. fMRI can also map brain areas subserving vital functions, which is significant for surgical planning in patients with neurological diseases and for minimizing the likelihood of post-surgical functional impairment. Diffusion tensor imaging, one specific application of MRI technology, is an important means of evaluating the integrity of white matter in the central nervous system. FA values derived from DTI provide quantitative data on microstructural changes in neural pathways associated with various neurologic diseases, particularly in disorders such as multiple sclerosis and cervical spondylotic myelopathy. Evidence also suggests that FA values can be linked to clinical measurements of function, making DTI a biomarker of disease severity and prognosis. For example, in one extensive study, preoperative FA measurements were shown to determine functional recovery in patients with cervical spondylotic myelopathy (Budde et al., 2018).

These findings highlight DTI's value in diagnosing and treating neurological disease and making rehabilitative interventions more targeted, with further patient benefit through evidence-based practice. Specifically, in some neurological disorders, DTI has shown promise for assessing structural pathology, even in orphan diseases such as mucopolysaccharidosis IVA (MPS IVA). MPS IVA patients often have widespread spinal involvement and associated neurological deterioration. Integration of DTI with standard imaging modalities may enhance the early identification of spinal cord involvement and permit timely interventions (Goel et al., 2013). Active intervention through such measures minimizes the worsening of neurological impairment, ultimately leading to a better long-term prognosis for patients. Furthermore, the inclusion of DTI in routine imaging protocols reinforces the need for continued monitoring in patients at risk of progressive neurological abnormalities, making it a valuable tool in today's neurological evaluation and management plans.

2.4.3. Contribution to Understanding Psychiatric Conditions

Research on psychiatric diseases has been considerably enhanced by advances in neuroimaging techniques, particularly fMRI and diffusion imaging. These imaging techniques make it possible for researchers to image brain activity and connectivity in real time, offering critical information on the neural mechanisms of mental illness disorders. With studies of structural and functional abnormalities of the brain, the research has facilitated the understanding of the biological mechanisms of various psychiatric diseases, such as schizophrenia, bipolar disorder, and major depressive disorder.

These imaging modalities not only enhance our understanding of the disorders' pathophysiology but also inform the formulation of targeted therapeutic approaches, a development increasingly relevant in a field where the heterogeneity of symptomatology makes diagnosis and treatment challenging. Together, fMRI and diffusion imaging are valuable portals of entry between clinical psychiatry and neuroscience. The ENIGMA Consortium is a pioneer that pools the excellence of large-scale neuroimaging research to propel our understanding of psychiatric disorders. The shared network of over 1,400 researchers all around the globe converged on an attempt to combine vast neuroimaging data and genetic data for well-established psychiatric disorders as well as for new areas of study (Figure 2.11).

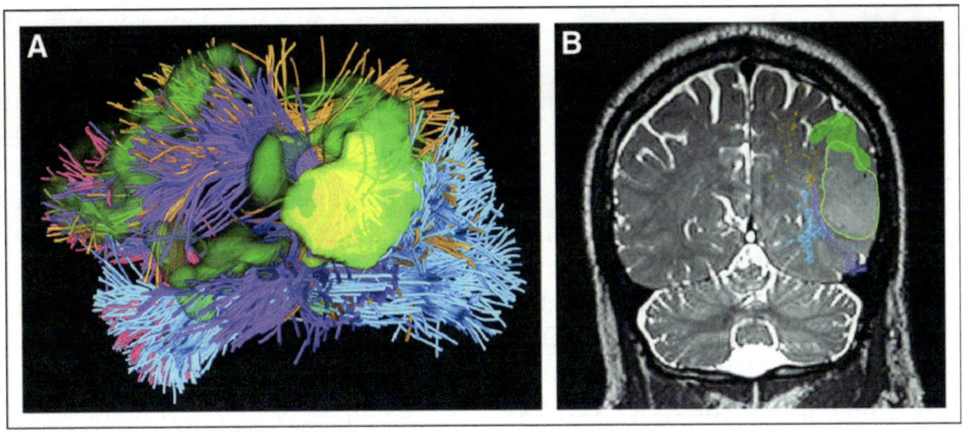

Figure 2.11. Visualization of multimodal diffusion magnetic resonance imaging (MRI) and functional MRI (fMRI) data for patient dataset 2. (A) Three-dimensional (3D) visualization of tractography using a two-tensor unscented Kalman filter method with free water modeling with fMRI (dark green) and tumor (bright yellow green); and (B) Intersection of the 3D visualization with a preoperative coronal T2-weighted MRI showing overlay of tracts, fMRI activations, and tumor surface. Recognition of the fMRI speech-related activations and the deeper subcortical arcuate fasciculus is important in tumors that are adjacent to the eloquent brain. Intraoperative visualization of these areas can aid the surgeon in preserving language and achieving gross total resection.

Source: https://www.researchgate.net/publication/340239803/figure/fig5/AS:873866662510593@1585357456660/sualization-of-multimodal-diffusion-magnetic-resonance-imaging-MRI-and-functional-MRI.png.

ENIGMA's approach has led to the identification of meaningful brain measures associated with disorders such as post-traumatic stress disorder, obsessive-compulsive disorder, and autism spectrum disorders. The collaborative infrastructure not only enhances the statistical power of the evidence but also enables researchers to examine several demographic and psychosocial factors leading to psychiatric disorders. These large-scale investigations point to the potential of big data aggregation with resultant replicable and reproducible findings, our insight into complex psychiatric syndromes is clear as in research by ENIGMA (Adhikari et al., 2020; Adhikari et al., 2020). Psychiatric disorder knowledge derived from functional neuroimaging is also informed by associations between genetic and environmental correlates and brain activity patterns. The range of disciplines within the ENIGMA Consortiums enables this question to be posed, exploring how life experience and biological traits interact to be expressed as mental illness. For instance, the exploration of genes associated with altered brain measurements has revealed heritable factors of psychiatric disease, alongside exploring how factors such as trauma and stress affect brain function. This holistic approach is a significant leap in psychiatric science, reaffirming the point that mental illness can never be fully understood without consideration of the complex interdependencies of the brain, genes, and environment. Thus, functional MRI and diffusion imaging, with their capability to enhance and enlighten interdisciplinary work, are significantly engaged in dismantling the complexity of psychiatric diseases, thereby paving the way for improved treatment and prevention strategies (Adhikari et al., 2020; Adhikari et al., 2020).

2.5. Clinical Applications of Diffusion Imaging

The clinical applications of diffusion imaging have now become revolutionary tools in investigating many varied neurological diseases. One of the most impressive applications of DTI is in the assessment of Alzheimer's disease (AD), whereby white matter integrity can be investigated to yield valuable information on disease progression. Studies have revealed that MCI and early AD have significant changes in specific white matter tracts, such as the splenium of the corpus callosum and thalamic pathways. These are significant because they are associated with cognitive impairment and may serve as good indicators for cerebral reserve capacity. Comprehending how diffusion imaging can illuminate such changes in structure has significant potential for the early diagnosis and ongoing monitoring of cognitive impairment, opening windows for the development of targeted therapeutic interventions aimed at correcting the causative neuroanatomical disruptions in AD. (Babiloni et al., 2016) Besides Alzheimer's, diffusion imaging is also of great clinical significance in the field of spinal cord injury (SCI). Advanced methods such as double diffusion encoding (DDE) have enhanced the ability to assess axonal injury severity quickly and precisely. In animal models, DTI has been reported to have high sensitivity for detecting acute alterations after injury, facilitating accurate evaluation of injury progression. Filter-probe diffusion MRI, an innovative application, has further augmented diagnostic strength, offering enhanced predictive power for functional outcome. These advances prove the strength of diffusion imaging as much of a diagnostic tool as a recovery and prognostic tool for the functional capacity in SCI patients, emphasizing its position as a vital tool within clinical practice. (Brian et al., 2017) Aside from neurodegenerative diseases and spinal injuries, diffusion imaging continues to advance in other fields of clinical application, including oncology and psychiatric diseases. For instance, diffusion imaging can, in tumor characterization, differentiate between malignant and benign tumors by examining the microstructural properties of tissue. Differences in the magnitude of restricted diffusion in tumors can provide insight into tumor aggressiveness and how they respond to treatment. In psychiatric illnesses, diffusion imaging has also been employed to understand changes in brain connectivity associated with diseases such as schizophrenia and major depressive disorder. This use of diffusion imaging on multiple levels makes it a vital instrument in clinical practice, providing enhanced diagnostic accuracy and a deeper insight into complex neurological and psychological diseases. The evolving nature of diffusion imaging continues to make it relevant and useful in the treatment of a variety of other health conditions.

2.5.1. Role in Diagnosing Acute Ischemic Stroke

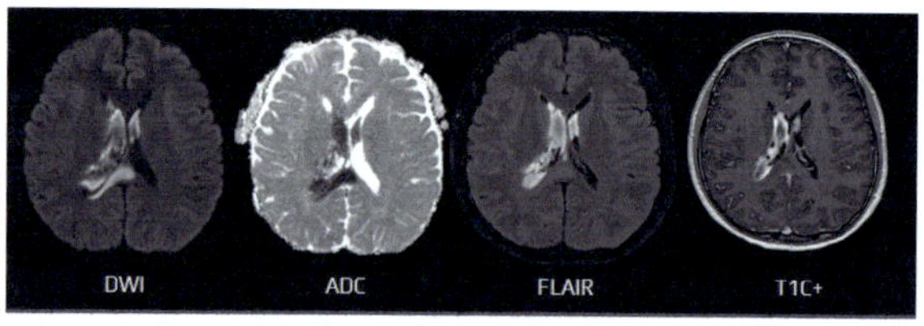

Figure 2.12. MR-DWI in the acute stroke diagnosis.

Source: https://www.stroke-manual.com/wp-content/uploads/2021/11/ischemie-v-corpus-callosum.jpg.

The value of fMRI and DWI in diagnosing acute ischemic stroke (AIS) has gained growing recognition since they can both detect underlying pathophysiological processes. Traditional imaging tools, such as CT, are insensitive to the identification of early ischemic changes. In contrast, fMRI and DWI provide information not only on hemodynamic brain conditions but also on the diffusion characteristics of water molecules in brain tissue. This function facilitates the identification of ischemic penumbra—high-risk but not infarcted regions—of utmost importance for therapeutic intervention at an early stage.

Current evidence also suggests that fMRI can delineate functional impairments, augmenting our understanding of axial patient profiles and guiding tailored treatment strategies. Such novel imaging modalities are thus central to optimizing therapeutic decision-making and outcomes in AIS treatment. Besides, integration of DWI in the diagnostic protocol for acute ischemic stroke has underscored its function in distinguishing core infarct from salvageable tissue. DWI represents water-molecule movement, which is restricted within infarcted tissue and can therefore be used to determine areas affected with great rapidity. Perfusion-diffusion mismatch theory has evolved as a critical tool for determining the viability of brain tissue after an ischemic insult, enabling effective interventions such as thrombolysis or thrombectomy. Further studies also provide evidence of a correlation between diffusion-weighted imaging and infarct volume in acute infarction, which could be interpreted as indicating that larger infarcts are associated with poorer outcomes, as demonstrated by recent analyses (Feldmann et al., 2013).

Thus, DWI is not only a diagnostic tool but also a prognostic indicator that guides clinical efforts to minimize neurological damage and maximize patient benefit in the acute setting. Clinical applications of fMRI and DWI in acute ischemic stroke are also complemented by research endeavors that aim to enhance imaging protocols and methods. Advanced research has investigated a range of factors in ischemic stroke, including how changes in signal intensity along intracranial arterial stenosis can represent hemodynamic severity, as outlined in the literature (Campbell et al., 2013). These findings are critical to enhancing our knowledge of treatment risks and benefits, particularly in the context of thrombolytic therapy. The use of rigorous imaging criteria in clinical trials has paved the way for the integration of perfusion-diffusion mismatch into therapeutic decision-making. With continued advances in fMRI and DWI technologies, their role in accurate AIS diagnosis and prognosis in patients becomes increasingly important. Collectively, these modalities lead the charge in stroke care innovation, ushering in a paradigm shift to more effective, evidence-based clinical practice (Figure 2.12).

2.5.2. Use in Tracking Neurodegenerative Diseases

The use of fMRI and diffusion imaging in the tracking of neurodegenerative diseases has generated increased attention within neuroscientific research. Both imaging techniques offer the potential of peering into the structural as well as functional changes of the brain with diseases such as Alzheimer's disease, Parkinson's disease, and multiple sclerosis. Functional MRI enables measurement of blood flow and oxygen levels following neuronal activity, and hence the identification of aberrant brain network connectivity characteristic of neurodegenerative diseases. Alzheimer's patients, for instance, are frequently found to have alterations in the default mode network, which illustrates the utility of fMRI as an early biomarker for diagnosis and disease progression monitoring. Combining these imaging modalities may provide clinicians with comprehensive data on the neuropathology underlying cognitive impairments associated with neurodegeneration, setting the stage for targeted interventions and improved patient care (Figure 2.13).

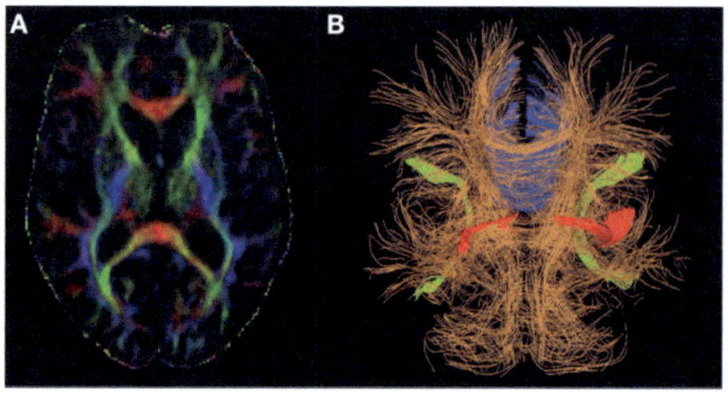

Figure 2.13. Diffusion tensor MRI in Alzheimer's research. Panel (A) shows the directional information encoded by diffusion tensor imaging by color (red: left-right, green: anterior-posterior, blue: head-foot) and fractional anisotropy (high intensity implies high fractional anisotropy). Panel (B) shows how the directional information may be represented in a deterministic tractography analysis. It shows the regions consistently identified and changing in AD (Blue: Corpus callosum, red: uncinate fasciculus, green: superior lateral fasciculus).

Source: https://www.researchgate.net/figure/Diffusion-tensor-MRI-in-Alzheimers-research-Panel-A-shows-the-directional_fig1_304009641.

Diffusion imaging, particularly DTI, is a continuation of fMRI, providing microscopic measurements of white matter integrity. DTI quantifies water-molecule motion along brain tissue, yielding critical information about changes that occur during structural alterations in neurodegenerative diseases. It has been observed that patients with mild cognitive impairment (MCI) and Alzheimer's disease exhibit wide-ranging disruption in certain white matter tracts, such as the splenium of the corpus callosum and anterior thalamic radiations. These findings point to the potential of DTI as a remarkable diagnostic tool that can image early changes in brain structure prior to the onset of apparent clinical symptoms. Real-time visualization of these changes provides an enhanced understanding of disease pathogenesis and enables the identification of individuals at risk, thereby translating into more informed clinical decision-making and targeted treatments (Babiloni et al., 2016). Increased focus on data-driven models of disease development further underscores the emergence of a new paradigm in neurodegenerative disease research. Integration of multiple data types—such as imaging findings from fMRI and DTI, as well as biochemical markers—enables scientists to build robust models that can predict disease courses and stratify patients based on their individual risks. Advances in differential equation techniques and spatiotemporal modeling have also proven promising for revealing subtle patterns of neurodegeneration that were not previously detectable; alterations in brain morphometry, for instance, may begin decades before overt neurodegeneration is apparent (Alexander et al., 2017). Consequently, the combination of functional MRI, diffusion imaging, and advanced modeling techniques not only sheds light on the processes underlying neurodegenerative diseases but also holds revolutionary potential for therapeutic applications, such as targeted therapies and optimized recruitment schemes for clinical trials.

2.5.3. Contribution to Understanding Traumatic Brain Injury (TBI)

Understanding of TBI has significantly been enhanced through the use of fMRI and diffusion imaging techniques. These new neuroimaging technologies play a pivotal role in revealing the intricacy of TBI pathology, enabling the identification of new biomarkers that accurately predict patient outcomes. By applying both fMRI, assessing brain function in blood flow, and DTI, which probes white matter integrity, researchers can construct a unified comprehension of brain alterations following injury. The multidisciplinary approach allows clinicians not just to map out structural impact but to quantify the functional impact of TBI on brain networks, radical understanding that enhances diagnosis and treatment strategies (Figure 2.14).

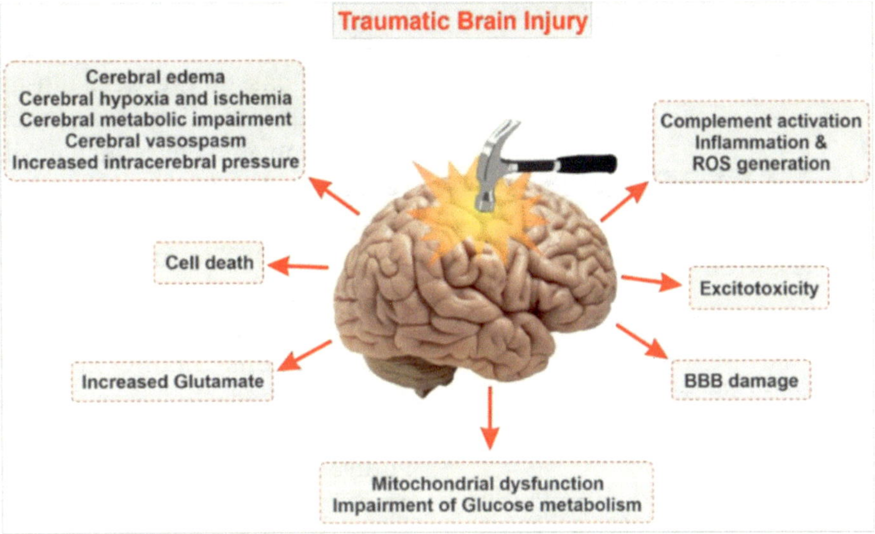

Figure 2.14. Role of diffusion tensor imaging in the diagnosis of traumatic axonal injury.

Source: https://pub.mdpi-res.com/ijms/ijms-21-02721/article_deploy/html/images/ijms-21-02721-g001.png?1586872285.

Consequently, the synergy of these imaging modalities continues to challenge conventional conceptualizations, underscoring the need for further investigation and validation in clinical and research settings (Aylward et al., 2012). Furthermore, the interplay between structural and functional changes post-TBI is central in comprehending the long-term effects of TBI on cognition and behavior. Recent studies using advanced MRI approaches have revealed new reorganizational patterns in brain connectivity. For instance, subsequent to injury, certain brain regions, particularly the prefrontal cortex, play a central role in linking remote networks involved in motor control and attention (Bonifazi et al., 2017). The reorganization of connectivity is a reflection of the brain's adaptive response to injury, but simultaneously makes it difficult to forecast the success of rehabilitation. Through the exploration of changes in the connectome, researchers can better understand how TBI affects local brain structure, but also large-scale brain networks responsible for cognitive and physical functions. An approach that underscores this perspective is the need to adopt a network-based approach to the study of TBI, which ultimately cascades into targeted intervention strategies for optimal outcomes. The ability of fMRI and DTI to provide precise information about the neural substrate of TBI has important implications for clinical practice and research. Neuroimaging-based biomarker identification enables improved prognostication and personalized intervention plans, leading to best practices for managing TBI patients. Recent advancements underscore the significance of volumetric and morphometric measurements using fMRI and DTI to provide a more robust understanding of structural pathology and its interrelationship with rehabilitation (Aylward et al., 2012). With the evolution towards using these techniques, there is scope for developing integrated models that move clinical assessment and imaging information closer together. Encouraging increased research in this area will not only fine-tune existing protocols but also create new therapeutic techniques able to address the complicated needs presented by traumatic brain injury. Ultimately, enhancing our understanding of TBI with sophisticated neuroimaging technologies reaffirms the wisdom of interdisciplinary cooperation in progressing both clinical and scientific endeavors within the discipline of brain injury.

2.6. Future Directions in Neuroimaging

Technological improvements in neuroimaging hold the promise of redefining the future of clinical diagnostics, with particular promise in the combination of fMRI and DTI. As researchers delve into the subtleties of traumatic brain injury (TBI), the combination of multimodal neuroimaging is being found to play a central role in the detection of prognostically significant biomarkers. Recent studies emphasize the need to harmonize structural and functional imaging modalities to reveal the brain's connectivity and network properties at the connectome level. These novel approaches not only enhance the sophistication of TBI outcome prediction but also pave the way for personalized medicine, in which treatment regimens can be tailored to individual neuroimaging traits. These advances highlight a pivotal shift in how neuroimaging is conceived and applied in research and clinical settings, underscoring its potential to alter patient management fundamentally (Aylward et al., 2012). Machine learning is a term used to describe artificial intelligence that can learn and improve itself. It is poised to revolutionize the analysis of neuroimages. The convergence of convolutional neural networks (CNNs) and neuroimaging technology offers an unprecedented horizon of diagnostic accuracy beyond standard imaging assessment. For instance, a recent study demonstrated the ability to rival or exceed human experts in MS diagnosis using advanced MRI scans and machine-learning-based approaches. However, challenges persist in the form of the opacity of machine learning models that can complicate clinical adoption. The creation of transparent frameworks such as layer-wise relevance propagation (LRP) is pivotal in breaking the black box of neural networks. By providing explanations of the decision-making process that underpin diagnoses, such frameworks make automated neuroimaging diagnostics more reliable and valid, enabling clinicians to accept and understand machine-made results (Asseyer et al., 2019). The future of neuroimaging will be marked by advancing technologies and a greater focus on collaboration. Multidisciplinary collaborations among neuroscientists, data scientists, and clinicians will be fundamental in defining novel approaches and applications. Future studies will be geared towards exploring new synergies between neuroimaging and sophisticated computational methods, such as big data analytics, to identify significant patterns in large datasets. By leveraging these collaborative energies, the field will be increasingly capable of confronting complex neurological diseases. Advances in imaging technologies and analytical techniques will uncover more about brain disease and how it operates, with the end goal of enhanced therapeutic interventions and outcomes. With these dynamic trends still in development, the broad range and transformative potential of neuroimaging in research and clinical applications are demonstrated.

2.6.1. Advances in Technology and Imaging Techniques

dvances in imaging technologies have significantly influenced neuroscience research, particularly in the deciphering of complex brain functions. The discovery of magnetic resonance imaging (MRI) in the early 1970s was one of the most significant breakthroughs in non-invasive imaging of the brain. MRI paved the way for more advanced methodologies, such as fMRI and diffusion tensor imaging (DTI), which enhanced our capacity to monitor brain activity and structural connectivity in real time. These imaging techniques have increasingly found applications in investigating various neurological diseases, for example, Alzheimer's disease (AD), yielding information on volumetric changes in brain regions as well as on specific patterns of activation observed during cognitive tasks. With such technologies, researchers can now analyze disease-specific cohorts, thereby opening the door to targeted therapeutic interventions based on measurable brain changes and functions (Camargo et al., 2015). Aside from their application in neurodegenerative diseases, recent advances in imaging technology have shed some light on the complexity of traumatic brain injury (TBI). Multimodal neuroimaging—comprises structural MRI, fMRI, and DTI—is now a powerful tool for identifying biomarkers of recovery and outcome following injury. Utilizing these strategies together enables the extensive examination of brain network properties at the connectome level, thereby providing insight into the pathological underpinnings of TBI. More current studies emphasize the role of advanced MRI processing techniques in conjunction with volumetric and morphometric analysis that can aid the identification of structural neuroimaging biomarkers that can be correlated with patient outcomes. By the integration of structural and functional assessments, researchers can form multivariate models that provide more precise predictions of outcomes, which would revolutionize clinical practice for TBI management (Aylward et al., 2012). Diffusion imaging techniques cannot be overstated, particularly their capacity to reveal changes in the brain's structural connectivity. Diffusion tensor imaging, as one aspect of diffusion imaging, can represent and quantify the orientation and coherence of white matter tracts and is therefore a highly valuable instrument for clarifying a variety of neurological disorders. As evidence mounts linking physical activity with neuroprotection, diffusion imaging has enabled increased understanding of how lifestyle interventions can promote brain health. Research indicating that enhanced cardiorespiratory fitness is related to beneficial changes in brain volumes illustrates the potential of diffusion imaging across research and clinical settings. Thus, the integration of functional MRI and diffusion imaging techniques allows for a more holistic examination of brain health and provides new directions for intervention and enhances our understanding of cognitive resilience against neurodegeneration (Camargo et al., 2015).

2.6.2. Integration of fMRI and Diffusion Imaging for Comprehensive Analysis

The integration of fMRI with diffusion imaging is a revolutionary advance in neuroimaging that makes the evaluation of brain activity and connectivity more comprehensive. While fMRI provides data on brain function by detecting alterations in blood flow and accompanying neural activity, diffusion imaging, specifically DTI, measures water-molecule diffusivity within brain tissue and maps the integrity of white matter tracts. This convergence enables researchers not only to investigate which areas of the brain are involved in specific tasks but also how these areas communicate with one another. This knowledge is valuable for describing complex neurological processes such as cognitive processing, emotional regulation, and how various disorders affect brain function (Basu et al., 2018). Using fMRI along with diffusion imaging is of great value in both research and clinical practice. The two-step process enables better understanding of neuroanatomical connections, which can shed light on brain function. For instance, examination of patterns of connectivity as well as functional activation can identify biomarkers for diseases such as Alzheimer's disease or schizophrenia, where disruptions in connectivity may become evident prior to functional deficits. Moreover, this integration aids assessment of treatment outcomes by real-time measurements of changes in function and microstructural integrity following therapeutic procedures. Quantification and visualization of such changes enhance the accuracy of clinical diagnostics and facilitate the development of site-specific therapeutic protocols (Avants et al., 2019). Further, the convergence of fMRI and diffusion imaging is amenable to multi-dimensional analysis, providing insight into the complexities of brain networks. Advanced techniques such as graph theory can exploit fMRI data to establish network efficiency and hub properties, while simultaneously using diffusion imaging to study structural connectivity patterns. This complementary approach not only increases functional network analysis but also allows for the examination of how anatomical characteristics influence functional behavior. As neuroimaging technologies improve, the conjunction of these methods is bound to yield profound insight into the architecture of brains and their connection to behavior and hence more insight into healthy and pathological states (Basu et al., 2018; Avants et al., 2019).

2.6.3. Potential for Personalized Medicine in Neurological Treatment

The use of fMRI and diffusion imaging in personalized medicine heralds a new age in the management of neurological disorders. These advanced imaging techniques provide essential information about the brain's structure and function, which is essential for individualizing treatment programs. For instance, fMRI allows researchers to observe brain activity after specific stimulation, while diffusion imaging monitors the integrity of white matter tracts. This convergence enables clinicians to gain a greater understanding of individual patients' distinct brain networks, leading to more accurate and effective interventions. Therefore, the ability to identify specific biomarkers of disease progression in conditions such as epilepsy or multiple sclerosis significantly enhances patient care. Advances in personalized brain network models reflect the need for data-driven approaches to neurological therapy. With the assistance of subject-specific data from structural and functional imaging, researchers can construct intricate models to investigate and predict brain dynamics. This new method not only enables the investigation of structure-function relationships in the brain but also enables one to simulate virtual experiments that might uncover critical information. These computer models have been shown to improve surgical outcomes in the management of epilepsy by enabling better localization of the affected tissue and directing stimulation for focused interventions. Therefore, the potential for individualized treatment planning to the individual's brain makes personalized medicine an exhilarating new area in neurology, encouraging more effective and subtle patient treatment. Secondly, the emergence of personalized medicine in neurology is fueled by growing evidence supporting the use of imaging data in clinical decision-making. The interplay among genes, environment, and brain structure underscores the complexity of neurological disorders, necessitating an individualized treatment strategy. Personalized treatment can be based on an individual's brain's response to various therapies, thereby optimizing therapeutic effect and minimizing side effects. For example, by employing personalized models from both structural and functional MRI data, it is possible to discover some areas of the brain that remain resistant or sensitive to treatment (Bansal et al., 2018). The results can help clinicians prescribe the most appropriate therapies to individuals, optimizing the overall effectiveness of neurological treatment and paving the way for future innovations (N/A, 2010).

SUMMARY

The combination of fMRI and diffusion imaging is a milestone in neuroimaging, particularly for understanding certain neurological conditions. In the major points discussed, both imaging modalities have shown tremendous promise for the detection of biomarkers of TBI. More importantly, multimodal neuroimaging techniques, combining structural MRI with fMRI and DTI, have helped forecast the outcome of TBI by linking brain networks and examining structural changes. Such multi-dimensional evaluation allows for a better understanding of brain function and connectivity, of crucial importance for clinicians to establish prognosis in the patient and tailor therapeutic interventions. These remarks emphasize the value of introducing new imaging techniques in clinical settings to optimize the efficacy and efficiency of neurological assessment (Aylward et al., 2012). Furthermore, advanced imaging in acute stroke treatment is increasingly being adopted, particularly in determining response to treatment. Although traditional imaging can effectively rule out non-stroke-related lesions, the incorporation of techniques like angiography and penumbral imaging can yield important information regarding the ischemic brain regions. These newer modalities enhance trial recruitment by involving more likely-to-benefit populations and reduce the sample size required for statistical precision. The inclusion of such sophisticated imaging strategies in clinical trials thus enhances research capability while optimizing resource utilization. Thus, stroke research demonstrates the potential for integrated comprehension to drive significant breakthroughs in patient treatment plans (Macrae et al., 2016). Moreover, the implications of applying functional MRI and diffusion imaging go beyond clinical utility to include additional information about underlying biology. The multimodal imaging data collection enables an accurate assessment of structural and functional alterations in the brain over time. This instant feedback can reveal how different interventions alter disease trajectories or recovery trends, providing a platform for future research. In addition, the ability to collect multiple metrics without invasion provides greater insight into neuroplasticity and its implications for rehabilitation after injury. Thus, the establishment of fMRI and diffusion imaging encourages current practices for the diagnosis and management of neurological disorders while paving the way for more targeted and potent therapeutic methods in the future (Aylward et al., 2012; Macrae et al., 2016).

The potential of diffusion imaging and fMRI to influence both clinical practice and research design is vast. Functional MRI, with ongoing research into ischemic stroke pathophysiology, can revolutionize treatment approaches by improving patient selection. This can be observed, especially in thrombolytic therapy, where fMRI measurements have already begun to optimize the risk-to-benefit ratio in decision-making. As new imaging technology is created and older methods are better validated, their incorporation into standard practice may enable clinicians to make more accurate decisions and, consequently, improve patient outcomes and reduce the burden of stroke-related morbidity and mortality. The development of fMRI techniques, thus, will increasingly lead to more targeted therapies and underpin the rationale for continued research in this essential area of medical imaging and therapy. In cancer, diffusion-weighted MRI (DW-MRI) is also emerging as a useful predictive biomarker of treatment response, particularly for advanced oropharyngeal squamous cell carcinoma. Research, including the MeRInO trial, aims to define threshold changes in the apparent diffusion coefficient (ADC) to differentiate responders from non-responders in radical chemoradiotherapy. By comparing ADC changes at multiple time points, researchers can develop tailored adaptive therapy plans. The data thus collected can significantly improve the therapeutic ratio in head and neck cancer therapy and provide chances of successful outcomes without unnecessary treatment-induced toxicity. Such a new application of imaging for real-time monitoring of therapy is a new paradigm in clinical oncology, where therapy can be tailored individually based on the patient's response. The integration of fMRI and diffusion imaging into routine clinical practice will also guide future research agendas, driving the development of personalized medicine across a multitude of medical disciplines. By employing these newer imaging modalities, scientists can identify biomarkers associated with various disease states or treatment responses. This could not only enhance our understanding of complex pathophysiologic mechanisms but also enable the development of tailored therapies for specific patient requirements. As these researches become established, the dialogue between clinicians and researchers will be essential to capture imaging advances in the clinic. The ultimate long-term goal shall be to build a holistic and responsive system of health care where ongoing imaging assessment directs therapy adjustments, pushes the envelope of treatment innovation, and leads to improved overall patient care outcomes, especially for previously challenging disease states highlighted by studies like those referenced in Campbell et al. (2013) and Allwood-Spiers et al. (2017).

CLOSER LOOK

THE SIGNIFICANCE OF FMRI AND DIFFUSION IMAGING IN NEUROSCIENCE

The face of neuroscience has been transformed with advancements in neuroimaging techniques, namely fMRI and diffusion imaging. These techniques enable one to view as well as measure brain function and structural components in vivo, thus providing critical information on neuroanatomical changes in various domains, ranging from development, neurodegenerative diseases, and psychiatric diseases. The ability of fMRI to measure dynamic changes in cerebral blood flow enables neuroscientists to formulate hypotheses about neuronal activation in real time, making it feasible to examine how the brain processes information and responds to stimulation. fMRI thus became a keystone of preclinical and clinical research, influencing cognitive neuroscience and psychopathology methodologies. The contributions of fMRI extend beyond mere identification of functional regions; they encompass integrative functions that elucidate the complex interplay between various neural circuits, informing therapeutic interventions and enhancing our understanding of brain health. In parallel, diffusion imaging has solidified its role in elucidating the brain's microstructure through the mapping of white matter integrity and fiber tractography. This approach is particularly vital for assessing the extent to which structural connectivity drives functional outcomes. Investigation with DTI has managed to demarcate abnormalities in white matter integrity that accompany such disorders as traumatic brain injury, schizophrenia, and autism spectrum disorders. For instance, in one study of BTBR mouse model of autism, diffusion imaging mapped extensive changes in white and gray matter, highlighting the translational significance of the results to human autism research and suggesting a potential line of intervention design. With the aid of advanced imaging techniques, researchers are better able to elucidate the underlying mechanisms of neurodevelopmental disorders and long-term diseases, setting the stage for improved diagnostic criteria and targeted therapy, as evidenced by the findings reported in Gozzi et al. (2013) and Aylward et al. (2012). Further, the fusion of fMRI with diffusion imaging also provides the opportunity to gain a greater insight into brain network dynamics. The application of both techniques offers a multi-dimensional approach, not only demonstrating the organization of neural tracts but also their functional ability and connectivity. The multimodal perspective is essential in the quest to identify new biomarkers for a wide range of conditions, including post-traumatic stress disorder and neurodegenerative illnesses. By adopting new, state-of-the-art analytic methods, such as network analysis and multivariate statistics, researchers are able to delve more deeply into the brain's connectome and uncover predictors of results for diseases like traumatic brain injury. Combining fMRI and diffusion imaging information not only improves the predictive power of clinical assessment but also further advances neuroscience by de-mystifying the complexity of brain function and its relationship to behavior, as with recent studies on TBI outcomes reported in Aylward et al. (2012).

REFERENCES

1. Thompson, P.M., Jahanshad, N., Ching, C.R.K. *et al.* ENIGMA and global neuroscience: A decade of large-scale studies of the brain in health and disease across more than 40 countries. *Transl Psychiatry* **10**, 100 (2020). https://doi.org/10.1038/s41398-020-0705-1Alexander, G. S., Bakas, S., Nikam, R., Palmer, J., et al. (2018). Advanced magnetic resonance imaging in glioblastoma: A review. https://core.ac.uk/download/155271644.pdf (accessed on 5th August 2025).
2. Allwood-Spiers, S., Chalmers, A., Duffton, A., Foster, C., et al. (2017). Study of diffusion weighted MRI as a predictive biomarker of response during radiotherapy for high and intermediate risk squamous cell cancer of the oropharynx: The MeRInO study. https://core.ac.uk/download/96882989.pdf (accessed on 5th August 2025).
3. Alves, C. E., Alves, G. S., Engelhardt, E., Fußer, F., et al. (2012). Different patterns of white matter degeneration using multiple diffusion indices and volumetric data in mild cognitive impairment and Alzheimer patients. https://core.ac.uk/download/14528092.pdf (accessed on 5th August 2025).
4. Asseyer, S., Bellmann-Strobl, J., Brandt, A. U., Eitel, F., et al. (2019). Uncovering convolutional neural network decisions for diagnosing multiple sclerosis on conventional MRI using layer-wise relevance propagation. https://core.ac.uk/download/300327855.pdf (accessed on 5th August 2025).
5. Avants, B., Avants, B., Caffo, B. S., Caffo, B., et al. (2019). Neuroconductor: An R platform for medical imaging analysis. https://core.ac.uk/download/287605316.pdf (accessed on 5th August 2025).
6. Aylward, S. R., Gerig, G., Hovda, D. A., Irimia, A., et al. (2012). Neuroimaging of structural pathology and connectomics in traumatic brain injury: Toward personalized outcome prediction. https://core.ac.uk/download/323078685.pdf (accessed on 5th August 2025).
7. Babiloni, C., Dyrba, M., Grothe, M. J., Sepulcre, J., et al. (2016). Measuring cortical connectivity in Alzheimer's disease as a brain neural network pathology: Toward clinical applications. https://core.ac.uk/download/98336520.pdf (accessed on 5th August 2025).
8. Baccari, P., Cappabianca, S., D'Andrea, A., Falcone, R., et al. (2016). Pancreatic tumors imaging: An update. https://core.ac.uk/download/98333045.pdf (accessed on 5th August 2025).
9. Bansal, K., Muldoon, S. F., & Nakuci, J. (2018). Personalized brain network models for assessing structure-function relationships. *arXiv*. http://arxiv.org/abs/1802.00473 (accessed on 5th August 2025).
10. Barchetti, G., Carano, D., Catalano, C., Catto, H., et al. (2017). An evaluation of morphological and functional multi-parametric MRI sequences in classifying non-muscle and muscle invasive bladder cancer. https://core.ac.uk/download/98341280.pdf (accessed on 5th August 2025).
11. Barkovich, A. J., Mukherjee, P., & Wahl, M. (2010). Diffusion imaging and tractography of congenital brain malformations. https://core.ac.uk/download/323074405.pdf (accessed on 5th August 2025).
12. Bassett, D. S., Betzel, R. F., Davis, K. A., Khambhati, A., et al. (2018). Genetic and neuroanatomical support for functional brain network dynamics in epilepsy. *arXiv*. http://arxiv.org/abs/1809.03934 (accessed on 5th August 2025).

13. Basu, N., Goni, M., Murray, A. D., Waiter, G., et al. (2018). Neural indicators of fatigue in chronic diseases: A systematic review of MRI studies. https://core.ac.uk/download/159067075.pdf (accessed on 5th August 2025).

14. Bonifazi, P., Cortes, J. M., Diez, I., Drijkoningen, D., et al. (2017). Enhanced pre-frontal functional-structural networks to support postural control deficits after traumatic brain injury in a pediatric population. https://core.ac.uk/download/84043245.pdf (accessed on 5th August 2025).

15. Breidthardt, G., Chowdhury, M., de Boer, R. A., Dinah, F., Dong, F., Fine, D., et al. (2016). Imaging the kidney using magnetic resonance techniques: Structure to function. https://core.ac.uk/download/76974984.pdf (accessed on 5th August 2025).

16. Brockhuis, B., Dąbrowska, M., Jamrozik, Z., Muraszko-Klaudel, J., et al. (1970). The role of neuroimaging in the diagnosis of the atypical parkinsonian syndromes in clinical practice. https://core.ac.uk/download/268477145.pdf (accessed on 5th August 2025).

17. Budde, M. D., Kaushal, M., Kurpad, S. N., Motovylyak, A., et al. (2018). Diffusion tensor imaging in a large longitudinal series of patients with cervical spondylotic myelopathy correlated with long-term functional outcome. https://core.ac.uk/download/213080007.pdf (accessed on 5th August 2025).

18. Cabarrus, M. C., & Westphalen, A. C. (2017). Multiparametric magnetic resonance imaging of the prostate–a basic tutorial. https://core.ac.uk/download/323063417.pdf (accessed on 5th August 2025).

19. Caffo, B., Crainiceanu, C., Du, Y., Goldsmith, J., et al. (2011). Nonlinear tube-fitting for the analysis of anatomical and functional structures. *arXiv.* http://arxiv.org/abs/1104.3005 (accessed on 5th August 2025).

20. Campbell, B. C. V., & Macrae, I. M. (2013). Translational perspectives on perfusion-diffusion mismatch in ischemic stroke. https://core.ac.uk/download/42352524.pdf (accessed on 5th August 2025).

21. Catana, C., Cherry, S. R., Jacobs, R. E., Judenhofer, M. S., et al. (2008). Simultaneous *in vivo* positron emission tomography and magnetic resonance imaging. https://core.ac.uk/download/4877262.pdf (accessed on 5th August 2025).

22. Chakravarty, M., Chen, A., Devenyi, G., Germann, J., et al. (2019). Investigating microstructural variation in the human hippocampus using non-negative matrix factorization. https://core.ac.uk/download/287607112.pdf (accessed on 5th August 2025). *(Note: If the URL is not provided in your original list, please add or confirm it.)*

23. Chao, L. L., Kaufer, D., Neylan, T. C., Tosun, D., et al. (2015). Preliminary evidence of increased hippocampal myelin content in veterans with posttraumatic stress disorder. https://core.ac.uk/download/323072028.pdf (accessed on 5th August 2025).

24. Cherry, S. R., Jacobs, R. E., & Louie, A. Y. (2008). The integration of positron emission tomography with magnetic resonance imaging. https://core.ac.uk/download/4877286.pdf (accessed on 5th August 2025).

25. Colonnese, C., Coppola, G., Di Lorenzo, C., Di Lorenzo, G., et al. (2016). Thalamo-cortical network activity between migraine attacks: Insights from MRI-based microstructural and functional resting-state network correlation analysis. https://core.ac.uk/download/74321594.pdf (accessed on 5th August 2025).

26. Dani, K. A., Goutcher, C., Moreton, F. C., Muir, K. W., et al. (2016). Respiratory challenge MRI: Practical aspects. https://core.ac.uk/download/42371355.pdf (accessed on 5th August 2025).

27. Destefani, V. C., Destefani, A. C., & Vitrio, B. (2024). Advancing neuroimaging frontiers: A comprehensive review of novel diagnostic techniques in neuroradiology and their clinical applications. https://core.ac.uk/download/617924644.pdf (accessed on 5th August 2025).

28. Goel, A., McDonald, A., Madawi, A. A., Brooks, A. L., McLaughlin, A. M., Montano, A. M., Ransford, A. O., et al. (2013). Spinal involvement in mucopolysaccharidosis IVA (Morquio-Brailsford or Morquio A syndrome): Presentation, diagnosis and management. https://core.ac.uk/download/323073297.pdf (accessed on 5th August 2025).

29. Gozzi, A., Turk, A. A., Stanfield, A. C., et al. (2013). Neuroimaging evidence of major morpho-anatomical and functional abnormalities in the BTBR T+TF/J mouse model of autism. https://core.ac.uk/download/18434871.pdf (accessed on 5th August 2025).

30. Halpern, E. J., Kim, S., Salmanoglu, E., Thakur, M., et al. (2018). A glance at imaging bladder cancer. https://core.ac.uk/download/227055407.pdf (accessed on 5th August 2025).

31. Macrae, I. M., & Muir, K. W. (2016). Neuroimaging as a selection tool and endpoint in preclinical and clinical trials. https://core.ac.uk/download/46164953.pdf (accessed on 5th August 2025).

32. N/A. (2010). *Focal Spot, Winter 2009/2010.* https://core.ac.uk/download/129069377.pdf (accessed on 5th August 2025).

33. N/A. (2018). *Full Issue: Volume 13, Issue 1–Winter 2018.* https://core.ac.uk/download/155271646.pdf (accessed on 5th August 2025).

34. Perea Camargo, R. D. (2015). The impact of aerobic exercise on brain's white matter integrity in the Alzheimer's disease and the aging population. https://core.ac.uk/download/213413301.pdf (accessed on 5th August 2025).

35. Pur, D. R. (2020). Structure-function relationships in the brain: Applications in neurosurgery. https://core.ac.uk/download/322920284.pdf (accessed on 5th August 2025).

36. Schallmo, M. P., Weldon, K. B., Burton, P., Sponheim, S. R., & Olman, C. A. (2021). Assessing methods for geometric distortion compensation in *7 T* gradient echo functional *MRI* data. *Human Brain Mapping, 42*, 4205–4223. https://doi.org/10.1002/hbm.25540 (accessed on 5th August 2025).

37. Schmit, B. D., Muftuler, L. T., Budde, M. D., Skinner, N. P., Skinner, N. P., & Kurpad, S. N. (2017). Optimizing filter-probe diffusion weighting in the rat spinal cord for human translation. https://core.ac.uk/download/213080947.pdf (accessed on 5th August 2025).

38. Vogelbacher, C. (2020). Development of quality standards for multi-center, longitudinal magnetic resonance imaging studies in clinical neuroscience. https://core.ac.uk/download/287653461.pdf (accessed on 5th August 2025).

39. You, Y. T., Hardiman, K. M., Bafford, A. C., Poylin, V., Francone, T. D., Davis, K. G., Paquette, I. M., et al. (2020). The American Society of Colon and Rectal Surgeons clinical practice guidelines for the management of rectal cancer. *Diseases of the Colon & Rectum, 63*, 1191–1222. https://doi.org/10.1097/dcr.0000000000001762 (accessed on 5th August 2025).

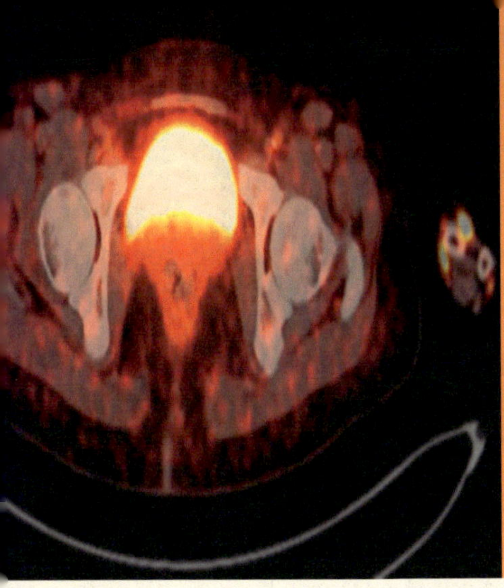

Chapter 3

HYBRID IMAGING: PET/CT AND PET/MRI

Contents

Introduction

Medical imaging has had extraordinary advancements over the last few years when it comes to hybrid imaging techniques that combine different modalities in order to offer better diagnosis. When combined, two of the top imaging devices, positron emission tomography (PET) and magnetic resonance imaging (MRI), provide a means for clinicians to assess a broad range of medical conditions. Hybrid modalities such as PET/CT and PET/MRI combine PET's functional imaging strengths with the high anatomical resolution of CT and MRI, respectively. This combination allows for simultaneous, complete assessment of both metabolic and structural abnormalities, leading to better diagnoses and more effective treatment planning in oncology, neurology, and cardiology. The arrival of these hybrid imaging techniques is transforming clinical practice, and there is a shift in the paradigm for patient management among healthcare workers. The major impetus of hybrid imaging lies in its ability to acquire complementary data from different sources. For instance, PET acquires radiotracers to assess metabolic activity, providing important information about tumor function and biology (Inglese et al., 2019). In contrast, MRI offers stronger soft-tissue imaging capabilities, providing high-resolution anatomical data without ionizing radiation exposure. By leveraging the benefits of both modalities, medical staff can gain a more comprehensive view of a patient's condition. This complementary relationship can be particularly valuable in oncology, where it is critical to assess tumor characteristics, such as perfusion and metabolism. The integration of these imaging modalities not only enhances diagnostic performance but also enables real-time monitoring of treatment response, facilitating a personalized model that adjusts interventions based on a patient's individual needs. As imaging continues to develop in medicine, new paths are opened for optimizing patient outcomes through novel hybrid strategies. This chapter addresses the intricacies of PET/CT and PET/MRI, laying down their individual contributions to imaging technologies and clinical use. Emphasizing the quantification of perfusion and tracer kinetics, this study explores how diagnostic performance can be enhanced by analyzing dynamic PET and MRI images (Joseph et al., 2015). Furthermore, the presentation will address the application of new models and approaches that allow precise measurements of perfusion in lesions at multiple anatomical sites, including lung, brain, liver, prostate, and breast cancers. This opening background sets the stage for a comprehensive examination of the revolutionary impact of hybrid imaging on today's medical practice.

3.1. Fundamentals of PET Imaging

The image acquisition principles of positron emission tomography (PET) follow those of nuclear medicine, in which radiotracers are used to image metabolic processes in the body. The technique enables clinicians to detect cellular-level abnormalities by introducing a radionuclide that emits positrons. The method is particularly valuable in oncology because cancer cells will have increased metabolic activity compared with normal tissues. Understanding the physical foundation of PET, namely annihilation events and the detection of gamma rays, will be vital to further developing imaging techniques. Moreover, the integration of PET with computed tomography (CT) or magnetic resonance imaging (MRI) enhances diagnostic precision by combining metabolic data with anatomical data to provide a comprehensive image of pathology relevant to treatment planning and follow-up. Integration of advanced computational techniques, such as machine learning, into PET imaging is fundamentally redefining diagnostic accuracy and workflow efficiency. Advances in deep learning emphasize the capability of deep learning algorithms to handle large datasets and to advance image reconstruction and interpretation. The advent of artificial intelligence here not only helps radiologists identify minute defects but also raises questions regarding the transparency and interpretability of machine decisions in critical medical diagnoses.

According to the recent literature, greater interpretability becomes more of a requirement in medical applications, as clinicians must understand the rationale behind algorithmic findings. This two-way interaction between technology research and clinical practice also underscores the need to develop standardized frameworks that enable informed decision-making on hybrid imaging platforms to advance PET in modern healthcare (Tjoa et al., 2020). Moreover, recent developments in machine learning are inducing more complex approaches in PET imaging, namely involving the integration of MRI. By employing deep learning techniques, researchers can now streamline image acquisition and processing, thereby optimizing the workflow. The ability of deep learning to analyze vast quantities of data is directly related to improved diagnostics and operational efficiency in hybrid imaging modalities. Despite all these advancements, the importance of acknowledging the issues that accompany such innovations cannot be overemphasized, including the importance of having stringent validation and verification processes for clinical validity. Closing the loop between innovative algorithms and real-world use still requires interdisciplinary collaboration across departments, which provides the environment for medical imaging experts to utilize such technologies responsibly and effectively (Selvikv et al., 2018).

3.1.1. Principles of Positron Emission Tomography

PET principles rely on the annihilation of positrons and electrons with the emission of gamma rays. This process occurs when a positron that has been liberated from a radioactive tracer collides with an electron within the body. It primarily involves injecting a radiopharmaceutical, most commonly 18F-FDG (fluorodeoxyglucose), which is taken up by metabolically active tissues. Understanding the biodistribution of this tracer allows clinicians to map and quantify metabolic activities in the body and, therefore, allows for the detection of abnormalities at the cellular level (Figure 3.1).

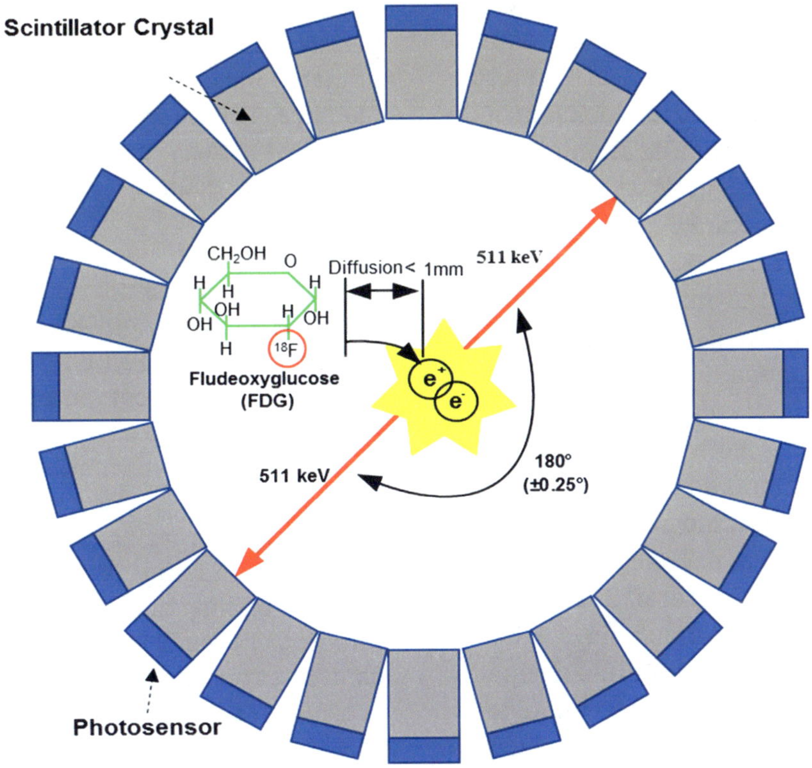

Figure 3.1. The basic principle of a positron emission tomography (PET) system.

Source: https://www.researchgate.net/publication/337325700/figure/fig1/AS:11431281390734114@1745285857206/The-basic-principle-of-a-positron-emission-tomography-PET-system-A-PET-detector-ring.tif.

This capability is particularly valuable in cancer, where metabolic function often precedes observable anatomical changes. The integration of PET with other imaging technologies, such as CT or MRI, leverages PET's strength in generating functional information while compensating for its weakness in anatomical detail, thereby providing greater diagnostic accuracy and clinical utility (Zaidi et al., 2017). While stand-alone PET is useful, its integration with computed tomography (CT) and magnetic resonance imaging (MRI) has had a profound impact on medical practice. By integrating PET and CT (PET/CT), diagnostic specificity is significantly enhanced, providing accurate anatomical localization of metabolic disease. This dual-modality platform is now commonplace in the evaluation and staging of numerous cancers because it combines functional imaging with superb high-resolution anatomical detail. However, while PET/CT mitigates some of the limitations of stand-alone PET, it still falls short of maximizing the soft tissue contrast offered by MRI. Therefore, the introduction of PET/MRI is another advancement in hybrid imaging technology. Simultaneous acquisition of PET and MRI data supplies both metabolic and structural tissue characteristics with true, accurate, and comprehensive examination, offering a better representation of pathologies, especially in demanding cases such as neurological conditions and soft tissue tumors (Zaidi et al., 2017). In some clinical situations, for instance, in evaluating diabetic patients' Charcot neuroarthropathy, the application of PET has been found to be categorical over traditional imaging procedures. A recent comparison of ring 18F-FDG PET, hybrid PET, and MRI in preoperative staging showed that although MRI is conventionally used for soft tissue analysis, PET provided complementary information in differentiating infectious from inflammatory lesions. The research validated that PET successfully identified Charcot lesions that MRI could not certainly characterize, thus providing important information to guide surgical treatment. Also, the ability of PET, particularly ring PET, to perform well in the presence of metallic implants increases its clinical utility in patients with such devices. This highlights the transformative potential of applying hybrid PET technologies to deliver more accurate diagnostic data and improve patient outcomes.

3.1.2. Radiotracers Used in PET

The use of radiotracers in PET has a central role in improving diagnostic accuracy in hybrid imaging modalities such as PET/CT and PET/MRI. Radiotracers, molecules tagged with positron-emitting isotopes, enable visualization of metabolic processes at the cellular level. For instance, 18F-fluorodeoxyglucose (18F-FDG) is the most widely used radiotracer in clinical practice, particularly for its ability to delineate areas of increased glucose metabolism that are characteristic of neoplasms. This ability not only contributes to the detection of cancer, but also to the staging and evaluation of treatment response. Coupling PET with magnetic resonance imaging (MRI) or computed tomography (CT) allows clinicians to correlate metabolic activity with anatomical information, thereby providing a comprehensive understanding of the patient's status and increasing the diagnostic value of standard imaging techniques. In vascular disease, adding the application of specialized radiotracers sheds light on the pathophysiologic context, especially in diseases such as peripheral artery disease (PAD). Hybrid imaging methods can utilize radiotracers to assess the biological activity of atheromatous plaques and vascular inflammation (Figure 3.2).

Next-generation PET radiotracers for molecular markers of inflammation and oxidative stress have been developed to provide a more effective imaging technique than traditional methods. Molecular-specific tracers are crucial for identifying high-risk plaques and thereby directing therapeutic intervention. The use of these radiotracers in hybrid imaging not only detects the anatomical changes involved in PAD but also provides information about function and molecular processes, improving the diagnostic process and patient outcomes significantly, as evident in recent literature on the topic (Chan et al., 2023). The advancement of hybrid imaging, including PET, also relies on the development of new imaging biomarkers. These biomarkers are essential for optimizing the sensitivity and specificity of radiotracers, particularly in the evaluation of cardiovascular disease. Hybrid devices that integrate PET with CT or MRI enable the patient to be evaluated in an integrated fashion by combining functional imaging with anatomical resolution. Notably, the diagnostic utility of these systems can be significantly improved by employing radiotracers that selectively target specific physiological processes, e.g., inflammation or neovascularization. This marriage not only simplifies the diagnostic process but also holds the key to personalized medicine, wherein hybrid imaging can guide therapeutic interventions based on individual patient needs. In the long run, the studies being carried out to develop novel radiotracers and the evolution of hybrid imaging technologies will continue to advance diagnostic imaging in clinical practice, enhancing decision-making and patient management (Ascione et al., 2021).

Radiotracer	Uptake Mechanism	Indications
Oxygen 15–water	Perfusion	Tumoral perfusion
Copper 60–diacetyl-bis(N4-methylthiosemicarbazone)	Hypoxia	High sensitivity to hypoxia
Carbon 11–acetate	Synthesis of fatty acids	Genitourinary and brain imaging
^{18}F-fluoromisonidazole	Hypoxia	Imaging of the prostate and cervix
^{18}F–fluoroazomycin arabinoside	Hypoxia	Hypoxic tumors
^{18}F-fluoride	Formation of fluoroapatite	Bone metastases
^{18}F-fluorotamoxifen	Estrogen metabolism	Breast imaging
^{18}F–fluor-17-estradiol	Estrogen metabolism	Breast imaging
^{11}C- or ^{18}F-acetate	Synthesis of fatty acids	Prostate imaging
^{11}C- or ^{18}F-choline	Phospholipid synthesis	Prostate imaging
^{18}F-fluorodopa	Metabolism of amino acids	Neuroectodermal tumors
^{18}F–fluoro annexin V	Apoptosis	Tumor follow-up

Figure 3.2. Radiotracers used in PET.

Source: https://www.researchgate.net/profile/Joan-C-Vilanova/publication/51799039/figure/tbl2/AS:668669948489739@1536434747836/Radiotracers-Used-in-PET.png.

3.1.3. Clinical Applications of PET

The clinical applicability of PET with hybrid imaging platforms such as PET/CT and PET/MRI constitutes a significant advancement in diagnostic medicine. Particularly in the oncology branch, PET imaging has been instrumental in tumor identification and characterization. The approach provides crucial molecular-level data on metabolic activity, enabling early detection of malignancy, assessment of treatment responses, and follow-up for recurrence. As reported in the literature, hybrid modalities integrate the anatomical precision of CT or MRI with the functional imaging ability of PET, thus enabling clinicians to achieve more accurate diagnoses and personalized treatment planning for patients. The visualization of structure and function in a single imaging procedure enhances diagnosis and, in turn, improves patient outcomes in cancer care (Aldahery, 2023). In addition, PET hybrid imaging is utilized outside of oncology and has a significant impact on healthcare in the fields of cardiology and neurology. In cardiology, PET is used to assess myocardial blood flow and viability and assist in the treatment of coronary artery disease. PET with MRI provides enhanced soft-tissue contrast, which is extremely beneficial for imaging cardiac structures (Figure 3.3).

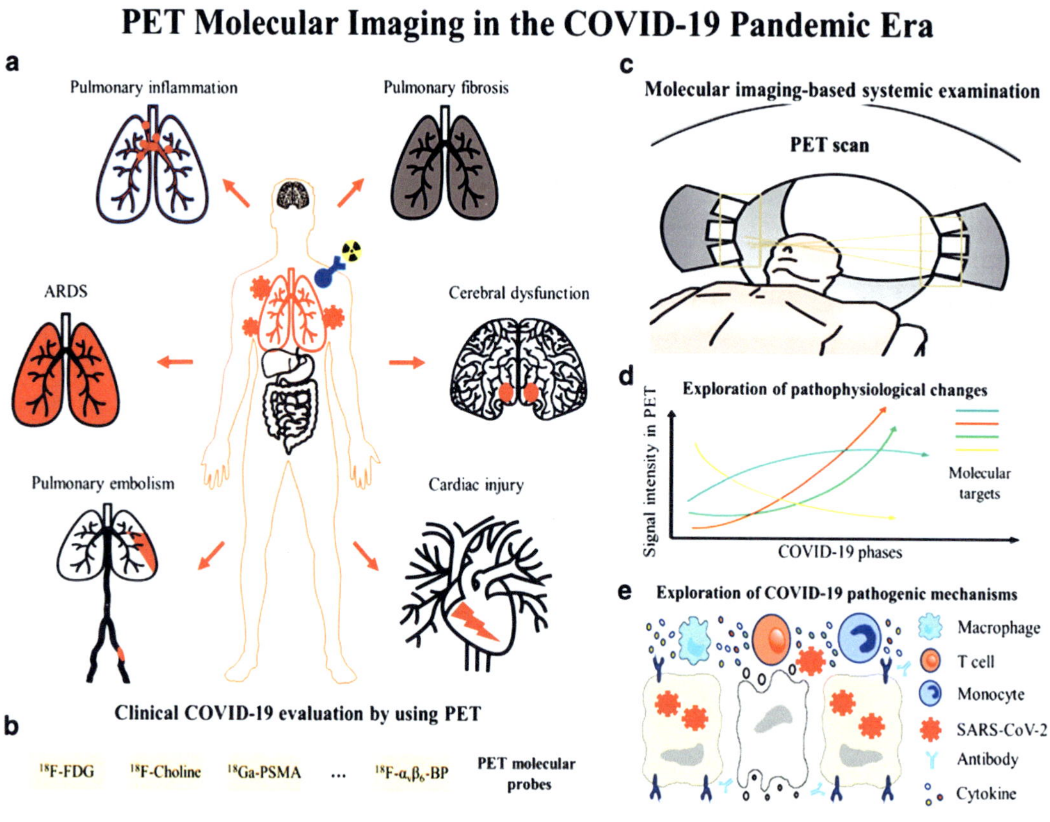

Figure 3.3. Schematic diagram illustrating the role of PET in the pandemic era. A variety of clinical applications of PET imaging have been reported, facilitating the evaluation of pulmonary inflammation, ARDS, pulmonary embolism, pulmonary fibrosis, cerebral dysfunction, and cardiac injury (a), by using various PET molecular probes (b). PET enables the whole-body evaluation for COVID-19 patients in molecular perspectives (c), helping the exploration of pathophysiological changes of molecular targets in different COVID-19 phases by using specific radiotracers (d), as well as the exploration of COVID-19 pathogenic mechanisms through the visualization of molecules involved in the occurrence and development of COVID-19 (e).

Source: Positron emission tomography in the COVID-19 pandemic era - Scientific Figure on ResearchGate. Available from: https://www.researchgate.net/figure/Schematic-diagram-illustrating-the-role-of-PET-in-the-pandemic-era-A-variety-of-clinical_fig1_351710086 [accessed 8 Aug 2025].

In neurology, PET/MRI has also been a very effective instrument for diagnosing and treating neurological disorders, including Alzheimer's disease and epilepsy. The ability to derive both neuroanatomical and functional data in a single examination helps in the differentiation between dementias and the assessment of brain function during seizure activity. These innovations demonstrate the revolutionary potential of hybrid imaging instruments to enhance diagnostic accuracy across a wide range of clinical contexts (Aldahery, 2023). Furthermore, the multi-potentiality of PET in diagnosing inflammatory disorders is another important use of the modality. With the ability to detect changes in glucose metabolism, PET has potential applications in detecting inflammatory conditions such as sarcoidosis, rheumatoid arthritis, and infections. Coupling of PET with CT or MRI makes it even more helpful since it allows for accurate localization of inflammation as well as disease activity monitoring, thus targeted therapy. Clinicians can differentiate between malignant and benign processes using this collective data, thereby delivering optimized patient management plans. Despite certain limitations of the technology used to fuse these imaging modalities, the medical significance of PET hybrid imaging across various areas of medicine is evident, underscoring the need for ongoing research and development in this area (Aldahery, 2023).

3.2. Fundamentals of CT Imaging

The rules of CT imaging make up one of the foundations of modern diagnostic radiology, significantly enhancing the visualization of internal body structures. X-ray technology enables CT scans to generate high-resolution cross-sectional images of patients, allowing clinicians to assess a wide range of conditions, from trauma to malignancies. The process is achieved by applying several X-ray images obtained from different angles and reconstructing them into a 3D image by a computer. The enhanced contrast resolution of CT scanning enables improved differentiation between soft tissues, an area of utmost importance for diagnosing diseases such as tumors and inflammatory conditions. Therefore, in addition to aiding correct diagnosis, CT scans also assist in treatment planning and follow-up, bridging the gap from initial detection to follow-up intervention. Furthermore, the advent of hybrid imaging modalities such as PET/CT and PET/MRI has had a profound impact on the range of CT imaging applications in clinical practice. By combining anatomical data from CT with functional data from PET and MRI, these hybrid scanners enhance diagnostic certainty and therapeutic planning. For instance, the interplay of metabolic data from PET enables cellular behavior to be comprehended, which is not apparent in routine anatomical imaging. This synergy allows for improved characterization of pathologies like cancers, particularly in oncology, where distinction between active tumor tissue and necrotic tissue is essential for effective treatment planning. The application of CT imaging thus transcends the confines of anatomical evaluation to provide a greater understanding of physiological events. In pediatric practice, the application of advanced imaging modalities, including CT, has presented dramatic advantages but must be accompanied by proper consideration of radiation exposure. Hybrid imaging in the guise of PET/CT offers promise for the evaluation of conditions in children, such as infection and inflammatory conditions. The advantages of using [18F]-FDG-PET to detect and follow conditions like Crohn's disease have been on the horizon in recent reports, where precise imaging may guide therapeutic strategies. In these circumstances, CT imaging not only serves as a source of anatomical reference but also aids in the functional assessment of illness, enhancing clinical care and patient well-being. Therefore, hybrid imaging that leverages CT's strengths has become a focal pillar in pediatric diagnostics, highlighting the technology's utility and effectiveness in modern clinical practice (Yuan et al., 2014; Signore et al., 2017).

3.2.1. Principles of Computed Tomography

CT principles form the foundation for the success of hybrid imaging modalities such as PET/CT and PET/MRI. CT generates cross-sectional images of the body utilizing X-rays, allowing precise visualization of body structures. The imaging process uses a gantry that rotates to record a set of projection images at various angles, which are reconstructed by sophisticated algorithms to produce three-dimensional images. The most fundamental benefit of CT is its ability to delineate anatomical structures with high spatial resolution, which is essential when co-registering functional imaging information from PET or MRI. As technology for hybrid imaging continues to progress, it is still important to know the fundamentals of CT since it not only contributes to the functional data obtained with PET but also enhances the general clinical usefulness in day-to-day practice, particularly in oncology, where accurate localization of tumors is required for effective treatment planning and follow-up (Dhafer et al., 2024). Hybrid imaging, in the way of PET-CT and other hybrids, utilizes the strengths of the respective modality to provide more comprehensive diagnostic data. By combining PET's ability to image metabolic activity with high-resolution anatomy provided by CT, lesion detection and characterization are improved. This synergy offers precise localization of hypermetabolic activity frequently associated with tumors to transform the process of diagnosis, especially in oncology application. Furthermore, technological innovation in CT, such as iterative reconstruction methods, enhances image quality while reducing radiation exposure. As clinicians increasingly rely on such hybrid modalities, it is important to understand how CT works and the implications of integrating it with PET imaging. This not only facilitates optimal utilization in clinical practice but also fosters research directions to enhance hybrid imaging methods for better patient outcomes (Prasad et al., 2024). Regarding the assessment of therapeutic response, CT imaging is significant in cases such as neuroendocrine tumors undergoing peptide receptor radionuclide therapy (PRRT). Current guidelines consider the combination of conventional imaging modalities, such as CT, with advanced modalities, such as SST PET/CT, for further differentiated assessment of treatment efficacy. When CT results are indeterminate, PET imaging is recommended to further characterize and differentiate pseudo-progression from true progression of disease. The combined approach improves diagnostic sensitivity, thereby enabling more tailored treatment strategies. Emerging expert opinion emphasizes the need for more sophisticated criteria in response assessment, underscoring the pivotal role of CT and PET imaging in complex clinical scenarios. As hybrid imaging technologies evolve, the principles of computed tomography remain crucial in informing patient care and treatment outcomes (Dhafer et al., 2024; Prasad et al., 2024).

3.2.2. Contrast Agents in CT Imaging

The use of contrast agents in CT imaging is a key aspect in enhancing the diagnostic capabilities of hybrid imaging modalities such as PET/CT and PET/MRI. Contrast agents, usually iodine-based for CT imaging, improve the visibility of internal structures by increasing the contrast between tissues. This high-resolution imaging is essential for evaluating complex diseases like atherosclerosis, where precise characterization of plaque morphology and distribution is required for patient management. The integration of CT imaging with PET provides an enhanced evaluation of anatomical and functional pathology and aids decision-making in a clinical setting. With the help of targeted contrast agents, doctors can overcome the limitations of conventional imaging and develop more specific treatment regimens that address each patient's individual needs (Kjær et al., 2015; Ahmed et al., 2019). The evolving context of molecular imaging also requires more sophisticated contrast agents to be developed continuously. Current CT contrast agents do not provide detailed information about the inflammatory components of atherosclerotic plaques, which are essential for assessing cardiovascular risk. New strategies, such as functionalizing contrast agents with targeting moieties, promise to enhance specificity and sensitivity in the detection of pathological changes at the molecular level. By incorporating such advances into hybrid imaging techniques, clinical professionals can gain vital information about the pathological processes underlying disease states. Such an improvement would lead to more precise therapeutic interventions aimed at countering vulnerabilities inherent to atherosclerotic lesions, thereby reducing the probability of catastrophic events such as myocardial infarctions (Kjær et al., 2015; Ahmed et al., 2019). The coupling of CT contrast agents with hybrid imaging modalities is a revolutionary time in medical imaging. In light of the increasing demand for precise diagnosis and intervention, research focused on developing optimized molecular probes is urgently required. Such probes can image not only structural abnormalities but also functional parameters of disease, such as inflammation in atherosclerotic plaques. Extensive molecular imaging would enable earlier diagnosis and improved surveillance of disease progression. Their successful integration into daily practice hinges on multidisciplinary collaboration, closing the gap among imaging science, molecular biology, and medical practice. Interdisciplinary collaboration can facilitate the progress of hybrid imaging methods that have the promise of raising standards in patient management and disease treatment (Kjær et al., 2015; Ahmed et al., 2019).

3.2.3. Clinical Applications of CT

Clinical applications of CT have expanded significantly, particularly in oncology, trauma assessment, and vascular imaging. CT technology provides high-resolution, cross-sectional images of organs and tissues within the body, making it very valuable for identifying and diagnosing many conditions. CT scans are applied in oncology to identify tumors, estimate their size and location, and monitor response to therapy. This is indispensable in guiding clinical decision-making and creating tailored treatment approaches. Moreover, rapid imaging acquisition combined with advanced image reconstruction software enhances the sensitivity and specificity of the scans to improve diagnostic accuracy. Consequently, CT plays a critical role in the multidisciplinary treatment of patients with cancer, allowing timely intervention that eventually affects clinical outcomes. In trauma, rapid acquisition of CT scans is critical as it allows for rapid assessment of injuries, especially in emergencies. Use of CT in acute cases provides for the detection of potentially life-threatening diagnoses such as intracranial hemorrhage, organ laceration, and fractures. Modern CT scanners use multi-slice technology that allows multiple anatomical structures to be visualized rapidly simultaneously, and it could be highly beneficial in the management of polytrauma patients. Furthermore, advancements in CT technology, including artificial intelligence and machine learning, are likely to further enhance diagnostic accuracy (Zhou et al., 2021). With the incorporation of such algorithms into clinical practice, radiologists will be assisted in interpreting challenging images, thereby streamlining the diagnostic process and enhancing the quality of patient care. The integration of CT with other imaging technologies, particularly in hybrid forms such as PET/CT and PET/MRI, has been a significant breakthrough in diagnostic imaging. The hybrid modalities exploit the strengths of each modality; for instance, PET provides metabolic information and CT provides anatomical information. This synergy allows clinicians to obtain rich information about the nature of diseases, especially cancers. However, there are issues in the interpretability field of advanced algorithms which underpin these technologies (Tjoa et al., 2020). As clinical practitioners increasingly rely on automated analysis techniques, understanding the reasoning behind these algorithms is central to ensuring trust and reliability in clinical practice. Overall, the clinical applications of CT continue to expand with further research focused on extending its role in hybrid imaging, which has tremendous potential to transform patient management across a variety of medical specialties.

3.3. Fundamentals of MRI Imaging

MRI is a valuable new technology in medical imaging that exploits the physics of nuclear magnetic resonance to produce extremely detailed images of internal body structure. Unlike all other imaging technologies, such as X-rays or CT scans, MRI employs no ionizing radiation and hence maintains patient exposure to the detrimental effects to a minimum. The fundamental MRI technique relies on the alignment of hydrogen nuclei, which are found in the greatest abundance in water and fat molecules, in a very strong magnetic field. When a radiofrequency pulse is applied to these nuclei, they oscillate and subsequently transmit signals that are received and interpreted by sophisticated algorithms to produce accurate images. This is its exceptional ability to produce multi-planar images, and it allows accurate characterization of soft tissues, making MRI a vital modality in neurology, orthopedics, and oncology. Another salient feature of MRI imaging is its ability to provide different types of contrast, which boosts the modality's diagnostic value. By varying scan parameters, radiologists can obtain T1-weighted, T2-weighted, and proton-density-weighted images, each with specific advantages for the representation of anatomical structures and pathologies. T1-weighted images, for instance, are best for assessing anatomical detail and the presence of fat, while T2-weighted images are optimal for detecting edema and fluid-related pathology. In addition, advances such as DWI and fMRI over the last few years have expanded the utility of MRI for quantifying tissue microstructure and brain activity. Built-in versatility in imaging protocols ensures that MRI can be tailored to meet the individual diagnostic requirements of different medical disorders. Coupling MRI with other imaging modalities, such as PET, has enabled hybrid imaging technologies that provide enhanced diagnostic confidence and support treatment planning. Hybrid imaging systems like PET/MRI merge the metabolic imaging of PET with the anatomical resolution of MRI, enabling a comprehensive understanding of disease processes, particularly in oncology. The confluence of such modalities enables precise localization of metabolic disturbances alongside structural information, resulting in improved diagnoses and patient care. Furthermore, developments in artificial intelligence promise to make MRI scan interpretation more efficient, whereupon AI algorithms can assist in image analysis, segmentation, and predictive modeling, all of which underscore the revolutionary nature of MRI utility in hybrid imaging environments (Dalmaz et al., 2022; Najjar, 2023).

3.3.1. Principles of Magnetic Resonance Imaging

MRI operates on the principle of nuclear magnetic resonance using the unique characteristics of specific atomic nuclei when they are exposed to a magnetic field. Hydrogen nuclei are of primary concern, owing to their prevalence in the human body, given the widespread presence of water. The hydrogen nuclei become oriented along the field direction when exposed to the magnetic field. A series of radiofrequency pulses is then released, which annihilate this alignment, causing the nuclei to absorb energy and release it when they resume equilibrium.

This released energy is captured and reconverted into detailed images that correspond to various tissue types. The ability of MRI to capture both anatomical and physiological data renders it a promising technique, particularly in the hybrid imaging situation where it supplements and augments modalities like PET by providing better resolution and contrast (Najjar, 2023). Combining MRI with hybrid imaging systems, particularly PET, enhances diagnostic capacity significantly. PET provides functional imaging by detecting metabolic activity, while MRI excels at providing high-resolution anatomical images. Such synergy brings to the table a more comprehensive image of numerous clinical conditions, like tumors, with the integration of metabolic activity and structural information. The absence of ionizing radiation in MRI compared with CT further underscores MRI's superiority in hybrid systems.

As can be observed from recent advancements, PET and MRI (PET/MRI) integration enables improved lesion localization, distinction between necrotic tissue and viable tumor tissue, and therefore improved patient outcomes and treatment planning (Zhou et al., 2021). As great as it sounds, different challenges still exist in the smooth integration of MRI with PET technology. One of the biggest challenges is the technical complexity of the physical principles underlying these modalities. For instance, the demand for high-strength magnetic fields in MRI can disrupt PET detector operation, and hence the design becomes challenging. In addition, the subtle interpretations of image—based contrast methodologies demand an advanced skill set from technologists as well as radiologists. Addressing these issues requires interdisciplinary collaboration, encouraging innovation in hardware and image analysis software. With the increasing spotlight on artificial intelligence in radiological practice, further progress could make integration easier, enhancing image quality and diagnostic accuracy in hybrid imaging (Najjar, 2023).

3.3.2. Advantages of MRI Over Other Imaging Modalities

The advantages of MRI over other modalities are numerous, particularly in the context of hybrid imaging modalities like PET/CT and PET/MRI. First and foremost, MRI offers enhanced soft-tissue contrast, which is of utmost significance for separating tissue types and identifying anomalies in complex anatomical structures. Compared to radiation-based CT, which produces less detailed images of soft tissues, MRI takes advantage of strong magnetic fields and radiofrequency pulses to provide a more nuanced characterization of tissues. This is particularly useful in tumor assessment, where precise demarcation is required to ensure effective management. Moreover, MRI's ability to visualize both structural and functional aspects of tissues enhances clinical decision-making, making it an indispensable tool in oncological imaging, as evidenced by advanced applications in neuroendocrine neoplasm assessment (Hubalewska-Dydejczyk et al., 2016). Another significant advantage of MRI is its non-ionizing nature, which makes it a safer alternative to modalities such as CT and PET that expose patients to ionizing radiation. This ability is especially beneficial for patient groups that must be imaged repeatedly, such as cancer patients being followed and treated. Even within the realm of hybrid imaging, the union of MRI and PET (PET/MRI) further leverages these strengths, combining the metabolic information of PET with the high-resolution anatomic data of MRI. This synergy not only increases lesion detection rates but also reduces radiation exposure, addressing one of the most significant challenges in imaging strategies today. Application of MRI in hybrid arrangements has been shown to increase sensitivity and specificity, particularly in the presence of small lesions or assessing intricate anatomical relationships within tumors (Bose et al., 2019). Finally, ' versatility in the assessment of a wide range of conditions refutes any argument against their superiority to other methods of imaging. Beyond imaging tumors, MRI plays a critical role in assessing neurological disorders, cardiac disease, and musculoskeletal disorders due to its high-resolution capabilities. MRI enables the study of metabolic activity and brain functional connectivity, several orders deeper than is possible with CT or ultrasound. The technical innovations in MRI, including fMRI and DWI, offer new avenues for diagnostic precision and therapeutic follow-up. Such capabilities not only broaden the areas of MRI application but also underscore its relevance to improving hybrid imaging models, particularly in diagnosing and treating cancerous conditions such as neuroendocrine tumors, where precise imaging is essential for optimal therapy follow-ups and patient management (Hubalewska-Dydejczyk et al., 2016).

3.3.3. Clinical Applications of MRI

In the last few years, the clinical application of MRI has expanded considerably, particularly in hybrid imaging frameworks such as PET/MRI. The complementarity between MRI's excellent soft tissue contrast and the metabolic data provided by positron emission tomography works to enhance diagnostic ability across suites of medicine. The coupling has been critical in oncology, where the ability to visualize both the form and function of tumors directly translates into improved patient management. For instance, DCE-MRI enables assessment of tumor perfusion and angiogenesis, which are significant in cancer diagnosis and therapeutic evaluation. When combined with PET, this imaging method yields a broad survey that enables clinicians to individualize treatment plans and optimize prognostic assessments, playing a significant role in advancements in oncologic imaging and therapeutic modalities (Aldahery, 2023). Besides oncology, MRI applications extend beyond the mentioned fields to neurology and cardiology. Progressive MRI techniques are increasingly making significant contributions to the early diagnosis and monitoring of neurodegenerative diseases like multiple sclerosis and Alzheimer's. Perfusion-weighted imaging allows cerebral blood flow to be measured and gives valuable information on pathophysiology in a variety of neurological disorders. In cardiology, MRIs non-invasive character for myocardial viability measurement and perfusion abnormalities detection significantly improves diagnosis accuracy. The integration of PET and MRI in these conditions enhances understanding of the disease process, enabling more efficient interventions. These hybrid imaging technologies are thus a reflection of the sustained development of diagnostic radiology, cementing MRI's essential role in clinical evaluation and treatment planning (Inglese et al., 2019). The clinical use of hybrid imaging modalities, such as PET/MRI, underscores the need to further explore them to establish them as the best in their applications across various clinical contexts. Description of the tissue's biochemical and functional properties through multimodal imaging has the potential to lead to improved treatments and more accurate predictive models. For example, correlations between the kinetics of contrast media used in MRI and radiolabeled tracers used in PET provide a multi-parameter view of tissue microenvironment dynamics. This multi-parameter view may identify biomarkers of therapeutic response, particularly in oncology and infectious disease, where perfusion dynamics may be altered by pathological conditions. With ongoing advances in MRI-based clinical applications in hybrid designs, the integration of new imaging modalities has the potential to reshape therapeutic and diagnostic frameworks, paving the way for precision medicine across diverse patient populations (Aldahery, 2023).

3.4. PET/CT Imaging

The possibility of hybrid imaging modalities, particularly PET/CT, has transformed the field of medical diagnostics by combining the functional data of PET with the anatomical resolution of CT. This combination allows for a close examination of most diseases, and especially cancer, where one must know both metabolic function and anatomical structure. PET imaging offers vital information about cellular activity and tumor metabolism by detecting radiolabeled tracers, while CT yields high-resolution, detailed images that outline the anatomical context of such abnormalities. The combination ensures that physicians have a complete perspective, improving diagnostic precision and enabling better treatment planning. Consequently, PET/CT scanning has become the norm in oncologic assessment, making not only initial diagnoses, but also monitoring for response to therapy and recurrence detection possible, and therefore a critical part of improving patient outcomes. In addition, one of PET/CT imaging's greatest strengths is the ability to reduce the number of invasive diagnostic tests. Traditional imaging modalities also require biopsies or surgery to determine final diagnoses, which pose a potential risk to patients and take a longer time to recover. In contrast, PET/CT provides non-invasive techniques to detect and characterize tumors and assess tumor sensitivity to therapy, thus minimizing patient discomfort as well as risk of complications. The higher accuracy of the hybrid method in diagnosis also led to cost reductions for healthcare systems, as it limited the need for many studies or follow-up interventions. Also, ongoing research and development of optimizing the imaging protocols and adding artificial intelligence are likely to maximize the capacity of PET/CT further in terms of even lesser doses of radiation without compromising on image quality and diagnostic precision, as implied in recent reviews (David-Olawade et al., 2025; Syahputra et al., 2025). Despite its many advantages, PET/CT imaging is never without restriction. One of the key issues is the radiation dose from both PET and CT components, which has caused concerns, particularly among vulnerable populations that may have to go in for repeated imaging. To balance such concerns, there must be a careful balance between optimizing diagnostic effectiveness and avoiding harm. Imaging devices and technologies with features like AI-driven low-dose imaging protocols have been regarded as efficient tools towards lowering radiation dose while preserving image integrity. These advances enable physicians to perform PET/CT scans using reduced radiation doses, thereby enhancing patient safety without reducing diagnostic accuracy. Therefore, ongoing monitoring of emerging technologies and adherence to current best practices in radiology are critical for optimizing the benefits of PET/CT imaging in clinical applications so that it can remain a valuable resource in modern medicine.

3.4.1. Technical Integration of PET and CT

The technological fusion of PET and CT has revolutionized imaging protocols in the health care field and has resulted in the development of hybrid PET/CT systems. These systems combine PET functional imaging with the anatomical precision of CT to offer a superior evaluation of many pathologies. The synergy of the process facilitates the correct localization of metabolically active areas by clinicians while simultaneously providing very precise anatomical information important for proper diagnosis and treatment planning. Furthermore, the hybrid technology enhances the detection capabilities of the clinicians to identify and differentiate between malignant and benign lesions, hence facilitating more appropriate decision-making for patient management. To this end, PET/CT technical integration is a significant move in radiology that addresses the need to deliver both morphological and functional information in a single scan. The integration not only enhanced diagnostic capabilities but also ensured patient safety by maximizing imaging protocols. With healthcare professionals increasing awareness of the potential risks of ionizing radiation, particularly in susceptible patients, innovation for low-dose imaging protocols is now most important. The application of artificial intelligence (AI) to PET/CT scanners enables the creation of low-dose imaging protocols with diagnostic quality, without compromising radiation exposure. AI-driven technologies are adept at noise reduction, removal of artifacts, and optimization of imaging parameters in real-time, as emphasized in recent studies. Consequently, the technical fusion of PET and CT not only enhances image quality but also underscores the need for patient health safeguarding by reducing radiation risks at the cost of diagnostic accuracy (Adeleke et al., 2025). In addition, ongoing progress in hybrid imaging modalities is charting new frontiers for therapeutic applications, particularly in oncology. As molecular imaging progresses, PET/CT integration enables quantitative assessments of disease course and treatment response. The ability of PET imaging to explain biological processes, coupled with the precise anatomical localization of CT scans, permits medical practitioners to modulate treatment regimens based on patient response. Theranostics, the new field in which imaging guides therapy, is also assisted by this customized approach. As reported in the literature, hybrid imaging provides greater insight into disease mechanisms and enables more tailored care in oncology and beyond (Augustynowicz et al., 2023). The technological merging of PET and CT is thus a step toward a more integrative patient-centered model of healthcare.

3.4.2. Advantages of PET/CT Over Standalone Imaging

The advantages of combining PET and CT through hybrid imaging are profound, particularly in oncology. Standalone traditional imaging techniques are likely to provide limited information primarily regarding anatomical shape without identifying functional characteristics of tumors. PET/CT compensates sufficiently for such a deficiency by integrating metabolic and anatomical data so that cancerous progression can be assessed comprehensively. Evidence shows that the positional and functional information provided by PET/CT enhances diagnostic specificity, thereby improving patient management strategies. Research shows that PET/CT plays a determinative role in treatment planning, underscoring the device's role as a cornerstone in oncology (Saad et al., 2015). The combined modalities enable physicians to diagnose malignancies earlier and with greater precision, thereby making therapeutic intervention timely. In addition to its greater diagnostic capability, PET/CT also has a strong role in therapeutic monitoring. Whereas isolated imaging can provide images of structural changes over time, PET/CT enables health professionals to observe metabolic changes in response to therapy, e.g., changes in tumor glucose metabolism. This enhances the ability to evaluate therapy effectiveness in real time, allowing oncologists to adjust therapeutic regimens accordingly. The integration of functional imaging data provides an immense contribution to prognostication, as it informs decisions about potential patient outcomes based on tumor response to various treatments. Moreover, studies have shown that the incorporation of PET/CT into clinical practice can reduce unnecessary surgical interventions, thereby enhancing patient care and the overall cost-effectiveness of treatment (Saad et al., 2015). In terms of nodule detection, PET/CT is superior to single-modality imaging, particularly in the lung. In a comparison study of CT images acquired for attenuation correction (AC) and diagnostic purposes, nodule detection was much better on the diagnostic images. This finding supports the use of optimized imaging techniques that prioritize diagnostic image quality to enable accurate evaluation of pulmonary pathology. In the clinical environment, PET/CT's improved visualization properties enable differentiation between benign and malignant nodules, thereby impacting treatment plans. Therefore, aside from increased diagnostic sensitivity, PET/

CT's advantages over stand-alone imaging include more profound implications for patient management and the effectiveness of oncologic treatments, and are worth continued application in contemporary medical practice.

3.4.3. Clinical Applications and Case Studies

Hybrid imaging modalities, PET/CT and PET/MRI, have revolutionized clinical applications in various fields of medicine. Complementary information can be combined using these modalities, incorporating anatomical details from CT and MRI and functional details from PET. One excellent example is in cancer medicine, where hybrid imaging improves tumor detection, staging, and monitoring of treatment response. PET/CT has proved central in imaging metabolic activity, and the structural information provided by CT improves lesion characterization. Additionally, uses in personalized medicine are growing, with clinicians able to identify specific metabolic pathways that suggest tumor behavior and adapt therapy accordingly. Case studies illustrate the value these imaging technologies add to patient care; for instance, patients with lung cancer receive more precise staging information and improved management options when imaged with PET/CT than with traditional imaging. In addition to oncology, hybrid imaging is also of significant importance in neurology, particularly for diagnosing neurodegenerative diseases. PET/MRI preferentially benefits the evaluation of dementia and Alzheimer's disease because of its excellent soft tissue contrast and functional imaging capabilities. Research indicates that PET/MRI neuroimaging provides simultaneous access to amyloid plaque deposition and glucose metabolism data, which provides better insight into the disease course. Case reports describe settings in which these hybrid modalities enabled earlier diagnosis and more accurate measurement, thereby informing treatment planning and patient care. For example, visualization of metabolic and physiological alterations within the brain allows distinguishing between types of dementia and thus maximizes therapeutic interventions and improves patient outcomes via evidence-based clinical decision-making. Moreover, in cardiac imaging, hybrid technologies such as PET/CT have evolved significantly in assessing heart disease. The combination of metabolic imaging with PET and the anatomical detail provided by CT provides clinicians with vital information on coronary artery disease (CAD) and myocardial viability. Clinical case histories demonstrate how PET/CT can effectively identify areas of ischemia and scarring in the myocardium and guide the management of patients who present with chest pain and risk factors for cardiac complications. Technological developments in hybrid imaging are promising, as they facilitate the evaluation of treatment effectiveness and more cautious post-intervention follow-up of patients. As clinicians grow to use these technologies, multimodal imaging integration will enhance diagnostic performance and enable the development of personalized treatment algorithms, with attendant improvements in cardiovascular medicine clinical outcomes.

3.5. PET/MRI Imaging

The combination of PET and MRI has been a huge breakthrough in hybrid imaging modalities, and today it is a powerful tool for research as well as for clinical applications. The technique employs metabolic and functional data from PET, paired with the high soft-tissue contrast of MRI. PET/MRI is emerging as a valuable modality for evaluating a variety of conditions, most notably in oncology and neurology. When integrated PET/MRI systems were developed, simultaneous data acquisition became feasible, allowing clinicians to correlate metabolic activity with anatomical structure more effectively than with other imaging modalities. Such a comprehensive approach may lead to more accurate diagnoses, better-informed treatment planning, and ultimately improved patient outcomes, despite the individual limitations of each stand-alone imaging technique (Dhami et al., 2008). As part of the advancement of hybrid imaging systems, PET/MRI has evolved significantly since its inception. Early on, the models were essentially tandem systems composed of separate PET and MRI subsystems, which created complex workflows and imposed major limitations on image registration. Advances since then have moved towards combined PET/MRI devices that optimize data acquisition and provide better image quality. Combined platforms allow for imaging sessions simultaneously, reducing the time for both tests and minimizing patient exposure to potential complications.

The technology capitalizes on improvements in PET detector materials and MRI gradient systems to provide high-quality images required for proper clinical evaluation (Dhami et al., 2008). But as this technology continues to progress, it will be necessary to continue researching and testing to grasp the long-term implications for patient care fully. New clinical data underscore the benefit of PET/MRI imaging while suggesting the need for further study in most diagnostic uses. The merging of high-resolution anatomical data from MRI and functional imaging of metabolism from PET creates a rich dataset that neither modality can provide alone. It is particularly promising in oncologic diagnostics, where accurate characterization of tumors is crucial for effective treatment planning. However, there are questions about standardizing protocols and merging findings across mixed patient populations, particularly where multi-comorbidity exists. To this end, although early results are promising, extensive clinical trials will be required to establish the utility of PET/MRI for broad diagnostic use and to confirm that this new technology can be utilized without interference with current clinical practice (Czepczyński et al., 2016).

3.5.1. Technical Integration of PET and MRI

The technical fusion of PET and MRI has transformed diagnostic imaging by enabling comprehensive evaluations of disease. By combining the metabolic data from PET with the sophisticated anatomical information from MRI, clinicians can better understand pathological processes.

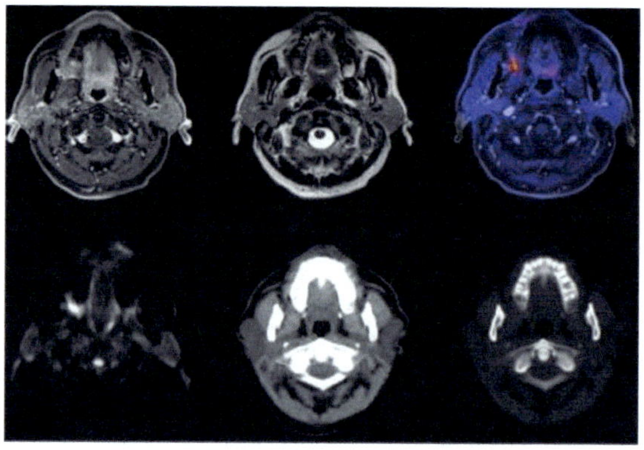

Figure 3.4. Whole-body PET/MRI in oncology. A 67-year-old male patient with squamous cell carcinoma of the upper alveolar ridge. From left to right, upper row: T1 TSE tra FAT SAT (after contrast), T2 TSE tra and PET/MRI fusion (FDG); lower row: DWI (b = 800), CT and CT (bone window). PET/MRI allows better lesion identification and anatomical location compared with PET/CT. In addition, bone marrow involvement was found, allowing correct T3 staging.

Source: https://media.springernature.com/lw685/springer-static/image/art%3A10.1007%2Fs40336-013-0012-4/MediaObjects/40336_2013_12_Fig1_HTML.jpg?as=webp.

This combined modality is beneficial in cancer, where tumor characterization and treatment assessment can be more accurately assessed, ultimately refining patient management. In addition, simultaneous imaging of both modalities facilitates greater spatial correlation, thereby reducing misregistration that generally occurs when these imaging methods are used separately. With continued hardware development, the processing and real-time coordination of imaging data become increasingly possible, which presents a critical step toward fully integrated imaging systems and the associated benefits in clinical applications of hybrid imaging technology (Figure 3.4).

One of the challenges in PET/MRI integration is the divergence in their working principles and supporting technologies. PET relies on detecting gamma rays from radiotracers, which requires specialized materials and detectors, whereas MRI uses magnetic fields and radiofrequency pulse sequences to generate images by exploiting the magnetic properties of hydrogen nuclei in tissues. This inherent difference makes the technical integration of the two modalities challenging, and advanced engineering techniques must be employed to achieve complete interoperability. Additionally, software platforms for image processing and visualization pose another challenge that calls for concerted collaboration between multimodal imaging researchers and engineers. Solving these problems is of great importance, as improved communication between the two modalities is not only important for successful workflow but also for increasing diagnostic accuracy and improving patient outcomes in hybrid imaging applications. Advancements in AI and deep learning technologies continue to influence the technical fusion of PET and MRI, inviting new solutions to common challenges. The deployment of AI algorithms can improve image quality and enhance interpretability, thereby assisting clinicians in making rational decisions based on hybrid imaging information. The application of AI to clinical practice, however, demands a thoughtful process to ensure machine learning models deliver repeatable, interpretable results, especially in high-risk environments such as medicine. As Zhou et al. (2021) also note, the particularities of medical imaging necessitate specialized solutions of deep learning addressing specific clinical needs and technology challenges. Additionally, Tjoa et al. (2020) also observe the importance of medical AI solution interpretability, noting that increased understanding of decision-making is needed to establish clinician trust and optimize patient treatment. Finally, the successful integration of PET and MRI, supplemented by AI developments, will significantly enhance diagnostic capabilities and treatment planning in medicine.

3.5.2. Advantages of PET/MRI Over PET/CT

The combination of PET with MRI offers several benefits compared to the conventional combination of PET and CT. Perhaps most important is the improved soft tissue contrast of MRI. Improved resolution enables more refined visualization of anatomical structures, a benefit especially in the assessment of soft tissue tumors and intricate anatomical areas where CT may be less effective. This enhanced contrast resolution enables better characterization of lesions and differentiation of benign from malignant processes by clinicians, as well as better tracking of response to therapy, potentially improving patient outcomes. Overall, the integration of MRI and PET maximizes the diagnostic capabilities of hybrid imaging and makes it a first-line modality in certain clinical conditions. One of the major advantages of PET/MRI is the reduced radiation dose that patients are exposed to compared with PET/CT. As there is greater awareness and concern about the total dose of ionizing radiation from imaging examinations, the reduced radiation dose of MRI is particularly crucial. PET/MRI exploits the non-ionizing nature of MRI to substantially reduce radiation exposure while still providing valuable diagnostic information (Figure 3.5).

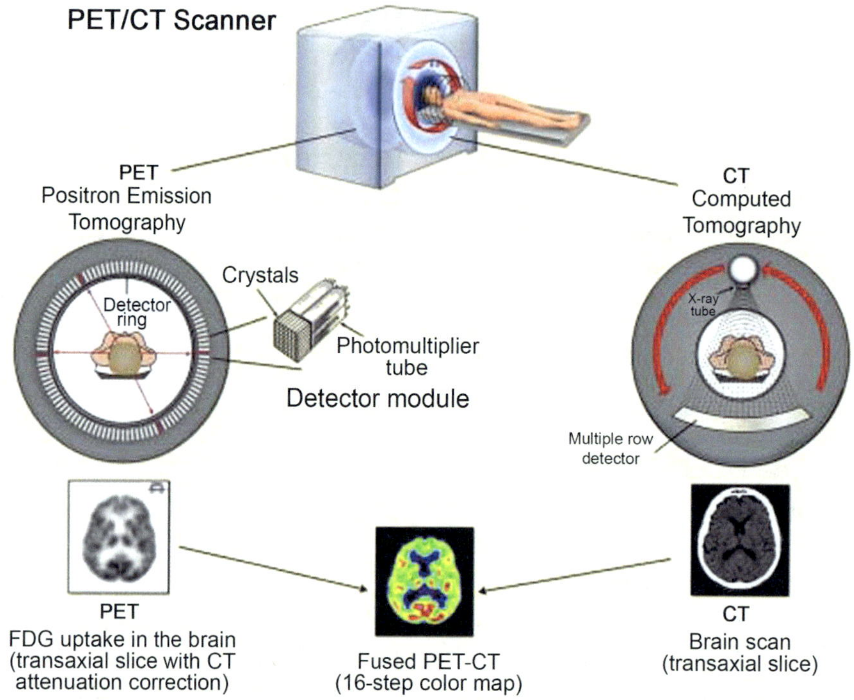

Figure 3.5. A combination of the PET and CT imaging systems for anatomic imaging.

Source: https://www.researchgate.net/profile/Zainab-T-Al-Sharify/publication/343048715/figure/fig4/AS:914811755966464@1595119527017/A-combination-of-the-PET-and-CT-imaging-systems-for-anatomic-imaging-55.jpg.

This is especially relevant to populations that require multiple scans, such as cancer patients who require repetitive follow-up scans. Secondly, this reduction in exposure to radiation fits into the overall objective of patient safety in imaging protocols. Therefore, PET/MRI is a highly promising alternative for repeated measurements under treatment monitoring or disease follow-up. PET/MRI also has a unique ability in functional imaging that PET/CT lacks. The integration of dynamic contrast-enhanced MRI imaging and PET allows simultaneous assessment of both metabolic and physiological parameters. This is of great value in assessing inflammatory diseases such as Charcot neuroarthropathy, where one needs to distinguish inflammatory from infectious processes for treatment. As new evidence indicates, PET can provide very valuable information regarding metabolic activity, whereas MRI can give an anatomic depiction of soft tissues with high sensitivity. Consequently, the combined data from PET/MRI can assist in enhanced clinical decision-making as an added value in clinical situations in a variety of domains, including oncology and neurology, where the understanding of both the functional and anatomical data is indispensable for successful treatment planning (Brinkbäumer et al., 2004; Bose et al., 2019).

3.5.3. Clinical Applications and Case Studies

The clinical applications of hybrid imaging, particularly PET/CT and PET/MRI, have completely revolutionized diagnostic techniques in various specialties of medicine. Such newer imaging techniques have unique advantages by unifying anatomical and metabolic data in a symphony of information, enabling clinicians to arrive at improved diagnoses and treatment strategies. For instance, PET/CT has been of immense value in oncology by facilitating tumor characterization and staging, as well as accurate evaluation of treatment response. In head and neck cancers, synergistic modalities distinguish residual viable tumors from post-treatment changes, thereby altering patient management strategies. Such integration enhances the role of hybrid imaging in improving diagnostic accuracy and, with potential, significantly improving patient outcomes. The most recent advancements in PET/MRI systems, particularly at institutions such as UZ Leuven, have underscored the clinical significance of using isotopes such as F-18, Ga-68, and Y-90 for specific pathological assessments (Figure 3.6).

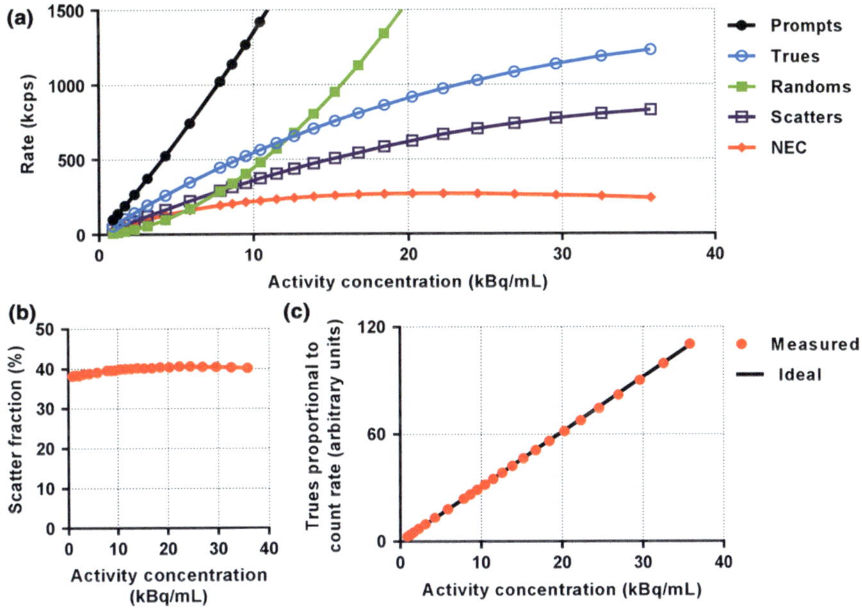

Figure 3.6. Representative results of NEMA performance testing on one 5-ring discovery MI scanner (MD Anderson). The figure shows results for counting rate performance (a), scatter fraction as a function of activity concentration (b), and accuracy (c). NEC, noise-equivalent counting.

Source: https://www.researchgate.net/publication/332970144/figure/fig2/AS:11431281255339577@1719418674699/Representative-results-of-NEMA-performance-testing-on-one-5-ring-Discovery-MI-scanner-MD.png.

NEMA performance tests illustrate differences in system characteristics when employing these different isotopes, which imply that the image quality and spatial resolution can become key factors in the clinical interpretations. Experiments have shown that even if Ga-68 may have smaller recovery coefficients for small lesions, PET imaging is still a highly useful tool for oncology applications, especially for tumor characterization, which involves the uptake of radiolabeled ligands. Thus, the clinical use of hybrid imaging systems must account for the intrinsic benefits and limitations of the isotopes employed, which influence diagnostic capability and treatment response, thereby justifying ongoing evaluation and adjustment of imaging protocols. Aside from oncology, the application of hybrid imaging is also extended to regenerative medicine, specifically for monitoring stem cell therapy. The introduction of molecular imaging techniques, such as PET and MRI, enables real-time imaging of the viability, distribution, and functionality of stem cells post-transplant *in vivo*. This is significant since clinical use of stem cell therapies is hampered by safety and efficacy concerns (Figure 3.7).

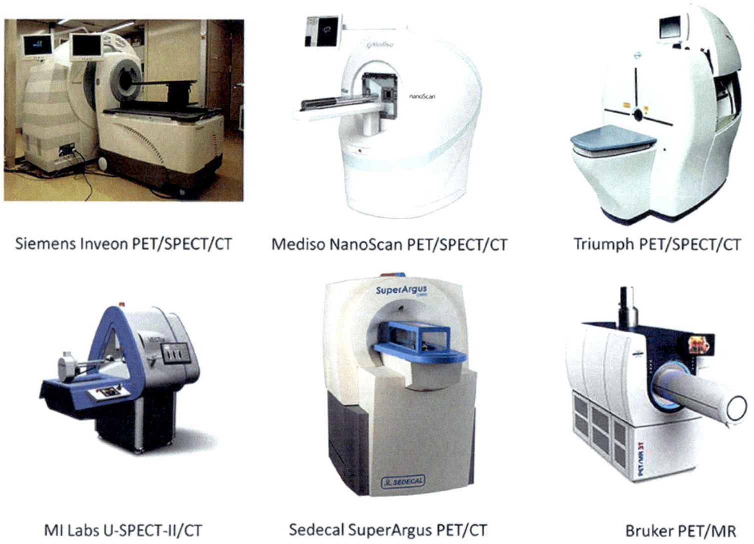

Figure 3.7. Shows hybrid imaging.

Source: https://www.frontiersin.org/files/Articles/345924/fphy-06-00047-HTML-r1/image_m/fphy-06-00047-g002.jpg.

By applying hybrid imaging modalities, researchers and practitioners can not only quantify the biodistribution of transplanted cells but also assess therapeutic effects in the target tissues. The focus of stem cell research, as reflected in recent research, relies heavily on the effective use of hybrid imaging technologies to trace cellular dynamics, with the aim of improving the efficacy of such new therapies in clinical settings (Bose et al., 2019).

3.6. Challenges and Limitations

The advent of hybrid imaging techniques, such as PET/CT and PET/MRI, has significantly enhanced diagnostic capability but has not been without difficulties and limitations. A major difficulty is the inherent complexity of standardizing imaging protocols within diverse clinical settings. Despite the advantages accruing from combining the metabolic information obtained with PET into a form of precise anatomical data provided by CT or MRI, differences in equipment, software, and reading techniques may introduce diagnostic variation. Subsequent treatment planning, particularly in oncology, where precise delineation of the tumor is essential to effective intervention, can be affected. The requirement of highly established guidelines and performance measures is paramount to ensure that clinicians can effectively interpret the information derived from these advanced image modalities to reach reliable patient management and outcomes (Alanazi, 2024). The second significant challenge concerns the problems of limited availability and high cost of hybrid imaging technologies. The technical complexity of PET/CT and PET/MRI necessitates significant investment in equipment and the training of medical personnel, which presents barriers to dissemination, particularly in low-resource settings. Further, operational expenses may limit access to these cutting-edge imaging modalities at reference centers, with most patients relying on conventional imaging techniques that may be less specific for effective cancer detection and tracking.

This disparity underscores the pressing need for interventions that can decrease costs or enhance the availability of hybrid imaging technologies to allow more patients to access their enhanced diagnostic yields, hence lessening the public health implications of unequal access to advanced medical care (Costin et al., 2024). Hybrid imaging also has technical limitations in effectively imaging certain pathological conditions. Though PET/CT can provide both structural and functional images, it has limited capability in detecting tumor hypoxia, which is crucial in the interpretation of treatment resistance and recurrence. Similarly, though PET/MRI has improved soft-tissue contrast and reduced radiation exposure, it must be properly calibrated to provide meaningful hypoxia-specific information. The marriage of functional and structural imaging modalities requires continuing research on tracers to enhance the specificity of hypoxia detection in tumors, particularly for cancers notorious for treatment resistance. Resolution of such technical challenges is imperative to realizing the full clinical potential of hybrid imaging and guaranteeing that diagnostic challenges are systematically diagnosed and overcome within routine clinical practice (Costin et al., 2024).

3.6.1. Technical Challenges in Hybrid Imaging

The union of PET and MRI is also fraught with technical challenges stemming from the different operating principles of the two modalities. While PET relies on detecting gamma rays emitted during positron annihilation, MRI uses a magnetic field and radiofrequency pulses to form images. Such fundamental disparity can pose challenges, particularly in spatial resolution and sensitivity when applying various PET isotopes. Notably, the performance of hybrid imaging systems varies considerably depending on the isotope employed. For instance, studies reveal that the spatial resolution of Gallium-68 (Ga-68) is approximately 1 mm lower than that of Fluorine-18 (F-18), resulting in lower image quality and diagnostic accuracy in oncological applications (D'Asseler et al., 2019) (Figure 3.8).

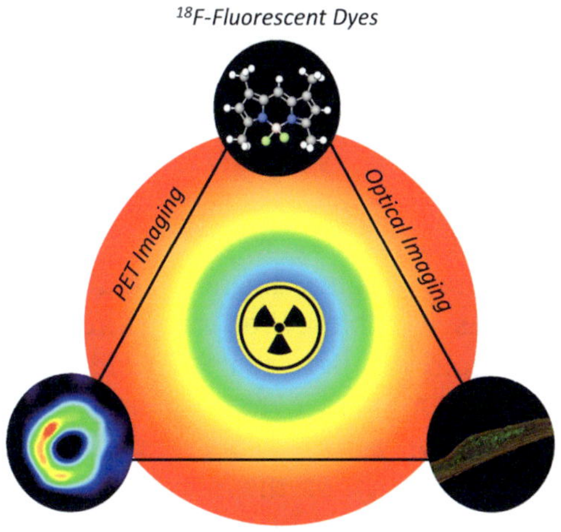

Figure 3.8. Fluorine-18-labeled fluorescent dyes for dual-mode molecular imaging.

Source: https://pub.mdpi-res.com/molecules/molecules-25-06042/article_deploy/html/images/molecules-25-06042-ag.png?1608688371.

These differences call for meticulous consideration of isotope selection for optimal hybrid imaging outcomes. Moreover, with the emergence of hybrid imaging machines such as PET/MRI, the problem of interactions among hardware, particularly in the presence of magnetic fields, becomes a concern. Insertion of conductive SPECT collimators into the MRI unit in SPECT/MRI configurations can induce eddy currents that degrade hybrid imaging performance. This is further exacerbated by the intimate needs of high-resolution imaging with the operational characteristics of MRI, which necessitate precise gradient fields to capture good images. Advances such as novel tungsten collimators produced with additive manufacturing have been observed to significantly reduce the impact of such eddy currents, eliminating over 50% of the impact. These developments point to a promising future for overcoming technical hurdles in integrating such modalities, thereby paving the way for enhanced imaging performance in clinical and research settings (Joseph et al., 2015). Besides spatial resolution and hardware interactions, calibration and alignment of hybrid modalities also introduce an additional layer of complexity. Efficient coordination between PET and MRI components is essential for successful integration. Alignment variation will create artifacts and inaccuracies, rendering the value of fused data in clinical diagnosis and treatment planning useless. Moreover, time differences in image acquisition between PET and MRI will create challenges in dynamic studies, where patient motion and temporal conditions will affect the validity of the results. Therefore, developing robust calibration protocols and synchronization strategies emerges as a high-priority goal for achieving high-quality hybrid imaging solutions. This is required to enhance the clinical usefulness of hybrid imaging systems by ensuring that they provide beneficial diagnostic information without compromising on a high degree of accuracy and reliability in patient treatment.

3.6.2. Limitations in Clinical Applications

The emergence of hybrid imaging devices such as PET/CT and PET/MRI has certainly transformed medical diagnostics. However, there are still inherent limitations in their clinical use that must be critically examined with caution. One of the major problems is the complexity and cost of integrating these technologies into routine clinical practice. The substantial financial outlays for high-end imaging equipment tend to result in unequal access across healthcare organizations. Less sophisticated hospitals may not be able to afford the high-technology equipment utilized in hybrid imaging. Thus, it may be challenging for patients to access such sophisticated diagnostic methods. Thus, this financial limitation exacerbates already present inequities in the provision of medical services, particularly in rural communities where precise imaging is severely needed. In addition to financial considerations, the varying properties of radiotracers used in PET imaging can significantly contribute to clinical efficacy. For instance, while F-18 is one of the most widely used isotopes in PET scans, its behavior can differ substantially from that of other isotopes, such as Ga-68 and Y-90, which are used more commonly for oncological applications. These differences have implications for spatial resolution and image quality measurements, which can lead to misinterpretation or error in diagnosis or treatment planning. Specifically, the spatial resolution of Ga-68 will be about 1 mm lower in the axial plane than F-18, thus lowering sensitivity in detecting small lesions (D'Asseler et al., 2019). Hence, the choice of radiotracer is critical, and its implications for clinical outcomes must be evaluated carefully to maximize patient outcomes. Another significant limitation lies in the complexities of data interpretation and the need for precise training of healthcare professionals. Combining data from more than one imaging modality necessitates sufficient knowledge of both modalities to diagnose ailments effectively. Because hybrid imaging combines anatomical and functional information, misinterpretation is possible if clinicians are not trained in both modalities. Further, the technical intricacies of attenuation and scatter correction can lead to variations in image quality, which in turn have implications for clinical decisions (Bose et al., 2019). Therefore, continuous training and education are the most important needs in overcoming these challenges, so that health care providers can overcome the complexities of hybrid imaging with confidence in improving patient care.

3.6.3. Cost and Accessibility Issues

The addition of hybrid imaging technologies such as PET/CT and PET/MRI to the clinical environment offers significant advantages in oncology diagnosis, but these advances are weighed against high cost and accessibility issues (Figure 3.9).

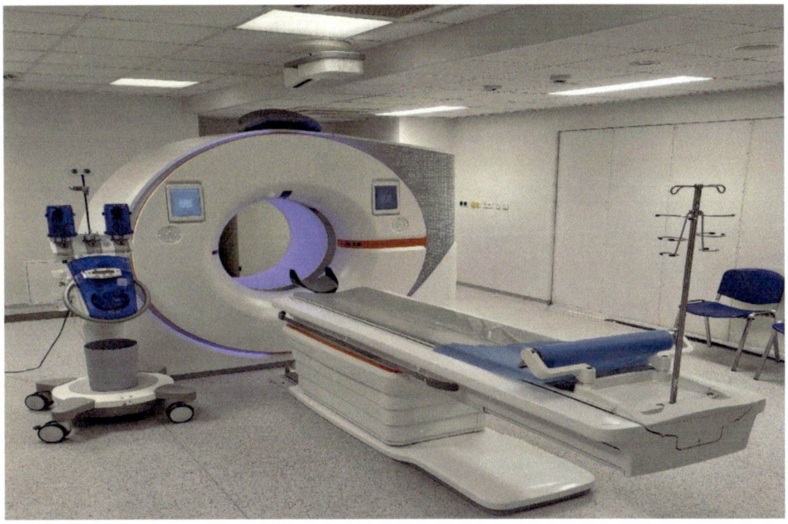

Figure 3.9. The initial capital expense of acquiring and maintaining these advanced imaging systems can be prohibitive for many healthcare facilities.

Source: https://img1.wsimg.com/isteam/ip/2842fe6f-7182-4d3e-9b3e-f4b3dbfae9d8/labdunia-pet%20ct%20machine-7683ea0.jpg.

For instance, the cost of PET/CT systems is considerable, including capital and operational/ maintenance costs for both the device and the required maintenance and operational procedures. The specialized technologists and radiologists required are also a factor in increasing the overall cost. As a result, some smaller or rural health organizations may not be able to afford the cost, potentially restricting access to advanced imaging technology to cities, creating uneven access across patient populations. Access to hybrid imaging technologies also intersects with insurance coverage policies, which vary widely. For insured patients relying on reimbursement, access to PET/ CT or PET/MRI is not always assured. These modalities are the current standards recommended for accurate staging and treatment follow-up in most cancers. Still, payment criteria and amounts do not necessarily align with clinical need and can lead to denial or to coverage being limited within practice. This variation is not only a challenge to the patient's financial means, but is also bound to slow down necessary diagnostic processes. Economic studies suggest that while hybrid imaging is more diagnostically accurate, insurance may lag behind in accepting such technologies and hence perpetuate unequal access for those patients in need of timely and effective treatment options, as identified in studies on cervical cancer treatment protocols that are not all advocating routine use of PET-CT despite potential benefits (Auguste et al., 2013). Moreover, the additive cost impacts extend beyond mere hardware and insurance coverage to affect patient outcomes and health care efficiency. Delay in access to hybrid imaging may retard early cancer detection and hence reduce cure rates. Health care systems are thus not only faced with ethical dilemmas in ensuring fair access but also with economic imperatives, including increased downstream expenditures due to late diagnoses. Efforts to become more cost-effective must be accompanied by solutions that enable hybrid imaging within established paradigms without worsening inequalities. Breakthroughs like artificial intelligence for imaging and the introduction of lower-cost imaging devices could offer pathways to fix some of these issues. Addressing the twin challenges of cost and accessibility is critical not only to improve patient care but also to spur the wider adoption and utilization of PET/CT and PET/MRI technologies (Carsrud et al., 2024).

SUMMARY

The addition of hybrid imaging modalities, such as Positron Emission Tomography/Computed Tomography (PET/CT) and Positron Emission Tomography/Magnetic Resonance Imaging (PET/MRI), addresses the urgent need for enhanced diagnostic accuracy in oncology and other clinical fields. PET/CT marries the functional data of PET with the anatomical data of CT to provide a comprehensive view of tumors and metastasis. Based on studies, this method shows 94.8% and 86.9% sensitivity and specificity, respectively, in cervical cancer recurrence (Auguste et al., 2013). Apart from its use in diagnosis, the combination technique is of great utility for preoperative planning, where precise knowledge of tumor extent is critical for any intervention. Therefore, PET/CT is unique in that it provides information that can significantly affect the patient's management. In contrast, PET/MRI is increasingly being highlighted by its unique superiority, particularly in soft tissue imaging, where MRI plays a superior role. The hybrid technique offers enhanced resolution and contrast, which are necessary for differentiating malignant from benign lesions. In addition, visualization of metabolic activity relative to highly detailed anatomical structures enables improved tumor characterization, which benefits particular therapeutic techniques. Although sensitivity and specificity vary by MRI alone, coupling with PET yields a more realistic diagnostic strategy (Auguste et al., 2013). In a few clinical applications, such as in cardiac imaging, the blending of PET and MRI unifies anatomical and functional information for a comprehensive appraisal that informs treatment modalities and interventions. With the advent of hybrid imaging, awareness of the sophistication of PET/CT and PET/MRI is paramount for clinicians and researchers to maneuver. Both modalities are impressive; however, the choice between them is typically based on specific clinical needs and the inherent strengths of each. Furthermore, while PET/CT has been more extensively studied and has more established protocols for various diseases, PET/MRI is gaining popularity, with ongoing research aimed at realizing its full potential. Future studies must bridge the existing evidence gaps regarding peak use, especially in surveillance studies and comparative effectiveness. A balanced understanding of the advantages and disadvantages of these hybrid imaging techniques will ultimately guide their use in the clinic, allowing clinicians to make informed decisions for patient care.

As hybrid imaging technology advances, the future of this field is toward greater integration of advanced methodologies to improve diagnostic accuracy and therapeutic interventions. Uses such as the development of novel radiopharmaceuticals are likely to be a focal point, allowing more targeted imaging of biological processes at a molecular level. These advances are particularly important in oncology, where precise imaging of tumor metabolism can have significant effects on treatment planning and follow-up. More sophisticated image reconstruction and analysis algorithms will enable PET/CT and PET/MRI modalities to be integrated more effectively, facilitating greater anatomical localization of functional abnormalities. The ongoing studies in machine learning and artificial intelligence technologies can potentially transform the interpretation of data via auto-automization of image analysis with less human error, making the clinical utility of hybrid imaging techniques higher in diverse medical settings (Carsrud et al., 2024). Patient-specific dosimetry and individualized treatment planning are other directions that future innovations using hybrid imaging can follow. Both PET/MRI and PET/CT have the ability to inform clinicians about the metabolic makeup of tumors and adjacent tissues, enabling individualized therapeutic strategies. Advances in radiomics, such as high-dimensional data extraction from medical images, will enable the enhancement of predictive modeling and patient stratification capabilities. In addition, the integration of hybrid imaging technologies into multimodal workflows has the potential to streamline diagnosis in cases with more than one pathology. This approach would ultimately lead to enhanced disease control, particularly in cardiology and neurology, whose timeliness of diagnosis and management is critical. The emphasis on personalized medicine underscores the need for sustained collaboration between imaging technologists, oncologists, and data analysts in optimizing the use of hybrid imaging modalities (Mishra, 2024). Finally, the correction of current hybrid imaging modalities' limitations will be the key to determining their future effectiveness. Challenges such as higher costs, access barriers, and safety concerns about radiation exposure must be addressed comprehensively. Studies aimed at enhancing spatial resolution and reducing radiation dose through improved imaging protocols will make PET/CT and PET/MRI safer and more effective. Furthermore, education and training programs for healthcare professionals on the evolution of these hybrid imaging systems will be crucial to their utilization in clinical settings. As hybrid imaging evolves, innovation, research collaboration, and education will guide the continued development of these technologies to deliver better patient outcomes and spur innovation in medical imaging (Carsrud et al., 2024).

CLOSER LOOK

IMPACT OF HYBRID IMAGING IN MEDICINE

With the evolution of medical imaging, the integration of hybrid imaging modalities such as PET/CT and PET/MRI is proving revolutionary for clinical practice. The modalities improve the visualization of both anatomical and functional tissue features, ultimately enhancing diagnostic accuracy and therapy planning. The synergy between anatomical imaging by CT or MRI and functional imaging by PET, due to their complementary strengths, improves the detection of malignancy, enabling earlier intervention and tailored treatment strategies. In addition, their ability to provide real-time data regarding disease processes makes these systems particularly valuable in oncological settings. The enhanced sensitivity and specificity of hybrid imaging have been recognized not just in the detection of cancer but also for the evaluation of treatment response and potential recurrences of disease, thus cementing their important role in modern medicine. In spite of the immense advantages offered by hybrid imaging, certain limitations still prevail that need to be addressed to fully harness its potential. These are concerns regarding radiation exposure with CT scans and limitations in image resolution and quality using several radiotracers. For instance, PET performance with isotopes such as Ga-68 and Y-90 has proved inconsistent relative to F-18, the most commonly used in clinical practice, and has affected spatial resolution and noise-equivalent count rate (NECR) measurements. Success in addressing these challenges is crucial to the creation of a safe environment for patients and to the successful integration of these new imaging modalities into mainstream clinical practice. Continued innovation in detector systems and image reconstruction algorithms will likely alleviate many of these issues and enhance hybrid system performance, leading to greater patient outcomes and satisfaction. In a word, the impact of hybrid imaging, through the utilization of PET/CT and PET/MRI, is a paradigm change in medical imaging and patient management. The ability to obtain anatomical and functional information simultaneously has revolutionized how physicians approach disease detection, treatment planning, and monitoring. Even though there are problems that accompany the use of diverse radiopharmaceuticals and the need for an optimal imaging protocol, progress in this instance still enables effective overcoming of these problems. Ultimately, as hybrid imaging systems become more widespread in the clinical environment, they will not only make diagnoses more accurate but also, overall, more effective and efficient for patient treatment, an important advance in the ever-more complicated world of medical imaging.

REFERENCES

1. Abdullah Dhafer, M., Alshehri, M., Balous, T. G., Refaei, M. Y., Hussein, H., Hakami, H., Hamzi, A. S., et al. (2024). Hybrid imaging technologies: The intersection of PET, CT, and MRI. *Power System Technology*. https://www.semanticscholar.org/paper/43946bee15cb3067a90ff9a65d16add1c4c8c7e5 (accessed on 5th August 2025).
2. David-Olawade, A. C., Olawade, D. B., Vanderbloemen, L., Rotifa, O. B., Fidelis, S. C., Egbon, E., Akpan, A. O., Adeleke, S., Ghose, A., & Boussios, S. (2025). AI-Driven Advances in Low-Dose Imaging and Enhancement—A Review. *Diagnostics, 15*(6), 689. https://doi.org/10.3390/diagnostics15060689Ahmad Saad, F. N., Fikri, F. F., Cheah, Y. K., Nordin, A. J., et al. (2015). Applications of 18(F) FDG PET/CT in oncology. https://core.ac.uk/download/153820314.pdf (accessed on 5th August 2025).
3. Ahmed, M. (2019). *Development of Probes for Molecular Imaging: Evaluation in Models of Inflammation and Atherosclerosis*. https://core.ac.uk/download/187429875.pdf (accessed on 5th August 2025).
4. Alanazi, M. M. (2024). Advancements in hybrid imaging techniques: Enhancing diagnostic accuracy with PET/MRI and PET/CT. *International Journal of Health Sciences*. https://www.semanticscholar.org/paper/ffc3d785df2be2dd52071419fd61b25aba276f60 (accessed on 5th August 2025).
5. Aldahery, S. (2023). The impact of PET/MRI fusion on the diagnostic imaging industry. https://core.ac.uk/download/581830877.pdf (accessed on 5th August 2025).
6. Ascione, R., Cuocolo, A., Cuocolo, R., Imbriaco, M., et al. (2021). Cardiac hybrid imaging: Novel tracers for novel targets. https://core.ac.uk/download/541678960.pdf (accessed on 5th August 2025).
7. Auguste, P., Barton, P., Borowiack, E., Davenport, C., et al. (2013). Evaluating PET-CT in the detection and management of recurrent cervical cancer: Systematic reviews of diagnostic accuracy and subjective elicitation. https://core.ac.uk/download/29140077.pdf (accessed on 5th August 2025).
8. Augustynowicz, K., Morawski, P., Ostaszewska, S., Pactwa, K., et al. (2023). Advancements in radiology and diagnostic imaging. https://core.ac.uk/download/587246519.pdf (accessed on 5th August 2025).
9. Belderbos, S., Cawthorne, C., Cleeren, F., Correcher, C., et al. (2020). Characterization of a preclinical PET insert in a 7 tesla MRI scanner: Beyond NEMA testing. https://riunet.upv.es/bitstream/10251/166819/3/Gsell%3bMolnos%3bCorrecher%20-%20Characterzaton%20of%20a%20preclncal%20PETnsertn%20a%207%20tesla%20MRI%20scanner%3a%20beyond%20NE....pdf (accessed on 5th August 2025).
10. Bose, R. J. C., & Mattrey, R. F. (2019). Accomplishments and challenges in stem cell imaging *in vivo*. https://core.ac.uk/download/287623865.pdf (accessed on 5th August 2025).
11. Boss, M., Eriksson, O., Mikkola, K., Eek, A., Brom, M., Buitinga, M., Brouwers, A. H., et al. (2024). Improved localization of insulinomas using 68Ga-NODAGA-Exendin-4 PET/CT. *Journal of Nuclear Medicine, 65*, 1959–1964. https://www.semanticscholar.org/paper/e94fa5c97c6d660f5f5a98769b8836048cce2ee0 (accessed on 5th August 2025).

12. Brinkbäumer, K., Dresel, S., Hahn, K., Höpfner, M., et al. (2004). Preoperative imaging of Charcot neuroarthropathy in diabetic patients: Comparison of ring PET, hybrid PET, and magnetic resonance imaging. https://core.ac.uk/download/12175339.pdf (accessed on 5th August 2025).

13. Carsrud, N. D. V., Flores, J. V., Holets, H. M., Kadivi, A., et al. (2024). Transformative precision: Investigative summary of PET/CT-guided radiation therapy simulation in comprehensive cancer management. https://core.ac.uk/download/603903713.pdf (accessed on 5th August 2025).

14. Chan, D. Y. S., Chong, T. T., Gan, J., Hausenloy, D., et al. (2023). Multi-modality imaging of atheromatous plaques in peripheral arterial disease: Integrating molecular and imaging markers. https://core.ac.uk/download/573841607.pdf (accessed on 5th August 2025).

15. Costin, I., & Marcu, L. (2024). Affinity of PET-MRI tracers for hypoxic cells in breast cancer: A systematic review. *Cells, 13*. https://www.semanticscholar.org/paper/b5e8aa11b13f48e1636de3b02321f0a312c56109 (accessed on 5th August 2025).

16. Czepczyński, R., Guzikowska-Ruszkowska, I., Ruchała, M., Sałyga, M., et al. (2016). PET/MR–A rapidly growing technique of imaging in oncology and neurology. https://core.ac.uk/download/268441052.pdf (accessed on 5th August 2025).

17. D'Asseler, Y., De Vasconcelos Caribé, P. R. R., Deller, T. W., Koole, M., et al. (2019). NEMA NU 2–2007 performance characteristics of GE Signa integrated PET/MR for different PET isotopes. https://core.ac.uk/download/222452323.pdf (accessed on 5th August 2025).

18. Dalmaz, O., Yurt, M., & Çukur, T. (2022). ResViT: Residual vision transformers for multimodal medical image synthesis. *IEEE Transactions on Medical Imaging, 41*, 2598–2614. https://doi.org/10.1109/tmi.2022.3167808 (accessed on 5th August 2025).

19. David-Olawade, A. C., Olawade, D., Vanderbloemen, L., Rotifa, O. B., Fidelis, S. C., Egbon, E., Akpan, A. O., et al. (2025). AI-driven advances in low-dose imaging and enhancement—A review. *Diagnostics, 15*. https://www.semanticscholar.org/paper/44051b152f1c9fdf0599bfc6f3bf4a45b07ac104 (accessed on 5th August 2025).

20. Dhami, S. (2008). Strategic analysis of the commercialization potential of a novel algorithm. https://core.ac.uk/download/638896345.pdf (accessed on 5th August 2025).

21. Gullberg, G. T., Liu, J., Ordovas, K., Segars, W., et al. (2019). Multiresolution spatiotemporal mechanical model of the heart as a prior to constrain the solution for 4D models of the heart. https://core.ac.uk/download/287622092.pdf (accessed on 5th August 2025).

22. Hogg, P., Szczepura, K., Thompson, J. D., Vinjamuri, S., et al. (2017). A JAFROC study of nodule detection performance in CT images of a thorax acquired during PET/CT. https://core.ac.uk/download/80694820.pdf (accessed on 5th August 2025).

23. Hubalewska-Dydejczyk, A., Opalińska, M., Sowa-Staszczak, A., Stefańska, A., et al. (2016). NEN–The role of somatostatin receptor scintigraphy in clinical setting. https://core.ac.uk/download/268441054.pdf (accessed on 5th August 2025).

24. Hvittfeldt, E., Hedeer, F., Thimansson, E., Sandeman, K., Minarik, D., Ingvar, J., Bjartell, A., et al. (2025). Semi-standardized evaluation of extraprostatic extension and seminal vesicle invasion with [18F]PSMA-1007 PET/CT: A comparison to MRI using histopathology as reference. *EJNMMI Reports, 9*. https://www.semanticscholar.org/paper/a2fe55d584397a968993594c38a966655ffd8344 (accessed on 5th August 2025).

25. Inglese, M. (2019). *Advanced Perfusion Quantification Methods for Dynamic PET and MRI Data Modelling.* https://core.ac.uk/download/188833355.pdf (accessed on 5th August 2025).
26. Joseph, W., Martens, L., Poole, M., Samoudi, A., et al. (2015). Analysis of eddy currents induced by transverse and longitudinal gradient coils in different tungsten collimator geometries for SPECT/MRI integration. https://core.ac.uk/download/55806647.pdf (accessed on 5th August 2025).
27. Joseph, W., Martens, L., Samoudi, M., Van Audenhaege, K., et al. (2015). Simulated design strategies for SPECT collimators to reduce the eddy currents induced by MRI gradient fields. https://core.ac.uk/download/55710178.pdf (accessed on 5th August 2025).
28. Kjær, A., & Ripa, R. S. (2015). *Imaging Atherosclerosis with Hybrid Positron Emission Tomography/ Magnetic Resonance Imaging.* https://core.ac.uk/download/269254845.pdf (accessed on 5th August 2025).
29. Lundervold, A. S., & Lundervold, A. (2018). An overview of deep learning in medical imaging focusing on MRI. *Zeitschrift für Medizinische Physik, 29*, 102–127. https://doi.org/10.1016/j.zemedi.2018.11.002 (accessed on 5th August 2025).
30. Mishra, A. (2024). PET/CT scan: Bridging metabolic and anatomical imaging. https://core.ac.uk/download/622189017.pdf (accessed on 5th August 2025).
31. Najjar, R. (2023). Redefining radiology: A review of artificial intelligence integration in medical imaging. *Diagnostics, 13*, 2760–2760. https://doi.org/10.3390/diagnostics13172760 (accessed on 5th August 2025).
32. Prasad, V., Koumarianou, A., Denecke, T., Sundin, A., Deroose, C. M., Pavel, M., Christ, E., et al. (2024). Challenges in developing response evaluation criteria for peptide receptor radionuclide therapy: A consensus report from the European Neuroendocrine Tumor Society Advisory Board Meeting 2022 and the ENETS Theranostics Task Force. *Journal of Neuroendocrinology, 37.* https://www.semanticscholar.org/paper/cf16a74f13ab51a0df741570338bd1116eda2778 (accessed on 5th August 2025).
33. Signore, A., Glaudemans, A. W. J. M., Galli, F., & Rouzet, F. (2015). Imaging infection and inflammation. https://core.ac.uk/download/54518572.pdf (accessed on 5th August 2025).
34. Signore, A., Glaudemans, A., Gheysens, O., Lauri, C., & Catalano, O. (2017). Nuclear medicine imaging in pediatric infection or chronic inflammatory diseases. *Seminars in Nuclear Medicine, 47*(3), 286–303. https://www.semanticscholar.org/paper/ab0bb5d336c7f10a80f712b357af4d274cab4f4e (accessed on 5th August 2025).
35. Syahputra, M. T., Rahman, Y., Rahman, R., & Zahra, R. (2025). Role of radiology in diagnostic metastatic disease: A comprehensive systematic review. *Journal of Advanced Research in Medical and Health Science* (ISSN 2208–2425). https://www.semanticscholar.org/paper/33f0cf052555ea7939dc1820a894b7dd35f4fd73 (accessed on 5th August 2025).
36. Tjoa, E., & Guan, C. (2020). A survey on explainable artificial intelligence (XAI): Toward medical XAI. *IEEE Transactions on Neural Networks and Learning Systems, 32*, 4793–4813. https://doi.org/10.1109/tnnls.2020.3027314 (accessed on 5th August 2025).
37. Yuan, Z., & Sar, M. (2014). Molecular imaging in clinical investigation of central nervous system. https://www.semanticscholar.org/paper/ea03b45d373114e7f38c9d5d50f192ac431567a2 (accessed on 5th August 2025).

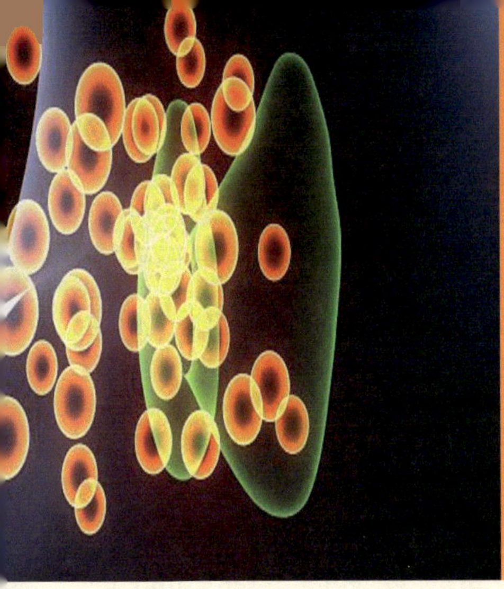

Chapter 4

MOLECULAR AND CELLULAR IMAGING MODALITIES

Contents

Introduction

The field of molecular and cellular imaging modalities is a breakthrough in biomedical research and clinical practice. It is an innovative approach that uses various imaging modalities to visualize biological processes at the cellular and molecular levels, providing essential information for understanding disease mechanisms, treatment response, and therapeutic advances. Through the application of modalities such as fluorescence imaging, magnetic resonance imaging (MRI), and positron emission tomography (PET), researchers can visualize living biological processes without causing harm. Merging modalities enhances resolution and specificity of imaging, so cellular structures and functions may be defined in detail. Therefore, advances in imaging technologies are making it possible for the emergence of a new age of precision medicine, in which medical therapies can be tailored to individual cellular responses. Advances in computational technology have significantly enhanced the capabilities of molecular and cellular imaging in recent years. Advances in image analysis algorithms and machine learning methods facilitate high-throughput handling of large-scale imaging data, leading to improved detection of disease and diagnostic accuracy. For example, the application of computer-aided diagnosis (CAD) algorithms is changing the role of the pathologist by bringing more insights to the diagnostic process. The technology has become increasingly significant with the advent of digitized tissue histopathology because it facilitates whole slide image analysis, which can be stored digitally. As outlined in earlier studies, CAD approaches have seen major improvements in application domains, particularly in disease diagnosis and prognosis, and in the context of creating histopathological complications in Europe and the United States (Boucheron et al., 2009). Further, the interdisciplinary nature of molecular and cellular imaging draws on a range of scientific disciplines, including biology, medicine, engineering, and computational sciences. This synergy is the foundation for the continuing development of imaging modalities, new methods, and technologies that have the potential to increase our understanding of complex biological systems significantly. Possible applications are widespread, ranging from the detection of early cancer to the assessment of treatment efficacy and cellular reaction to therapies. Due to the revolutionary potential of these technologies, integration of new imaging modalities is essential to the progress of personalized medicine. It is crucial that, as the science progresses, scientists are equipped with the latest state-of-the-art equipment and methods that increase imaging ability and diagnostic precision, thus laying the stage for future health care breakthroughs (N/A, 2006).

4.1. Principles of Molecular Imaging

The basic principles of molecular imaging are critical to advancing knowledge and treatment of many diseases. Molecular imaging is a range of techniques that enable scientists and clinicians to visualize, characterize, and quantify molecular and cellular processes in the intact organism. With the aid of specific imaging agents that interact with distinct molecular targets, it is now feasible to track biological processes such as gene expression and cell signaling non-invasively. This skill not only enhances diagnosis but also allows tracking of treatment efficacy over time, especially in illnesses with multiple variables, such as rheumatoid arthritis (Figure 4.1).

The creation and optimization of molecular imaging agents are important because they must be highly specific and exhibit favorable pharmacokinetics to yield accurate results in live animals. These developments have the potential to advance patient care through the ability to give real-time information regarding pathophysiological alterations and treatment effects in a clinical environment (Funk et al., 2017). One key aspect of molecular imaging is the development of imaging agents that enhance the diagnostic capabilities of imaging devices. Over the last few years, researchers have been working to overcome the limitations of conventional imaging agents with low specificity and binding affinity. The employment of multivalent ligands offers a promising solution, in which a set of ligand copies is used to increase binding interactions with target molecules. This approach has been reported to significantly improve the efficacy of imaging agents by enhancing their affinity for targets, thus enabling improved imaging and localization of disease processes. It is also vital to recognize the challenges inherent to the design of efficient imaging agents, as greater insight into such principles largely impacts the development of highly effective imaging modalities that can meet the many-sided needs of modern medicine (Bohmer et al., 2021). Furthermore, the influence of molecular imaging on the practice of clinical medicine is of particular importance, particularly on early diagnosis and individualized medicine. By creating information about the biological substrates of illness, molecular imaging has the potential to guide optimal treatment strategies based on an individual's molecular profile. This is most relevant to oncology, in which imaging of metastases and tumor microenvironments can direct therapy. Furthermore, the ability to monitor changes in molecular targets over time enables dynamic adjustment of the regimen based on an individual's response. Consequently, the principles of molecular imaging not only enhance understanding of disease mechanisms but also form a basis for advancing targeted therapy and patient care more broadly. Through the combination of various imaging methods with robust molecular markers, the horizon of molecular imaging continues to expand, presenting avenues for future disease management (Funk et al., 2017).

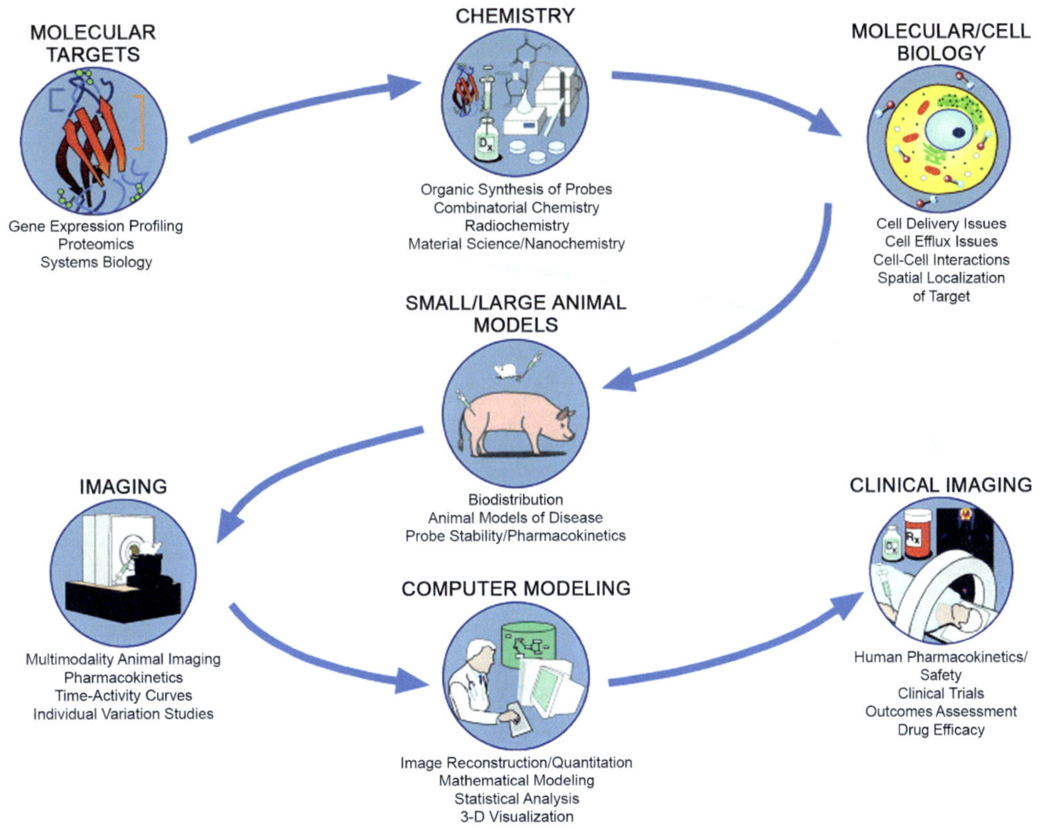

Figure 4.1. General principles of molecular imaging.

Source: https://ars.els-cdn.com/content/image/3-s2.0-B9780128163863000028-f01-01-9780128163863.jpg.

4.1.1. Basic Concepts of Molecular Imaging

Molecular imaging is an emerging technology in biomedical research that provides information at the cellular and molecular levels not attainable with conventional imaging modalities. It combines different imaging modalities to represent biological processes in real time, permitting researchers to study disease processes, monitor therapy response, and develop targeted therapies. Molecular imaging uses binding agents specific to biomolecules such as receptors or enzymes to detect and describe tissue based on biochemical and molecular content rather than anatomical structure (Figure 4.2).

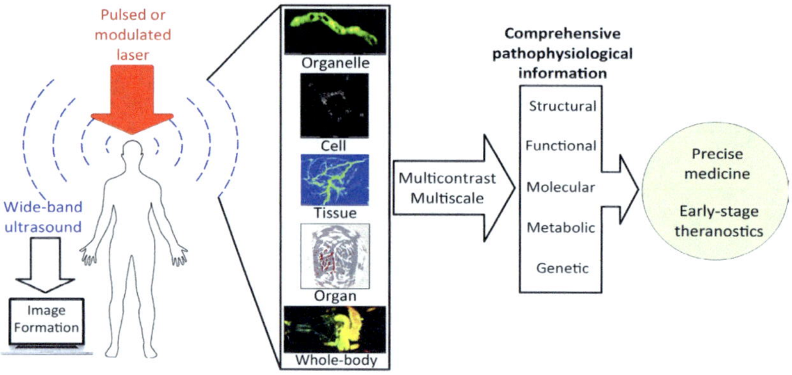

Figure 4.2. Photoacoustic molecular imaging.

Source: https://www.cell.com/cms/10.1016/j.tibtech.2016.02.001/asset/665a3262-65b5-46f9-a4cb-a455b8b12196/main.assets/gr1_lrg.jpg.

This shift in focus allows for a more nuanced understanding of disease progression and the effectiveness of treatments (Figure 4.3).

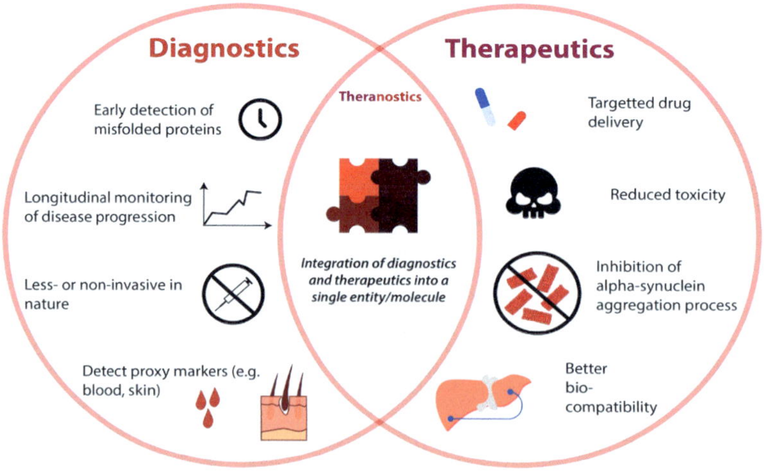

Figure 4.3. Venn diagram depicting attributes of diagnostics and therapeutics for the detection and reduction of alpha-synuclein aggregates. A union of diagnostic and therapeutic capabilities has given rise to the booming field of "theranostics," whose properties are also illustrated.

Source: https://www.researchgate.net/publication/354029906/figure/fig3/AS:1058868532637696@1629465339052/Venn-diagram-depicting-attributes-of-diagnostics-and-therapeutics-for-detection-and.png.

Thus, molecular imaging stands at the threshold of diagnostics and therapeutics, with future personalized medicine strategies which have the potential to significantly improve patient outcomes. Among the cutting-edge technologies of molecular imaging, PET and MRI are two modalities that have seen spectacular progress in the last few years. The creation of hybrid imaging systems that combine PET and MRI, an imaging scheme in which both modalities can be collected simultaneously, illustrates progress in expanding imaging capacity. Although PET yields essential information on metabolism, MRI is superior for anatomical information. Such a combination provides a more complete description of the biological activity taking place in the body. But combining the two technologies is not easy; most importantly, to obtain artifact-free images requires meticulous calibration and inventive engineering solutions. With ongoing research, these hybrid modalities will also be central to clinical applications, offering novel platforms for disease diagnosis and treatment monitoring, particularly in cancer. Uses of molecular imaging are not restricted to cancer diagnostics and research but also include cardiovascular diseases, neurodegenerative diseases, and inflammatory conditions. Visualization of distinct molecular targets in vivo enables a better understanding of pathophysiological mechanisms. For example, in cardiovascular disease, molecular imaging can reveal plaques or inflammation, which are critical for cardiovascular risk stratification. In addition, the development of imaging agents, such as those designed for PET/MRI platforms, is enhancing the sensitivity and specificity of these imaging tests. With the development of the science of molecular imaging, there is the promise further to increase understanding of cellular behavior and disease development, leading eventually to more effective therapeutic interventions and improved patient care. The present work discussed imaging agent optimization and technological improvements in imaging modalities as an essential milestone in the quest for precision medicine, making molecular imaging an indispensable element of modern healthcare (Brinkley et al., 2002; Cherry et al., 2008).

4.1.2. Contrast Agents and Their Role

Contrast agents play a vital role in molecular and cellular imaging modalities for delineating internal anatomy and processes within the body. The agents, which are administered into the body through different routes, optimize imaging modalities like MRI, CT, and PET. Contrast agents improve the definition of anatomical structures and pathological changes by altering the imaging characteristics of tissue. For instance, gadolinium contrast agents employed in MRI enhance signal differences between pathologic and normal tissues to facilitate better diagnosis of diseases such as tumors and inflammation. Importantly, the successful application of contrast agents can lead to better assessment of disease progression and response to therapy, with a subsequent effect on patient management and outcome (Figure 4.4).

The inclusion of contrast agents in emerging imaging modalities is central to advancing molecular and cellular imaging. Researchers continue to develop new imaging agents that not only show more but also provide specific biological information pertinent to disease. As an illustration, targeted contrast agents could be designed to bind to specific receptors on cancer cells, enabling precise definition of tumor margins. This is particularly pertinent for examples such as stem cell therapy (SCT), where imaging must track the position and viability of implanted cells post-implantation. As cited in more recent studies, imaging is a crucial tool throughout SCT, both for monitoring cell delivery and assessing treatment effectiveness over the long term (Jokerst et al., 2016). These advances underscore the role of contrast agents in optimizing the functional potential of imaging modalities. Furthermore, the integration of newer imaging modalities, such as PET and MRI, presents unique opportunities to develop integrated imaging systems that utilize contrast agents to their full potential. The integration of these technologies enables simultaneous acquisition of anatomical and functional data, leading to a deeper understanding of disease processes. In this context, advanced contrast agents can improve the quality of real-time imaging, alleviating imaging artifacts caused by the inherent complexity of hybrid systems. Recent literature suggests that advances in PET/MRI technology have spurred studies of new contrast agents intended for use with combined modalities (Cherry et al., 2008). These developments not only enhance imaging performance but also enable a range of biomedical applications, maintaining the primacy of contrast agents in molecular and cellular imaging modality development.

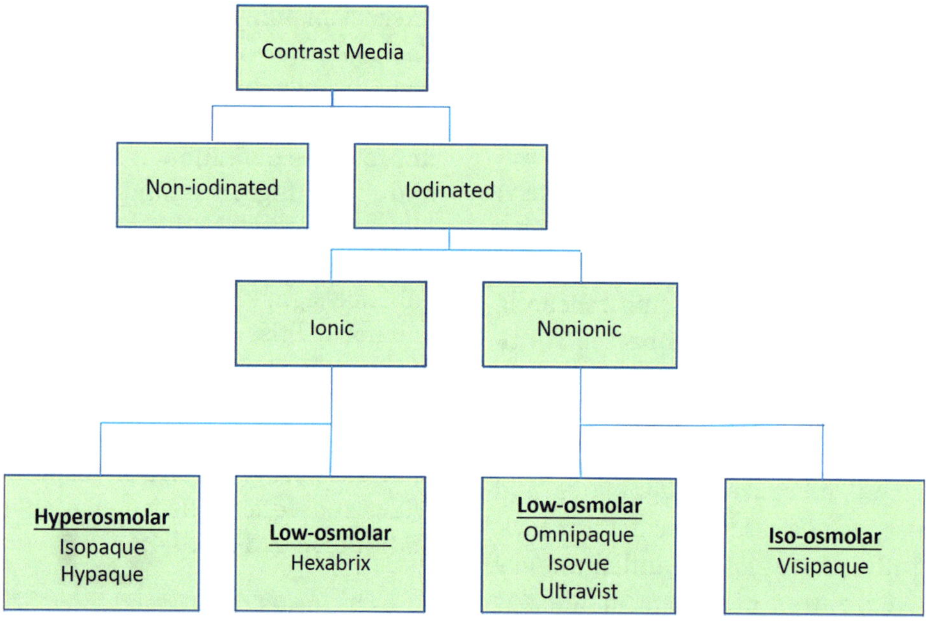

Figure 4.4. Types of contrast media.

Source: https://www.researchgate.net/profile/Richard-Josephson-2/publication/324235534/figure/fig1/AS:658535536930816@1534018515445/FigureTypesof-contrast-media.png.

4.1.3. Imaging Resolution and Sensitivity

The relationship between imaging sensitivity and resolution underpins further innovation in molecular and cellular imaging modalities. Imaging resolution measures the ability to resolve closely spaced objects, which is valuable for accurate anatomical and functional measurements. Increased resolution allows finer localization of cellular structures, enabling detection of even subtle pathological changes. Conversely, sensitivity is the ability of an imaging system to detect low concentrations of signals emitted by molecular probes or tracers. This duality becomes very important when the diagnostic potential of imaging modalities is contemplated; an optimum balance between resolution and sensitivity enhances the overall efficiency of imaging modalities in clinical as well as research applications. In recent years, innovations in hybrid imaging technologies have emerged, promising to significantly improve both metrics and to facilitate advanced visualization of cellular events beyond traditional imaging frameworks (Figure 4.5).

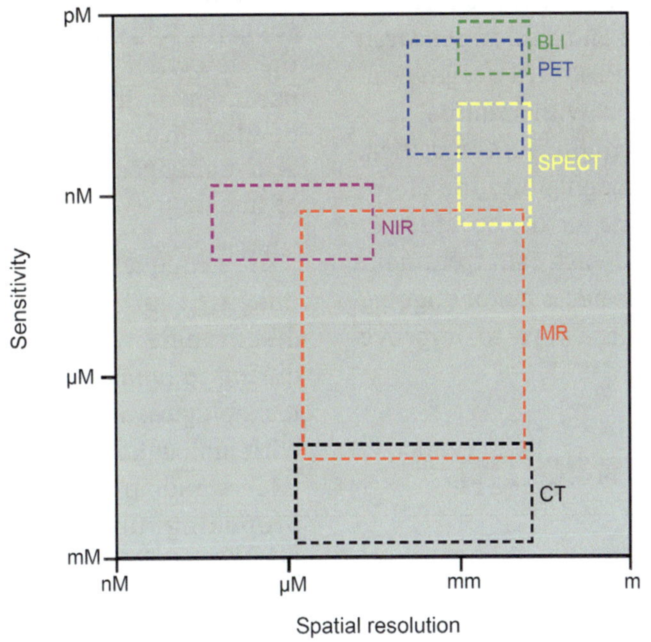

Figure 4.5. Sensitivity and spatial resolution ranges of the different imaging modalities (figure adapted from Cassidy et al. (Cassidy and Radda, 2005). Efforts by various groups are focused on extending the current sensitivity and spatial limits of each modality.

Source: https://www.researchgate.net/profile/Jinzi-Zheng/publication/225828094/figure/fig1/AS:302658138198023@1449170731725/Sensitivity-and-spatial-resolution-ranges-of-the-different-imaging-modalities-figure.png.

The fusion of PET and MRI is one of the most significant improvements in imaging resolution and sensitivity. MRI is optimally suited to provide high-resolution, high-contrast images of soft tissue, which is crucial for accurate anatomical studies. PET, conversely, is sensitive and can image biologically targeted radiotracers, but has historically been limited by reduced spatial resolution (Catana et al., 2008). The combined functionality of both modalities enables temporally correlated data acquisition, allowing PET radiotracer distributions to be properly co-registered with the anatomic context provided by MRI. Current technical developments in PET/MRI technology aim to overcome the traditional disadvantages of both modalities and to develop a consolidated framework for the characterization of metabolic processes alongside structural imaging. With this cooperation, the hybrid modality improves prognostic and diagnostic potential in neurology and oncology. There are remaining issues in achieving high imaging sensitivity and resolution, including the challenge posed by hybrid PET/MRI systems. While new systems have promise, problems of image artifacts during simultaneous data acquisition are highly pertinent (Cherry et al., 2008). Artifacts can result from hardware interactions, protocol mismatches, or heterogeneity in the sensitivity profiles of imaging modalities. Moreover, it is more difficult to achieve a high signal-to-noise ratio when combining different imaging paradigms. Yet, preclinical and clinical research have proven that modern PET/MRI designs can maintain spatial resolution with minimal loss of imaging quality. This equilibrium is critical to translating advanced imaging into the clinic, as it has direct implications for the accuracy of diagnostic findings and downstream treatment planning, underscoring the necessity of ongoing innovations in imaging hardware to improve resolution and sensitivity.

4.2. Optical Imaging Techniques

Methods of optical imaging have evolved into key tools within the platform of molecular and cellular imaging, offering unique advantages in their high resolution and ability to interrogate biological processes at the cellular level. Traditional modalities such as fluorescence and bioluminescence have been extensively employed, but the paradigm is shifting toward the use of a variety of new techniques. Techniques such as optical coherence tomography (OCT) and reflectance confocal microscopy are gaining momentum for their ability to image biological structures in real time without requiring extensive sample preparation. These imaging techniques leverage the properties of light to interrogate both morphological and functional aspects of cells, hence illuminating complex biological processes more vividly. With continued advances in research, new nonbioluminescent and nonfluorescent molecular probes have the potential to further broaden the scope of optical imaging applications, with improved detection and diagnostic capabilities (Boppart et al., 2005). The development of coherent optical modalities for imaging is a significant milestone toward imaging molecular interactions within living systems. Instead of using fluorescence only to be exploited, more recent advances focus on controlling local optical properties through sophisticated probe design, thereby enabling the detection of endogenous molecules. This paradigm shift permits not only a wider range of biological questions to be addressed but also enhances the sensitivity and specificity of imaging.

Techniques such as nonlinear interferometric imaging, for instance, allow scientists to disentangle complex dynamics occurring during cellular events. The integration of these technological advancements in coherent imaging with molecular probes will most likely advance understanding of disease mechanisms, eventually propelling therapeutic approaches toward personalized medicine. With their development over time, they can make new frontiers in the investigation of cellular phenomena (Boppart et al., 2005). In regenerative medicine, particularly in stem cell therapy (SCT), optical imaging technologies play a pivotal role throughout the entire therapeutic course. Imaging aids precise cell tracking from harvesting to purification and implantation protocols, such that health care practitioners can monitor cell function and cell distribution following therapy. Research on hand pinpoints the significance of imaging in quantifying therapeutic success and in establishing parameters that predict regenerative success. By facilitating real-time visualization of cell behavior and interactions in host tissues, optical imaging not only aids the evaluation of SCT efficacy but also informs the optimization of therapeutic approaches. The promise of SCT grows with each passing day, and as imaging technology continues to advance, it is well placed to make significant contributions to the field and spur further innovation and improved patient outcomes.

4.2.1. Fluorescence Imaging

Fluorescence imaging has emerged as a key modality within the umbrella of cellular and molecular imaging and offers immense strength for imaging biological functions at the molecular level. The fluorescence principle, wherein a chemical absorbs light at one wavelength and emits light at a longer wavelength, has been utilized in this imaging technique to perform specific imaging of proteins, cells, or tissue. Its ability to provide high spatial resolution and contrast makes it very useful in fields such as neuroscience and oncology (Figure 4.6).

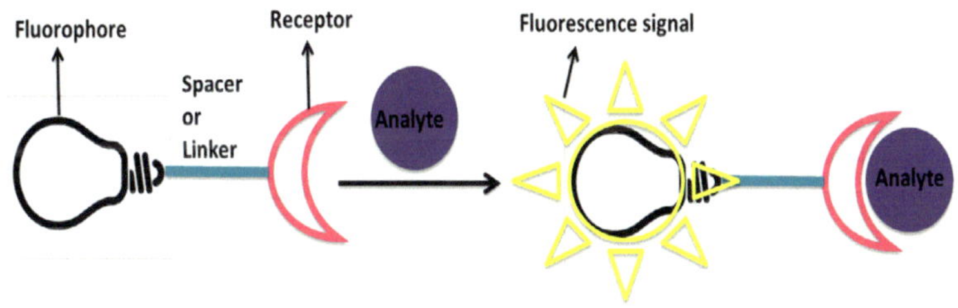

Figure 4.6. The use of fluorescent probes has significantly advanced our understanding of cellular mechanisms and interactions, thereby illuminating dynamic processes such as protein aggregation, cell signaling, and metabolic activities.

Source: https://www.researchgate.net/profile/Wafa-Mazi/publication/335756650/figure/fig2/AS:802219507085312@1568275443657/A-schematic-illustration-of-a-typical-fluorescent-probe.png.

Such skills not only facilitate basic research but also have potential clinical applications, including tracking disease course and measuring therapeutic response. New advances in fluorescence imaging technologies have further broadened their utility and potency, particularly in neuroscience. Conventional microscopy techniques are generally poor at capturing the elaborate network of neuronal activity, particularly when examining large populations across several brain regions. In these aspects, highly sensitive new optical calcium imaging technologies have been developed, enabling researchers to image the activity of cohorts of neurons in parallel at suitable temporal and spatial resolutions. These advances would allow researchers to gain a greater appreciation for how neural circuits implement information processing and can be instrumental in elucidating complex neurobiological phenomena. With the need for more advanced imaging modalities, fluorescence techniques are being combined with other imaging modalities to generate hybrid modalities that leverage the relative strengths of each, paving the way for revolutionary discoveries in neuroscience and other fields (Vaziri et al., 2018). The versatility of fluorescence imaging is further demonstrated by its integration with multimodal imaging approaches, which enhance the evaluation of therapeutic response in preclinical models. A great example is the assessment of novel chemotherapy constructs like HerDox, where fluorescence imaging played a crucial role in providing drug distribution and cellular uptake data. This multimodal imaging integrates high-frequency ultrasound and fluorescence and spectral imaging to facilitate an integrated assessment of treatment response beyond the standard outcome of tumor shrinkage. By employing fluorescence imaging to monitor cellular apoptosis in live cells and probe drug localization at the subcellular scale, researchers can obtain crucial information on the efficacy and behavior of therapeutic agents. These complementary methods may improve the efficiency of the drug discovery process, ultimately facilitating the faster translation of effective therapies from the laboratory to the clinic (Chu et al., 2012).

4.2.2. Bioluminescence Imaging (BLI)

BLI represents a cutting-edge modality within the broader context of molecular and cellular imaging (Figure 4.7).

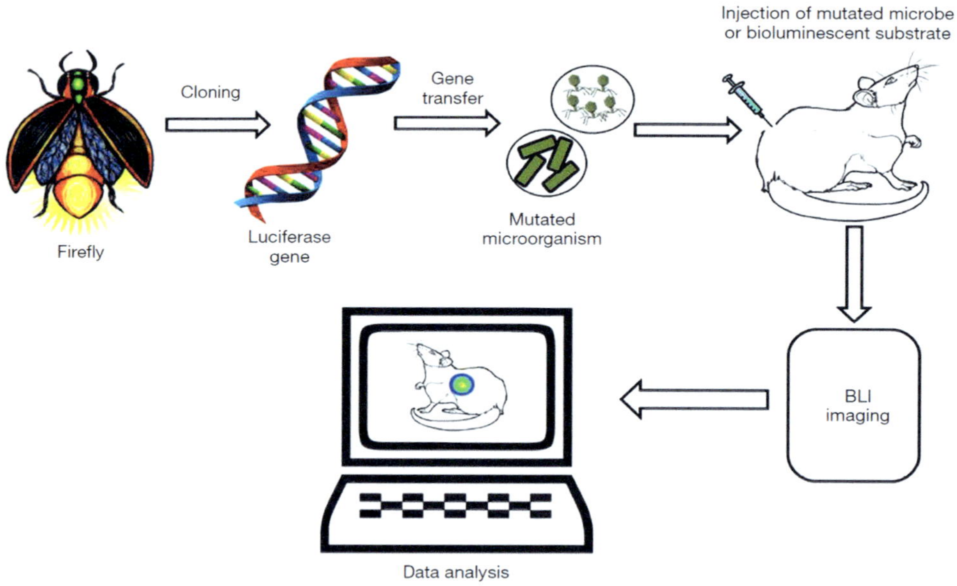

Figure 4.7. Schematic representation of bioluminescent imaging.

Source: https://www.researchgate.net/profile/Pala-Rajasekharreddy/publication/327973539/figure/fig2/AS:679473879977986@1539010605297/Schematic-representation-of-bioluminescent-imaging-BLI-bioluminescence-imaging.png.

By capitalizing on the inherent luminescent property of certain living things, BLI offers a non-invasive way to image and study biological processes in real time. The technique employs luciferase enzymes and their substrates, such as luciferin, to produce light in living organisms. This way, researchers can study cellular processes such as gene expression and cancer growth with excellent sensitivity and specificity. The potential applications of BLI extend into numerous fields, including cancer disease modeling, infectious disease, and stem cell therapy, where monitoring cellular behavior is relevant for therapeutic success and understanding the mechanism of action. The merging of BLI with other imaging technologies enhances its use in the exploration of complex biological systems. For instance, in combination with modalities such as magnetic resonance imaging (MRI) or positron emission tomography (PET), BLI can provide complementary information that complements knowledge of cellular dynamics. BLI is unique in that it can provide functional information and facilitate in vivo imaging of real-time cellular processes. It is particularly significant in regenerative medicine and stem cell therapy, where researchers aim to examine stem cell survival, distribution, and function following transplantation. The integration of BLI with other imaging technologies compensates for the shortcomings in translating preclinical findings to clinical applications, significantly advancing molecular imaging. Evolving technologies in bioluminescence imaging continue to provide new windows in biomedical research and clinical applications. The development of new luciferase variants and substrates has expanded the spectrum of emitted light, resulting in enhanced detection and multiplexing opportunities. Furthermore, BLI permits longitudinal analysis, allowing researchers to study the same animals sequentially over time without the adverse effects of repeated surgery. As evidenced by applications in stem cell therapy, the ability to identify the viability and functionality of implanted cells without an invasion is crucial for the development of therapeutic strategies. Given the limitations of existing imaging methods, BLI presents a promising avenue for real-time imaging of biological processes, as established by Jokerst et al. (2016) and Bose et al. (2019), underscoring its potential to enhance the efficacy and safety of new therapeutic strategies.

4.2.3. Near-Infrared Imaging (NIR)

NIR has emerged as an indispensable tool in the realm of molecular and cellular imaging modalities, making use of the unique properties of infrared light. This imaging mode operates within the wavelength range of approximately 700 to 1000 nanometers, allowing deeper penetration into biological tissues than visible light. The most important advantage of NIR imaging is its ability to produce high-resolution images with minimal background interference, which is critical for imaging molecular interactions and cellular processes deep within tissues. Furthermore, NIR imaging uses fluorescent probes selectively targeted to specific biomarkers, thereby increasing specificity and sensitivity. These attributes make NIR imaging an essential modality for researchers and clinicians who wish to examine disease mechanisms and monitor responses to therapy in the living organism. Near-infrared imaging is not only employed in straightforward research, but it also finds major applications in the clinic, particularly in oncology. NIR approaches enable detection and delineation of tumors by visualizing the augmented vascularization characteristic of malignant tumors (Figure 4.8).

By using targeted NIR fluorescent probes, surgeons can obtain real-time tumor imaging in the operating room, enabling more precise resections and reducing the risk of residual disease. Additionally, integration of NIR imaging with other modalities, such as MRI or CT, can offer integrative biological information, significantly enhancing diagnostic accuracy. This multimodal approach is particularly valuable in preclinical and clinical drug development settings, where practical imaging can inform therapy and monitor therapeutic efficacy, thereby contributing to personalized medicine. Enhanced computational processing and machine learning have also amplified the promise of near-infrared imaging, both in data interpretation and in enhancing diagnostic performance. Recent developments in NIR image automatic evaluation algorithms facilitate high-level pattern detection and quantitative measurement of molecular markers, supporting a more nuanced understanding of disease pathology. These developments run concurrently with those occurring in digital pathology, with computer-aided diagnosis (CAD) systems now being explored as possible adjuncts to human pathology evaluation, as noted in recent reviews of CAD technologies in histopathology (Boucheron et al., 2009). Moreover, by combining NIR imaging with techniques such as fluorescence molecular tomography (FMT), researchers can image fluorescent probes in three dimensions, providing data on biomolecular distributions in tissues (Ripoll et al., 2011). These advances not only supplement NIR imaging capability but also advance its status as a fundamental building block of molecular and cellular imaging modalities.

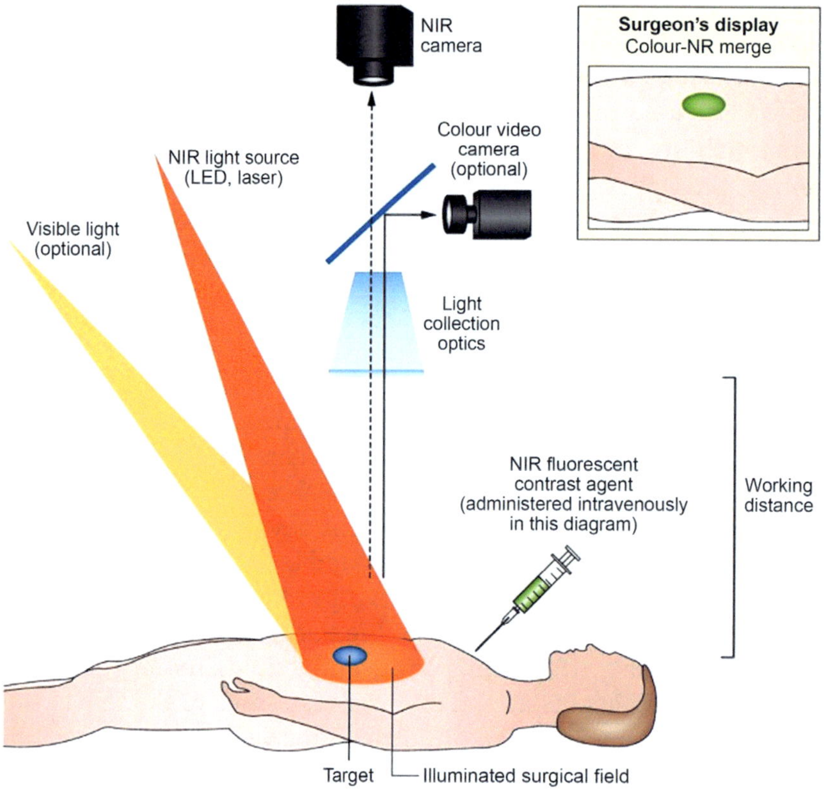

Figure 4.8. Image-guided cancer surgery using near-infrared fluorescence.

Source: https://media.springernature.com/m685/springer-static/image/art%3A10.1038%2Fnrclinonc.2013.123/MediaObjects/41571_2013_Article_BFnrclinonc2013123_Fig1_HTML.jpg.

4.3. Ultrasound Imaging

Ultrasound imaging has become a cornerstone modality in the arsenal of molecular and cellular imaging techniques, offering a non-invasive method for visualizing structures and tissues within the body. High-frequency sound waves are sent and received via transducers in this imaging process, creating real-time images formed by the echoes from various tissue densities. The strengths of ultrasound imaging, in particular, are its availability, cost-effectiveness, and safety, as it is not an ionising radiation system. Further, advances in high-frequency ultrasound technology have improved spatial resolution, enabling scientists and clinicians to detect structural and functional changes at the cellular level. As a result, ultrasound has increasingly been utilized in biomedical research, for example, in stem cell therapy, where monitoring cellular dynamics and response to treatment is crucial (Jokerst et al., 2016). The inclusion of ultrasound imaging in therapeutic assessment is particularly important for cancer treatments. For instance, new studies have confirmed that high-frequency ultrasound can effectively monitor tumor response to therapies using areal evaluations of tumor mass and function. The imaging technique is helpful in longitudinal studies, where the evaluation of the effectiveness of new drug combinations is highly essential. A multimodal approach with ultrasound and fluorescence imaging has also been recommended, where, through modulation assessment, the effectiveness of treatment at the molecular level can be made. For instance, in the case of HerDox chemotherapy construct testing, the spatial dynamics of tumor cell apoptosis along the treatment timeline were unveiled through ultrasound imaging (Chu et al., 2012). Thus, the synergy of ultrasound with other imaging technologies presents an intriguing avenue of boosting the efficacy and precision of anticancer therapy. In addition to its applications in oncology, ultrasound imaging plays a central role in regenerative medicine, particularly in stem cell therapy. Because it is non-invasive, ultrasound facilitates real-time monitoring of cell grafts and the dynamics of their integration into host tissue. Imaging the location and viability of transplanted stem cells enables clinicians to assess treatment success and tailor treatment strategies accordingly. Furthermore, novel applications of ultrasound include its use together with contrast agents that improve the quality and sensitivity of detection in imaging. With advancing technology, the contribution of ultrasound imaging to the development of customized treatment protocols and to improved patient outcomes across numerous therapeutic procedures becomes increasingly evident. By bridging gaps in cell and molecular imaging, ultrasound can potentially provide significant advances in the understanding and management of disease (Jokerst et al., 2016).

4.3.1. Principles of Ultrasound Technology

In the field of molecular and cellular imaging modalities, ultrasound technology offers a unique approach that leverages the behavior of sound waves to generate images of internal structures. By using high-frequency sound waves, ultrasound creates images from wave reflection and scattering as the waves encounter different tissue types. This ability to visualize real-time images makes ultrasound extremely useful relative to other imaging modalities; it is low expense, non-invasive, and offers dynamic assessment capabilities needed to monitor changes in tissues or lesions (Figure 4.9).

The viscoelastic nature of soft tissues played an influential role in ultrasound imaging, as elastic variations could affect the resolution and contrast of the image. Notably, a greater understanding of such mechanical properties further enhances the diagnostic utility of ultrasound, especially when employed clinically to detect pathologies that are difficult to diagnose using standard palpation methods (Bajwa et al., 2018). With improvements in ultrasound technology, innovative methods such as elastography are being devised to exploit tissue mechanical properties increasingly. Elastography enables quantitative measurement of tissue stiffness and provides data on disease processes, as well as discrimination between malignancies and benign disease. This imaging modality supplements routine ultrasound by analyzing changes in viscoelasticity and is therefore a cornerstone in oncology and hepatology. For instance, discrimination between various tissues, such as the gallbladder and liver, can be effectively achieved through the integration of elastographic approaches in ultrasounds. Such advancements implicate added importance to creating a cogent framework under which ultrasound's fundamental principles can lead to improved diagnostic practices based on tissue mechanical contrast (Bajwa et al., 2018). In addition, combining ultrasound with advanced data fusion algorithms can potentially enhance image performance. Data fusion, which integrates data across different imaging systems, integrates heterogeneous datasets into a multimodal description of biological structures. This can be done in ultrasound by combining ultrasound images with molecular markers or other imaging modalities to enhance diagnostics. Current studies indicate that the most prevalent data fusion method is image-to-image fusion, particularly when integrated with machine learning methods. This integration not only increases the precision of imaging results but also reduces uncertainty, thereby enhancing clinical diagnosis and prognostics. As the boundaries of ultrasound technology continue to expand, the principles of ultrasound will be at the epicenter of future molecular and cellular imaging development.

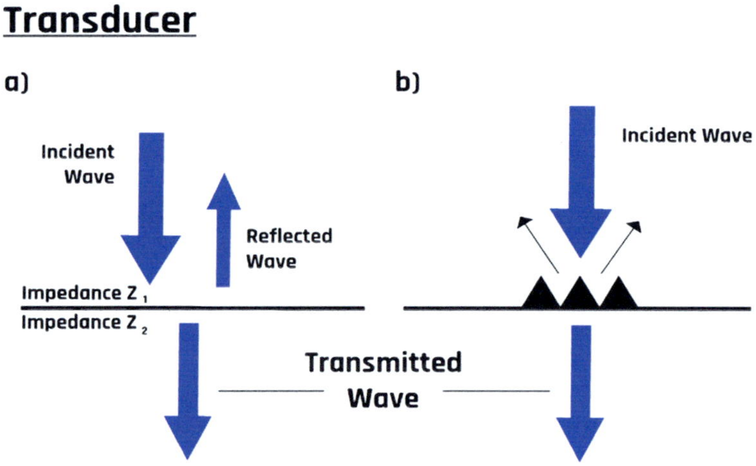

Figure 4.9. Basic principles of ultrasound.

Source: https://pressbooks.palni.org/ultrasoundphysicsanditsapplicationinmedicine/wp-content/uploads/sites/65/2024/02/image1-5.png.

4.3.2. Applications in Molecular Imaging

Molecular imaging has remapped the ability to visualize and understand biological processes at the cellular level, greatly enhancing diagnostic capabilities across a wide variety of medical specialties. A primary use is in the combination of synthetic biology and molecular imaging technologies. With advancements in synthetic biology enabling the engineering of cells to perform novel functions, molecular imaging becomes essential for in vivo tracking of these engineered systems. For instance, the application of reporter gene technologies can allow for noninvasive, real-time imaging of therapeutics. This technology is critical in cancer and neurodegenerative disease, where precise targeting and tracking of treatment effectiveness can realistically determine the course of treatment for a patient (Gilad et al., 2017) (Figure 4.10). The ability to track these engineered cells not only gives information regarding the therapeutic efficacy but also information regarding biological mechanisms. Another significant use of molecular imaging is the rational design of imaging agents (IAs) to augment diagnostic performance. Although there has been remarkable progress in the rational design of IAs, issues such as low binding affinity and specificity often undermine their imaging performance in vivo. Addressing such challenges, researchers have begun exploring the principle of multivalency, in which multiple copies of a ligand are employed to create more stable interactions with the target (Bohmer et al., 2021). The new approach is designed to optimize the diagnostic performance of molecular imaging modalities by tuning the pharmacokinetics and binding affinity of the imaging probes.

As IA design progresses further, multivalent compounds promise to provide progressively finer imaging of disease processes to achieve earlier diagnosis and better treatment planning in various diseases. Application of molecular imaging modalities in personalized medicine is yet another promising horizon. Personalized treatment regimens require an in-depth understanding of a patient's individualized biological milieu, which can be achieved by advanced imaging protocols. For example, molecular imaging can provide information about tumor heterogeneity, allowing clinicians to tailor treatment based on specific molecular signatures of the tumors. By employing modalities such as magnetic resonance imaging and bioluminescence imaging, health professionals can assess the effectiveness of various treatment approaches in real time (Gilad et al., 2017). With the acceleration of personalized medicine, the incorporation of molecular imaging will be crucial in the enhancement of patient management, optimization of therapeutic effectiveness, and ultimately, the enhancement of patient outcomes across various clinical applications.

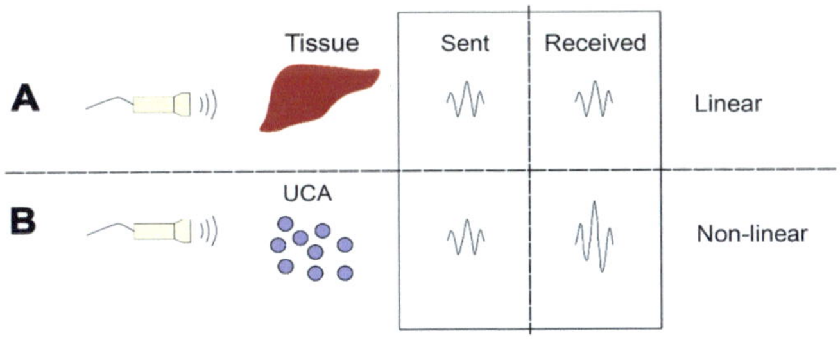

Figure 4.10. Molecular ultrasound imaging.

Source: https://www.mdpi.com/nanomaterials/nanomaterials-10-01935/article_deploy/html/images/nanomaterials-10-01935-g001.png.

4.3.3. Advantages and Limitations of Ultrasound

Ultrasound imaging is extremely highly prevalent medical diagnosis modality, and it has various benefits, particularly for molecular and cellular imaging. One of its fundamental benefits is that the method is non-invasive and thus offers real-time visualization of soft tissues without the use of ionizing radiation. This is particularly beneficial for assessing embryonic development and in vivo tracking of various physiological processes. In addition, ultrasound has high temporal resolution, enabling clinicians to observe dynamic changes in cellular and molecular targets over time (Figure 4.11).

Advantages	Disadvantages
Real-time visualization of vessel	Equipment expense
Improved pre-procedure planning	Equipment availability
Increased success rates	Training of practitioners
Reduced complications	Requirement for skilled practitioners for training
Reduced time spent placing the catheter	

Figure 4.11. Advantages and disadvantages of ultrasound guidance.

Source: https://www.researchgate.net/profile/Andrew-Miller-84/publication/287151411/figure/tbl1/AS:614155128147969@1523437401501/Advantages-and-Disadvantages-of-Ultrasound-Guidance.png.

These capabilities are useful in imaging studies such as stem cell tracking, where the behavior and dissemination of implanted cells must be known to establish therapeutic efficacy and safety (Bose et al., 2019). Furthermore, ultrasound is less costly than other imaging technologies and, therefore, more feasible for regular clinical use, especially in developing nations. However, despite its advantages, ultrasound imaging also has certain drawbacks. One of the most significant limitations is its reliance on acoustic properties, which can be affected by the intervening medium, leading to inconsistent image quality. This is particularly apparent in obese patients or with the presence of excessive bone or gas, which can limit the passage of ultrasound waves and lead to distal attenuation and poor visualization of the internal structures. In addition, while ultrasound provides high spatial resolution, its ability to analyze molecular-level tissue data remains incomplete, even relative to advanced imaging modalities like PET or MRI. This lowers its relevance to high-accuracy molecular imaging applications, i.e., quantifying stem cell viability and function following transplantations, where great detail on cellular dynamics is important for study and therapeutic aims (Jokerst et al., 2016). In general, ultrasound imaging is a valuable part of molecular and cellular imaging modalities with significant advantages of non-invasive assessment and real-time identification. Nevertheless, its limitations in image quality and molecular information pose challenging reflections for researchers and clinicians. The fine line between the urgent benefits and limitations of ultrasound should be achieved, particularly in advanced indications like stem cell therapy. With advances in imaging technology, the integration of ultrasound with other imaging modalities may unlock new ways to overcome its limitations and to better understand cellular dynamics in therapeutic applications (Bose et al., 2019; Jokerst et al., 2016). Through synergistic innovation, the future of molecular imaging, with the potential to deliver improved results, may transform patient treatment and regenerative medicine.

4.4. Clinical Applications of Imaging Modalities

The clinical application of imaging modalities is, in turn, being reoriented to address technological advances in molecular and cellular imaging techniques. The modalities provide invaluable windows into biology, enabling clinicians to make more precise diagnoses of disease. For instance, the coupling of imaging technologies with designed biological systems, in the form most closely associated with synthetic biology, enables monitoring of the therapeutic impact of treatment at the cellular level. It is particularly pertinent now that novel therapies are becoming apparent; for example, treatment with bacteria and immunotherapy can be reviewed continuously with non-invasive imaging methods. The creation of imaging agents tailored for specific cellular functions has precipitated the demand for rigorous preclinical assessment to confirm that such modalities are capable of accurately representing the tissues' in vivo pathological and physiological conditions, thus enhancing patient outcomes through targeted monitoring (Gilad et al., 2017). In addition to established imaging standards, emerging paradigms in molecular imaging have expanded the ability to detect complex diseases. At the core of the discipline is the application of compatible IAs, which are built in order to image particular cellular processes and interactions. Although knowledge of how they should be designed effectively has been enhanced, several challenges remain, particularly regarding their in vivo efficiency and specificity. Many IAs struggle with low binding affinity, which limits their use in clinical situations. But there are already innovations such as multivalency, where multiple copies of a ligand bind to increase efficacy. With advances in pharmacokinetics and target binding of such agents, physicians can significantly increase the diagnostic value of molecular imaging and make it an essential tool in contemporary medicine (Bohmer et al., 2021). The intersection of novel imaging modalities is also critical in enabling individualized medicine. By employing techniques such as PET, MRI, and ultrasound, doctors gain a thorough understanding of tumor characteristics and treatment-induced physiological effects. Furthermore, visualization of intricate interactions at the molecular level assists in predictive biomarker identification for the effects of therapy. With such a tailored strategy, doctors can optimize therapeutic interventions based on patient-specific profiles. With advances in the field, collaboration among imaging scientists, clinicians, and biomedical engineers is also advancing. All of them can contribute to strengthening the clinical applications of imaging modalities, ensuring that innovations translate into better diagnostic and therapeutic devices for numerous diseases across diverse patient populations (Gilad et al., 2017; Bohmer et al., 2021).

4.4.1. Cancer Detection and Monitoring

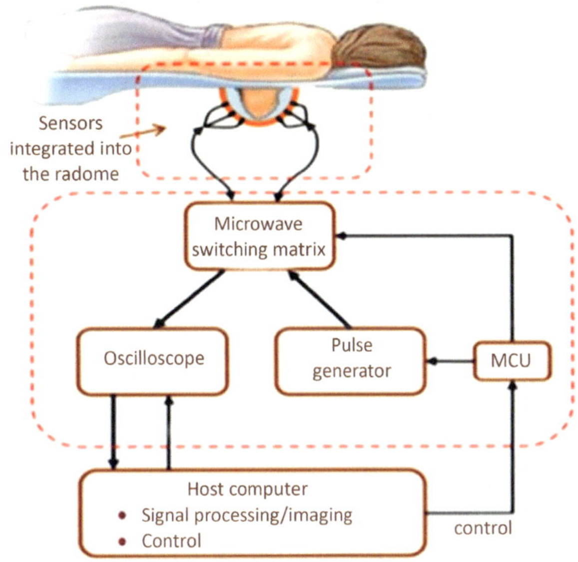

Figure 4.12. Various modalities in breast imaging.

Source: https://media.springernature.com/lw685/springer-static/image/art%3A10.1186%2Fs43055-020-00175-5/MediaObjects/43055_2020_175_Fig26_HTML.png.

The field of cancer detection and monitoring has evolved considerably with the advent of molecular and cellular imaging modalities (Figure 4.12). These technologies offer the potential to assess tumors visually and quantitatively at multiple biological levels, from cellular function to tissue structure. For instance, traditional imaging equipment such as MRI and CT scans is often limited in its ability to discriminate between tumor types or to assess the specific cellular response to therapy. In contrast, advanced modalities such as high-frequency ultrasound and confocal microscopy enable real-time monitoring of therapeutic response at the microscopic scale. Through multimodal imaging, scientists can provide extensive information on tumor dynamics, which results in personalized medicine strategies to tailor treatment to patients' specific needs. One of the notable advancements in this field is the use of targeted drug delivery systems, such as HerDox, that contain doxorubicin within a viral-like particle specifically targeted at HER2+ tumor cells. Not only does this maximize therapeutic effect, but it also minimizes systemic toxicity, a precise illustration of how molecular imaging can make cancer therapy effective. In a multimodal imaging investigation, the researchers demonstrated that apoptosis in cancer cells can be monitored in vivo during therapeutic treatment using high-frequency ultrasound imaging. The method allows clinicians to assess response to therapies in real time and adapt accordingly based on real-time data, maximizing treatment outcomes and patient prognoses, such as in the notable findings of multimodal imaging methods in preclinical testing (Chu et al., 2012). Moreover, the multimodality integration is not only limited to therapeutic monitoring but also to preclinical assessments that determine the translation of therapy from the bench to the clinic. Techniques such as spectral imaging enable quantitative discrimination between drug fluorescence and tissue autofluorescence, enabling accurate assessments of drug distribution in tumors. Imaging is a pivotal aspect of the procedural steps of cell harvesting, purification, and implantation in stem cell therapy. With the use of imaging modalities, practitioners cannot only visualize stem cells but also accurately assess their therapeutic impact following implantation in cancer treatment (Jokerst et al., 2016). Continuing optimization of these imaging modalities will significantly alter cancer detection and monitoring, ultimately benefiting patient outcomes and treatment efficacy.

4.4.2. Cardiovascular Imaging

Cardiovascular imaging has seen unprecedented progress, evolving from conventional anatomical evaluation to methods that enable the thorough interrogation of underlying molecular and cellular mechanisms. In the past, imaging modalities emphasized the visualization of structural pathologies, but advances in cardiovascular biology over the last few years have shifted the focus towards the identification of particular molecular targets associated with disease processes like atherosclerosis. There have been some probable imaging targets identified from preclinical studies, thereby enabling new imaging technologies to probe cellular activities and metabolic processes involved in the onset and progression of plaque. While the advancements have been immense, there is, however, a significant hurdle for the widespread clinical use of these molecular imaging methods, much of which entails sensitivity, standardization, and cost issues. Addressing these barriers is necessary for the successful incorporation of advanced imaging modalities into routine clinical practice, where they can provide valuable information on disease pathophysiology and contribute to patient management (Camici et al., 2017) (Figure 4.13). Among the numerous modalities utilized in cardiovascular imaging, cardiovascular magnetic resonance (CMR) has emerged as a noninvasive modality of particular use. CMR is effectively capable of detecting complications such as microvascular obstruction (MVO) and intramyocardial hemorrhage (IMH), both of which are common sequelae of reperfused myocardial infarction (MI). Prompt detection of MVO is particularly important, considering it is linked with poor prognosis and adverse ventricular remodeling. Similarly, the occurrence of IMH after revascularization underscores the importance of precise diagnostic imaging modalities in understanding these pathophysiologic complications. Though various studies have investigated the patterns of late gadolinium enhancement in different CMR sequences, the development of standardized protocols for the evaluation of IMH is still challenging. This underscores the need for continued research to refine imaging methods so they can reliably elucidate the intricacies of myocardial healing and guide treatment approaches (Calvieri et al., 2015). Not only does the progression of advanced imaging modalities enhance diagnosis, but it also holds the potential to allow for the tailoring of therapeutic strategies in cardiovascular disease. Molecular imaging techniques may enable better understanding of disease processes, thereby supporting clinical decision-making. Visualization of molecular interactions and cellular activity in real time permits physicians to assess the effectiveness of treatment regimens and alter therapies accordingly. Furthermore, future evaluation and standardization of such imaging modalities across multinational networks can further advance clinical practice by ascertaining their added value and facilitating broader applications. Lastly, the convergence of molecular data and new-generation imaging modalities is a critical frontier in cardiovascular medicine with the potential to translate precision medicine into better patient care and increased diagnostic accuracy (Camici et al., 2017).

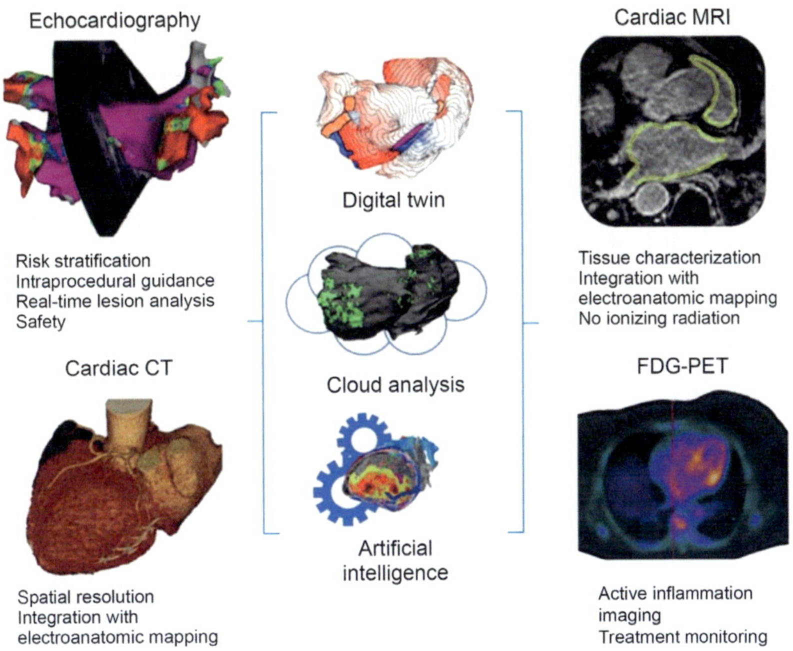

Figure 4.13. Cardiovascular imaging techniques for electrophysiologists.

Source: https://media.springernature.com/m685/springer-static/image/art%3A10.1038%2Fs44161-025-00648-8/MediaObjects/44161_2025_648_Fig1_HTML.png.

4.4.3. Neurological Applications

The application of molecular and cellular imaging techniques in neurology has revolutionized the diagnosis and conceptualization of neurologic brain diseases. Techniques such as PET and MRI enable researchers and clinicians to visualize structural alterations and metabolic activity within the brain with unparalleled precision. These imaging techniques enable clinicians and researchers to offer early diagnosis of neurological diseases such as Alzheimer's disease and Parkinson's disease by highlighting metabolic abnormalities years before the detection of clinical symptoms. For instance, amyloid PET imaging is now a standard diagnostic modality for Alzheimer's, enabling clinicians to visualize amyloid plaque deposition in the living patient, a feature of the disease. Such ability not only enhances diagnostic accuracy but is also the basis for patient management approaches targeted at underlying neurobiologic mechanisms rather than clinical symptoms per se. Moreover, high-resolution imaging techniques have been instrumental in assessing treatment response and monitoring disease course in neurological disorders. In conditions such as multiple sclerosis, magnetic resonance spectroscopy (MRS) is employed to study biochemical changes in brain tissue, with relevance to neuronal integrity and metabolic shifts. Such information can guide therapeutic decisions and stratify patient groups based on predicted disease patterns (Figure 4.14).

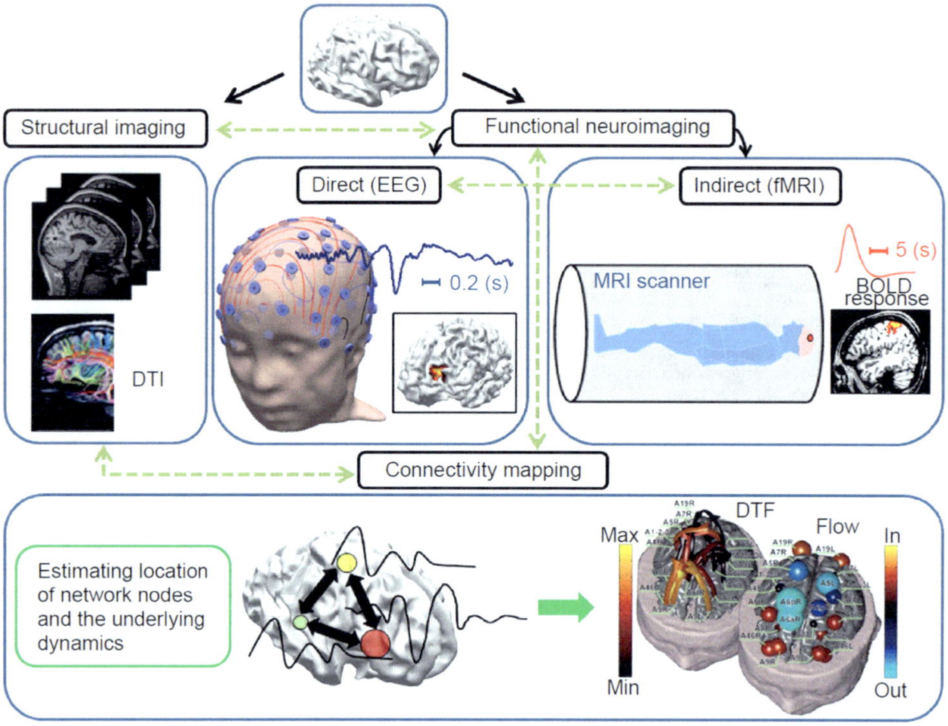

Figure 4.14. Neuroimaging at a glance: Different neuroimaging modalities interact with each other to delineate underlying brain networks (not inclusive of all modalities).

Source: https://www.researchgate.net/publication/283753260/figure/fig1/AS:613949510783015@1523388378589/Neuroimaging-at-a-glance-Different-neuroimaging-modalities-interact-with-each-other-to.png.

Additionally, fMRI is a robust neuroimaging technique to construct brain activity maps based on the identification of changes in blood flow, which is highly useful in the pre-surgical evaluation of patients with epilepsy. Defining functional brain elements for necessary functions, fMRI enhances the accuracy of surgery and diminishes the risk of postoperative complications, thereby significantly impacting clinical outcomes and patient quality of life. In science, molecular and cellular imaging modalities have been crucial for revealing the pathophysiological mechanisms of neurological illnesses and for developing new therapeutic paradigms. Advances such as in vivo imaging of transgenic animal models allow scientists to track disease progression and evaluate the effectiveness of experimental treatments in real time. For example, imaging modalities have been instrumental in assessing the impact of new drug leads on neurodegenerative phenomena and thereby paving the way for the development of targeted therapies. Moreover, multimodal imaging approaches that integrate dissimilar modalities maximize the scope of neurological assessment by synergistically combining structural, functional, and molecular data. The integration of these modalities not only contributes to individualized medicine but also to an enhanced understanding of complex neurological conditions, ultimately leading to improved patient care and outcomes, as seen in studies presented in N/A (2004, 2006).

SUMMARY

Molecular and cellular imaging modalities encompass a broad array of techniques that play significant roles in advancing biomedical research and clinical investigations. Each technique, whether MRI, PET, or fluorescence microscopy, offers unique characteristics that allow us to comprehend biological events at the molecular and cellular levels. For instance, MRI is primarily used for anatomical imaging to visualize internal anatomy in intact organisms, while techniques such as PET enable researchers to study metabolic processes by monitoring biochemical changes. Combining these modalities enables researchers to perform in-depth analysis of disease and normal states, thereby accelerating the discovery of novel therapeutic interventions and enhancing diagnostic specificity in individualized medicine. One of the primary research areas in current imaging is the integration of high-resolution multimodal data, which combines different imaging modalities to provide a fuller picture of biological processes. The INCF Digital Atlasing Program is itself one such project insofar as it facilitates the standardization and provision of multidimensional data pertaining to the rodent brain. This effort aims to create a common platform to manage information flow across different imaging modalities, enabling researchers to harness and interpret data to promote cooperation and innovation. With robust standards in place, imaging modalities can image not only biological complexity but also enable interdisciplinary approaches that combine molecular biology, neuroimaging, and data science to enhance our understanding of the intricate networks that regulate physiological processes. Patient-derived xenograft (PDX) models are also becoming immensely useful tools for measuring cancer biology, particularly with advanced imaging techniques. The work discussed in Altschuler et al. (2019) underscores the imperative need to understand cellular heterogeneity in tumors, as variation among PDX models significantly impacts research and treatment outcomes. Through multi-modal imaging—conventional ones, as well as immunofluorescence and proteomic assays—researchers are able to comprehensively profile intratumor heterogeneity, acquiring insight into the spatial dynamics of tumor growth. This critical review underscores the potential of synergistic coordination of molecular and cellular imaging modalities to further advance cancer research, paving the way for more efficacious targeted therapies that are sensitive to the subtle dynamics of tumor biology. With progress to come, the fine details obtained by these techniques will continue to inform both scientific investigation and clinical practice.

CLOSER LOOK

THE IMPACT OF IMAGING MODALITIES ON HEALTHCARE AND RESEARCH

Imaging modalities have revolutionized health care and research, providing the essential imaging technologies for disease diagnosis and monitoring at the molecular and cellular levels. Developments in imaging technologies as modalities such as MRI, PET, and CT scanning have significantly enhanced the precision with which clinical status of patients can be assessed. Enhanced patient care is the direct consequence of this enhanced capability in the sense that early and precise diagnoses allow timely intervention. For instance, in oncology, being able to see tumor characteristics has shifted treatment plans from generic therapies to more customized regimes in terms of patient profiles. There has been an important shift towards predictive, preventive, and personalized medicine (PPPM) emphasizing the need to include advanced imaging techniques in treating conditions appropriately and improving quality of life, as emphasized in the cancer predisposition and risk assessment strategy discussion presented in Bubnov et al. (2015). Research, particularly in molecular biology and pharmacology, greatly benefits from the application of advanced imaging modalities. These technologies enable a comprehensive understanding of physiological function and biochemical processes involved in various diseases. With the application of molecular imaging modalities, researchers can observe highly interconnected cellular interactions that take place in real time, making it possible to examine action mechanisms in novel therapeutics. This information is critical for the development of drugs, allowing for the identification of potential biomarkers and therapeutic targets. As imaging technology advances, its integration into research paradigms becomes increasingly essential for hypothesis development and experimentation. Interactive interplay between imaging and research not only becomes increasingly crucial for developing the scientific rationale for understanding disease but also for accelerating innovation to discover new ways of addressing shared health issues, as also illustrated under preterm labor and associated issues in Kriete et al. (2007). Furthermore, the policy and public health implications of imaging modalities are significant since they are engaged in epidemiological research and implementation of screening programs. Techniques capable of providing population-based screenings can identify risk factors among individuals, thereby complementing preventive healthcare planning. The combination of such modalities, however, would have to be pragmatic and guided by ethical concerns, including data privacy and cost-benefit analysis of screening interventions. Effective public health program implementation of imaging is dependent on robust systems with the right balance of patient data protection and optimization of health benefits to populations. Both the ongoing controversy regarding population screening and the solution pathways will remain informed by the effects of advanced imaging, and its role will remain pivotal in defining effective healthcare provision systems and augmenting overall public health outcomes, thereby supporting the initial assumptions of Bubnov et al. (2015).

REFERENCES

1. Kerna, N. A., Ngwu, D. C., Kadivi, K., Carsrud, N. V., Pruitt, K. D., Flores, J. V., Holets, H. M., Jomsky, B. M., Chawla, S., Azi, C. I., McKee, D., Nwokorie, U., Anderson, J., II, Dugeri, J. L., Hammam, H. S. H., Chiedozie, O. B., Nnake, I., David, C. O., & Adadzi, J. (2024). Transformative advancements in diagnostic imaging: reducing risks, enhancing accuracy, and promoting sustainability. *European Journal of Medical and Health Research*, *2*(5), 153–172. https://doi.org/10.59324/ejmhr.2024.2(5).16Altschuler, S. J., Atreya, C. E., Hann, B., Malato, C., et al. (2019). A multi-modal data resource for investigating topographic heterogeneity in patient-derived xenograft tumors. https://core.ac.uk/download/323079314.pdf (accessed on 5th August 2025).
2. Azam, K. S. F., Bocklitz, T., & Ryabchykov, O. (2022). A review on data fusion of multidimensional medical and biomedical data. https://core.ac.uk/download/553461045.pdf (accessed on 5th August 2025).
3. Bajwa, N., Grundfest, W., Maccabi, A., Namiri, N., et al. (2018). Quantitative characterization of viscoelastic behavior in tissue-mimicking phantoms and *ex vivo* animal tissues. https://core.ac.uk/download/323077188.pdf (accessed on 5th August 2025).
4. Bohmer, V. I., Elsinga, P. H., Feringa, B. L., Szymanski, W., et al. (2021). Multivalent probes in molecular imaging: Reality or future? https://core.ac.uk/download/518777332.pdf (accessed on 5th August 2025).
5. Boonzaier, N. R., Piccirillo, S. G. M., Price, S. J., Watts, C., et al. (2015). Assessing and monitoring intratumor heterogeneity in glioblastoma: How far has multimodal imaging come? https://core.ac.uk/download/35278890.pdf (accessed on 5th August 2025).
6. Boppart, S. A., Marks, D. L., Oldenburg, A. L., Xu, C., et al. (2005). Optical probes and techniques for molecular contrast enhancement in coherence imaging. https://core.ac.uk/download/582227201.pdf (accessed on 5th August 2025).
7. Bose, R. J. C., & Mattrey, R. F. (2019). Accomplishments and challenges in stem cell imaging *in vivo*. https://core.ac.uk/download/287623865.pdf (accessed on 5th August 2025).
8. Boucheron, L. E., Can, A., Gurcan, M. N., Madabhushi, A., et al. (2009). Histopathological image analysis: A review. https://core.ac.uk/download/46378.pdf (accessed on 5th August 2025).
9. Brinkley, J. F., & Rosse, C. (2002). Imaging informatics and the Human Brain Project: The role of structure, review. https://core.ac.uk/download/pdf/9412262.pdf (accessed on 5th August 2025).
10. Bubnov, R., Danesi, R., Desiderio, D. M., Grech, G., et al. (2015). EPMA position paper in cancer: Current overview and future perspectives. https://core.ac.uk/download/293881196.pdf (accessed on 5th August 2025).
11. Burger, A., Verbeek, F., Johnson, G. A., Zaslavsky, I., Nissanov, J., Boline, J., Puelles, L., et al. (2009). The INCF Digital Atlasing Program: Report on digital atlasing standards in the rodent brain. https://core.ac.uk/download/pdf/288929.pdf (accessed on 5th August 2025).
12. Calvieri, C., Fedele, F., Gualdi, G. F., Masselli, G., et al. (2015). Intramyocardial hemorrhage: An enigma for cardiac MRI? https://core.ac.uk/download/54514955.pdf (accessed on 5th August 2025).

13. Camici, P. G., Gaemperli, O., Libby, P., Rimoldi, O., et al. (2017). Non-invasive anatomic and functional imaging of vascular inflammation and unstable plaque. https://core.ac.uk/download/85219371.pdf (accessed on 5th August 2025).

14. Catana, C., Cherry, S. R., Jacobs, R. E., Judenhofer, M. S., et al. (2008). Simultaneous *in vivo* positron emission tomography and magnetic resonance imaging. https://core.ac.uk/download/4877262.pdf (accessed on 5th August 2025).

15. Chan, D. Y. S., Chong, T. T., Gan, J., Hausenloy, D. J., et al. (2023). Multi-modality imaging of atheromatous plaques in peripheral arterial disease: Integrating molecular and imaging markers. https://core.ac.uk/download/573841607.pdf (accessed on 5th August 2025).

16. Cherry, S. R., Jacobs, R. E., & Louie, A. Y. (2008). The integration of positron emission tomography with magnetic resonance imaging. https://core.ac.uk/download/4877286.pdf (accessed on 5th August 2025).

17. Chu, D., Farkas, D. L., Hwang, J. Y., Kang, J., et al. (2012). Multimodality imaging *in vivo* for preclinical assessment of tumor-targeted doxorubicin nanoparticles. https://core.ac.uk/download/323077463.pdf (accessed on 5th August 2025).

18. Ehrlich, S., Frank, G. K. W., King, J. A., Thompson, P. M., et al. (2018). Structural neuroimaging of anorexia nervosa: Future directions in the quest for mechanisms underlying dynamic alterations. https://core.ac.uk/download/288432964.pdf (accessed on 5th August 2025).

19. Erturk, A., Labate, A., Seehaus, A., Silva, A. C., Khan, A. R., Jeurissen, B., Yang, B., et al. (2018). Voxel-wise comparisons of cellular microstructure and diffusion-MRI in mouse hippocampus using 3D Bridging of Optically-clear histology with Neuroimaging Data (3D-BOND). https://core.ac.uk/download/160499868.pdf (accessed on 5th August 2025).

20. Funk, J., Gay, S., Müller-Ladner, U., Straub, R. H., et al. (2017). Molecular imaging: Novel tools in visualizing rheumatoid arthritis. https://core.ac.uk/download/85212391.pdf (accessed on 5th August 2025).

21. Gilad, A. A., & Shapiro, M. G. (2017). Molecular imaging in synthetic biology, and synthetic biology in molecular imaging. https://core.ac.uk/download/84314121.pdf (accessed on 5th August 2025).

22. Jokerst, J. V., & Wang, J. (2016). Stem cell imaging: Tools to improve cell delivery and viability. https://core.ac.uk/download/323064235.pdf (accessed on 5th August 2025).

23. Kriete, A., Lopez Bernal, A., Blanks, A., Holden, A., Wang, B., Devedeux, D., Kell, D., et al. (2007). Towards understanding the myometrial physiome: Approaches for the construction of a virtual physiological uterus. https://core.ac.uk/download/48928.pdf (accessed on 5th August 2025).

24. Miller, H. G. (2023). Classification of cancer cell surface proteins by gold-based hybrid nanoparticles and optical spectroscopy. https://core.ac.uk/download/618308804.pdf (accessed on 5th August 2025).

25. N/A. (2004). *Focal Spot, Spring 2004*. https://core.ac.uk/download/129069329.pdf (accessed on 5th August 2025).

26. N/A. (2006). *Focal Spot, Winter 2005/2006*. https://core.ac.uk/download/129069348.pdf (accessed on 5th August 2025).

27. Ripoll, J., Rudin, M., & Stuker, F. (2011). Fluorescence molecular tomography: Principles and potential for pharmaceutical research. https://core.ac.uk/download/19079757.pdf (accessed on 5th August 2025).

28. Vaziri, A., & Weisenburger, S. (2018). A guide to emerging technologies for large-scale and whole brain optical imaging of neuronal activity. http://arxiv.org/abs/1805.03197 (accessed on 5th August 2025).

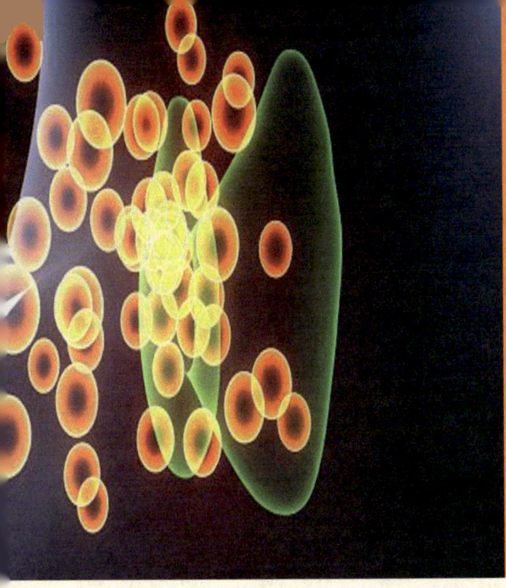

Chapter 5

IMAGE-GUIDED BIOPSY AND ABLATION TECHNIQUES

Contents

Introduction

In modern medicine, the development of image-guided biopsy and ablation technology is a milestone in therapeutic and diagnostic interventions. Image-guided treatment enhances tissue-targeting accuracy, thereby optimizing biopsies to their fullest potential and limiting risks. The integration of imaging technologies such as ultrasound, computed tomography, and magnetic resonance imaging facilitates real-time visualization, enabling clinicians to navigate complex anatomy with precision. These developments not only lead to improved patient outcomes but also reduce the time and resources required for care and diagnosis significantly. As medicine continues to progress, these newer techniques are at the cutting edge of minimal invasiveness and redefining traditional paradigms of patient management. Among the imaging modalities employed in these techniques, optical coherence tomography (OCT) is an important advance, supplementing existing modalities with its high-resolution imaging. In contrast to traditional ultrasonography with sound, OCT employs light to generate highly detailed and depth-resolved images with near-microscopic resolution. This novel imaging ability is of particular promise in the diagnosis of diverse gastrointestinal diseases, encouraging enhanced diagnostic precision in the clinic. Based on the endoscopic OCT review, the technology can be combined with conventional endoscopic techniques to provide a stratified view of pathological changes, as required in disease conditions such as Barrett's esophagus and inflammatory bowel disease.

The potential of OCT underscores the integration of cutting-edge imaging technologies into contemporary biopsy and ablation techniques, further underscoring their significance. Ongoing exploration of image-guided ablation and biopsy is continuing to bring important advancements to personalized medicine. By enhancing diagnostic precision and enabling targeted therapeutic interventions, these techniques are transforming management choices in numerous medical domains. Evidence of this transformation can be observed in developments in interventional imaging systems, with more sophisticated technologies being incorporated to improve efficacy and reduce patient risk. Though these techniques are being further refined by clinicians and researchers, understanding their basic principles and impacts is relevant. Through an in-depth examination of these innovations, the essay aims to illuminate the critical role image-guided techniques play in the pursuit of better patient care, with an emphasis on the necessity for continued research and development in this dynamic field of medicine.

5.1. Types of Image-Guided Biopsy Techniques

A number of image-guided biopsy techniques are now invaluable tools within the diagnostic process, particularly in cancers and other complex lesions. One such common technique is computed tomography (CT)-guided biopsy, particularly for lung lesions. It enables precise needle placement with minimal complications and is important in clinical settings due to its effectiveness. By enabling real-time positioning and imaging, CT-guided lung biopsy enhances precision and reduces the risk of procedural error. In addition to diagnosing malignancies, it also guides further treatment planning based on the acquired tissue. It is thus critical to promote practitioners' proficiency in CT-guided biopsies, as complications, however minor, can significantly affect patient outcomes and overall procedure success, underscoring the need for rigorous training and best practices in this domain (Fujimoto et al., 2018) (Figure 5.1).

Another promising approach is OCT, which is increasingly being applied in endoscopic biopsies. This advanced imaging modality relies on light to generate high-resolution cross-sectional images of tissue in real time during minimally invasive therapies. Its use in the clinical setting is most notable in the assessment of gastrointestinal diseases, allowing for the precise characterization of lesions, such as Barrett's esophagus or inflammatory bowel disease. By integrating OCT into standard endoscopic practice, clinicians can significantly enhance diagnostic sensitivity and support precise, targeted biopsies, thereby optimizing patient management strategies. With its ability to delineate microscopic features, aiding in the identification of malignancies and monitoring therapeutic response longitudinally, OCT is not only an important tool in clinical practice but also one from which any practice can become well-staffed (Fujimoto et al., 2018).

Ultrasound-guided biopsy is yet another significant technology in image-guided diagnostic interventions. During ultrasound-guided biopsy, high-frequency sound waves are used to create real-time images of internal anatomy, allowing clinicians to visually inspect regions of interest for biopsy.

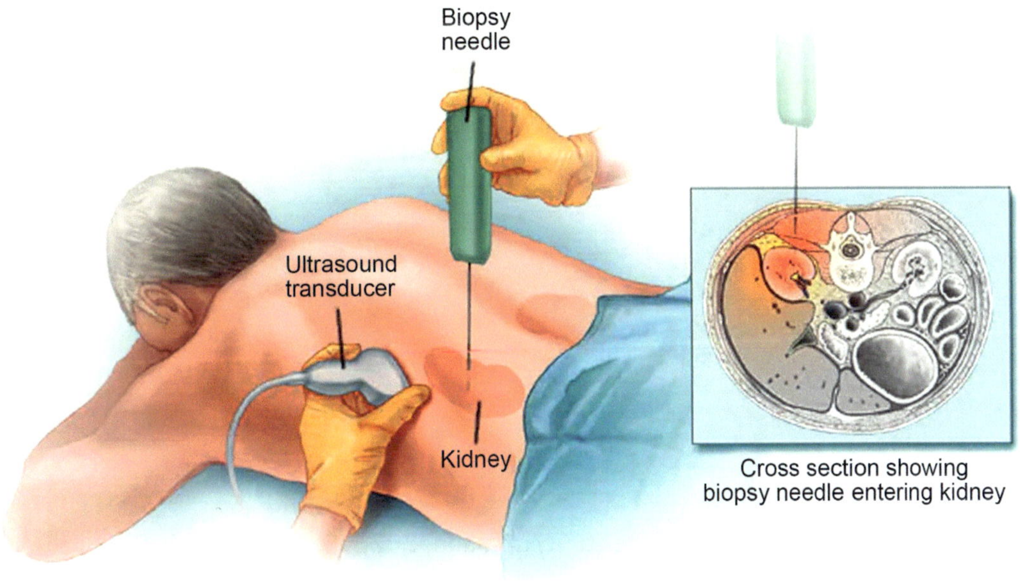

Figure 5.1. Biopsy and drainage procedure.

Source: https://www.cirse.org/wp-content/uploads/2018/08/Biopsy600x460.jpg.

Particularly ideal for soft-tissue lesions, the procedure is non-invasive and often associated with increased patient comfort. Sonographically guided biopsies are especially beneficial for lesions located within the abdomen or breast, where the procedure can enhance visibility and access. Furthermore, ultrasound guidance reduces exposure to ionizing radiation and makes it a safer alternative for certain patient populations. The effectiveness of this technique, paired with safety and simplicity, once again underscores the role of ultrasound in modern diagnostic techniques, with a focus on the added value of optimizing patient outcomes during biopsy procedures (Ascenti et al., 2024).

5.1.1. Fine Needle Aspiration (FNA)

FNA is an essential technique in image-guided biopsies, particularly because it provides cytological samples with minimal invasiveness. FNA allows clinicians to access tissue samples from various anatomical sites under imaging guidance, such as ultrasound and computed tomography. The primary advantage of FNA is its ability to provide quick results, enabling instant clinical decision-making in the context of suspicious lesions. However, there are still restrictions, particularly concerning inconclusive cytological findings (Figure 5.2).

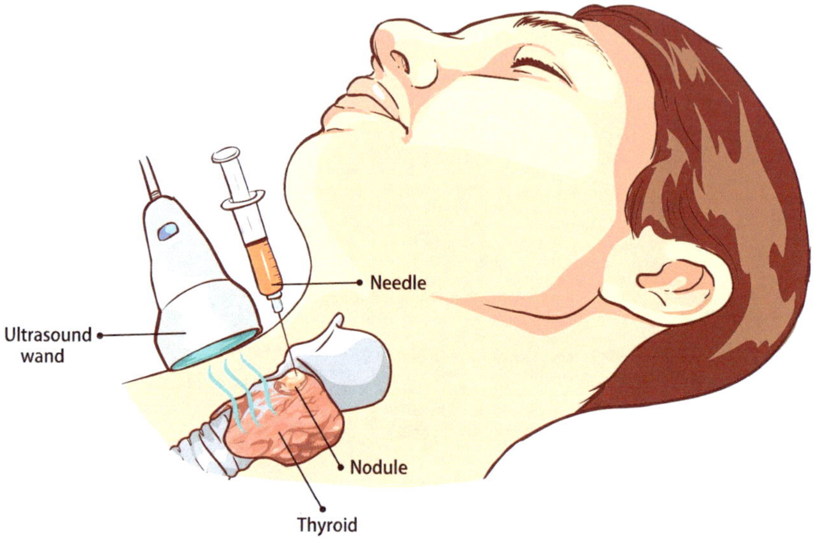

Figure 5.2. Fine needle aspiration.

Source: https://www.enthealth.org/wp-content/uploads/2022/03/ENThealth_ConditionsGraphic-FineNeedleAspiration.jpg.

It has been observed that up to 22.83% of primary EUS-FNA samples may be deemed inconclusive, underscoring the need to refine methods to maximize diagnostic precision while minimizing patient anxiety and treatment delays (Bacsur et al., 2023). Therefore, it is paramount to develop methods and technologies in FNA for elevating over-all diagnostic efficacy in clinical practice. Technical aspects of FNA are vital to avoid complications and achieve optimal results. Needle size and technique are critical considerations in sample adequacy; the use of larger-diameter needles is shown to reduce the likelihood of inconclusive results. Also, multiple punctures during the sampling process enhance the quality of cytologic specimens. Research underscores the use of slow-pull and standard suction techniques to achieve higher sample recovery rates and lower rates of inconclusiveness (Bacsur et al., 2023). As a result, these procedural parameters are most important for reducing complications and improving patient satisfaction during the biopsy process. Careful planning and implementation of each FNA process optimizes diagnostic quality, as well as upholding the quality of care required in the modern medical setting. One of the most significant advantages of FNA is that it can be used on a wide variety of tissue types, including lymph nodes, thyroid nodules, and breast lesions. As a method within the broad category of image-guided biopsies and interventions, FNA can lead to earlier diagnosis and timely treatment of malignancies and therefore has a significant impact on patient care. In addition, improvements in imaging modalities, including the technology behind fusion imaging, enable more accurate lesion targeting during FNA, hence fostering both the safety and effectiveness of the procedure. Although it has many benefits, existing challenges demand ongoing assessment and training for healthcare workers performing FNA to effectively address the intricacies of different anatomical locations and complications. With the evolution of imaging modalities, the potential for FNA to be increasingly utilized as an integral part of diagnostic and therapeutic schemes is growing.

5.1.2. Core Needle Biopsy (CNB)

CNB is now an integral part of image-guided biopsies, providing a minimally invasive option for histological evaluation of suspicious lesions. It's done using a hollow needle, directed by imaging methods such as ultrasound or CT, to the intended target. CNB is preferable to fine-needle aspiration because with it, one can obtain larger tissue samples, thus accurate assessment and reduce sampling errors (Figure 5.3).

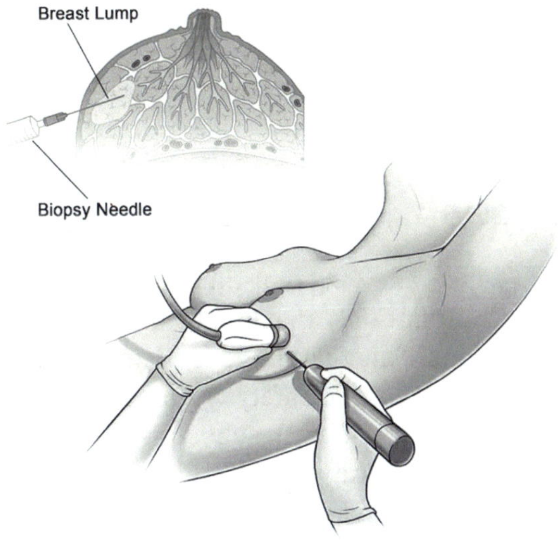

Figure 5.3. Core needle biopsy.

Source: https://andrewleebreastclinic.sg/wp-content/uploads/2024/03/core-needle-biopsy.jpg.

With the growing demand for accurate diagnostic procedures, the role of CNB has also become more prominent, especially in handling cancer cases and other critical pathologies. With the integration of reliable imaging techniques, CNB not only enhances the accuracy of pathological diagnoses but also improves patients' comfort and safety, as it is less invasive. Among the premium imaging applications, robotic-assisted CNB is a noteworthy advancement. The current technology has given rise to a premium robotic arm with a 7 7-degree-of-freedom (DOF) setup for application in CT-guided percutaneous biopsies. It provides precise needle placement by minimizing human error. The integration of robot technology enhances targeting precision to under 1 mm, which is particularly handy for targeting peripheral lung lesions or other challenging sites within the body. The robots' design also provides ample room to move without compromising the small size required for insertion, further adding to the technique's versatility for other biopsies beyond those it is specifically recommended for, such as lung cancer. The application of this technology represents a paradigm shift toward safer, more efficient, and more reliable medical interventions. Moreover, the complementary effects of core needle biopsies and ultrasound guidance reflect another level of improvement in this field. Ultrasound has proven not only to be a diagnostic modality but also an intrinsic guide to therapeutic interventions, particularly in pancreatic disease, where CNB plays a pivotal role in diagnosis. Recent technological developments in ultrasound techniques, including contrast-enhanced imaging and multimodality fusion imaging, have significantly improved the accuracy of CNB procedures. Technological innovations are most important in reducing complications from biopsies as well as improving patient outcomes. As experts recognize the advantages that accompany such advancements, reliance on image-guided methods like CNB will most likely rise, promising a future where accurate diagnosis and treatment can navigate the complexity of complex pathologies without compromising care.

5.1.3. Vacuum-Assisted Biopsy (VAB)

The VAB procedure is a critical advance in the practice of image-guided breast biopsies, and it plays a critical role in the diagnosis of breast cancer. Through its application of negative pressure, VAB can excise larger tissue samples than conventional core needle biopsies. This is a critically important point, as there must be sufficient tissue for appropriate histopathological examination, which, in turn, dictates treatment strategies (Figure 5.4).

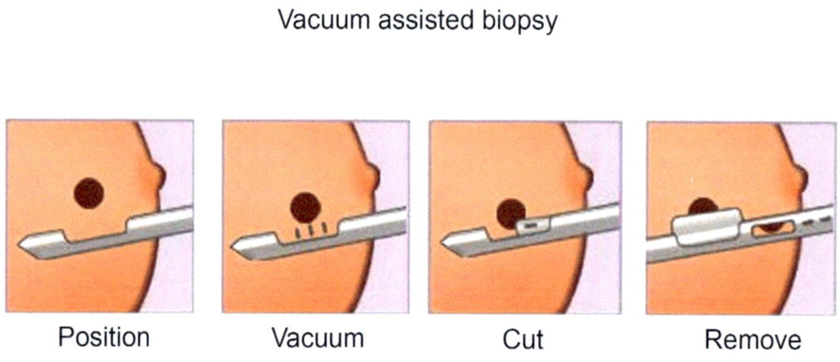

Figure 5.4. Vacuum-assisted breast biopsy.

Source: https://medicaldialogues.in/wp-content/uploads/2015/11/Vacuum_Assisted_Biopsy.jpg.

Notably, VAB is usually performed under ultrasound guidance, allowing real-time visualization of the target lesion and enabling accurate targeting. This precision not only maximizes the diagnostic yield but also minimizes the risk of biopsy-related complications. This technique is in line with the trend towards less invasive procedures that prioritize patient comfort and safety without sacrificing effectiveness in diagnosing breast carcinomas. The synergistic use of VAB with subsequently applied minimally invasive treatments such as laser interstitial thermal therapy (LITT) has come under the spotlight in recent years as being promising for treating early-stage cancer. The potential to merge VAB with therapeutic ablation techniques suggests a paradigm shift in treatment approaches, particularly for unifocal ductal breast carcinomas smaller than 1 cm. According to an early study, VAB usage in tissue sampling followed by immediate LITT has shown promising outcomes with a reported ablation rate of 90.9% on tested patient cases (Anemona et al., 2021). These results reiterate the twin benefits of VAB as both a diagnostic tool and an assistant to therapeutic maneuvers, thereby substantiating the hypothesis that image-guided interventions could help transition from diagnostic to therapeutic roles in oncology. Ultrasound and other imaging technologies have made tremendous contributions towards maximizing the use of VAB. Technologies such as computer-aided detection (CAD) and elastography have improved ultrasound imaging to a significant extent, thereby making biopsies and subsequent treatment interventions more accurate (Marks et al., 2017). These technologies assist in the easy detection of small cancers with high growth potential in a timely manner so that appropriate intervention is taken. Alongside VAB, ultrasound's enhanced capabilities make image-guided biopsy techniques more effective overall. The synergism of these modalities not only aids in the accurate diagnosis of breast lesions but also optimizes patient outcomes by enabling targeted delivery of therapies. As the technology continues to evolve, the combination of VAB with advanced imaging technologies has huge potential to improve further the prognosis and quality of life of patients who present with breast cancer diagnoses.

5.2. Indications for Image-Guided Biopsy

The role of image-guided biopsy has increasingly become pivotal in the diagnosis and management of most malignancies. The technique employs advanced imaging modalities such as ultrasound, CT, and MRI to enable precise targeting of lesions that are otherwise inaccessible to standard biopsy procedures. The applications for image-guided biopsies are diverse, ranging from the evaluation of masses suspicious for cancer within organs such as the breast, liver, and prostate, to the diagnosis of disease that is not easily accessible via conventional means. For instance, ultrasound-guided biopsy is most frequently used to evaluate thyroid nodules and liver lesions, with real-time imaging that improves the specificity of tissue sampling. By using such targeted approaches, clinicians can minimize complications while maximizing diagnostic yield, thereby setting a solid foundation for future treatment. In prostate cancer, image-guided biopsy techniques have revolutionized diagnostic paradigms. Transrectal ultrasound (TRUS)- guided biopsy was the most commonly used technique; however, its limitations have prompted the development and use of more sophisticated imaging approaches. With the evolution of multiparametric magnetic resonance imaging (mpMRI), the detection and characterization of prostate lesions have been made simpler, and clinicians can now get higher-resolution images to target biopsies more accurately. This change is particularly important given the fact that prostate cancer is plagued with complications in its heterogeneity in growth patterns and overdiagnosis of slow-growing forms. The enhanced capacity for localizing provided by mpMRI facilitates personalized patient care, enabling active surveillance protocols and individually tailored treatment regimens for patients with potentially aggressive forms of the disease (Cabarrus et al., 2017). In addition, the use of fusion imaging modalities is a bright outlook in the practice of biopsy techniques. By adding real-time ultrasound to other imaging methods, such as MRI or CT, fusion imaging enhances the capacity of clinicians to target abnormalities that might be difficult to differentiate in isolation. The technique has been beneficial in gynecologic and obstetric practice, where it aids in the investigation of conditions such as cervical cancer and benign pathologies (Bellati et al., 2018). Ultimately, the dynamic nature of image-guided biopsies underscores the need for continual refinement of indications and methodologies, as technologies evolve and our understanding of various diseases deepens. By embracing these innovations, the medical community can improve diagnostic accuracy and treatment outcomes, ultimately providing superior patient care across diverse clinical contexts.

5.2.1. Diagnosis of Tumors

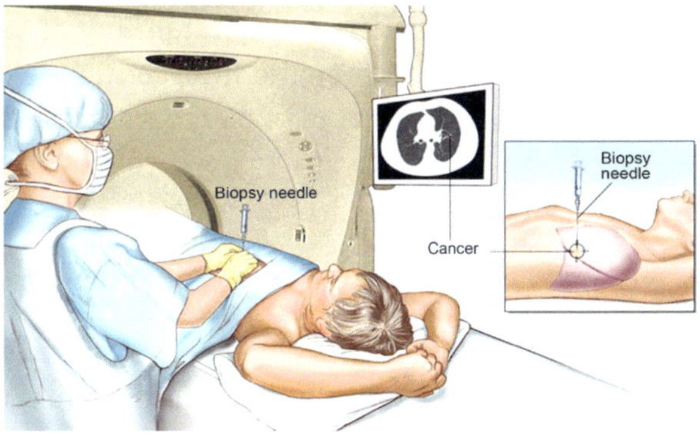

Figure 5.5. Image-guided biopsy for diagnosis of tumors.

Source: https://virclinic.com/wp-content/uploads/2025/01/biopsy.png.

Tumor diagnosis is a very intricate process that is based mainly on high-technology imaging techniques to detect malignancies accurately. Tumor diagnosis, particularly in the case of prostate cancer, in recent decades has undergone a total transformation with the introduction of high-technology imaging equipment (Figure

5.5). TRUS-guided biopsies have been the mainstay; however, low resolution and inferior tissue characterization can obviate precise diagnosis. These have prompted the need for more effective imaging modalities and have led to the advent of multiparametric magnetic resonance imaging (mpMRI). Evidence has shown that mpMRI not only has a higher detection rate but also improves localization and staging, thereby playing a vital role in personalized treatment plans such as active surveillance protocols (Cabarrus et al., 2017). In the diagnosis of breast cancer, the use of image-guided technology has also demonstrated phenomenal breakthroughs. The combination of ultrasound-guided vacuum-assisted excisions and follow-up laser interstitial thermal therapy (LITT) has been an effective way of treating localized tumors. In an initial study employing this treatment, the results showed promising outcomes, including a high ablation rate of 90.9% immediately after the procedure, with no complications. This dual therapy allows physicians to resect the lesion effectively and simultaneously destroy any remaining tumor cells by thermal ablation (Anemona et al., 2021). Thus, this method not only targets tumor resection but also makes the possibility of cosmetic gain available for patients, marking a drastic shift toward minimally invasive oncology. Apart from this, the contribution of imaging to tumor diagnosis extends beyond detection to include ongoing monitoring of treatment response. With each advance in imaging technology, its application in evaluating the response of tumors to therapies becomes increasingly important. The radiographic and histopathologic correlations have been shown to give valuable information on ablation outcomes, which are crucial to optimizing patient management. Enhanced imaging studies, such as enhanced magnetic resonance and CESM, demonstrate their value in quantifying treatment results and determining ablation effects. This new synergy of treatment and diagnosis not only propels clinicians understanding of tumor dynamics but also improves patient outcomes with personalized therapeutic interventions, validating the place of ongoing innovation in cancer diagnostics (Cabarrus et al., 2017; Anemona et al., 2021).

5.2.2. Evaluation of Lymph Nodes

Lymph node assessment is highly important in the diagnosis and treatment of some malignancies, especially in evaluating the spread of disease. Advances in imaging modalities have enabled accurate evaluation of lymphatic involvement, which is important for cancer staging and treatment planning (Figure 5.6). For instance, ultrasound (US) has established itself as a common modality for lymph node assessment due to its non-invasiveness and real-time imaging. The US can easily demonstrate lymph node morphology, which may aid in the distinction of malignant from benign disease. This is especially so in light of the changing clinical presentation of cancers with smaller and localized tumors now preponderating, as seen in the case of differentiated thyroid cancers (DTCs) (Deandreis et al., 2016). Coupled with high-resolution imaging modalities, patient care can be made more personalized by ensuring complete and accurate assessment of lymph nodes. Furthermore, the new context of lymph node evaluation has been revolutionized by the development of image-guided biopsy techniques. These techniques allow for the sampling of suspicious nodes identified on imaging. As an example, ultrasound-guided FNAB is now widely employed to biopsy lymph nodes that may harbor metastatic disease. This minimally invasive technique not only confines patient morbidity but also provides rapid results, which can impact immediate management directly. There is sufficient evidence to recommend the use of image-guided biopsy to improve diagnostic accuracy and facilitate the mapping of disease extension (Kornecki et al., 2011). With real-time feedback during biopsy, these techniques reduce the risk of false-negative results, thereby ensuring that therapeutic treatment of the correct type can be initiated promptly based on lymph node evaluation findings. With ongoing progress in image-guided ablation techniques, their use in evaluating lymph nodes is increasingly important. Ablation therapies, such as radiofrequency ablation or cryoablation, destroy tumors and can also be applied to lymphatic tissue, providing a minimally invasive alternative to surgery. Imaging, in particular ultrasound, is responsible for guiding such interventions, enabling precise targeting while avoiding close-by normal tissue. The recent research on the efficacy of these treatments shows their potential to manage metastatic lymph nodes, especially in patients who may not be good surgical candidates (Kornecki et al., 2011). As the cancer treatment paradigm continues to evolve towards more targeted and minimally invasive interventions, evaluation of lymph nodes using image-guided modalities is at the forefront of modern oncologic practice. It paves the way for enhanced patient outcomes and monitoring protocols.

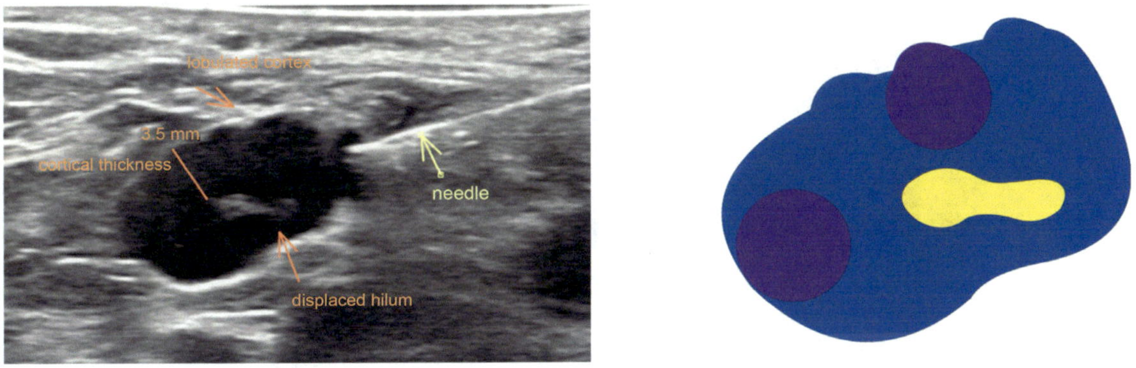

(a) (b)

Figure 5.6. The value of fine needle aspiration biopsy in the pre-operative assessment of the axilla in breast cancer.

Source: https://www.mdpi.com/jmp/jmp-03-00020/article_deploy/html/images/jmp-03-00020-g001.png.

5.2.3. Assessment of Inflammatory Conditions

Assessment of inflammatory disease is crucial within image-guided biopsy and ablation interventions in that proper identification of inflammation directly affects clinical results. Inflammatory illness exists at multiple levels of complexity, requiring precise imaging modalities to differentiate malignant from benign processes (Figure 5.7).

Other methods, such as OCT, have subsequently come to be used as key instruments in the evaluation of inflammation throughout tissues, particularly the gastrointestinal tract. This imaging method provides near-microscopic resolution that enables the evaluation of subsurface regions and facilitates diagnostics over the conventional modalities. This comes in particularly handy in conditions such as Barrett's esophagus and inflammatory bowel disease, where early identification of inflammatory change can trigger timely interventions and better patients' chances for recovery

(Fujimoto et al., 2018). Therefore, integrating advanced imaging techniques into the assessment process is imperative for developing a comprehensive picture of inflammatory disorders. The US is also critical in the assessment and management of inflammatory disorders, particularly of the pancreas. Its use extends beyond mere diagnosis; US is an interventional imaging guide for all types of percutaneous interventions to treat pancreatic diseases. Through techniques such as fine-needle aspiration, core-needle biopsy, and tumor ablation, ultrasound not only ensures accuracy but also safety in intervention. Developments such as contrast media and multimodality fusion imaging have enhanced diagnostic evaluation accuracy and interventional therapy accuracy, thereby minimizing the risk of complications from invasive procedures (Bele et al., 2019).

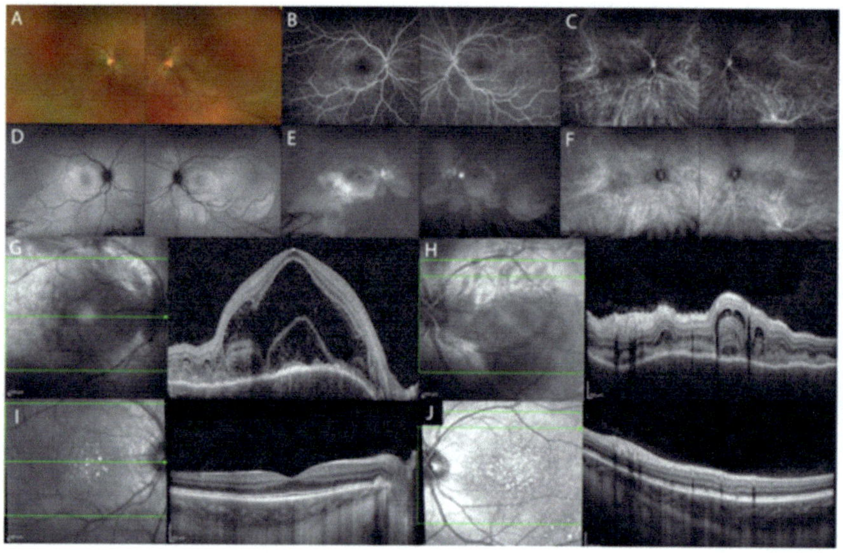

Figure 5.7. Multimodal imaging (MMI) of the acute uveitic phase of VKH disease. Ultra-wide field (UWF) pseudocolor fundus image (Optos PLC, Dunfermline, Scotland, UK) with multifocal ERD (A). FA showing peripapillary and posterior pole hyperfluorescence, indicating pooling of the ERD and hyperfluorescence of the optic disc (B,E). Fundus autofluorescence imaging (FAF) highlighting the ERD (D). ICGA hyperfluorescence with leakage from the choroidal vessels and multiple hypofluorescent dots (C,F). EDI-OCT (Spectralis OCT, Heidelberg Engineering, Heidelberg, Germany) showing multifocal ERD (G), RPE undulation (H), and diffuse thickening of the choroid, which all reduce post-treatment (I,J).

Source: https://www.mdpi.com/diagnostics/diagnostics-13-01991/article_deploy/html/images/diagnostics-13-01991-g001-550.jpg.

This ability to combine assessment and treatment decisions makes ultrasound an essential tool for managing dynamic inflammation. Therefore, the entire scope of ultrasound's utility has the ability to enrich the clinician's toolset in the management of pancreatic inflammatory conditions considerably. Moreover, integration of image-guided techniques into the assessment of inflammatory conditions enables more directed planning of patient management. The complementarity of advanced imaging modalities, such as OCT and US, allows for the detailed evaluation necessary to identify and characterize inflammation with precision. This information is used to tailor treatment plans, which, in turn, optimally reengineer the disease process. As technology and research in image-guided interventions advance, novel approaches to treating inflammatory diseases are likely to be developed. Ultimately, the integration of imaging, biopsy, and ablation not only enhances diagnostic accuracy but also creates a more cohesive treatment approach, thereby improving patient outcomes across numerous inflammatory disorders. The continuing evolution in this direction holds much promise in further advances of clinical practice and patient care.

5.3. Overview of Ablation Techniques

Ablation modalities are now focal technologies in the practice of interventional radiology, providing minimally invasive methods for the therapy of virtually all diseases, with tumors as the most prominent. Ablation modalities use multiple energy sources—heat, cold, or chemicals—to destroy diseased tissue without extensive surgical exposure. One of the most common modalities is radiofrequency ablation (RFA), microwave ablation (MWA), and cryoablation, each of which has a distinct mechanism by which cell death occurs. RFA produces heat with high-frequency electromagnetic waves that induce thermal coagulation of cancer cells, while MWA uses microwave energy that heats more quickly to higher temperatures. Cryoablation, on the other hand, is cold-induced tissue necrosis achieved by freezing, providing another alternative for certain tumor types and anatomical locations. Imaging guidance is critical to the success and safety of the procedure, providing maximum accuracy and minimal patient risk. Techniques such as US and MRI are commonly utilized to image the site in real time, enabling clinicians to target precisely during the procedure. The newer technical advances not only improve the accuracy of tumor ablation but also treatment effect imaging. For instance, the US can provide real-time feedback to the proceduralist during RFA or MWA by indicating the area of heat distribution. At the same time, MRI helps by providing accurate anatomical information and determining the extent of tissue necrosis following ablation. Accordingly, the integration of image guidance and ablative modalities enhances patient outcomes and enables better stratification of patients based on specific tumor characteristics and risks across techniques. Emerging technologies in image-guided ablation therapies continue to expand applications for cancer therapy and beyond. Focused ultrasound (FUS) is one technology that has been increasingly highlighted for its non-surgical nature. FUS allows for selective treatment with sparing of the surrounding tissues, and it has been effective in both malignant and benign tumors, particularly in the treatment of breast carcinoma. The success rates in complete tumor necrosis after FUS have been non-discriminate, ranging from 20% to 100%, depending on factors such as tumor size and type and the imaging method used during the intervention (Gelet et al., 2008). Furthermore, the evolving landscape of interventional radiology welcomes newly developed imaging technologies that enhance therapeutic capabilities, enabling precise, high-accuracy interventions that define the future of ablation therapy (Brock et al., 2023). This continuous progress highlights the importance of continuous research and development in this evolving field.

5.3.1. Radiofrequency Ablation (RFA)

Radiofrequency ablation (RFA) is now a dominant technique in image-guided therapy, particularly for the treatment of tumors in organs such as the liver, lungs, and kidneys (Figure 5.8). RFA is not a surgical intervention; it uses thermal energy to ablate diseased tissue with minimal damage to surrounding normal tissue. Combining imaging modalities, such as computed tomography and ultrasound, is pivotal for guiding RFA. Through real-time imaging of tumor location and nearby structures, these imaging modalities enhance the accuracy of needle placement and overall efficacy of optimal treatment. As evidence of the effectiveness of tumor control continues to accumulate, RFA is increasingly appreciated not only for its therapeutic applications but also for its potential to increase patient quality of life by reducing recovery periods and complications compared with traditional surgical resection. Furthermore, the viability of RFA is supported by advances in imaging technology that have enhanced its specificity and safety. Techniques such as contrast-enhanced ultrasound have supplemented RFA's therapeutic benefit by enabling more precise tumor and nearby vascular structure delineation. Such capability is crucial to prevent damage to adjacent tissues during ablation therapy. Additionally, innovations in multimodal imaging fusion technologies, which combine various imaging modalities, have further enabled the selection and preparation for intervention. These developments not only enhance operator confidence but also have been linked to improved patient outcomes by allowing quicker and more efficacious procedures. RFA, as a result, has gained popularity as the standard-of-care procedure for the majority of patients, reflecting its effectiveness and the shifting dynamics of minimally invasive intervention. The efficacy of RFA is supported by an increasing body of evidence demonstrating its use in the treatment of neoplasms, particularly in non-surgical patients. A multi-center registry documented improved diagnostic yield and treatment results with RFA procedures guided by advanced imaging modalities. For instance, studies have shown that tumor necrosis can be extremely high with the application of ultrasound-guided RF ablation, which yields good survival rates in liver tumor patients. Also, evidence has confirmed that RFA can be used as a bridge to transplantation for patients awaiting liver transplantation. Among the several advantages of RFA, such as reduced hospitalization stays and overall healthcare costs, its application underscores the importance of imaging guidance to enhance treatment efficacy while addressing the clinical needs of different patient groups, thereby positioning it as one among many image-guided biopsy and ablation techniques.

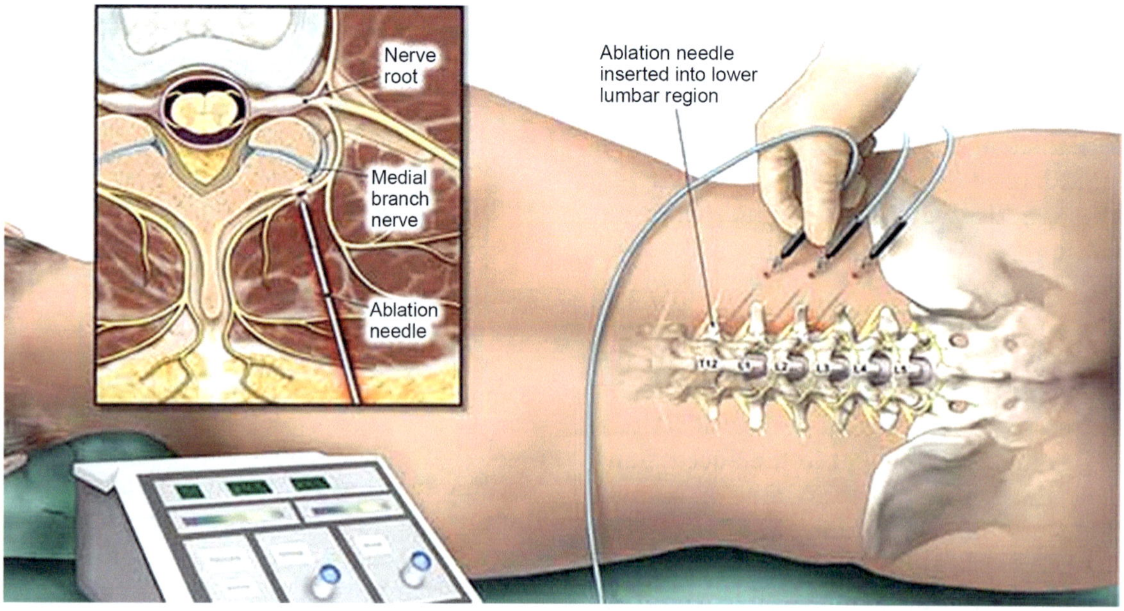

Figure 5.8. Radiofrequency ablation.

Source: https://ispinect.com/wp-content/uploads/2021/07/radiofrequency-ablation1.jpg.

5.3.2. Microwave Ablation (MWA)

One of the key advancements in minimally invasive treatments is MWA, which has also emerged as a promising alternative to traditional surgical procedures for the management of a vast array of tumors. MWA employs microwave energy to generate localized heat and effectively incinerate malignant tissue with little harm to surrounding healthy tissue. MWA is particularly effective in treating patients with renal masses of small size (less than 4 cm), especially those to whom surgery cannot be attempted due to comorbidities. Its ability to be performed with high technical success makes it increasingly acceptable to the medical fraternity and, hence, MWA a valuable alternative in the therapeutic armory for renal tumors and beyond. The findings of clinical application indicate an auspicious path for MWA, which encompasses its efficacy in targeted tumor elimination when performed under imaging guidance (Figure 5.9).

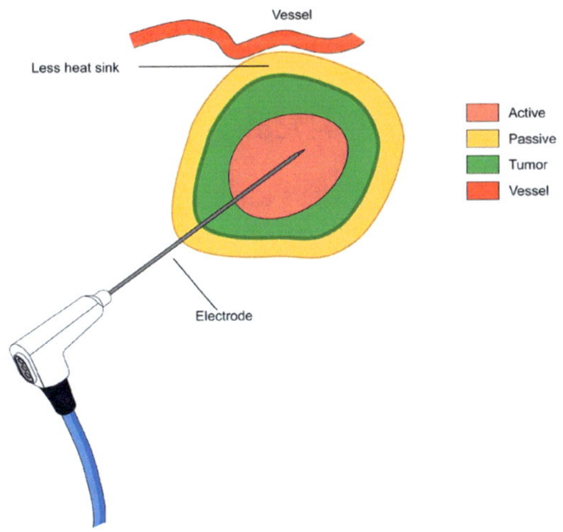

Figure 5.9. Technique of MWA ablation.

Source: https://www.researchgate.net/publication/359296185/figure/fig1/AS:1156764447834112@1652805544237/Technique-of-MWA-ablation-MWA-microwave-ablation.png.

A comparative analysis of radiofrequency ablation and microwave ablation reveals that both procedures achieve excellent technical success rates for treating small renal masses. Results of studies indicate that MWA has the ability to attain a primary efficacy rate of 89.3%, which is better than the 81.3% efficacy rate associated with radiofrequency ablation. Thus, MWA can be considered a powerful technique that not only enables efficient tumor ablation but also offers a favorable safety profile. However, it is important to acknowledge that MWA is associated with a higher rate of minor complications, cited at 18.5%, compared to its counterpart procedures. Although graded as low-grade, these complications require close monitoring and underpin the need for pre-procedure evaluation and patient education to manage probable adverse effects (Alduk et al., 2023). As technology continues to advance, the application of microwave ablation is guaranteed to grow in most oncological procedures. The evolution of imaging modalities has made MWA accessible and accurate as well, making it possible to perform the procedure under real-time imaging, which is crucial to achieving perfect results. The benefits of MWA are not only shorter procedure times but also enhanced patient satisfaction, primarily due to its minimally invasive procedure and less general anesthesia used. Because patients undergoing MWA require only local anesthesia and conscious sedation, the procedure can lead to shorter hospital stays and quicker recovery times. Overall, as borne out in recent research, MWA is an auspicious choice, further solidifying its place in broader treatment models for renal tumors and possibly other cancers as well (Zadravec et al., 2018).

5.3.3. Cryoablation

Cryoablation is increasingly being seen as a valuable tool in the practice of image-guided biopsy and ablation technologies, with special reference to the targeted destruction of unwanted tissue. This minimally invasive procedure employs extreme cold to create ice crystals in targeted cells, leading to cellular necrosis without damaging adjacent healthy structures. This precision is valued in delicate anatomical sites where preservation of the neighboring structures is crucial. In urology, for instance, cryoablation has gained popularity as an effective tumor therapy modality, supplemented by advances in imaging technologies, allowing real-time monitoring and guidance throughout the procedure (Figure 5.10).

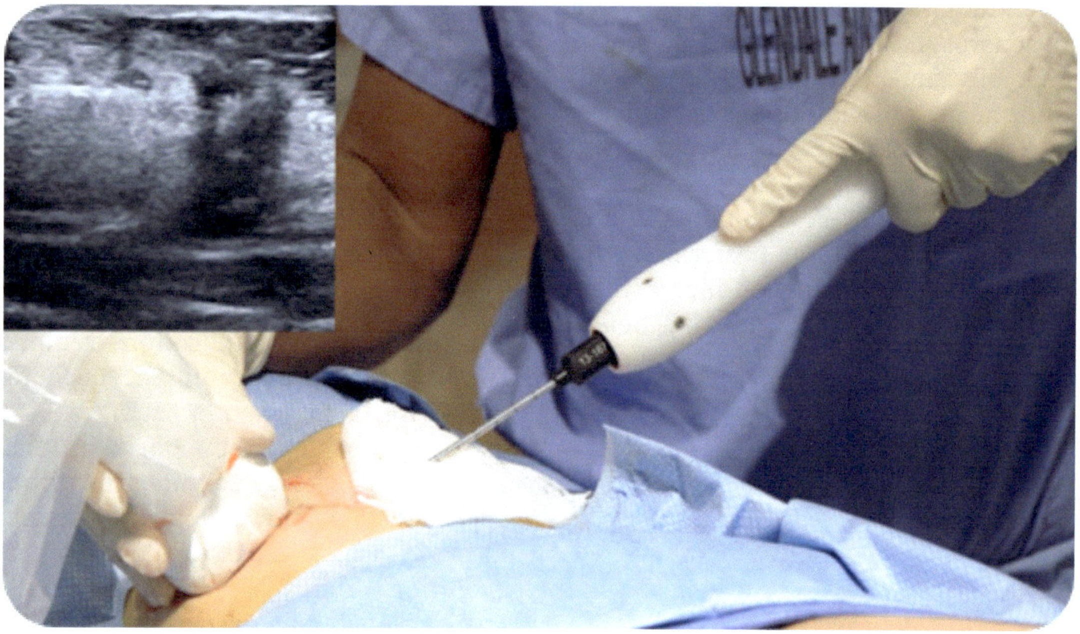

Figure 5.10. Cryoablation for breast cancer.

Source: https://www.icecure-medical.com/wp-content/uploads/2023/04/download-1-1.png.

The integration of these imaging modalities enables clinicians to address anatomical complexity, thereby enhancing the efficacy and safety of cryoablation procedures (Bart et al., 2006). Procedural adaptability of cryoablation extends beyond urology to others, including breast surgery, where it has been found to be effective in the treatment of lesions such as fibroadenomas. These benign breast masses are frequent, particularly in teenagers, and present unique challenges in terms of treatment due to psychological as well as aesthetic considerations in their management (Sherwani et al., 2016). Cryoablation is an interesting alternative compared to traditional operative resection, especially among young patients who may prefer conservative strategies with minimal physical trauma. By ensuring precision-guided techniques, cryoablation not only reduces recovery times but also decreases the aesthetic impact that can follow surgery. Such is the argument for using cryoablation that it is altering the discourse on lesion management with emphasis on patient comfort and outcomes. Its advantages aside, the widespread use of cryoablation is tempered by the intricacies of its application. Of these, the use of sophisticated imaging technologies that can accurately target lesions and cause no complications to the surrounding tissues is a key consideration. Development and research in computer-assisted medical interventions have focused on enhancing these imaging techniques, thereby making cryoablation procedures more effective (Bart et al., 2006). Additionally, given the growing popularity of minimally invasive methods in most clinical settings, continuous education and technique refinement are essential to their successful application. Continued research into cryoablation as an initial treatment option illustrates its potential to modernize biopsy and ablation procedures, staying ahead of growing demands for patient-oriented care and customized treatment protocols.

5.4. Indications for Ablation Techniques

Ablation techniques are increasingly well known for their value in the management of many diseases, predominantly in oncology. The first indications for applying these techniques typically encompass the development of tumors deemed to be not suitable for surgical resection due to anatomic site, tumor size, or patient comorbid conditions. For instance, imaging-guided ablation may be judiciously used in the case of a small focal cancer with a size less than 3 cm, for which preservation of the surrounding tissues is preferable. Furthermore, these techniques offer a minimally invasive approach to tumor control in sensitive locations, reducing overall recovery time and improving patient quality of life. The uses are not restricted to oncology, however. They can be applied in non-oncologic pathology, like vascular malformations or chronic pain disorders, and illustrate the effectiveness of ablation techniques in modern medicine practice. In the treatment of prostate cancer, the use of ablation technology has been increasingly accepted, especially as screening and diagnostic imaging escalate. Prostate ablation procedures, including cryoablation and radiofrequency ablation, are being used more frequently to treat low to intermediate-risk localized prostate cancer and avoid the complications of standard surgery. Multiparametric magnetic resonance imaging (mpMRI) ability has played an important role in this regard, as it enhances detection, localization, and assessment of tumor extension, leading to improved decision-making regarding whether the patient is a suitable candidate for ablation. These targeted approaches allow therapists to individualize treatments based on tumor-specific properties and patient preferences, representing an advancement toward individualized medicine in cancer treatment. The use of new imaging technologies like fusion imaging is also central in defining indications for ablation. By combining ultrasound with computed tomography or magnetic resonance imaging, this new imaging technique provides enhanced visualization and improved lesion targeting. In obstetrics and gynecology, for instance, fusion imaging is able to detect benign and malignant pathologies and guide ablation intervention accordingly. Its function is to refine ablation indications so that clinicians can work more effectively within complex anatomy. As highlighted in systematic reviews, while the findings are promising, additional studies are required to define the full potential of fusion imaging across various clinical scenarios and to create standardized protocols for its use, hence enhancing treatment outcomes among patients who receive ablation therapies.

5.4.1. Treatment of Malignant Tumors

The treatment of cancerous tumors has significantly enhanced with advances in imaging technology, particularly for image-guided biopsy and ablation procedures. These techniques are vital to the accurate diagnosis and proper treatment of various cancers. For instance, image-guided biopsies enable physicians to obtain tissue samples from poorly accessible or difficult-to-see tumors, facilitating timely and accurate diagnoses essential for the development of targeted therapeutic regimens. The intersection of imaging modalities such as CT and ultrasound with the biopsy process enhances precision in needle placement, reducing sampling error and hence complications. These imaging modalities not only help confirm malignancy but also allow one to assess tumor characteristics that can inform future management strategies and treatment plans (Figure 5.11).

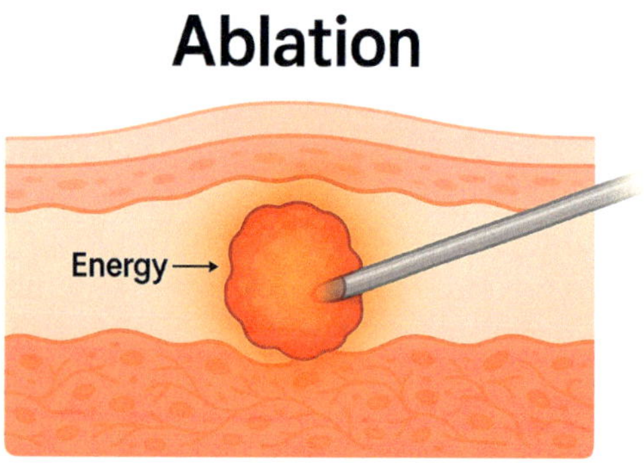

Figure 5.11. Ablation therapy for cancer.

Source: https://oncodaily.com/pub/uploads/2025/05/Ablation_Energy_OncoDaily.jpg.

Apart from their applications in diagnosis, image-guided techniques also serve as effective modalities in the treatment of cancerous tumors directly through ablation procedures. Thermal ablation techniques such as radiofrequency ablation (RFA) and microwave ablation (MWA) are particularly effective for treating small tumors, especially those located in the kidney, liver, or lung. These technologies achieved excellent treatment success rates for small renal masses in a comparative analysis. With respect to patients who may not be ideal candidates for surgical management, these modalities by MWA and RFA are reliable, thus making their efficacy considerable. Considering imaging follow-ups as an indicator of these technologies' efficacy, the findings suggest an encouraging treatment modality that offers tremendous control over the tumor. However, development of low-grade complications of the procedures, particularly in MWA, needs ongoing optimization and monitoring to deliver the best possible patient outcomes and limit adverse events (Alduk et al., 2023). In addition, use of advanced imaging modalities such as needle-based confocal laser endomicroscopy (nCLE) is emerging as an impending adjunct to standard biopsy methods. nCLE enables real-time visualization of cancer cells within the site of the biopsy, potentially increasing diagnostic yield by confirming cellular malignancy. The technique has also been found to be feasible and safe for scanning peripheral lung nodules with suspected lung cancer, paving the way for more precise targeting of tumor sites. Furthermore, improvements in the optimization of needle placement with nCLE criteria can avoid mistakes generally inherent in conventional methods, hence enhancing diagnostic precision. Future use of artificial intelligence and fluorescent tracers holds great potential to further improve these imaging technologies and enhance diagnostic efficiency and therapeutic applications in the treatment of malignant tumors (Kramer et al., 2024).

5.4.2. Management of Benign Lesions

Therapy for benign lesions is typically a multidisciplinary effort, best administered using imaging modalities capable of characterizing and assessing these abnormalities. In breast imaging, ultrasound has emerged as a central player, particularly when used as an adjunct to mammography. This is especially the case in younger women and pregnant or lactating women, where there is less risk of malignancy. The use of the Breast Imaging Reporting and Data System (BI-RADS) in the US enhances diagnosis by allowing clinicians to classify results more accurately as benign or malignant (Figure 5.12).

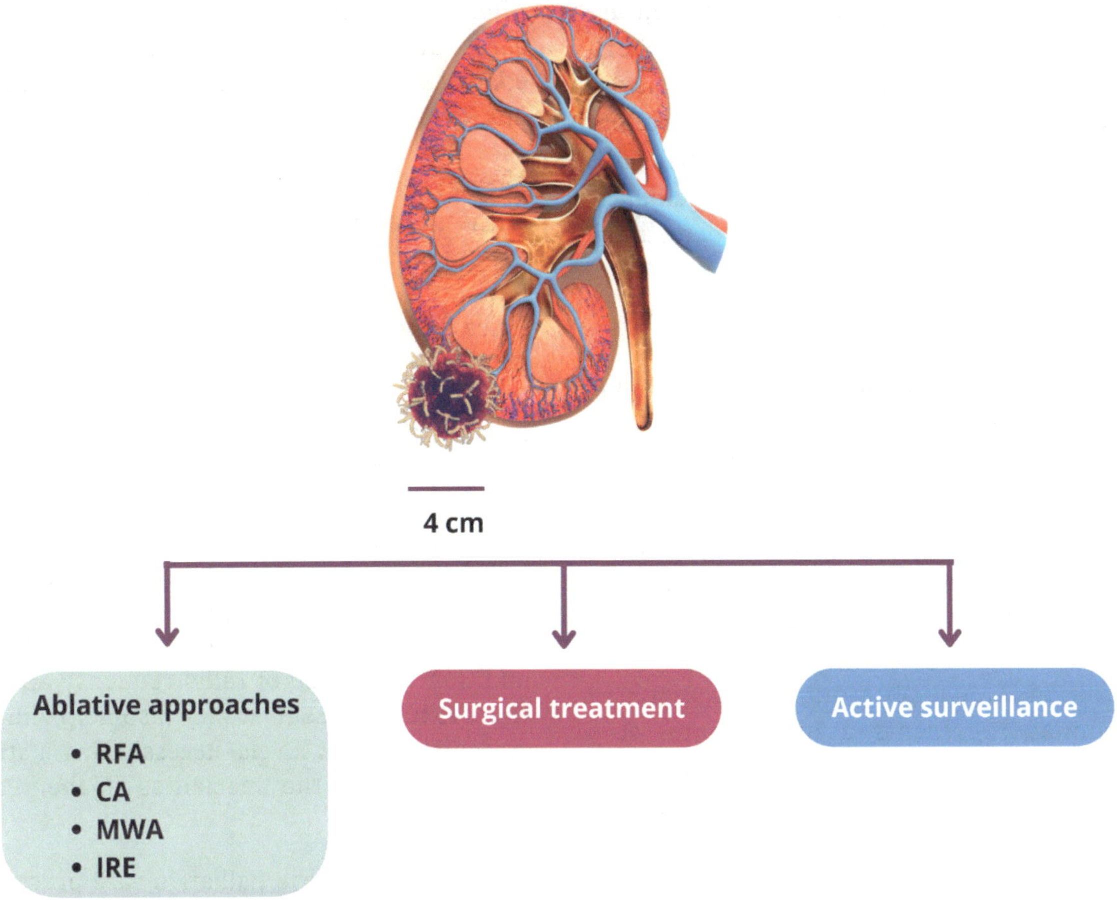

Figure 5.12. Ablative treatments for small renal masses and management of recurrences.

Source: https://pub.mdpi-res.com/life/life-14-00450/article_deploy/html/images/life-14-00450-g001.png?1711951122.

The presence of suspicious features or the absence of benign features can make biopsy inevitable to avoid an inappropriate management plan and diagnose them in error. The ability of US to guide interventional breast procedures underscores its indispensable role in managing benign lesions. It ultimately ensures personalized choices of therapy for the ultimate good and safety of the patient (Kornecki et al., 2011). Beyond ultrasound, fusion imaging modalities also offer promising advantages in the management of benign lesions, particularly in urology and gynecology. This new diagnostic modality combines standard imaging modalities such as ultrasound and MRI to improve lesion visualization. By integrating information from multiple imaging modalities, fusion imaging improves characterization of benign abnormalities, particularly in complex anatomy, thereby enhancing diagnostic accuracy and treatment planning. While current applications have primarily focused on prenatal disease and benign pathologies, there is strong potential for broader applications. Studies have shown that fusion imaging can augment diagnostic value for many gynecological diseases, providing information critical to successful treatment. Further research is, however, essential to confirm its usefulness and solidify its place in clinical practice (Bellati et al., 2018). Image-guided interventions, including biopsy and ablation, are in the treatment protocol for benign tumors, providing the advantages of a minimally invasive approach with a significant reduction in patient morbidity. These procedures can be performed with high precision under imaging guidance, such as ultrasound, which not only detects the lesion but also facilitates real-time monitoring during the procedure. In atypically presenting or symptomatic benign lesions, minimally invasive ablation, such as radiofrequency or cryoablation, is able to offer therapeutic solutions without sacrificing the integrity of adjacent tissue.

This is an intervention that becomes explicitly effective in settings where lesions are not amenable to surgical resection, thus avoiding patients having to undergo more aggressive procedures with prolonged recovery times. Overall, additional progress in image-guided techniques represents a fundamental step forward in benign lesion treatment, balancing clinical practice and the goal of maximizing patient outcomes through greater accuracy and reduced intervention burden (Kornecki et al., 2011; Bellati et al., 2018).

5.4.3. Palliative Care Considerations

In the practice of interventional oncology, the palliative care concerns are becoming paramount in the planning of treatment among patients with metastatic cancers. Integration of image-guided biopsy and ablation treatments must be complemented by a multidisciplinary approach that addresses symptom management and quality of life. As patient-centered care becomes more of a focus in oncology, it is critical that not just the physical manifestations of the disease are addressed, but also the emotional and psychological aspects of the patient's experience. It is essential to do this holistically, especially with the recognition that many patients with advanced cancer are unlikely to gain much benefit from aggressive treatments. Thus, the timely development of palliative care pathways can provide timely symptom control and prevent unwarranted interventions, allowing patients to receive evidence-based care that aligns with their values and wishes. Furthermore, integrating palliative care teams with interventional radiology practitioners can maximize the treatment paradigm for patients undergoing image-guided procedures. Since interventional radiology may now be the cornerstone of cancer complication management treatment, as indicated by reports from a number of NHS trusts, the important issue is that supportive and disease-modifying therapy should be made available to those who require it. The success of interventional techniques in relieving pain and treating complications, for example, organ obstruction, is directly relevant to the aims of palliative care. For instance, in addition to the use of radiofrequency ablation to treat tumor tissue, it may also help enhance patients' comfort levels, necessitating a strong synergy among the specialties (Maher et al., 2011).

Importantly, the palliative care practice in interventional oncology is presently being held back by the necessity for enhanced pathways and systems to provide integrated support for patients. As noted in recent studies, while many NHS trusts have established interventional oncology services, the gap remains significant in terms of formal referral pathways for palliative interventions. To bridge this gap, healthcare systems must establish collaborative networks between interventional radiology services and palliative care resources. This dependence is essential to ensure that patients not only receive disease-altering treatment but also the right supportive care that addresses pain management and psychosocial concerns. Ultimately, creating a seamless collaboration between disciplines will enhance patient outcomes and maximize quality of life through their cancer journey (Alcorn et al., 2017).

5.5. Risks and Complications

Image-guided biopsy and ablation technologies possess vast potential in the realm of diagnostic precision and targeted therapy, but carry risk and complications as well. One of the risks to such techniques is infection, either developing at the site of biopsy or arising from thermal ablation. Insertion of devices through the skin or other protective barriers necessarily carries the risk of introducing pathogenic organisms into the body.

Complications range from localized mild infections to systemic severe reactions necessitating further medical interventions. Bleeding is also a risk, which may happen during the biopsy or ablation procedure, particularly in vascular-rich tissues. Kidney mass management is a case in point, where renal mass biopsy (RMB) may provide diagnostic information but is also risky, and whose risk balance must be carefully weighed by clinicians in making patient management plans (Lim et al., 2012).

One important aspect of image-guided procedures has to do with the risk of procedure errors. These can occur due to a localization error in the needle or suboptimal image resolution, leading to poor sampling or accidental damage to nearby tissues. They could have a major impact, even causing more harm than benefit in some cases. One such case is lung biopsies, where improper targeting could result in pneumothorax (i.e., air leakage in the space between the chest wall and the lung), necessitating further interventions.

Moreover, complications related to anesthesia, though sometimes taken for granted, can also pose a risk to patients during procedures. Therefore, strict patient selection and thorough pre-procedure evaluations are also crucial for effectively mitigating such risks and improving patient outcomes (Ng et al., 2020). Finally, the long-term psychosocial impact of complications related to image-guided biopsies and ablation procedures should also be considered.

These patients can experience anxiety related to health and the risk of unfavorable outcomes. Adverse experiences during the early treatment periods may generate suspicion against medical providers, affecting future healthcare-seeking behavior unconsciously. The lingering effect of complications, such as functional impairment or chronic pain, can lead to severe emotional distress and lowered quality of life. Hence, in managing technical and physical risks, medical practitioners must place the utmost importance on a holistic care approach through counseling and psychological support for patients, ensuring they are thoroughly informed and prepared for the physical and emotional implications of their treatments (Lim et al., 2012).

5.5.1. Potential Complications of Biopsy Procedures

Biopsy procedures, particularly image-guided procedures, have grown in popularity as diagnostic procedures. Despite their utility in determining pathologies, these procedures are not complication-free. Some of the most frequent side effects encountered include bleeding and infection. Hemorrhage can be observed during or after the biopsy, and its risk depends on tissue vascularity and the biopsy modality employed. Other variables, such as the site of the biopsy, near large blood vessels, can significantly influence this risk. Infection, though less common, is also a severe complication, particularly in immunocompromised individuals or those with underlying comorbidities (Figure 5.13).

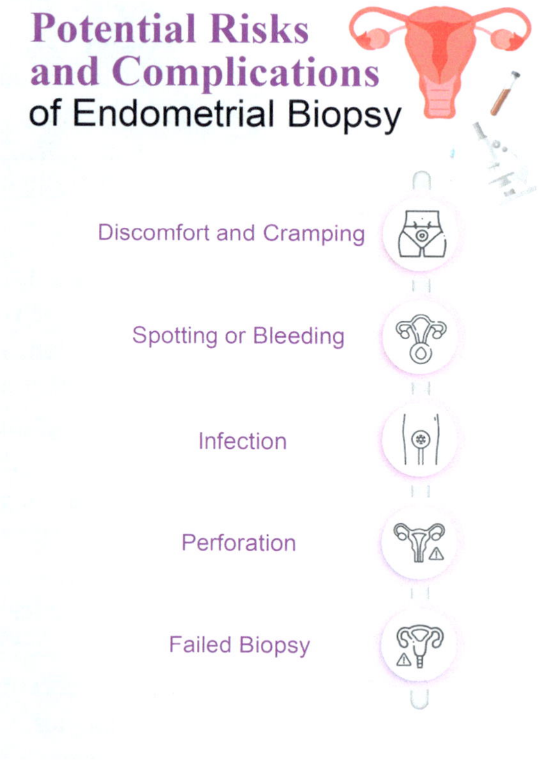

Figure 5.13. Endometrial biopsy.

Source: https://images.ctfassets.net/eexbcii1ci83/5TGnz2n0LZCmmhNLezVNUa/de827b07956ce21325d0e90e137ed5c7/Potential_Risks_and_Complications_of_Endometrial_Biopsy.jpg.

With precise imaging modalities making biopsies possible, it is imperative to weigh these complications against the benefits of certain tissue diagnosis for optimal patient outcome. Pain at the biopsy site represents another potential complication that must be weighed. Pain can occur from the puncture itself or from subsequent manipulation of the instrumentation used during the procedure. While most patients to tolerate image-guided biopsies well, with the advent of local anesthesia, there are some who will find it significantly painful, and this will color their overall assessment of the procedure's effectiveness. In addition, the specific technique used—fine-needle aspiration, core needle biopsy, etc.—can affect the degree of pain reported. As addressed in literature, advancements in imaging technologies, including the incorporation of high-resolution ultrasound, are intended to minimize pain and anxiety during such interventions, thus enhancing patient satisfaction and preventing possible complications (Bele et al., 2019). Moreover, biopsies taken within sensitive anatomical regions such as the liver or pancreas also pose unique challenges and risks. Complications such as organ injury or puncture have serious consequences and need careful planning and execution before undertaking the procedure. As a case in point, percutaneous ablation procedures, now commonly performed to treat tumors, reduce some of the risks associated with standard surgery but create their own set of possible complications, including necrosis of tissue or damage to surrounding structures caused by heat. The dynamic nature of image guidance, e.g., real-time imaging advancements, can be a critical determinant in reducing these risks and enabling a shift toward more individualized, patient-specific approaches to the selection of biopsy techniques (Filippiadis et al., 2019). Therefore, while biopsy techniques are indispensable to diagnostic medicine, the medical practitioner must be acutely aware of potential complications to optimize therapeutic outcomes and patient safety.

5.5.2. Risks Associated with Ablation Techniques

Ablation procedures, increasingly utilized in the management of other cancers, entail a variety of complications and risks that need to be considered seriously. Ablation procedures, intended to ablate abnormal tissue through multiple mechanisms—radiofrequency, microwave, and cryoablation—may result in side effects that complicate patient care. Of significant concern, during and after procedures, are hemorrhage, infection, and damage to adjacent organs. Furthermore, even if these treatments are less aggressive than traditional surgery, they remain under close imaging guidance to maximize accuracy and avoid such possible harm.

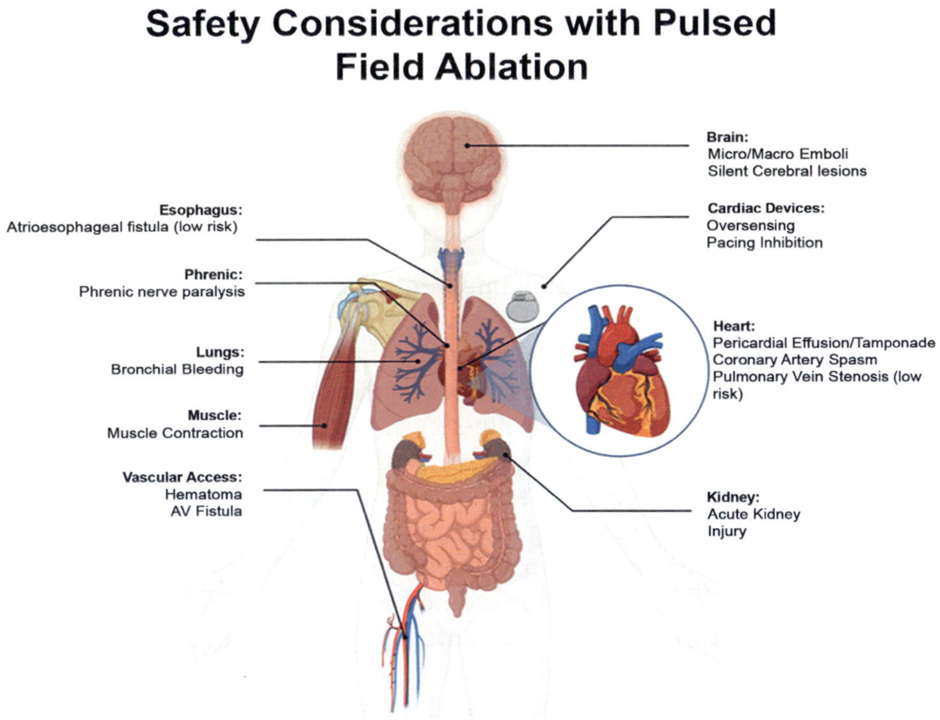

Figure 5.14. Considerations for safety with pulsed-field ablation for atrial fibrillation.

Source: https://encrypted-tbn0.gstatic.com/images?q=tbn:ANd9GcS92TYP9sRPZ1bG9fc-heqgpuYstzfV_jllAw&s.

The rising prevalence of small renal masses detected by high-technology imaging modalities has resulted in increased utilization of image-guided biopsy and resultant ablation. Highlighted, therefore, is the need to know the intrinsic risks inherent in these treatments (Lim et al., 2012).

The effectiveness of ablation treatments, particularly for cancers such as differentiated thyroid cancer (DTC), relies on advances in imaging technologies, but the same technologies generate new problems. Although imaging allows for accurate targeting of cancerous tissue for ablation, potential risks are thermal injury to neighboring healthy tissues, causing such complications as hypothyroidism or parathyroid gland injury. In addition, recurrence of malignancy in ablated tissue is a concern for the long-term efficacy of such techniques (Figure 5.14).

As the face of DTC management changes, the integration of risk stratification becomes paramount by the use of imaging, both for treatment guidance and counseling the surveillance modalities (Deandreis et al., 2016). The combination of therapeutic advantages and risks underscores the need for informed decision-making by both clinicians and patients. The psychological impact of exposure to an ablation procedure must also be considered in any discussion of potential risks. Patient anxiety is experienced over the efficacy of the treatment and fear of complications or recurrence. Psychological responses to these events can arise from the inherent uncertainties of the diagnosis and the treatment process itself, most notably in cases where ablation is chosen over more traditional surgical options. As well as these emotional considerations, physical complications such as post-surgery pain and recovery time contribute to the patient experience. Therefore, it is very important that pre-procedure counseling by clinicians be adequate, addressing the potential benefits and limitations of ablation technologies and providing reassurance to dispel patients' anxieties. Such an integrative strategy is likely to contribute positively not only to patient satisfaction but also to follow-up compliance, ultimately affecting long-term treatment outcomes.

5.5.3. Strategies for Minimizing Risks

In the case of image-guided biopsy and ablation interventions, risk reduction is essential to enhance procedural safety and effectiveness. A good solution uses advanced imaging technologies to enable real-time visualization of anatomy and tumor margins. High-resolution imaging, such as MRI or CT scans, allows precise localization of lesions, hence increasing the possibility of preventing targeting errors. Additionally, advances in needle-steering technologies, as presented in Audette et al. (2020), can substantially improve needle placement accuracy. The use of curvilinear robots and multiple steering strategies can guide needles along optimized trajectories while minimizing avoidance of key structures, thereby reducing harm to surrounding healthy tissue during biopsies or thermal ablations. These advancements constitute an important step towards managing risks to both patients and healthcare workers. Another method of minimizing risks is the pre-procedural planning process, the primary secret of which is planning for potential complications. Comprehensive risk analyses that integrate patient-specific factors, such as underlying medical conditions and anatomical variations, can inform personalized procedural approaches. Also, applying machine learning algorithms and deep learning models can enhance risk stratification and decision-making. The pre-training and meta-fine-tuning methods presented by Colantonio et al. (2024) are likely to yield robust predictive models that will help clinicians gauge lesion aggressiveness and adapt ablation techniques accordingly. With data-driven insights, medical professionals can implement protocols that not only reduce the frequency of adverse outcomes but also improve overall patient results for minimally invasive treatments. Lastly, post-procedure monitoring plays a key role in minimizing the risks of image-guided ablation and biopsy procedures. Adhering to strict follow-up procedures allows early detection of complications such as infection, bleeding, or failure of tumor ablation. Telemedicine can facilitate the use of continued patient monitoring and instant intervention on cancer-related issues, thereby enhancing patient safety. In addition, training and education of healthcare professionals on procedure-related risks and mitigation measures are crucial. Continuing professional development courses can equip practitioners with the latest information and expertise necessary to address the complexities of these advanced techniques to the best of their capabilities. By instilling an organizational culture of awareness and readiness, the overall risk profile with respect to image-guided interventions can be significantly diminished, culminating in better patient care and outcomes.

SUMMARY

The incorporation of sophisticated imaging methods into biopsy and ablation therapy has consequently revolutionized the treatment and diagnosis of numerous medical diseases. The creation of image-guided biopsies, particularly when performed with a CT or MRI, is highly advantageous in terms of accuracy and precision. For instance, the development of the mechatronic needle guidance system, as presented by Cepek et al. (2013), has demonstrated improved tumor targeting in prostate cancer during MRI-guided focal laser ablation therapy. The system allows clinicians to deliver needles through angulated paths, resulting in better treatment with fewer complications compared to whole-gland therapies. In addition to this, CT-guided biopsies have historically had spatial referencing problems to deal with, which directly impact on procedure accuracy. The proposals developed by Shar et al. (2017) aim to address these problems with an infrared navigation system intended to enable more accurate needle placement. Through real-time visualization and navigation with a proprietary graphical user interface, clinicians can significantly reduce the need for repeated scans and enhance patient safety. This innovation not only streamlines biopsy procedures but also promotes greater clinician confidence in procedure techniques. In general, the introduction of image-guided biopsy and ablation procedures is a significant advance in medical technology, yielding improved patient outcomes. The advances in needle guidance, as addressed in the reviewed studies, highlight the critical interplay between efficacy and safety in procedures and the need for continued innovation. The present research on training settings for clinicians, as described in Shar et al. (2017), lends traction to the establishment of best practices in the field. As a collective, these developments represent a revolutionary shift in how target therapy is implemented, ensuring that patients benefit from timely and accurate diagnosis and treatment.

CLOSER LOOK

THE ROLE OF TECHNOLOGY IN IMPROVING PATIENT OUTCOMES

Medical technology has revolutionized the diagnosis and treatment process in many fields, significantly enhancing patient outcomes. With image-guided biopsy procedures, this technology enables more accurate targeting of lesions, thereby reducing collateral injury to surrounding tissue. With the use of sophisticated imaging modalities such as MRI and ultrasound, accurate tumor localization is facilitated, specifically for small renal masses as well as other non-ideal targets. This accuracy is significant in enabling patients to undergo less invasive treatment that not only shortens recovery time but also lessens the risk of complications. With an increasing body of evidence supporting the benefits outlined here, selective incorporation of imaging technology into biopsies underscores their indispensable role in personalized patient management and care, underscoring the need for continued development of biomedical imaging systems to further enhance diagnostic accuracy (Lim et al., 2012). While enhancing the promise of diagnosis, improvement in biopsy techniques also makes significant contributions to the management of prostate cancer. Traditional biopsy is not without limitations, particularly in separating clinically significant from insignificant cancers, leading to overdiagnosis and overtreatment. The introduction of mpMRI has transformed the management of prostate biopsies by facilitating targeted sampling of suspicious lesions. Existing evidence indicates that mpMRI-directed targeted biopsies improve clinically significant tumor detection while minimizing unnecessary treatment for less aggressive tumors, with a favorable influence on patient outcomes. By providing a more accurate application of biopsies, physicians can craft individualized treatment protocols, reducing both patient anxiety and the emotional burden of prostate cancer diagnosis and therapy (Barbiero et al., 2024). Merging advanced technology imaging modalities with biopsy protocols underscores the necessity for an interdisciplinary patient management model that integrates diagnostic radiology and therapeutic approaches. This kind of collaboration is necessary for refining techniques such as image-guided ablation, for which real-time imaging is used to monitor ablation procedures and assess effectiveness. With evolving technology, healthcare providers must be continually educated to use these developments to their full potential, leading to more informed decision-making. This kind of balanced system not only facilitates patient protection but also significantly optimizes outcomes, ensuring that therapeutic objectives and patient-specific requirements are aligned. Finally, the technology comes center stage, as it forms the setting in which precision medicine thrives, ultimately leading to improved patient satisfaction and quality of life across every medical specialty (Lim et al., 2012).

REFERENCES

1. Zhong, J., Atiiga, P., Alcorn, D. J., Kay, D., Illing, R., Breen, D. J., Railton, N., McCafferty, I. J., Haslam, P. J., & Wah, T. M. (2017). Cross-sectional study of the provision of interventional oncology services in the UK. *BMJ Open*, *7*(10), e016631. https://doi.org/10.1136/bmjopen-2017-016631Alduk, A. M., Grbanović, L., Hudolin, T., Kaštelan, D., et al. (2023). Usporedba kratkoročnih ishoda perkutane radiofrekventne i mikrovalne ablacije u liječenju malih tumora bubrega. https://core.ac.uk/download/591677285.pdf (accessed on 5th August 2025).
2. Anemona, L., Buonomo, O. C., De Stasio, V., Di Stefano, C., Ferrari, D., Lamacchia, F., Manenti, G., et al. (2021). Ultrasound-guided laser ablation after excisional vacuum-assisted breast biopsy for small malignant breast lesions: Preliminary results. https://core.ac.uk/download/576883213.pdf (accessed on 5th August 2025).
3. Ascenti, V., Biondetti, P., Carrafiello, G., Carriero, S., Ierardi, A. M., Lanza, C., Piacentino, F., et al. (2024). Computed-tomography-guided lung biopsy: A practice-oriented document on techniques and principles and a review of the literature. https://core.ac.uk/download/614044153.pdf (accessed on 5th August 2025).
4. Audette, M. A., Blatt, J. E., & Bordas, S. P. A. (2020). Robotically steered needles: A survey of neurosurgical applications and technical innovations. https://core.ac.uk/download/346493042.pdf (accessed on 5th August 2025).
5. Bacsur, P., Bor, R., Bálint, A., Bősze, Z., Farkas, K., Fábián, A., Molnár, T., et al. (2023). Risk factors and interpretation of inconclusive endoscopic ultrasound-guided fine needle aspiration cytology in the diagnosis of solid pancreatic lesions. https://core.ac.uk/download/587082410.pdf (accessed on 5th August 2025).
6. Barbiero, M., Claps, F., Giaimo, R., Pavan, N., Rebez, G., Simonato, A., Simonato, F. A., et al. (2024). Targeted prostate biopsy: How, when, and why? A systematic review. https://core.ac.uk/download/638995763.pdf (accessed on 5th August 2025).
7. Bart, S., Baumann, M., Berkelman, P., Bolla, M., et al. (2006). Medical image computing and computer-aided medical interventions applied to soft tissues. Work in progress in urology. http://arxiv.org/abs/0712.2100 (accessed on 5th August 2025).
8. Bele, A., D'Onofrio, M., & De Robertis, R. (2019). Ultrasound-guided percutaneous procedures in pancreatic diseases: New techniques and applications. https://core.ac.uk/download/217591693.pdf (accessed on 5th August 2025).
9. Bellati, F., Caserta, D., Costanzi, F., De Marco, A., et al. (2018). Real-time virtual sonography in gynecology & obstetrics: Literature analysis and case series. https://core.ac.uk/download/195777140.pdf (accessed on 5th August 2025).
10. Berzin, T., Cash, B., Chang, K., DeMeester, S., et al. (2019). Volumetric laser endomicroscopy and its application to Barrett's esophagus: Results from a 1,000-patient registry. https://core.ac.uk/download/286362760.pdf (accessed on 5th August 2025).
11. Brock, K. K., Chen, S. R., Sheth, R. A., Siewerdsen, J. H., et al. (2023). Imaging in interventional radiology: 2043 and beyond. https://core.ac.uk/download/622991664.pdf (accessed on 5th August 2025).
12. Cabarrus, M. C., & Westphalen, A. C. (2017). Multiparametric magnetic resonance imaging of the prostate: A basic tutorial. https://core.ac.uk/download/323063417.pdf (accessed on 5th August 2025).

13. Cepek, J. (2013). New technology and techniques for needle-based magnetic resonance image-guided prostate focal therapy. https://core.ac.uk/download/61657739.pdf (accessed on 5th August 2025).

14. Colantonio, S., Pachetti, E., & Tsaftaris, S. A. (2024). Boosting few-shot learning with disentangled self-supervised learning and meta-learning for medical image classification. http://arxiv.org/abs/2403.17530 (accessed on 5th August 2025).

15. Deandreis, D., Durante, C., Filetti, S., Lamartina, L., et al. (2016). Endocrine tumours: Imaging in the follow-up of differentiated thyroid cancer: Current evidence and future perspectives for a risk-adapted approach. https://core.ac.uk/download/74318453.pdf (accessed on 5th August 2025).

16. Filippiadis, D., De Cobelli, F., Charalampopoulos, G., Mauri, G., Gennaro, N., & Marra, P. (2019). Percutaneous ablation techniques for renal cell carcinoma: Current status and future trends. https://core.ac.uk/download/322793232.pdf (accessed on 5th August 2025).

17. Fujimoto, J. G., Mashimo, H., & Tsai, T. H. (2018). Endoscopic optical coherence tomography for clinical gastroenterology. https://core.ac.uk/download/157613508.pdf (accessed on 5th August 2025).

18. Gelet, A., Khiat, A., Shiraishi, A., Schmitz, A. C., Schouten van der Velden, A. P., Fisher, B., Daniel, B. L., et al. (2008). Image-guided focused ultrasound ablation of breast cancer: Current status, challenges, and future directions. https://core.ac.uk/download/pdf/8103328.pdf (accessed on 5th August 2025).

19. Kornecki, A. (2011). Current status of breast ultrasound. https://core.ac.uk/download/pdf/82627972.pdf (accessed on 5th August 2025).

20. Kramer, T. (2024). Bronchoscopic confocal laser endomicroscopy for lung cancer diagnosis: Shining light on advanced needle techniques. https://core.ac.uk/download/604743947.pdf (accessed on 5th August 2025).

21. Lim, A., O'Neil, B., Dechet, C., Heilbrun, M. E., & Lowrance, W. T. (2012). The contemporary role of renal mass biopsy in the management of small renal tumors. https://core.ac.uk/download/pdf/82846186.pdf (accessed on 5th August 2025).

22. Maher, M. M., O'Connor, O. J., O'Neill, S. B., Ryan, D., et al. (2011). Interventional radiology and the care of the oncology patient. https://core.ac.uk/download/pdf/8631075.pdf (accessed on 5th August 2025).

23. Marks, C. G., & Rapelyea, J. A. (2017). Breast ultrasound past, present, and future. https://core.ac.uk/download/322432873.pdf (accessed on 5th August 2025).

24. N/A. (2002). Focal Spot, Summer 2002. https://core.ac.uk/download/129069324.pdf (accessed on 5th August 2025).

25. N/A. (2021). Advancements and Breakthroughs in Ultrasound Imaging. https://core.ac.uk/download/478140644.pdf (accessed on 5th August 2025).

26. Ng, C. S. H., & Yuan, E. Q. (2020). Role of hybrid operating room: Present and future. https://core.ac.uk/download/322446162.pdf (accessed on 5th August 2025).

27. Norbash, A. M., Schreiber, D. A., Shak, D. B., Yip, R., et al. (2019). An open-source 7-axis, robotic platform to enable dexterous procedures within CT scanners. http://arxiv.org/abs/1903.04646 (accessed on 5th August 2025).

28. Shar, B. (2017). Dual-camera infrared guidance for computed tomography biopsy procedures. https://core.ac.uk/download/211502416.pdf (accessed on 5th August 2025).
29. Sherwani, A. M. (2016). Comparison of management and treatment options for recurrent breast fibroadenomas in adolescent females. https://core.ac.uk/download/142068381.pdf (accessed on 5th August 2025).
30. van Riel, L. A. M. J. G. (2024). Illuminating the pathway: For image-guided prostate cancer care. https://core.ac.uk/download/604736714.pdf (accessed on 5th August 2025).
31. Zadravec, D., Tomašković, I., Pezelj, I., & Novosel, L. (2018). Početna iskustva u usporedbi CT-vođene radiofrekventne i mikrovalne ablacije u terapiji karcinoma bubrega. https://core.ac.uk/download/481944651.pdf (accessed on 5th August 2025).

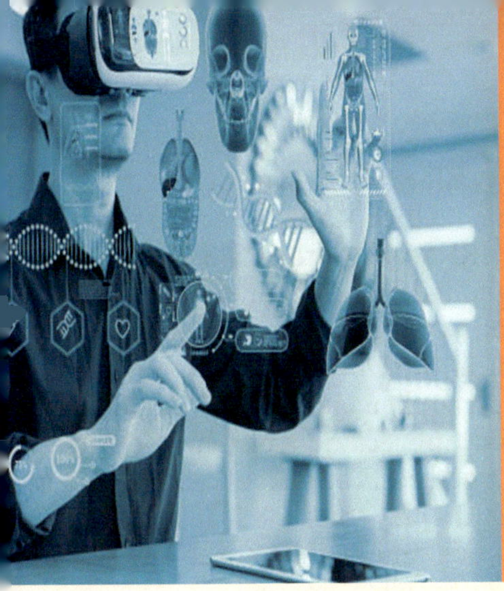

Chapter 6

3D RECONSTRUCTION, PRINTING, AND VIRTUAL REALITY IN MEDICAL IMAGING

Contents

Introduction

In the last couple of years, the use of technology in healthcare has experienced dramatic advances, particularly in medical imaging, 3D reconstruction, and printing. These technological developments have transformed how medical professionals receive, interpret, and use patient data, enhancing diagnostic and treatment processes. 3D reconstruction facilitates the development of highly accurate three-dimensional images from two-dimensional image data, making complex anatomical structures easier to comprehend for clinicians and patients alike. Such a change is also essential for personalizing medical procedures, as it yields deeper insight into the individual patient's anatomy. In addition, the use of virtual reality (VR) technologies alongside 3D models enhances the relationship between healthcare professionals and patients, enabling improved education and preoperative planning. 3D printing has become a cutting-edge technology in medicine, and even more so in the production of personalized medical devices, implants, and anatomical models. The ability to produce personalized products can positively influence patient outcomes because the devices will be tailored to patients' individual needs. For instance, in dentistry, technological advancements have enhanced practices in prosthodontics and oral implantology, enabling the manufacture of patient-tailored implants with flawless integration (Tian et al., 2021). Efficient material use and geometric complexity underscore the relevance of 3D printing in the clinical environment. While it holds great promise, issues such as high cost and post-processing requirements remain, necessitating ongoing technological advancements. Another technology with a novel aspect in medical technology convergence is augmented reality (AR), which enhances real-world observations by combining virtual information. Its application in medical robotics has gained traction in recent years, particularly under the umbrella of robot-assisted surgery and rehabilitation systems. AR provides surgeons with enhanced visualization and spatial awareness during intricate operations, making it possible for more precise interventions (Makhataeva et al., 2020). The integration of AR with 3D imaging modalities is an exciting field for augmenting surgical and therapeutic interventions. Issues such as environment mapping and camera localization are still barriers. Overcoming these barriers is essential to the continued evolution of AR in medical imaging. With further research and development, the potential for these technologies to revolutionize healthcare delivery and patient outcomes is vast.

6.1. The Role of 3D Reconstruction in Medical Imaging

The advent of 3D reconstruction technology has transformed the practice of medical imaging, enabling unparalleled visualization and interaction with anatomical structures. The technology allows the transformation of two-dimensional medical images, such as those from CT and MRI scans, into full 3D models that offer enhanced insight into patient-specific anatomy. The reconstruction will become critical in both preoperative planning and intraoperative management by enabling a more detailed appreciation of complicated physiological structures. For instance, surgeons will move and display these 3D models to practice operations, thus reducing the risks of operative procedures while improving outcomes for the patient (Figure 6.1).

As the medical field is progressively embracing this technology, it is clear that 3D reconstruction is not only an evolution but, in fact, a significant modality in offering precision medicine and increasing surgical accuracy. Beyond its application in surgical planning, 3D reconstruction is also extremely important in diagnostic imaging and treatment planning. The ability to create accurate, patient-specific models allows clinicians to assess complex conditions such as congenital heart defects more effectively. Not only do such models improve the assessment of anatomical malformations, but they also enable the simulation of various treatment interventions and help healthcare practitioners select the most appropriate therapy. For example, patient-specific three-dimensional models in congenital cardiac surgery facilitate prediction of the complexity of each case, enabling optimized interventions to accommodate patient-specific anatomical diversity. Through enhanced diagnostic effectiveness, 3D reconstruction enables improved, tailored treatment planning, thereby improving patient care. Also, with continuous technological progress, the application of virtual reality (VR) and augmented reality (AR) in 3D reconstruction holds massive potential to yet further revolutionize medical imaging. For instance, computer programs like ARBrain apply advanced AR technologies to 3D visualize brain tumors, enhancing interaction and accuracy in medical assessments and interventions. Such advancements indicate more interactive and immersive research approaches in surgical procedures. As pointed out, 3D reconstruction integrated with AR and VR technologies redefines how doctors engage with spatial anatomy to visually examine and manipulate structures in real time. The engagement not only enhances education access for medical practitioners but also improves patient understanding and involvement in treatment processes. The synergic association between 3D reconstruction and virtual reality technologies thus promises to redefine medical imaging's future horizon.

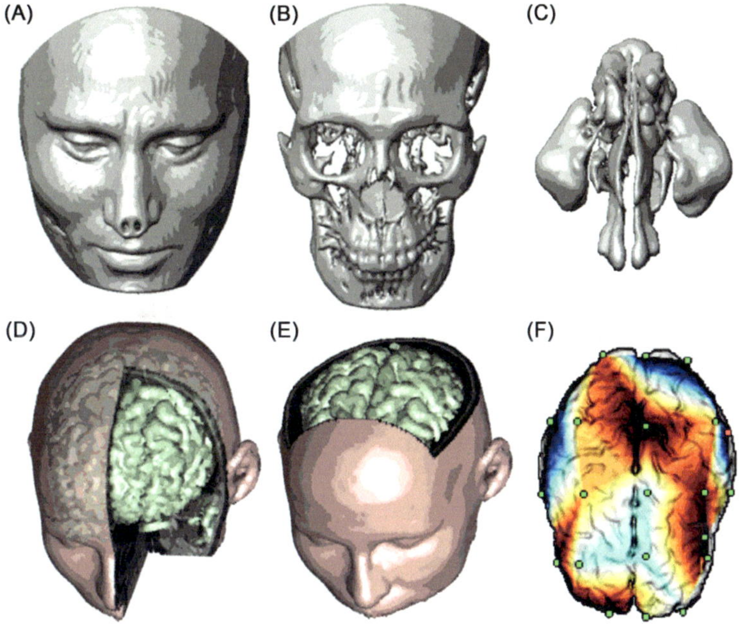

Figure 6.1. Three-dimensional visualization of medical images and signals.

Source: https://www.bem.fi/bem/research/medimag/image6.gif.

6.1.1. Techniques Used in 3D Reconstruction

The techniques applied in 3D reconstruction are diverse and application-specific, catering to the needs of various medical imaging applications. Volume rendering is one of the primary methods that produces a 3D image based on a stack of 2D cross-sectional images obtained through modalities such as computed tomography (CT) or magnetic resonance imaging (MRI). This technique allows visualization of internal structures in a detailed and perceptive manner, making it particularly valuable for diagnosing complex diseases. Also, algorithms for image segmentation have significantly improved the accuracy of 3D models, enabling more precise separation of anatomical structures. Medical professionals can gain a deeper understanding of spatial relationships within the body using these techniques, leading to improved surgical planning and patient outcomes. In 3D printing, several technologies facilitate the transformation of computer models into physical objects, with significant benefits for healthcare. Stereolithography and selective laser sintering are two of these with unique strengths based on material properties and resolution (Figure 6.2).

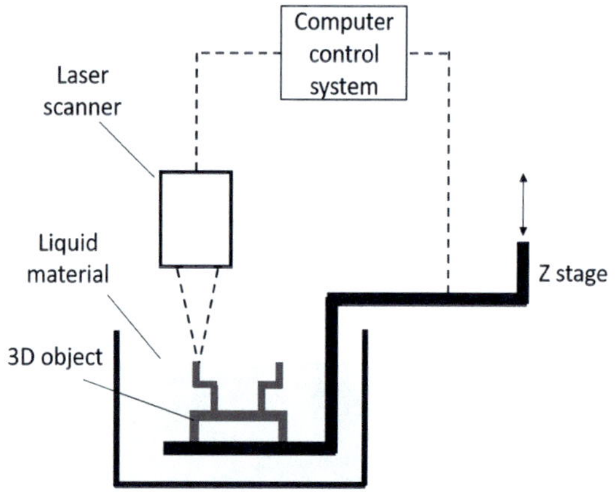

Figure 6.2. A review of stereolithography: processes and systems.

https://pub.mdpi-res.com/processes/processes-08-01138/article_deploy/html/images/processes-08-01138-g001-550.jpg?1602280180.

Stereolithography utilizes photopolymerization methods to produce high-resolution, precise models well suited for intricate structures, which can be critical in applications such as dentistry and prosthetics. Selective laser sintering, on the other hand, utilizes powdered materials to form solid and durable structures that can potentially withstand functional loading. As discussed, 3D printing methods have strengths of high material utilization and the ability to create a single complex geometry, but are linked to weaknesses of high cost and labor-intensive post-processing (Tian et al., 2021). This complex interplay of processes places the innovative potentiality of 3D reconstruction and printing on the pedestal of an accelerator of medical progress. A second essential aspect of 3D reconstruction is the use of advanced visualization techniques that enable more detailed interpretation of medical data. These techniques employ both 3D and 2D visualizations, each tailored to different audiences and applications. For instance, 2D visualizations can be more appropriate for experts performing detailed radiological examinations as they emphasize delicate details in anatomy relevant to diagnosis. On the other hand, 3D visualizations give more anatomical context and are therefore more suitable for non-specialists in forensic analysis or in a court of law. Annotation and layering methods further enhance such visualizations, making key conclusions easy to emphasize. The application of 3D printing and virtual reality helps make this process smoother, enhancing comprehension and understanding among stakeholders and making complex medical information more useful (Ebert et al., 2021). Through a combination of these techniques, medical imaging can transform raw data into valuable, informative information.

6.1.2. Benefits of 3D Reconstruction for Diagnosis

Applying 3D reconstruction technology to medical imaging significantly improves diagnostic capabilities, providing physicians with detailed anatomical images that surpass those of standard 2D imaging. By transforming volumetric data into interactive 3D models, physicians can better visualize complex anatomical structures, which aids in the precise positioning of abnormalities. The reconstructed images allow physicians to make a more comprehensive diagnosis of conditions such as tumors, fractures, and congenital deformities, thereby facilitating timely and correct diagnoses (Figure 6.3).

The ability to visualize and manipulate these models improves image interpretation, enabling more effective communication among medical teams and more informed clinical decision-making. These developments emphasize the paradigm shift in diagnostic practice enabled by 3D reconstruction, ultimately improving patient outcomes and reducing treatment options. Secondly, the use of 3D reconstruction advances personalized medicine through the ability to provide tailored diagnostic strategies based on anatomy within individual patients. By reconstructing each patient's anatomical data, physicians can create models that closely match the condition's idiosyncrasies. This level of detail not only aids diagnosis but also serves a crucial role in pre-surgical planning. Surgeons can use these accurate models to plan operations, anticipate complications, and refine surgical approaches, making surgery safer and more efficient. The insights gained from customized models are directly correlated with enhanced surgical precision and improve understanding of complex pathologies, making treatment strategies more patient-specific and ultimately leading to improved healthcare outcomes. In addition to improving diagnostic and surgical precision, 3D reconstruction can enhance educational and training procedures in the medical field. Medical professionals apply 3D models to visualize better and understand human anatomy, facilitating greater learning opportunities for medical students and doctors. Interactive training devices enable students to explore anatomical variations not visually apparent in traditional textbooks or 2D illustrations, thereby enriching the learning process. Furthermore, the development of virtual reality technology, when combined with 3D reconstruction, allows for interactive training spaces in which health professionals can practice procedures in artificial settings. Through the application of this new technique, not only is confidence boosted, but the future generation of clinicians is also capable of managing complex cases, revolutionizing medical diagnostics and treatment education as well as applied applications, thus becoming an essential component of modern medical imaging practice.

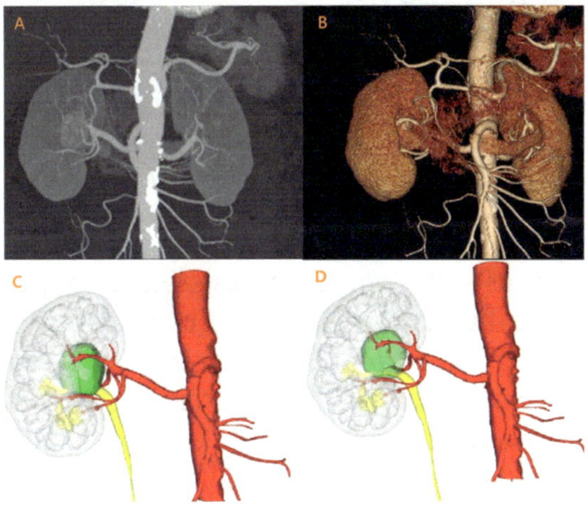

Figure 6.3. Conventional CTA and 3D reconstruction demonstrated a tumor located at the renal hilum. (a); Conventional CTA image could identify extrarenal arteries and the tumor, and sometimes the intrarenal artery branches, but failed to illustrate the relationship between tumor and its feeding arteries (b); Conventional 3D reconstruction based on the CTA could reveal the relationship between kidney, tumor and extrarenal arteries, but it typically present kidney, tumor and renal vessels as opaque, which makes it impossible to visualize the intrarenal anatomy and tumor feeding arteries. c-d the 3D reconstruction images in our study included transparent kidney and 3D course of extra- and intrarenal tumor feeding arteries (c); and 3D surface rendered semitransparent renal tumor, which makes it possible to show the target feeding arteries all around the tumor (d).

Source: https://www.researchgate.net/publication/341191129/figure/fig1/AS:962870569340977@1606577641815/Conventional-CTA-and-3D-reconstruction-demonstrated-a-tumor-located-at-the-renal-hilum-a.png.

6.1.3. Case Studies Showcasing Successful Applications

In recent years, the integration of 3D reconstruction and printing in medical imaging has revolutionized treatment planning and surgical outcomes, particularly in orthopedic applications (Figure 6.4).

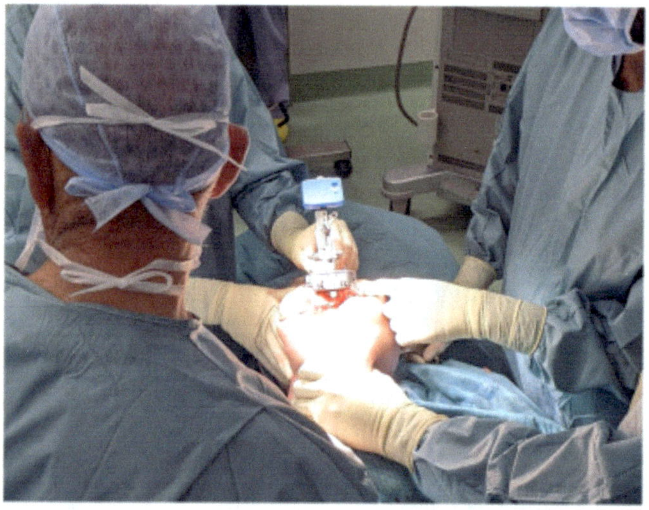

Figure 6.4. Computer-assisted orthopedic surgery (CAOS) system.

Source: https://ars.els-cdn.com/content/image/3-s2.0-B978012824481400010X-f27-11-9780128244814.jpg.

One such instance involved the use of Computer-Assisted Orthopedic Surgery (CAOS) systems that enhance precision in the treatment of musculoskeletal disorders. In one instance, surgeons used advanced volumetric imaging data from CT scans to create customized surgical guides and implants that were anatomically compatible with the patients' structures. The customized approach significantly reduced surgery times and improved post-operative recovery. The effectiveness of such applications further validates the high potential of CAOS technology, as it enables practitioners to use surgical navigation systems and mechanical instruments that adapt to individual patient anatomy, resulting in more effective treatment outcomes and, ultimately, enhanced patient safety and satisfaction (Kalová et al., 2019). Another remarkable case study illustrating the effectiveness of 3D printing in medical imaging involves the field of congenital heart disease. As death rates for this patient population continue to fall, requiring innovative solutions capable of enhancing surgical planning as well as patient management remains a pressing concern. A strong example reveals how engineering patients' hearts into 3D replicas helped cardiothoracic surgeons see intricate anatomical details before surgery. Such accurate models improved inter-team communication and significantly improved surgical precision. In one instance, a model was created to replicate a patient's unique cardiac malformations, enabling the operating team to develop an improved intervention plan. This groundbreaking use of 3D printing not only enhances training and education for healthcare professionals but also makes the experience more interactive and informed for patients and caregivers (Anwar et al., 2018). The impact of VR technology also contributes to advances in 3D reconstruction and printing. Case studies show how VR has been utilized for preoperative planning and intraoperative navigation in providing surgeons with a profound and interactive comprehension of intricate anatomy. For instance, one surgical team employed VR simulations to practice cardiovascular procedures with intricate blood vessel courses. This training phase was immensely beneficial as it improved the general performance of teams in actual surgery, yielding higher success rates and less complication. The evolution of these technologies has driven a significant paradigm shift in surgical practice, medical education, and patient interactions. Through improved visualization and real-time engagement with anatomical structures, VR can transform how healthcare professionals prepare for surgical interventions and optimize treatment approaches (Anwar et al., 2018).

6.2. Advances in 3D Printing Technology

The practice of medical imaging has been revolutionized by the most recent advancements in the 3D printing technology, allowing for increasingly accurate patient-specific models to be created. The use of various imaging modalities, i.e., MRI and CT scans, enables highly informative 3D reconstructions with precise delineation of pathological anatomy. These models have revolutionized surgical planning by providing surgeons with a tool to hold their hands while representing complex anatomy, thereby improving their understanding and management of surgical procedures. With these tailored models, clinicians can simulate surgical procedures, thereby enhancing their confidence and precision during surgery. This has a critical bearing in neurosurgery, where the complexity of cranial anatomy can complicate interventions (Figure 6.5).

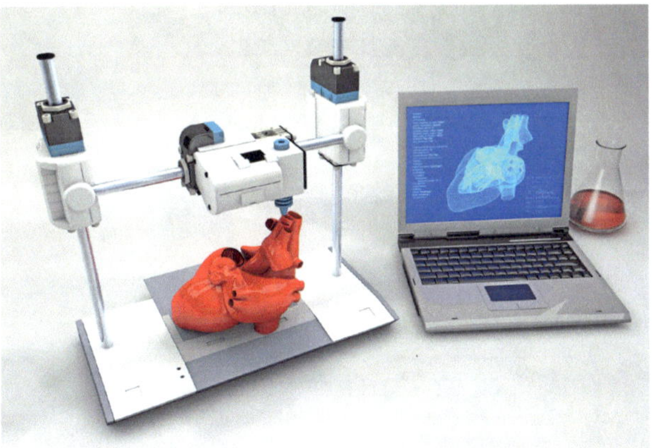

Figure 6.5. Medical 3D printing.

Source: https://www.3ds.com/assets/invest/2022-06/medical-3d-printing-tiny.jpg.

As highlighted by recent research, realistic visualization of neuroanatomical features has been proven to be beneficial in outcomes and reducing complications, further underlining the revolutionary capabilities of 3D printing technology in clinical use (İlkay et al., 2024). Further, the combination of artificial intelligence (AI) with 3D printing technology further raised the limits of clinical use. Artificial intelligence computer codes facilitate real-time analysis of imaging data and enhance the accuracy of 3D model development, leading to tailored individualized solutions for patients. The advances enable high-definition holography that is interactive and responsive to user input, thereby making interactive medical education and patient interactions possible. With the integration of AI and 3D printing, healthcare professionals can not only improve surgical education but also improve patient education through interactive and comprehensible 3D models. The uses are not restricted to surgery but extend to patient education and rehabilitation, where technologies such as these can be used to visualize the progression of disease or healing, ultimately leading to more well-informed decision-making within clinical practice (Reddy et al., 2024). Despite these promising developments, challenges remain to the widespread adoption of 3D printing technologies in healthcare. Among the biggest of these are defining standard operating procedures for model creation, regulations about how printed products will be used in the clinic, and the need for complete integration of the technology into existing workflows. The cost of buying and maintaining advanced 3D printing machines and artificial intelligence applications is a significant hurdle to adoption for some facilities. Surmounting these hurdles requires co-operation among surgeons, engineers, and regulatory bodies to develop a platform that offers safety and effectiveness. Research and development is key to surmounting these shortcomings, offering the optimal environment in which to implant such advancements into standard medical procedures, instilling improved surgical outcomes and patient care outcomes, as proven in groundbreaking uses in neurosurgery and beyond (İlkay et al., 2024).

6.2.1. Materials Used in Medical 3D Printing

The advent of 3D printing in the medical field has been propelled by the development of a diverse array of materials, each tailored to meet the specific requirements of various applications (Figure 6.6).

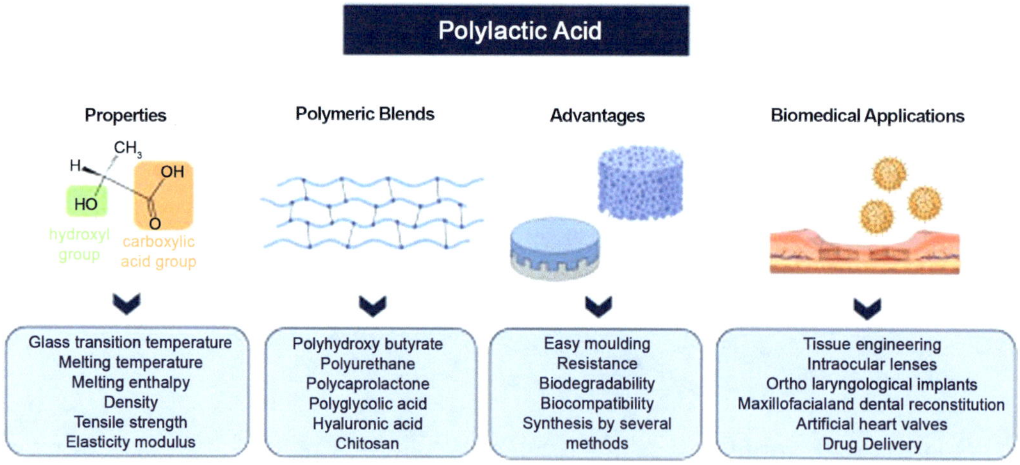

Figure 6.6. Polylactic acid (PLA) for biomedical applications.

Source: https://ars.els-cdn.com/content/image/1-s2.0-S0022286024007634-ga1.jpg.

Biocompatible polymers such as PLA and PCL are commonly used to manufacture anatomical models and surgical guides due to their ease of printing and non-toxicity. These enable visualization of complex anatomical details, thereby facilitating preoperative planning and patient communication. Further, advances in materials science have enabled the introduction of tailored compounds that provide additional functionalities, such as enhanced mechanical performance or tailored degradation rates, in tissue engineering. Such a choice is particularly valid in cardiovascular applications, where biomaterials' compatibility with body tissues and structural integrity are key parameters for successful surgery. Metallic materials, specifically titanium and its alloys, are gaining traction in medical 3D printing, especially for orthopedic implants and dental purposes. Their improved mechanical strength, wear resistance, and biocompatibility offer several advantages in load-bearing conditions, offering longevity and stability when implanted in the human body. Technological advancements in powder bed fusion have enabled manufacturing with high precision, enabling intricate geometries that closely emulate the unique anatomical details of individual patients. Further, the ability to selectively control porosity in these implants enhances biointegration and osseointegration, thereby improving implant functionality. This congruence of material and application underscores the necessity for further research into customized materials in line with the dynamic processes of repair and regeneration within the human organism, particularly in complex surgical interventions, as described in new research in cardiac anatomy and allied operations (Chen et al., 2025). Furthermore, the use of advanced composite materials, such as ceramic and polymer hybrids, is also opening new possibilities in 3D printing in medicine. The composites could mimic the mechanical properties of bone, which would be ideally suited for reconstructive surgery or trauma repair. Incorporating bioactive ceramics, for instance, enables cell adhesion and differentiation, thereby enhancing the healing process. These combination materials leverage the strengths of each component and deliver greater performance and flexibility across a broad array of clinical scenarios. Additionally, resin materials, particularly stereolithography materials, are also gaining wider use for creating highly detailed models that enable surgeons to view and rehearse complex cases in a virtual environment before actual surgery. As can be seen from the materials used in medical 3D printing, innovation is the only constant, and customization, biocompatibility, and innovation remain at the center of both research and applications aimed at enhancing patient outcomes (Hsia, 2021).

6.2.2. Customization of Medical Devices Through 3D Printing

Customization of medical devices through 3D printing is a groundbreaking advancement in medicine, particularly for patient-specific therapies. Conventional manufacturing techniques typically rely on generic models that may not fully meet a patient's unique anatomical needs. 3D printing, on the other hand, allows the creation of intricate structures tailored to the precise measurement of a patient's anatomy, enhancing the performance of medical devices and implants (Figure 6.7).

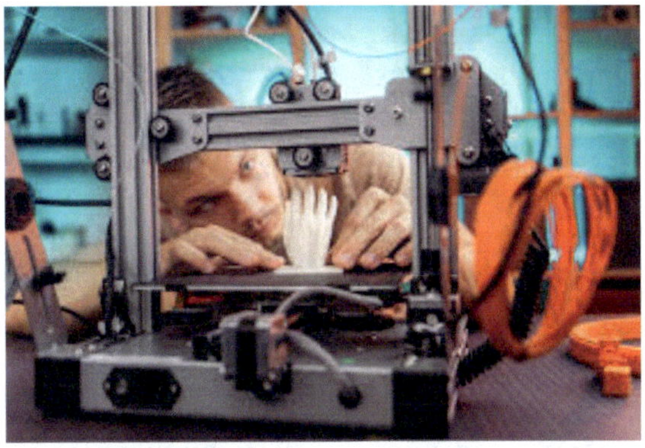

Figure 6.7. 3D printing in medical device design.

Source: Vantage Medtech.

This modernization is especially noteworthy in fields such as oral and maxillofacial surgery, where precision medicine ideas are the focal point. With the medical field embracing these new technologies, medical device customization not only optimizes patient outcomes but also streamlines surgery, resulting in enhanced care delivery systems and overall patient satisfaction (Zoabi et al., 2022). Additionally, 3D printing technology enables the creation of point-of-care treatment facilities, where surgical teams can engage directly in medical device design and production. The close coupling of clinical workflows with surgical teams enables faster prototyping of specialized devices for real-time surgical environments. Trauma surgery, orthognathic correction, and total joint arthroplasty are such classic examples of surgeries where this technology can significantly impact treatment protocols. The flexibility and speed of additive manufacturing allow practitioners to adjust their techniques to meet patients' current needs, ensuring each treatment is as effective and specific as possible. Such advancements indicate the extent to which 3D printing has a fundamental impact on not just single-patient care but on the medical model in general (Zoabi et al., 2022). In addition to reforming surgical practice, customization of medical devices using 3D printing-based technology supports pre-procedural planning, training, and education. By creating accurate anatomical models from patient-specific information, medical practitioners can conduct effective preoperative assessment and practice complex procedures prior to surgery. This rehearsal method not only improves surgical accuracy but also maintains the surgical team's morale, ultimately resulting in improved clinical outcomes. Secondly, the use of 3D-printed models in medical education enables hands-on training, allowing students and residents to practice procedures in risk-free conditions. Combined, these advances constitute a shift towards more personalized medical education and procedural training, being a prime example of the revolutionary potential of 3D printing to transform medical practices and improve patient care.

6.2.3. Regulatory Considerations for 3D Printed Medical Products

The emergence of 3D printing technology in the medical field poses significant regulatory challenges that must be addressed to ensure patient safety and product efficacy. The regulatory bodies, such as the Food and Drug Administration (FDA), have stipulations under which 3D-printed medical devices are classified based on their use and the hazards they present. The integration of this technology requires a holistic regulatory strategy that addresses the complexities of producing personalized medical devices, such as patient-specific implants or anatomical models. Compliance is not only about demonstrating safety and effectiveness through rigorous pre-market testing but also about continued post-market monitoring to ensure products align with evolving standards (Figure 6.8).

As 3D printing technologies evolve, so will the need to reform regulatory systems to facilitate innovation while keeping patient welfare as a priority. In examining the regulatory framework for 3D-printed healthcare products, the use of quality management systems is a sine qua non. These systems govern the practices and procedures that manufacturers must use to make their products conform to stated safety and quality standards at all times. The regulatory authorities emphasize good manufacturing practices for the fabrication of 3D printed devices. This includes significant documentation of design, manufacturing, and test protocols, as well as a defined risk management process to assess and mitigate the recognized hazards of new medical technologies. In handling specific applications, such as those within cardiovascular medicine, companies must also handle the unique challenges associated with bioprinting technologies, whose introduction necessitates new regulatory pathways towards the management of living tissues and their complexities, thus emphasizing the necessity to maintain high levels of strict quality controls throughout the product lifecycle (Chachques et al., 2020). Moreover, the large-scale deployment of 3D-printed medical devices necessitates collaboration among regulatory agencies, manufacturers, and clinicians to adopt a common approach to safety and performance. Incorporating healthcare professionals from the early stages of product development ensures that regulatory frameworks reflect the real-world experience and clinical needs that determine device performance. This joint effort not only enables the effective commercialization of new medical products but also helps develop guidance documents that clearly lay out regulatory requirements for different 3D printing applications. As the technology continues to advance, regular dialogue among stakeholders will be essential to addressing emerging issues such as intellectual property rights, data security, and the potential for counterfeiting along the supply chain. With this multifaceted dialogue, stakeholders can ensure that 3D printed medical devices are given regulatory attention corresponding to technological advancements and the evolving nature of medical therapy (Burity et al., 2014).

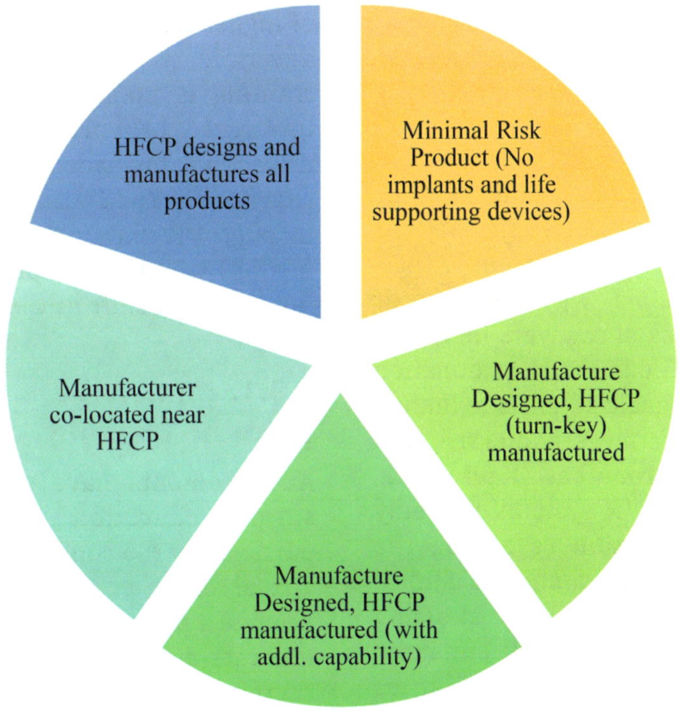

Figure 6.8. 3D printing and regulatory considerations.

Source: https://media.springernature.com/lw685/springer-static/image/chp%3A10.1007%2F978-3-031-34119-9_3/MediaObjects/525940_1_En_3_Fig3_HTML.png.

6.3. Virtual Reality in Medical Training

In the context of medical education, the integration of VR technologies is a paradigm shift from traditional learning models. The technology is sufficiently advanced to immerse students in realistic simulations of anatomy and surgery that enhance their understanding of anatomy and surgery, without the accompanying ethical and logistical challenges of cadaveric dissection, traditionally the cornerstone of anatomical training (Figure 6.9).

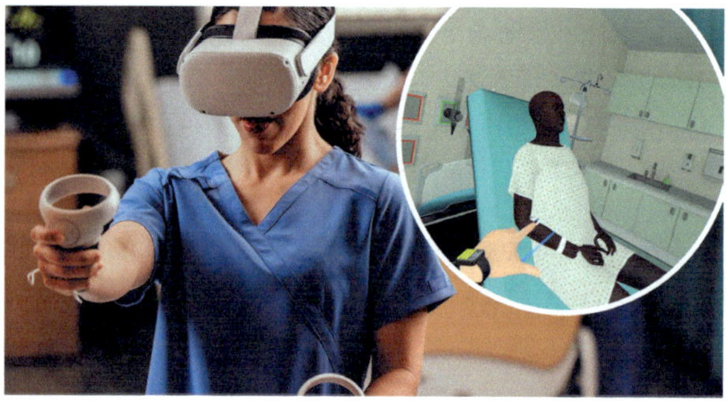

Figure 6.9. Virtual reality in healthcare.

Source: https://smarttek.solutions/wp-content/uploads/vr-for-medical.jpg.

For instance, virtual dissection tables offer students an interactive surface on which they can manipulate and explore 3D anatomical shapes, an interaction not feasible with diagrams or static images. As the lack of cadavers increases due to ethical considerations as well as donation rates, VR and AR are valuable adjuncts to human dissections and create a more immersive and inclusive learning environment (Ravi et al., 2022). Apart from that, VR systems not only offer anatomical information regarding the human body but also offer training in clinical skills within a risk-free setting. By allowing repeated practice of procedures, VR enhances students' psychomotor skills and solidifies muscle memory, an important factor for success in real-world clinical situations. Augmented reality technology is also being implemented in robotic surgical training, enabling learners to visualize and interact with the operating scene in real time. Through this interactive platform, complicated surgeries can gain training methods that might otherwise not have sufficient depth perception and spatial relations required (Makhataeva et al., 2020). The ability to use VR in simulated settings not only improves students' surgical competencies but also boosts their confidence upon transferring to actual patient scenarios. In addition, VR modalities of training cover a significant section of group learning, facilitating joint working among medical professionals. Virtual settings can support multiple users, enabling real-time communication and interaction, which is essential in healthcare, where interprofessional collaboration is paramount. Since medical teams often must operate under high pressure, training in unison in a managed VR environment cultivates a sense of group dynamics and prepares them for collective decision-making in real operations. With schools and institutions of higher learning continuing to embrace these advanced technologies, the future of medical training is poised for a revolution, moving toward a hybrid practice that values traditional dissection alongside modern virtual substitutes (Ravi et al., 2022). In the end, its optimization through VR may yield better results for both medical training and patient care, indicating a fundamental shift in the practice of medicine.

6.3.1. Immersive Simulations for Surgical Training

Advancements have significantly influenced surgical education in immersive simulating, particularly the combination of augmented and virtual reality technologies. These developments provide a platform for surgeons to engage with intricate anatomy in three-dimensional space, thereby enhancing their understanding and expertise across varied surgical procedures. Previous techniques primarily employ cadavers or two-dimensional imaging, which could confine an overreaching appreciation of fine details. Using 3D reconstruction techniques, individual patient-specific models can be created to facilitate patient-specific training for medical educators. Not only does this breakthrough in training technique improve surgical skill, but it also advances patient safety by reducing the occurrence of procedural errors, underscoring the value of immersive simulation as a key educational tool for modern surgical practice (Figure 6.10).

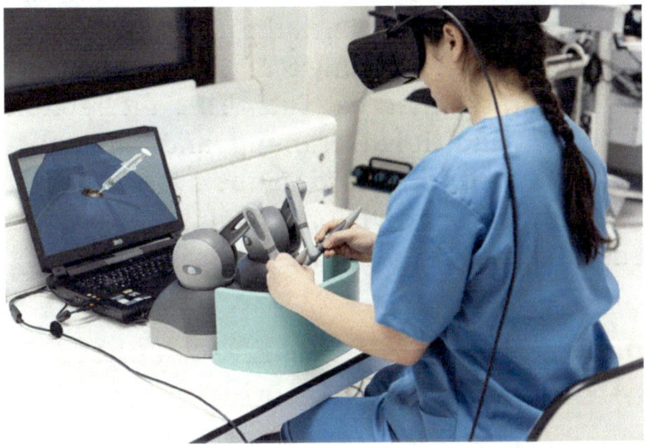

Figure 6.10. Immersive simulations for anatomical exploration.

Source: https://smarttek.solutions/wp-content/uploads/vr-for-surgical-training-1920x1280.jpeg.

The application of immersive simulation extends beyond mere anatomical exploration, serving as a key component in surgical planning and execution. For instance, in oral and maxillofacial surgery, augmented reality enables the superimposition of digital imaging onto a patient's anatomy, facilitating unambiguous surgical navigation during procedures. This technology enables surgeons to see the surgical field, improving their spatial understanding and decision-making during challenging procedures. The very immersive quality of these simulations not only enables a more profound knowledge of the surgical terrain but also sharpens technical skills through repeated practice in a risk-free setting. Studies have proven that virtual reality platform-based training can significantly improve hand dexterity and overall performance, making it a valuable and efficient alternative to traditional training in surgical education (Ayoub et al., 2019). Furthermore, immersive simulations hold promises not only in education but also in patient education and in surgical consultation. Using augmented reality apps, patients can view their planned surgery more tangibly, enhancing understanding and confidence in the operation. This interactive approach also reduces patient fear and increases compliance, as the patient learns the steps involved in their treatment. Moreover, the approach was demonstrated in creating accessible augmented reality programs for veterinary training, as noted in current research, which highlights the versatility of these technologies in medicine education (Christ et al., 2018). As patient and surgical education continue to improve, the inclusion of immersive simulations holds promise for the future, poised to change the landscape of medical practice.

6.3.2. Enhancing Patient Education Through VR

The incorporation of VR into the study of medicine has the potential to transform how patients understand their medical conditions and treatments. By placing patients in a simulated environment, healthcare professionals can easily demonstrate complicated medical concepts in an easy-to-understand format. This simulated experience enables the patient to see anatomical structures and surgical nuances within a 3D system, making them more participative and active in the healthcare process. As technology continues to grow, VR platforms are becoming more advanced and providing individualized scenarios that specifically tackle personal patient concerns. Personalized education has the potential to improve patient satisfaction and treatment plan adherence, ultimately leading to better health outcomes. By altering traditional learning mechanisms, VR not only enhances patient understanding but also enables individuals to play an active role in their healthcare experience. Secondly, VR enables greater communication between doctors and patients, reducing gaps inherent in descriptions based on word-of-mouth. This new approach to education enables a shared visual language, allowing clinicians to explain ailments such as congenital heart disease using detailed animations and simulations. As highlighted by research, the great synergy between visuals and experiential learning helps greatly enhance patient understanding (Anwar et al., 2018). Patients are better positioned to recall and have confidence in their treatment options when they can experience procedures virtually (Figure 6.11).

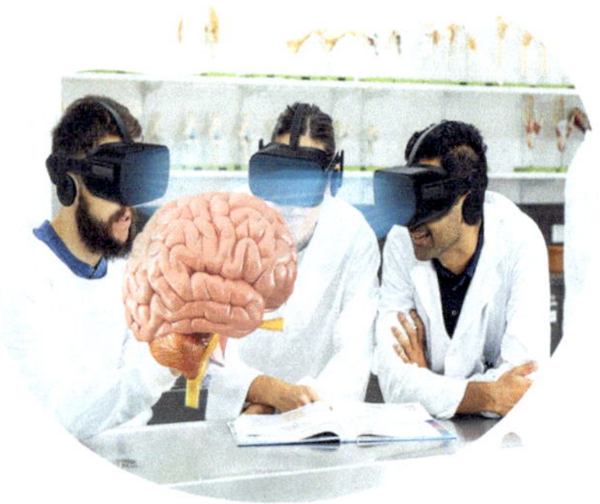

Figure 6.11. Virtual reality applications in medical education.

Source: https://www.ixrlabs.com/blog/assets/admin/uploads/Virtual-Reality-Applications-in-Medical-Education.png.

This is particularly significant in the more complicated cases, where easy explanations are insufficient. The end result is an educated patient group, more capable of having meaningful conversations with their caregivers. Through this mutualistic process, VR enables more participatory care aligned with patient preferences and supports shared decision-making. In addition to one-to-one patient education, VR holds high potential for training the next generation of healthcare providers. Simulation of real-world clinics gives healthcare trainees a chance to practice communication and ethical decision-making without risk, removing the harm associated with real experiences. Incorporating VR-based problem-solving, learners can engage with top-level visualization tools to support their learning of anatomy and procedural approaches. The application of 3D modeling in VR offers unprecedented insights into medical pathology, thereby enhancing the learning process (Anwar et al., 2018). With each of these new technologies supplementing the skill sets of upcoming healthcare professionals, they are becoming more and more efficient at educating their patients. This interaction between additional training and enhanced patient education improves the overall quality of healthcare provision, moving toward an educated and collaborative medical community.

6.3.3. Evaluating the Effectiveness of VR in Medical Training

The integration of VR into medical education is a paradigm shift in teaching practices. With the placement of students in virtual 3D worlds, VR technology enhances learning and offers the potential for experiential learning, which is crucial for skill acquisition. Immersive learning provides learners with an opportunity to practice diagnostic and surgical interventions in a safe environment, where mistakes can be made without patient safety at stake.

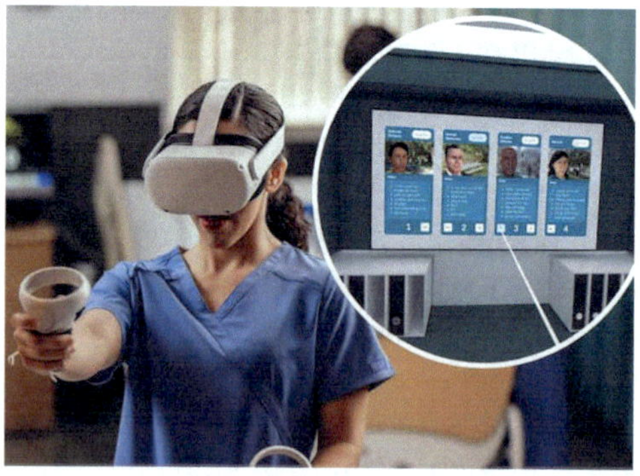

Figure 6.12. Benefits of VR simulation training for hospitals.

Source: https://laerdal.com/cdn-cgi/image/width=610,height=435,fit=crop,quality=60,format=auto/cdn-49bcb0/globalassets/images--blocks/products/virtual-products/vrclinicals-for-nursing/vrclinicals-beta-mutlipatient-prioritization.jpg.

In addition, the initial ability to replicate diverse clinical scenarios fosters critical thinking and decision-making skills, which are of paramount importance for future practitioners in high-stakes settings. Our measurement of VR's effectiveness relies on observations of learner outcomes, motivation, and retention, especially in comparison to traditional training methodologies, which may not generate equal confidence and proficiency in skills among medical learners. Another essential aspect of assessing VR in medical education is its ability to enable individualized learning experiences (Figure 6.12).

Personalized simulations, responsive to an individual learner's abilities, can enhance learning effectiveness and retention. With technology advancing alongside imaging procedures such as 3D reconstruction and printing, students may be able to engage with complex anatomy. This is paralleled by advancements in terahertz technology, which can enhance imaging capabilities and provide realistic models for VR simulations. The continued development of these technologies provides a vast training ground where students can observe complex systems before hands-on practice. The method fits the principles of healthcare 4.0 that highlight intelligent, integrated solutions that evolve in response to new educational imperatives while also presenting solutions for the difficulties of successfully integrating VR into regular curricula. In addition, challenges in applying VR to medical training must be given the attention they deserve. High development costs, the need for specialized technological infrastructure, and potential opposition from deeply rooted traditionalists within medical facilities can dampen the mass adoption of VR. While preliminary studies report encouraging findings in the skill acquisition and learner satisfaction, additional empirical evidence is necessary to solidify VR's position in the curricula of medical schools. Research needs to examine long-term outcomes, including skill retention and clinical performance in real-world practice settings. As evident from the illustration of 3D printing and augmented reality application in surgery, a proper study of VR's teaching value is essential. Strong evaluations could determine tremendous value added to customized patient care and innovation solutions in clinical training and thus enhance healthcare delivery results, as defined by Gezimati et al. (2023); José et al. (2022).

6.4. Integration of 3D Reconstruction and Printing

The integration of 3D printing and reconstruction in medical imaging is a paradigm shift for clinicians in diagnosis and treatment planning. This paradigm interaction enables clinicians to create precise anatomical models from imaging data and visualize complex structures in previously unknown ways. The transition from two-dimensional visualizations to three-dimensional perspectives enhances the understanding of anatomical relationships and pathological processes. Hence, surgeons can engage in more precise preoperative planning, tailoring their procedures to the unique morphology of individual patients. Not only does this tailored strategy accelerate surgical procedures, but it also maximizes the outcome for patients by virtue of decreased potential complications and improved overall quality of care rendered. Furthermore, 3D printing technology also supports the field of medical imaging by physically creating 3D reconstructed models. Such integration provides tangible benefits in surgical education and training, where trainees and clinicians can practice and refine their techniques using patient-specific anatomical models. By closing the gap between theoretical knowledge and practical application, 3D models printed by 3D printing technology facilitate a better understanding of complex surgical procedures and the overall proficiency of future professionals in the medical field (Figure 6.13).

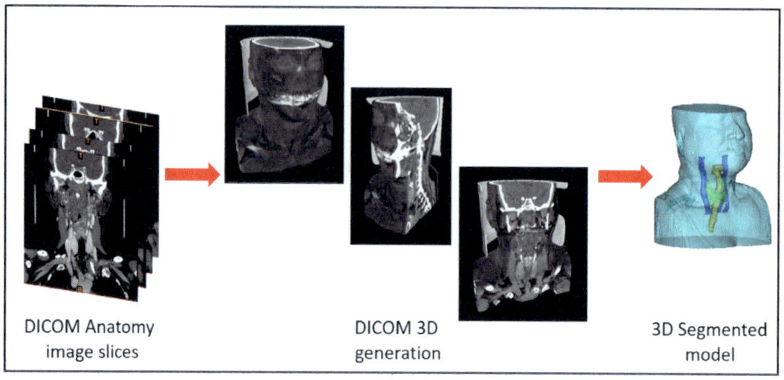

Figure 6.13. Representation of the DICOM anatomy imaging slices, illustrating the generation of the anatomy 3D generation and the correspondent segmented 3D model.

Source: https://www.mdpi.com/sensors/sensors-23-01610/article_deploy/html/images/sensors-23-01610-g003-550.jpg.

This interactive learning has the potential to increase retention and equip medical professionals with appropriate preparation for actual challenges. With increasing advances in 3D printing, the future of medical education and training holds huge and promising possibilities. Beyond surgical practice and training, the integration of augmented reality (AR) technologies with 3D reconstruction and printing is a landmark in medical imaging. AR applications will increase the perception of real-world environments by overlaying digital information on the actual world, thereby creating interactive experiences for medical professionals. For instance, AR can be applied to the use of 3D-printed models during surgery to provide real-time visual guidance based on preoperative imaging information. The convergence of technologies improves surgical precision by providing end-to-end visualization of internal structures, enhancing spatial understanding during delicate procedures. Also, as healthcare continues to rely more on such technologies, technologies for addressing challenges such as camera localization and environment mapping will be necessary to make them most effective in hospitals (Makhataeva et al., 2020). Overall, the combination of 3D reconstruction, printing, and AR holds limitless potential for medical imaging (Raul et al., 2019).

6.4.1. Workflow From Imaging to 3D Printed Models

The medical imaging-to-3D-printed model process is a sophisticated process that places great emphasis on the need for advanced imaging modalities. Data acquisition is typically an introductory process that uses high-resolution imaging technologies such as CT or MRI. Such technologies play a significant role in facilitating the acquisition of delicate anatomical structures, providing the initial data required for subsequent reconstruction. The fidelity of the resultant 3D models is greatly influenced by the quality of the imaged data, which is essential in most clinical applications. For instance, in mitral valve disease, not only is 3D imaging important for diagnostic accuracy, but also for surgical planning and construction of patient-specific models for better comprehension of intricate morphologies (Preethi et al., 2022). Hence, practical imaging is a critical first step in producing models that accurately reflect patient anatomy and pathology (Figure 6.14).

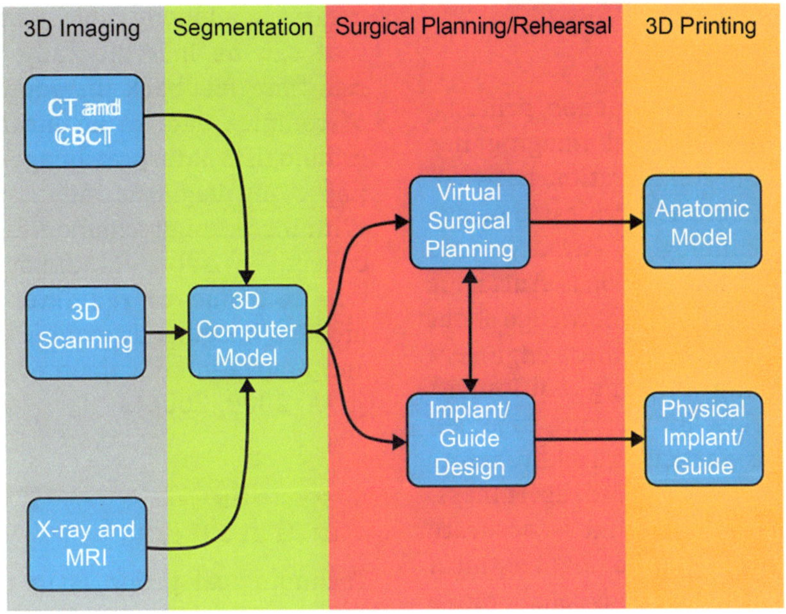

Figure 6.14. Overview of workflow from imaging to 3D printed model/implant.

Source: https://www.researchgate.net/publication/364613770/figure/fig1/AS:11431281241621623@1715203408767/Overview-of-workflow-from-imaging-to-3D-printed-model-implant.tif.

Following the acquisition of imaging data, the second process involves sophisticated reconstruction algorithms that translate the 2D image into comprehensive 3D models. The procedure involves segmentation, in which certain anatomical structures are separated from the remaining tissue and then reconstructed into three-dimensional form. Sophisticated algorithms enable the doctors to visualize precise information, which is essential for preoperative planning and simulation surgery. For instance, in pediatric heart surgery, the use of these reconstruction techniques enables surgeons to perform virtual manipulation of patient-specific cardiac structures, reducing uncertainty during actual procedures. Moreover, incorporating 3D printing capability gives such digital models a physical presence for tactile examination, enhancing preoperative planning (Hsia, 2021). Such merging of imaging, reconstruction, and printing maximizes the degree of personalization in patient treatment. The last step in this process results in the creation of the actual 3D-printed models available for use in surgical planning, education, and patient consultations. By translating digital constructs into physical form, clinicians can better understand the anatomical variations that will not be apparent with traditional imaging. For example, sophisticated models created from accurate imaging data enable new surgical methods, particularly in complex situations such as double-outlet right ventricle. This modeling, aside from promoting understanding of potential surgical alternatives, also has a dual value of facilitating patient education and participation in their own treatment procedures. With improvements in 3D printing technology, their roles in the clinical setting expand, offering new imaging modalities and preoperative surgical planning, and reducing surgical risks through detailed anatomical reconstructions (Preethi et al., 2022; Hsia, 2021). The whole process is a demonstration of how advances in medical imaging make their way into real-world applications that ultimately reach patient care.

6.4.2. Collaborative Efforts Between Radiologists and Engineers

The convergence of 3D reconstruction, printing, and virtual reality in medical imaging has increasingly relied on collaboration between radiologists and engineers. It is critical to bridge the gap between technological advancements and clinical needs, and cooperation is crucial for this purpose. Radiologists offer knowledge about patient anatomy and disease, which engineers need when designing imaging equipment and software platforms. By working together, they can dictate the particular requirements that enhance image quality and usefulness, facilitating easier creation of more accurate 3D models. Aside from improving technical proficiency in medical imaging, this collaborative process ensures that resulting innovations are appropriate to address real clinical cases. In addition, the integration of engineering principles and radiological competencies forms a symbiotic alliance that drives innovation in medical applications. For instance, when developers design new software for 3D printing, they must ensure that it effectively translates complex radiologic information into accurate physical models. This will require prompt feedback from radiologists who can provide critiques based on their experience with existing technology. Collaborative projects often lead to novel solutions, such as producing custom surgical guides or personalized prosthetics that are both feasible and clinically relevant. These technologies can significantly improve surgical outcomes, demonstrating the power of interdepartmental cooperation in advancing the frontiers of medical imaging and its uses. Moreover, the use of VR has transformed co-working between radiologists and engineers, delivering more interactive experiences and higher comprehension and interaction. Clinicians and engineers can see complex anatomy using VR models, enabling real-time discussion of design stages or technical problems. This shared virtual space enables greater innovation and creativity, allowing rapid prototyping of models that can be incrementally refined based on real-time feedback. In addition, visualization of complex data in an intuitive format helps radiologists interpret images more effectively, improving diagnosis and intervention planning. With increasing technological convergence, the collective wisdom of radiologists and engineers will continue to redefine the landscape of medical imaging, as evidenced by the research and innovation documented in studies such as (N/A, 2000, 2004).

6.4.3. Impact on Surgical Planning and Outcomes

Technological progress in three-dimensional reconstruction, printing, and virtual reality has now revolutionized surgical planning and outcomes across nearly every branch of medicine. These technologies provide visualization of intricate anatomical structures with previously unseen detail; now, surgeons can preoperatively model what occurs during real procedures. The ability to integrate preoperative 2D imaging into an immersive 3D model enables clinicians to develop tailored surgical plans that account for each patient's unique anatomy. This tailored modality not only enhances the accuracy of surgical interventions but also minimizes the risk of complications, ultimately leading to improved patient outcomes. The integration of these technologies in surgery ensures surgeons are better equipped, resulting in a more enhanced sense of confidence when operating in complex anatomical settings. Moreover, the input of 3D printing in surgical planning is even carried forward to improve surgical team communication. With 3D-printed models, tactile communication and group conversation are facilitated, allowing a mutual understanding of the surgical process required for complex cases. Emphasized in current literature is that the use of 3D printing has greatly influenced patient care by allowing surgical teams to talk in detail, facilitating an integrated solution customized based on the unique needs of every patient. Besides, the models can also act as teaching aids for surgical trainees to bridge the gap between theory and practice. By enhancing the learning process, these technologies empower future surgeons to deal with diverse clinical conditions. Moreover, the implementation of 3D technologies has demonstrated revolutionary potential in the management of congenital heart disease, with a widespread impact on surgical outcomes. With improvement in mortality rates for congenital heart disease over several decades, technologies such as 3D printing have taken center stage in creating tailored surgical possibilities, considering the complexity of every patient's case. Research has established that these technologies not only improve surgical accuracy but also streamline intraoperative decision-making with intraoperative real-time feedback. By using 3D models, surgeons can treat congenital malformations with an improved framework, hence improving their capability and patient recovery after surgery. This trend of moving forward in adopting 3D technologies is a milestone for surgical operations, reflecting the ongoing need for new inventions in caring for patients, as highlighted in today's discourse in surgical innovation (Burity et al., 2014; Anwar et al., 2018).

6.5. Challenges and Limitations

The integration of 3D reconstruction, printing, and virtual reality (VR) in medical imaging is faced with significant limitations and challenges that must be acknowledged. Perhaps the most significant limitation is the variability in imaging data quality that directly affects reconstructed 3D model accuracy and reliability. For instance, the success of computer-assisted orthopedic surgery (CAOS) systems is highly reliant on high-quality volumetric images obtained by modalities such as CT or MRI. This dependence identifies that any lack of image resolution or processing can have adverse effects on surgical planning and performance, finally causing potentially harmful outcomes in patient treatment (Kalová et al., 2019). Keeping the image quality consistent on platforms is therefore vital as variability in data can downscale the integration of advanced technologies and thereby lower their overall clinical efficacy. Another major limitation exists in the very process of 3D printed construct fabrication for medical use. While rapid prototyping technologies have advanced significantly, enabling high-accuracy prototypes in multiple materials, it is challenging to scale these processes to the point where they can be used clinically. The transition from conceptual models to fully functional medical devices requires extensive testing and verification to ensure that the 3D-printed constructs can withstand long-term biological interactions. This is particularly significant because the success of such devices would typically depend on their mechanical durability and biocompatibility. As noted, design decisions in bioengineering must be thoroughly scrutinized to address problems related to device operation within live biological systems (Andrés et al., 2012). This ongoing requirement for extensive analysis reflects the complexities involved in effectively applying 3D printing technologies in medical settings. Finally, the adjunct use of virtual reality in medical imaging also faces some challenges. Its first limitation is that it requires highly sophisticated hardware and software, which might not be readily available everywhere in healthcare settings. The availability of VR technology can vary widely, thereby creating disparities in training and procedure simulation experiences among healthcare providers. Moreover, while VR can potentially enhance visualization and interaction with the patient, the acquisition curve in using such systems might deter some practitioners from leveraging them at all levels. These factors all serve to highlight that while the promise of VR in enhancing the practice of medical imaging remains substantial, issues of adoption, accessibility, and usability remain the main hurdles to realizing the fullest extent of its potential within clinical use.

6.5.1. Technical Challenges in 3D Reconstruction and Printing

3D reconstruction and printing technology problems in medical imaging are intricate, typically being the result of hardware problems as well as software issues. Anatomical modeling accuracy is a crucial aspect in the generation of reliable prototypes. The use of high-resolution imaging techniques, e.g., CT scans and MRI, is needed to capture detailed anatomical data. Nonetheless, they tend to generate tremendous volumes of data that need very high processing abilities to construct good 3D models. Low computational power may result in an incomplete or inaccurate depiction of anatomical details, limiting its future use in surgical planning and medical education (Jarosław et al., 2022). As pointed out by numerous studies, the accuracy of such models directly affects the effectiveness of simulations used in pre-procedural training and planning, underscoring the utmost need to advance processing algorithms and hardware capabilities. Additionally, the integration of 3D printing into clinical practice introduces another set of challenges in terms of material choice and biocompatibility. Various 3D printing technologies like FDM, SLA, and SLS employ dissimilar materials like thermoplastics, photopolymers, and metal powders. Various materials possess their own mechanical properties and responses when processed in a biological tissue environment. Selecting appropriate materials that are resistant to surgical conditions and facilitate tissue compatibility is essential for creating functional implants or medical instruments (Ravi et al., 2022). Additionally, post-processing techniques required to obtain a better surface finish on printed models or to sterilize models intended for clinical use can add further layers of complexity, demanding considerable time and resource expenditures. This underscores the imperative need for standardized procedures to streamline the selection and preparation of materials used in medical 3D printing processes. Lastly, regulatory matters complicate the landscape of 3D reconstruction and printing for medical purposes. Given the patient-specific nature of 3D models and implants, there is a need to develop stringent validation and quality assurance procedures. Proof of safety and efficacy must be provided before permission for clinical use is granted by regulatory bodies, which can require time-consuming and costly testing and validation procedures. Taking research prototypes to the clinical product stage must comply with quality practices and safety standards, which may vary across jurisdictions. Thus, the evolving landscape of digital medicine demands collaboration between industry, clinicians, and regulators to establish appropriate frameworks to support innovation while ensuring patient safety and product integrity (Jarosław et al., 2022; Ravi et al., 2022). The convergence of such technical and regulatory issues highlights the complexities that must be addressed as the field of 3D reconstruction and printing continues to evolve in medical imaging.

6.5.2. Ethical Considerations in Virtual Reality Applications

The rapid development of VR technologies for medical training and imaging raises significant ethical concerns that must be scrutinized. One of the primary concerns is the desensitization of medical practitioners to highly realistic virtual simulations. The interactive nature of such simulations, as useful as it may be in training sessions, has the side effect of dulling practitioners' emotional responses to real medical cases. This desensitization can also carry over into patient interactions, diminishing empathy and compassion in critical care situations. Further, informed consent from the individuals participating in VR applications must be obtained. Participants, whether students or patients, should be clearly informed of the potential psychological impact from exposure to simulated environments and of the importance of open communication about the nature and purposes of the VR exposure, as well as any associated risks to mental health and emotional well-being. Alongside the psychological effects, data privacy and security need to be given high consideration when implementing VR in the healthcare sector. Most VR applications gather sensitive health-related data, which is stored in order to customize experiences, thereby increasing risks of data breaches. It is the developers' and healthcare providers' responsibility to implement robust data protection practices to safeguard patient data. Secondly, the threat of VR data abuse—whether through unauthorized access or interference—calls for a general ethical framework that addresses data ownership and consent. All parties need to join hands to develop standards that regulate the use of patient data in virtual reality settings to avoid privacy invasions, which can lead to losses of trust between health providers and patients. Moreover, the socioeconomic impact of applying VR technology in healthcare imaging must not be overlooked. Access to sophisticated VR applications may be limited by financial constraints, leading to inequalities in healthcare delivery. Such disparities will exacerbate existing disparities in medical training and the care of patients, particularly among marginalized communities. Ethical considerations demand that measures be instituted to make access to VR technologies available on a fair and equitable basis so that all stakeholders can benefit from enhancements in medical imaging. As applications of VR continue to expand, there is an even more urgent need to address these social determinants of health by implementing policies that promote inclusivity. This responsibility not only ensures that the advantages of virtual reality are widely accessible but also underscores the need to pursue methods that mitigate potential inequalities in the health care setting, demonstrating a commitment to ethical practice and social justice in medical care.

6.5.3. Financial Barriers to Widespread Adoption

The extended use of 3D reconstruction, printing, and virtual reality in medical imaging is limited by huge financial barriers that restrict universal adoption in health systems. Initial investments in good-quality printers and sophisticated software can be astronomical, particularly for small healthcare facilities and low-income countries. Materials cost, such as biocompatible filaments applied in 3D printing, is another element of cost that comprises mainly of budget concerns in restricting access to new imaging solutions. The financial barriers can thus further perpetuate inequalities in healthcare delivery, as less resource-constrained institutions are unable to utilize the potential benefits of advanced imaging technologies, for instance, improved diagnostics and personalized treatment plans. Furthermore, training and maintenance costs are recurring expenses that increase the economic burden of adopting these technologies. For instance, doctors and technicians need to be well-qualified to effectively use advanced software and hardware, which is an added cost and diverts time from patient care. As is evidenced across numerous industries, effective integration of technology often demands a shift in culture and operations within organizations, also straining financial resources. Organizations with limited budgets or the ability to allocate funds toward implementing technology may not sustain the momentum needed for effective implementation, eventually leading to underutilization of the potential offered by 3D reconstruction, printing, and virtual reality. Finally, the ROI of implementing 3D technologies remains questionable for most healthcare providers, particularly given the high priority placed on cost-effectiveness today. While gains might lead to better patient outcomes and process effectiveness in the long term, the short-term bottom-line impact serves as a disincentive for most organizations. Without clear signs of cost reductions and increased efficiency, decision-makers may be hesitant to invest in such cost-intensive technologies. As revealed in various studies, for instance, when examining the financial impacts of advanced technologies in forensic science and their integration challenges (Llerena et al., 2024), the healthcare sector also faces similar reluctances and uncertainties. Therefore, bridging such financial barriers is critical to enabling the widespread uptake of ground-breaking technologies in medical imaging practice (Ewart et al., 2019).

6.6. Future Trends in Medical Imaging Technologies

The evolution of medical imaging technology is significantly driven by the application of three-dimensional (3D) reconstruction techniques. They facilitate a more precise and refined observation of complex anatomical structures, thereby enhancing diagnostic accuracy. Medical professionals can more accurately evaluate patient conditions by transforming traditional two-dimensional images into 3D models, thereby improving treatment planning and surgical accuracy. One of the most important applications of 3D reconstruction is computer-assisted orthopedic surgery (CAOS) where it permits individualized surgical procedures on the basis of specific anatomical data derived from various imaging modalities like CT and MRI. This type of technology points to a significant trend in medical imaging, as the transition toward immersive and interactive systems is reshaping standards of patient care across orthopedics and other areas (Kalová et al., 2019). Further, the introduction of 3D printing into medical imaging exemplifies a transformative trend with potential for personalized medicine. With patient-specific anatomical models, healthcare professionals can perform more precise pre-surgery simulations to enhance surgical education and inter-professional communication. Not only does 3D printing help produce replicas of organs or body parts, but it also makes it possible to generate personalized implants that reduce risks from surgery and enhance overall patient experience. The technology enables rapid prototyping and iteration, allowing healthcare solutions to be customized to address the unique needs of every patient. As it continues to evolve, 3D reconstruction integrated with printing will be a key indicator of developments in medical imaging, ultimately leading to improved surgical outcomes and reduced recovery times (Burity et al., 2014). VR is another frontier on which medical imaging technologies are advancing, with groundbreaking potential for visualization and interaction with complex data. By putting healthcare professionals into a virtual environment, VR facilitates enhanced understanding of anatomical relationships and pathology and is therefore a valuable asset for training and clinical applications. The technology can enable virtual operations, allowing specialists to rehearse procedures in a risk-free environment, leading to improved confidence and performance in actual operations. Virtual reality applications also include patient participation, offering a platform for individuals to visualize their condition and planned interventions in a straightforward manner. The emergence of VR systems that allow real-time blending of imaging data from modalities such as CT or MRI heralds a new era in medical imaging, fostering collaboration among providers and patients while refining clinical decision-making (Kalová et al., 2019).

6.6.1. Innovations in 3D Reconstruction Algorithms

Advances in 3D reconstruction algorithms have significantly influenced the field of medical imaging, particularly by enhancing the accuracy and effectiveness of anatomical visualizations. The traditional methods, the majority of which were manual segmentation, are now supplemented by automated processes that employ machine learning and deep learning techniques. Such innovations facilitate more rapid processing of large data sets, for instance, from high-resolution imaging modalities such as CT or MRI scans.

Multiple, disparate data inputs can be processed by algorithms that can fuse them and produce detailed 3D reconstructions to facilitate further understanding of anatomical relations and structures, ultimately leading to better educational resources within medical education. This advancement not only simplifies healthcare practitioners' workflows but also provides more advanced graphical tools that are essential for surgical planning and diagnostics, paving the way for more innovative applications in the medical sector (Anderson et al., 2014). Recent studies have introduced new techniques, such as combining topographical 3D laser scanning with high-definition digital photography. This method captures a complete data set of anatomically relevant features without long processing times for conventional cross-sectional imaging.

The use of such techniques addresses the challenge of accurately describing complex anatomical structures and the burden of labor-intensive segmentation protocols. Combining these cutting-edge scanning technologies with advanced algorithms enables scientists to create even the most sophisticated and realistic 3D models for various applications, including educational instruction and preoperative simulation. Not only do these technologies have the capability to raise the level of fidelity within anatomical reconstructions, but a modifiable form of customizations may be created based on particular end-user needs in medical education and elsewhere (Anderson et al., 2014). Moreover, multidisciplinary teams are increasingly crucial to the development of 3D reconstruction algorithms, as evidenced by projects that combine principles of art history, archaeology, and forensic science. For example, applying 3D scanning technology to analyze ancient relics and human facial anatomy demonstrates how these diverse areas can collaborate to refine algorithmic methods. These multidisciplinary efforts enable the design of algorithms capable of handling sophisticated datasets effectively, thereby fostering in-depth exploration of contemporary and historical subjects. With the development of 3D reconstruction, it is increasingly important to leverage knowledge from various disciplines to transcend challenges such as dimension precision and feature detection. Innovations in these joint efforts not only enhance academic research but also have deep implications for practical applications in fields such as forensic analysis, biometrics, and beyond.

6.6.2. The Potential of Bioprinting in Regenerative Medicine

The discovery of bioprinting technology is a milestone in regenerative medicine with unforeseen potential for tissue engineering and organ transplantation. Bioprinting employs advanced 3D printing to create complex, living tissue by sequentially depositing cells and biomaterials. This breakthrough could help address the critical shortage of donor organs by enabling the fabrication of structures that closely resemble the intrinsic architecture of human tissues. Using patient-specific cell types, bioprinting not only yields higher compatibility but also reduces the risk of rejection, a common problem with conventional transplants. Thus, the integration of bioprinting into regenerative medicine is a groundbreaking approach, providing individualized solutions and new avenues for research and clinical practice that could radically redefine therapeutic approaches. In addition, bioprinting can potentially build complex vascular networks that are essential to the viability of engineered tissues. In addition to what was demonstrated in the last studies involving human thyroid construct bioengineering, the intricate vasculature topology has a decisive impact on nutrient diffusion and cellular performance. The study shows the successful construction of a three-dimensional bioartificial thyroid gland by exploiting the application of sophisticated computational templates in determining the development of vasculature and scaffold design.

These technologies complement ongoing developments in bioprinting techniques, enabling the fabrication of increasingly intricate tissue structures that can deliver more effective regenerative outcomes. With its ability to replicate biologically relevant microenvironments, bioprinting can offer solutions for organ replacement and the repair and regeneration of damaged tissues, providing a comprehensive approach to many diseases (Barbaro et al., 2023). In the case of reconstructive surgery, bioprinting methods have solutions for the shortcomings of traditional methods. Fibula free flaps, well-established for mandible and facial reconstructions, are complicated by donor-site morbidity and the need for precise planning. Use of bioprinted prostheses and personalized surgical templates can significantly improve patient outcomes by tailoring interventions to individual anatomical and clinical needs.

Moreover, the preoperative virtual planning and real-time intraoperative guidance would transform the field of reconstructive surgery. Reframing the routine and clinical concerns of such procedures through the lens of new bioprinting technologies could not only improve surgical accuracy but also minimize the risks associated with reconstructive procedures. With bioprinting growing its wealth of information, it potentially paves the way for revolutionary advancements in aesthetic as well as functional reconstructive applications (Alfertshofer et al., 2023).

6.6.3. Expanding the Role of VR in Patient Care and Rehabilitation

VR application for patient rehabilitation and care is an up-and-coming field that exploits technology to optimize the impact of therapy. Traditional methods of rehabilitation are stationary and cannot offer the dynamic level of interaction needed to encourage patients and keep them on track with therapy regimens. VR presents virtual spaces where patients can perform simulated activities applicable to the needs of rehabilitation. This shift not only makes the rehabilitation process more engaging but also allows for activity customization in tasks involving complex motor skills or cognitive functions. Through this, patients are exposed to rehabilitation in an interactive form that may positively contribute to physical recuperation and mental well-being. This application illustrates the capability of VR in reconceptualizing the patient experience, making a rehabilitative space where rehabilitation is engaged with more zeal and activity. In addition, VR can track large volumes of data on patient performance throughout rehabilitation exercise completion, providing healthcare professionals with valuable feedback. With improved data collection methods, VR systems can monitor progress in real time, enabling quick and accurate adjustments. When patients navigate virtual space, their movements are tracked and quantified, providing therapists with detailed information about their physical capabilities and limitations. This data-driven approach aligns with the shift in treatment models toward personalized health care interventions. Such insights are poised to enable more effective strategic planning within therapeutic programs, so that therapists can tailor treatment on an individual basis and thereby optimize recovery channels. Overall, these advances in VR technology represent a step forward in the integration of advanced medical imaging processes, such as 3D reconstruction and printing, into personalized rehabilitation schemes. Also, the ability to replicate complex surgical settings within VR can prove beneficial for patient education and pre-surgery preparation. Patients usually feel anxious when waiting for surgery; hence, placing them in a virtual simulation of what they are undergoing can help alleviate their fear and improve their overall experience. By offering an in-situ experience of surgery and potential recovery paths, VR facilitates informed consent and patient autonomy in healthcare. This educational tool can easily enhance comprehension, allowing patients to visualize treatment options that may involve intricate processes augmented by 3D images. Ultimately, as VR continues to expand in healthcare settings, its role will no longer be solely to alter the method of rehabilitation but also to how patients engage with and understand their medical care, ultimately resulting in better outcomes and satisfaction.

SUMMARY

The use of 3D technologies in the medical field has revolutionized several areas of healthcare, delivering better clinical outcomes and operational effectiveness. One of the most spectacular of these advancements is in surgical disciplines, where 3D printing has been used to create patient-specific implants and surgical devices tailored based on individual anatomy. Not only does this technology reduce the risk of complications associated with generic implantable medical devices, but it also provides the ability for a more personalized treatment approach. For instance, in oral and maxillofacial surgery, the precision afforded by 3D printing is directly correlated with improved patient recovery times and surgical success rates, changing the model of how clinicians treat and plan. The shift towards customized solutions highlights the central role played by technology in modern medical practice and foresees the potential for innovations in the treatment of patients. Beyond manufacturing, 3D printing also offers advantages in other areas, playing a key role in enhancing medical education and surgical simulation. By leveraging high-resolution medical imaging data from modalities such as CT and MRI, 3D printing can produce highly complex anatomical models for preoperative planning and education. This attribute is particularly valuable while training novice surgeons because it provides an in-vitro opportunity to practice on realistic models before operating on actual patients. The combination of advanced imaging technology and 3D printing creates a learning-and-application cycle that benefits both instructors and learners. Such practical experience leads to confidence and proficiency, eventually translating into higher levels of patient safety and quality of care in operating rooms, demonstrating the multidimensional benefits of 3D technology in medicine. Aside from surgical application, the synergy of 3D technologies also extends to preoperative and intraoperative planning, significantly enhancing the surgery. Three-dimensional reconstruction of a patient's individual anatomy allows surgeons to visualize complex structures in three dimensions, thus better understanding the unique challenges faced with specific procedures. This level of preparation is most valuable in complex cases, such as those involving the cardiovascular or musculoskeletal systems, where precision is critical. In addition, the development of augmented and virtual reality tools aids this process, providing immersive planning interfaces in which interaction with 3D models occurs in real time. Application of such advanced technologies not only optimizes the surgical process but also facilitates collaborative decision-making among multidisciplinary teams, ultimately improving patient outcomes and procedural efficiency. The transformational impact of 3D technologies in healthcare is thus monumental, ushering in a new era in healthcare delivery.

The course of development in 3D reconstruction, printing, and VR in medical imaging promises a revolutionary future of medicine, especially for the understanding of complicated anatomical structures. Digitized, high-resolution anatomical datasets are increasingly sought for their ability to explain complex anatomical changes associated with various pathologies, particularly myocardial infarction (MI). These advances enable not only greater visualization of cardiovascular anatomy but also the potential for new applications in computational simulation and individualized medicine. Reconstruction and segmentation of cardiac and other anatomical objects will enable new educational resources and further promote preoperative planning, ultimately leading to improved clinical outcomes across medical specialties and underscoring the vast significance of such technologies in an evolving healthcare environment (Chen et al., 2025). Along with this, VR technology holds powerful promise for augmenting surgical training and preoperative planning. The use of immersive environments allows surgeons to get accustomed to complex anatomical arrangements and perform virtual procedure simulations. Immersion not only enables surgical precision but also increases awareness of patient-specific anatomical variation, which is essential for achieving surgical efficacy to its full potential. Next-generation improvements to this tool can be made by integrating AI, which would analyze data patterns to offer predictive capabilities for surgical interventions. The possibility of using 3D-printed models with VR for accurate intraoperative navigation further underscores the complementarity of these technologies, making them essential tools in contemporary surgical practice (Kasai et al., 2024). As the medical field continues to explore the uses of 3D printing and VR, burgeoning progress in AR has the potential to revolutionize intraoperative guidance. By projecting important anatomical information onto the operating field itself, AR can help surgeons more accurately locate tissue structures during complex procedures, ensuring greater procedural efficacy. Secondly, AR has the potential to become invaluable in-patient communication, enabling patients to comprehend their clinical status through interactive 3D visualizations. These advancements hold potential for a future in which medical imaging frees itself from traditional methods, establishing new paradigms for diagnosis, treatment, and patient engagement. Continued research and collaboration between technologists, clinicians, and regulatory organizations will be required to leverage these innovations productively, finally enhancing the quality of care for patients in an ever-evolving medical world (Kasai et al., 2024; Chen et al., 2025).

CLOSER LOOK

INTEGRATION OF 3D RECONSTRUCTION, PRINTING, AND VIRTUAL REALITY (VR) IN HEALTHCARE

The use of 3D reconstruction, printing, and virtual reality technologies in healthcare represents a promising paradigm for enhancing patient care, education, and surgical outcomes. These technologies provide new approaches to simulating complicated anatomical details, with which medical professionals can conduct advanced surgical planning and practice. For instance, 3D printed models allow surgeons to practice on patient-specific replicas, which increases procedural accuracy and reduces operation time. The virtual reality-powered immersive environments can improve medical education to allow students and residents to practice realistic simulations that increase preparedness for real clinical scenarios. These advances highlight the need to integrate technology into the development of precision medicine and to improve healthcare delivery, introducing a scenario in which patient outcomes are significantly improved through tailored interventions and advanced surgical techniques. Although 3D technologies have the potential to deliver benefits, various barriers discourage their use in healthcare provision. Higher implementation costs and technical difficulties discourage health facilities from integrating these innovations into their care. Further, there is a disconnect between what developers and doctors perceive and how they feel about the actual use and satisfaction with these technologies. The research cited by Yun et al. (2024) reported that satisfaction levels differed between developers and medical students, suggesting that developers may not perceive end-users' practical requirements. Bridging this gap is essential for ensuring that these technologies are not only innovative but also meet the real-world demands of healthcare practitioners. Consequently, addressing this discrepancy is vital for refining the tools and enhancing their functionality in patient care settings. To fully realize the potential of 3D reconstruction, printing, and virtual reality, there must be collaborative efforts among developers and doctors to gear these technologies toward the specific needs of professionals. As discussed in the findings of Bhatti et al. (2025), the integration of artificial intelligence and user-friendly design can improve performance in the healthcare sector. Moreover, ongoing clinical trials are needed to establish the long-term benefits of these technologies to facilitate widespread adoption and integration into clinical practice. By focusing on accessibility, cost-effectiveness, and interoperability with existing systems, the healthcare industry can capitalize on these front-line innovations to not only alleviate diagnostic mistakes but enhance the quality of patient care overall. As they evolve, they can potentially redefine the interface between technology and patient-centered clinical practice.

REFERENCES

1. Aithal, P. S. (2023). Advances and New Research Opportunities in Quantum Computing Technology by Integrating it with Other ICCT Underlying Technologies. *International Journal of Case Studies in Business IT and Education*, 314–358. https://doi.org/10.47992/ijcsbe.2581.6942.0304Aleef, T. A., Hagos, Y. B., Khawaldeh, S., Minh, T., et al. (2017). Complete end-to-end low-cost solution to a 3D scanning system with integrated turntable. http://arxiv.org/abs/1709.02247 (accessed on 5th August 2025).
2. Alfertshofer, M., Baecher, H., Hoch, C. C., Kauke-Navarro, M., et al. (2023). From bench to bedside–current clinical and translational challenges in fibula free flap reconstruction. https://core.ac.uk/download/590331043.pdf (accessed on 5th August 2025).
3. Amara, K., Guerroudji, M. A., Kerdjidj, O., Zenati, N., Atalla, S., Mansoor, W., & Ramzan, N. (2025). A mobile AR computer-aided diagnosis: 6 DoF brain tumor pose estimator using a fine-tuned EfficientPose-based model. *IEEE Access, 13*, 41571–41589. https://www.semanticscholar.org/paper/d836ea0656ccaec9bde4a27332733fcd8951b0cd (accessed on 5th August 2025).
4. Anderson, M., Davy-Jow, S., Lorenz, K., Schofield, T., et al. (2012). Roman portraiture and biometric identification. https://core.ac.uk/download/42505482.pdf (accessed on 5th August 2025).
5. Anderson, P., Rea, P., & Welsh, E. (2014). A novel method of anatomical data acquisition using the Perceptron ScanWorks V5 scanner. https://core.ac.uk/download/141204718.pdf (accessed on 5th August 2025).
6. Anwar, A., Barach, B., Bhatla, A., Biglino, G., et al. (2018). 3D printing is a transformative technology in congenital heart disease. https://core.ac.uk/download/212858839.pdf (accessed on 5th August 2025).
7. Ayoub, A., & Pulijala, Y. (2019). The application of virtual reality and augmented reality in oral & maxillofacial surgery. https://core.ac.uk/download/237397848.pdf (accessed on 5th August 2025).
8. Barbaro, F., Spaletta, G., Di Conza, G., Sofroniou, M., Toni, R., & Mosca, S. (2023). A computational template for three-dimensional modeling of the vascular scaffold of the human thyroid gland. https://core.ac.uk/download/573435210.pdf (accessed on 5th August 2025).
9. Bhatti, H., Moeed, M., Bhatti, A., Ali, M., Shahid, S., Javed, M., Ali, S., et al. (2025). Augmented and virtual reality in radiology: A comparative analysis of clinical applications and outcomes. *Journal of Medical & Health Sciences Review*. https://www.semanticscholar.org/paper/6970f5a361f418f10ab30bd58d61657b5337b988 (accessed on 5th August 2025).
10. Burity, J., Fonte, I. B. da, & de Melo, P. B. (2014). Radiological Society of North America (RSNA) 3D printing Special Interest Group (SIG): Guidelines for medical 3D printing and appropriateness for clinical scenarios. https://core.ac.uk/download/212867900.pdf (accessed on 5th August 2025).
11. Chachques, J. C., Ferroni, L., Gardin, C., Latremouille, C., et al. (2020). Recent applications of three-dimensional printing in cardiovascular medicine. https://core.ac.uk/download/296232907.pdf (accessed on 5th August 2025).
12. Chango Llerena, X., Flor Unda, O., Gil Jiménez, P., Gómez Moreno, A., et al. (2024). Technology in forensic sciences: Innovation and precision. https://core.ac.uk/download/622341556.pdf (accessed on 5th August 2025).

13. Chen, W., Kuniewicz, M., Aminu, A. J., Karaesmen, I., Duong, N. C., Proniewska, K. K., van Dam, P. M., et al. (2025). High-resolution 3D visualization of human hearts with emphases on the cardiac conduction system components—a new platform for medical education, mix/virtual reality, computational simulation. *Frontiers in Medicine, 12*. https://www.semanticscholar.org/paper/f8f65fd8930e008d2383613045db9af5e09e5d41 (accessed on 5th August 2025).
14. Christ, R., Guevar, J., Poyade, M., Rea, P., et al. (2018). Proof of concept of a workflow methodology for the creation of basic canine head anatomy veterinary education tool using augmented reality. https://core.ac.uk/download/156870626.pdf (accessed on 5th August 2025).
15. Cornejo, J., Cornejo, J., Vargas, M., Helguero, C. G., Andrade, R. M., Torres, S., Asensio-Salazar, J., et al. (2022). Anatomical engineering and 3D printing for surgery and medical devices: International review and future exponential innovations. *BioMed Research International, 2022*, 1–28. https://doi.org/10.1155/2022/6797745 (accessed on 5th August 2025).
16. Czerny, M., Grabenwöger, M., Berger, T., Aboyans, V., Della Corte, A., Chen, E., Desai, N. D., et al. (2023). EACTS/STS guidelines for diagnosing and treating acute and chronic syndromes of the aortic organ. *European Journal of Cardio-Thoracic Surgery, 65*. https://doi.org/10.1093/ejcts/ezad426 (accessed on 5th August 2025).
17. Díaz Lantada, A., De Laurentis, K. J., Díaz Lantada, A., Gerrits, A., Ghosh, S. K., Guo, X., et al. (2012). Rapid prototyping for biomedical engineering: Current capabilities and challenges. https://core.ac.uk/download/148664608.pdf (accessed on 5th August 2025).
18. Ebert, L., Franckenberg, S., Sieberth, T., Schweitzer, W., Thali, M. J., Ford, J., & Decker, S. (2021). A review of visualization techniques of post-mortem computed tomography data for forensic death investigations. *International Journal of Legal Medicine, 135*, 1855–1867. https://doi.org/10.1007/s00414-021-02581-4 (accessed on 5th August 2025).
19. Ewart, P. (2019). A comparison of processing techniques for producing prototype injection molding inserts. https://core.ac.uk/download/322841895.pdf (accessed on 5th August 2025).
20. Gezimati, M., & Singh, G. (2023). Terahertz imaging and sensing for healthcare: Current status and future perspectives. *IEEE Access, 11*, 18590–18619. https://doi.org/10.1109/access.2023.3247196 (accessed on 5th August 2025).
21. Hsia, T. (2021). Invited commentary: Form and function in surgical planning. *World Journal for Pediatric and Congenital Heart Surgery, 12*, 244–245. https://www.semanticscholar.org/paper/e83675d52b71a5265d8a380600ff0c1d5ee51c73 (accessed on 5th August 2025).
22. Işıkay, İ., Çekiç, E., Baylarov, B., Tunc, O., & Hanalioğlu, Ş. (2024). Narrative review of patient-specific 3D visualization and reality technologies in skull base neurosurgery: Enhancements in surgical training, planning, and navigation. *Frontiers in Surgery, 11*. https://www.semanticscholar.org/paper/331095816fc59dd84e70bc37fabe9881884b4fd4 (accessed on 5th August 2025).
23. Kalová, M., Kubíček, J., Oczka, D., Tomanec, J., et al. (2019). Recent trends, technical concepts and components of computer-assisted orthopedic surgery systems: A comprehensive review. https://core.ac.uk/download/287649034.pdf (accessed on 5th August 2025).
24. Kasai, M., Aihara, T., & Yamanaka, N. (2024). Enhancing liver surgery and transplantation: The role of 3D printing and virtual reality. *Artificial Intelligence Surgery*. https://www.semanticscholar.org/paper/bba0d564271e2b69106840697dc96b77e29638e8 (accessed on 5th August 2025).

25. Makhataeva, Z., & Varol, H. A. (2020). Augmented reality for robotics: A review. *Robotics, 9*, 21–21. https://doi.org/10.3390/robotics9020021 (accessed on 5th August 2025).

26. Meyer-Szary, J., Souza Luis, M., Mikulski, S., Patel, A., Schulz, F., Tretiakow, D., Fercho, J., et al. (2022). The role of 3D printing in planning complex medical procedures and training of medical professionals—Cross-sectional multispecialty review. *International Journal of Environmental Research and Public Health, 19*, 3331–3331. https://doi.org/10.3390/ijerph19063331 (accessed on 5th August 2025).

27. N/A. (2000). *Focal Spot, Summer 2000*. https://core.ac.uk/download/129069318.pdf (accessed on 5th August 2025).

28. N/A. (2004). *Focal Spot, Summer/Fall 2004*. https://core.ac.uk/download/129069330.pdf (accessed on 5th August 2025).

29. Ohkohchi, N., & Oshiro, Y. (2017). Three-dimensional liver surgery simulation: Computer-assisted surgical planning with three-dimensional simulation software and three-dimensional printing. https://core.ac.uk/download/87200836.pdf (accessed on 5th August 2025).

30. Pathak, K., Saikia, R., Das, A., Das, D., Islam, M. A., Pramanik, P., Parasar, A., et al. (2023). 3D printing in biomedicine: Advancing personalized care through additive manufacturing. *Exploration of Medicine*. https://doi.org/10.37349/emed.2023.00200 (accessed on 5th August 2025).

31. Preethi, C., Sathik, M., & Nisha, S. (2022). An impact of three-dimensional techniques in virtual reality. *International Journal of Health Sciences*. https://www.semanticscholar.org/paper/673f4d398fbe04b30bea817adb23e181d290260b (accessed on 5th August 2025).

32. Ravi, K. S., Patra, A., & Pushpa, N. B. (2022). Future of cadaveric dissection in anatomical science education. *National Journal of Clinical Anatomy, 11*, 123–123. https://doi.org/10.4103/njca.njca_126_22 (accessed on 5th August 2025).

33. Reddy, B. V., Kulkarni, S., Kumar, N., Gosavi, V., & Khatri, R. (2024). An exploration of artificial intelligence (AI) integration with real-time three-dimensional holography to enhance visual quality, optimize processing efficiency, and facilitate interactive applications. *International Journal of Inventive Engineering and Sciences*. https://www.semanticscholar.org/paper/6b86ababd8839be1c9fb1f630eae0a7e4575792c (accessed on 5th August 2025).

34. Tian, Y., Chen, C., Xu, X., Wang, J., Hou, X., Li, K., Lu, X., et al. (2021). A review of 3D printing in dentistry: Technologies, affecting factors, and applications. *Scanning, 2021*, 1–19. https://doi.org/10.1155/2021/9950131 (accessed on 5th August 2025).

35. Uppot, R. N., Laguna, B., McCarthy, C. J., De Novi, G., Phelps, A., Siegel, E. L., & Courtier, J. (2019). Implementing virtual and augmented reality tools for radiology education and training, communication, and clinical care. *Radiology, 291*, 570–580. https://doi.org/10.1148/radiol.2019182210 (accessed on 5th August 2025).

36. Yun, Y., Shin, D. H., & Choi, H. (2024). Perspectives of medical students and developers regarding virtual reality, augmented reality, mixed reality, and 3D printing technologies: Survey study. *JMIR XR and Spatial Computing*. https://www.semanticscholar.org/paper/a4ad1935067f11101a755b7baed1e29cd1ac1494 (accessed on 5th August 2025).

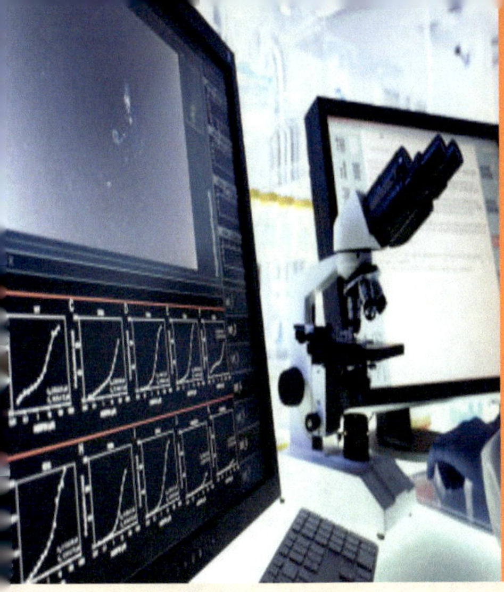

Chapter 7

ARTIFICIAL INTELLIGENCE AND MACHINE LEARNING IN DIAGNOSTIC IMAGING

Contents

Introduction

The arrival of machine learning (ML) and artificial intelligence (AI) technologies is transforming the diagnostic imaging industry, promising unprecedented precision and productivity. In the past, diagnostic procedures primarily relied on subjective evaluation by clinicians with limited supporting histopathological examination. Despite being rudimentary, such processes are accompanied by inherent limitations, such as scope for misinterpretation and invasiveness in certain diagnostic procedures, e.g., biopsies. With greater complexity in dermatological conditions, there is a rising demand for diagnostic innovation to minimize morbidity and maximize healthcare outcomes. Newer technologies, more specifically AI, thus become precious assets in seeking solutions to dermatological diagnostic issues and, in fact, even further afield, enriching the diagnostic arsenal of imaging modalities in a new direction (Gold et al., 2021). Artificial intelligence systems are now prominently featured not only because of their ability to manage large volumes of imaging data, but also because of their potential to enhance diagnostic accuracy. With the help of algorithms trained on big data sets, AI has been shown to have the capacity to detect patterns lost to human clinicians, thus introducing a paradigm shift in practice. This growth of AI, however, rests on a double-edged sword, with attendant ethical concerns (Figure 7.1).

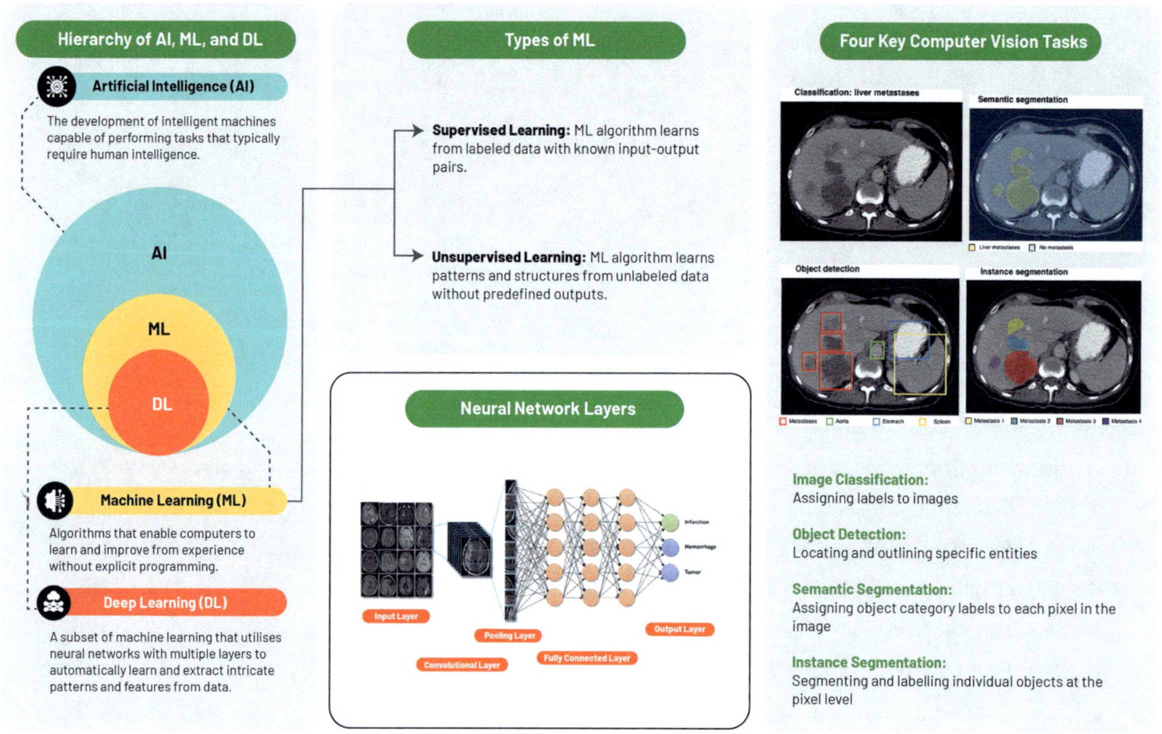

Figure 7.1. Schematic illustration of artificial intelligence and machine learning frameworks.

Source: https://www.mdpi.com/diagnostics/diagnostics-13-02760/article_deploy/html/images/diagnostics-13-02760-g003.png.

As more and more complex AI technologies function more or less like "black boxes," clinicians may find it challenging to align with the transparency of decision-making that is a natural application for these kinds of technologies. This poses severe tension to maintaining the core concepts of patient-centered care, which focus on shared decision-making and informed consent, as explained in recent debate over the implications of black-box medicine (Bjerring et al., 2020). Furthermore, the integration of AI and ML into diagnostic imaging requires reconsideration of the healthcare practitioner's role. As these new technologies improve, clinicians will need to modify not only how they diagnose but also how they interpret and use AI-suggested conclusions in practice. The balance lies between reliance on AI systems and maintaining clinical expertise and the ability to comprehend the rationale behind diagnostic data. This form of cooperative interaction will help optimize patient outcomes while limiting the risks associated with reliance on black-box algorithms. Therefore, creating a symbiotic relationship between clinical acumen and AI advancements will be paramount to the future of diagnostic imaging, enabling an integrated approach to patient care that optimizes the accessibility and effectiveness of medical diagnostics (Gold et al., 2021).

7.1. Current Applications in Diagnostic Imaging

The marriage of machine learning and artificial intelligence in diagnostic imaging has transformed the clinicians' interpretation process of medical images. Clinicians are increasingly relying on AI-based algorithms to enhance diagnostic performance, particularly in recognizing abnormalities on imaging modalities such as X-rays, MRIs, and CT scans. These advanced algorithms are trained on vast amounts of data, where they can recognize patterns that human eyes may not be able to see. By assisting the diagnostic process, AI improves accuracy and efficiency, ultimately yielding better patient outcomes. However, with emerging technologies, their implications for complexity cannot be disregarded (Figure 7.2).

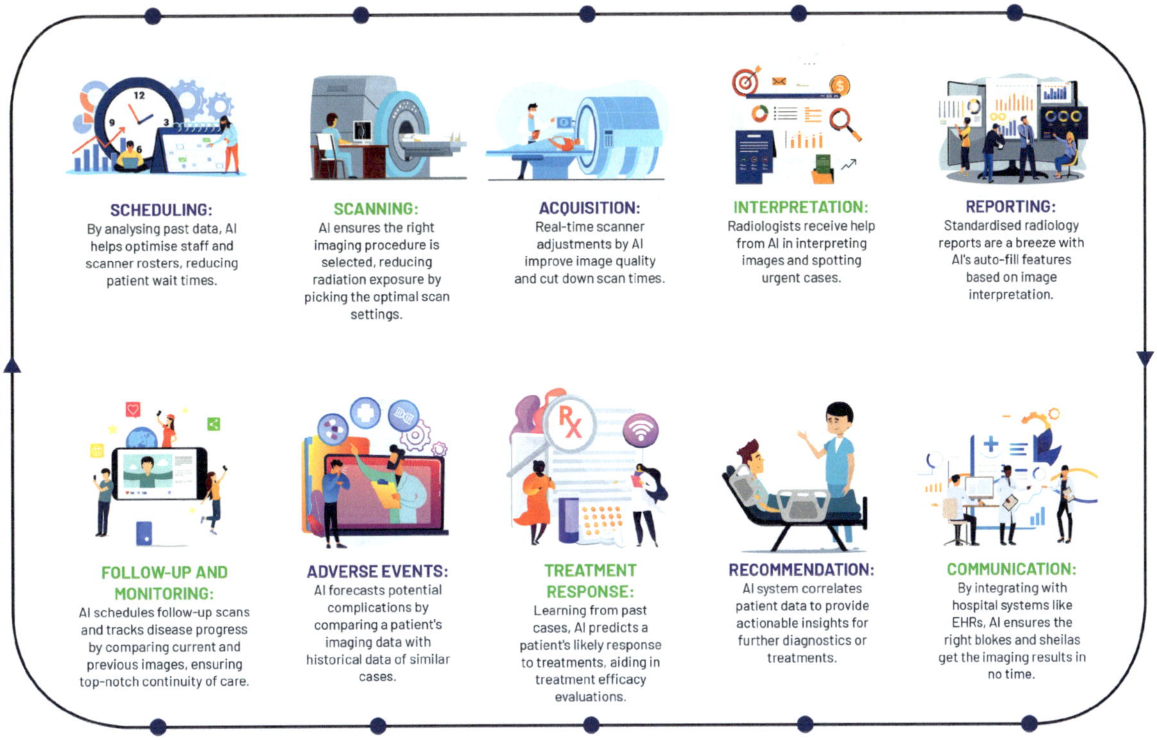

Figure 7.2. A streamlined workflow diagram illustrating the role of artificial intelligence in radiological practice.

Source: https://www.mdpi.com/diagnostics/diagnostics-13-02760/article_deploy/html/images/diagnostics-13-02760-g004.png.

The increasing application of AI is one component of the black-box medicine phenomenon, as the process of decision-making becomes opaque to practitioners, thereby eroding the very foundations of patient-centered care (Bjerring et al., 2020). In addition to enhancing image analysis, AI and machine learning technologies are also being used for patient prediction and risk stratification. Based on a review of historical patient data, AI systems can recognize risk factors for certain conditions. The predictive aspect is the ability to offer personalized medicine plans, in which treatment protocols are tailored to distinct patient characteristics, improving the quality of care. Furthermore, AI solutions also include automation of repetitive tasks such as image acquisition and workflow management, thus allowing radiologists to utilize their abilities on more complex cases. Not only does such a change make operational efficiency simpler, but it also minimizes burnout among physicians exposed to increasing workloads (Harwood et al., 2019). These advances underscore the transformative promise of AI in diagnostic imaging for a future where care is more effective and patient-centered. Even as the grand promises of AI in diagnostic imaging are significant, there remain ethical and practical issues that are paramount. The most significant of these pertains to the transparency and interpretability of AI algorithms, which can hinder their deployment by physicians. As artificial intelligence technologies become increasingly more sophisticated, they are likely to be black boxes that produce outputs without seeming reasons. This lack of understanding can be a hindrance to well-informed decision-making, as clinicians would not be able to explain to patients the recommendations developed by AI (Bjerring et al., 2020). It is therefore imperative that these ethical concerns be addressed, as gaining trust in AI technology is the key to effective integration of such technology into clinical practice. Furthermore, as those technologies progress, ongoing education and training will be important so that healthcare professionals can use AI effectively while maintaining the core tenets of patient-centered medicine. Above all, additional research into AI applications in diagnostic imaging needs to give precedence to ethical issues in an effort to deliver the utmost patient care and informed clinical practice.

7.1.1. Image Analysis and Interpretation

The marriage of AI and ML with diagnostic imaging has revolutionized the analysis and interpretation process of images. The shift is driven by advanced AI algorithms' ability to analyze large volumes of medical imaging data to detect patterns and abnormalities that could go unnoticed even by skilled practitioners. This capability improves the speed and accuracy of diagnoses, particularly in fields such as radiology and dermatology, where visual inspection is the norm. The reliance on such sophisticated systems, however, raises questions about the transparency and interpretability of their decision-making process. In an era when AI is increasingly autonomous, the term "black-box medicine" has to be read. The challenges posed by such a lack of transparency require a closer examination of how AI is working to fulfill patient-centered principles, which prioritize informed choice and collaborative healthcare for patients and practitioners (Bjerring et al., 2020) (Figure 7.3). The success of AI in imaging diagnosis is also explained by its use for specific medical conditions, such as identifying skin cancer. Deep learning-based classifiers have been shown to be highly successful in diagnosing melanocytic naevi, melanoma, and seborrheic keratosis, indicating that such classifiers are likely to outperform traditional methods. Even so, computer-aided diagnosis (CAD) systems have not gained much traction in clinical practice because their decision-making process is transparent. Existing work is beginning to address this challenge via mapping AI types to human-understandable concepts through techniques like CAVs. This not only achieves a broader interpretability of AI results but also builds the needed trust among healthcare professionals and these systems, ensuring that nuances of diagnostic reasoning are preserved and understood (Ahmed et al., 2020). As the potential of AI expands, so too does our approach to image analysis and interpretation in diagnostic imaging. Where the intersection of AI technology and medical expertise is called for is an architecture that enhances the principles of transparency and intelligibility. While AI can identify complex patterns in medical images, practitioners must still be involved in interpretation. This exchange fosters mutual understanding and enhances patient communication, ultimately leading to healthier, more informed healthcare decisions. The imaging diagnostics of the future will rely not only on technological progress but also on the development of more robust systems that harmonize AI interpretations with human experience, without compromising the foundations of patient-centered care in automated settings (Bjerring et al., 2020).

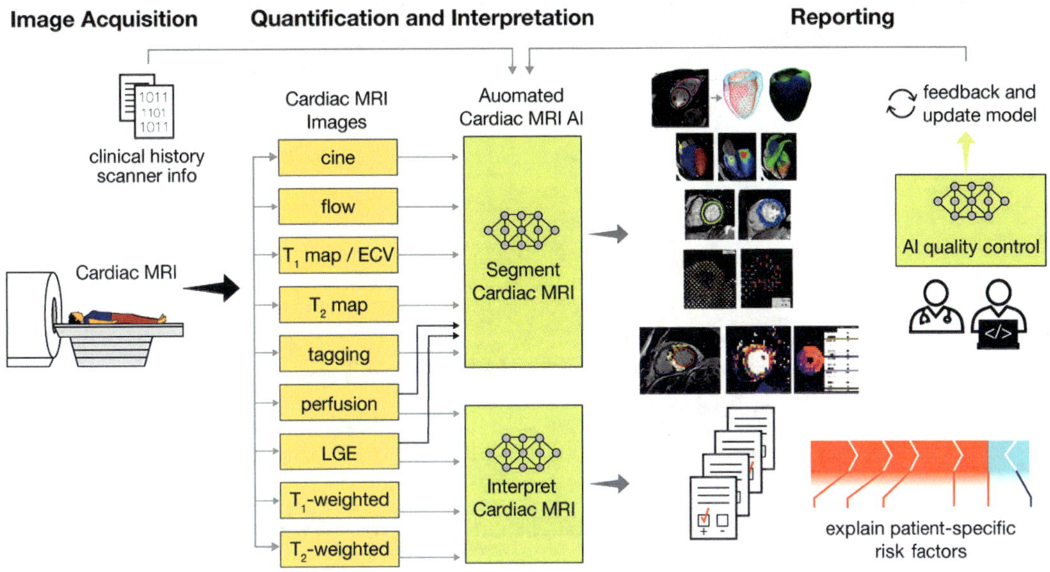

Figure 7.3. Diagram shows artificial intelligence (AI)-enabled cardiac MRI analysis, interpretation, and reporting. In cardiac MRI, images are collected to characterize function (ie, cine and tagging images), flow, tissue properties, and fibrosis (i.e., T1 and T2 maps and T1-weighted, T2-weighted, and extracellular volume [ECV] images), and scarring (i.e., late gadolinium enhancement [LGE] images). AI can substantially impact the analysis workflow after imaging. The clinical reading includes quantification (e.g., functional assessment on cine images) and clinical interpretation of individual sequences (e.g., the presence and location of scarring on LGE images). AI can assist in both the analysis and interpretation of clinical readings and can change the role of imagers to oversight.

Source: https://www.researchgate.net/profile/Manuel-Morales-50/publication/377270016/figure/fig5/AS:11431281248672815@1717257038556/Diagram-shows-artificial-intelligence-AI-enabled-cardiac-MRI-analysis-interpretation.ppm.

7.1.2. Automated Detection of Anomalies

Automated anomaly detection by artificial intelligence and machine learning-based approaches in diagnostic imaging is a paradigm shift in the practice of medicine. The evolution of machine learning algorithms in recent years has enabled systems to handle humongous datasets more effectively than their predecessors, resulting in more accurate diagnoses. Such technologies employ pattern comparison to match suspected anatomical or physiological deviations against normative benchmarks to identify anomalies in real time. Apart from enhanced diagnostic precision, the application of these technologies also reduces radiologists' workload, thereby enabling specialists to focus on complex cases requiring human intervention. As the technology of automated systems improves, health care professionals begin to integrate these technologies into routine practice, paving the way for improved patient outcomes through earlier treatment and more personalized care (Figure 7.4).

In particular, the integration of machine learning into obstetric and maternity care reflects the profound impact of automated diagnosis of abnormalities in these fields. Intelligent software applications designed for processing magnetic resonance imaging and ultrasound results can predict and diagnose conditions such as gestational diabetes or pre-eclampsia based on characteristics detected in imaging scans.

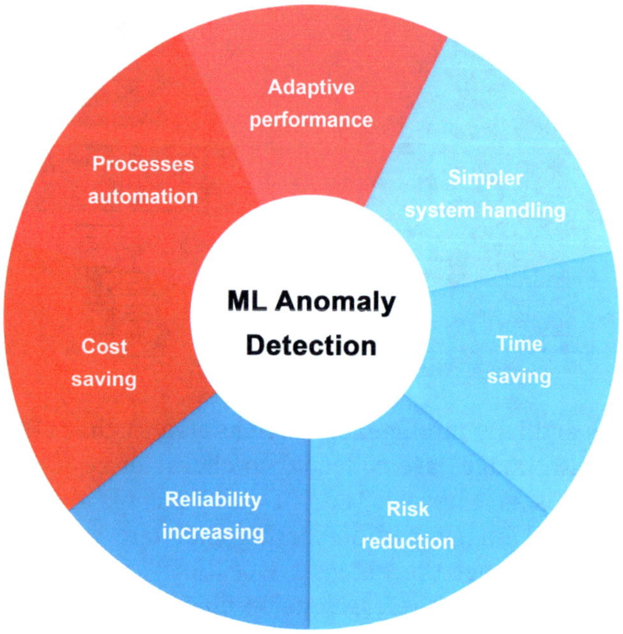

Figure 7.4. Anomaly detection with machine learning (ML).

Source: https://nix-united.com/wp-content/uploads/2021/10/3.1-2.jpg.

The creation of such predictive devices demonstrates the capability of artificial intelligence to enhance patient safety and clinical efficacy by rendering early detection of fetal abnormalities. Additionally, the use of AI in assessing fetoplacental and cervical function illustrates the versatility of automated systems, as they adjust to any modality of imaging. Such developments highlight the revolutionary nature of machine learning in clinical diagnosis and, by extension, towards improved paradigms in patient care for obstetric practice (Arain et al., 2023). The application of deep learning models for identifying precancerous conditions is just as intriguing, as demonstrated in diagnosing colorectal cancer. Routine colonoscopy practices are often plagued by problems, including difficulty identifying polyps because of their size and shape. However, with the advent of convolutional neural networks, the detection of polyps during colonoscopies has been significantly enhanced with high sensitivity and specificity. In raising adenoma detection rates, AI systems not only reduce the risk of missing precancerous lesions but also endoscopist fatigue, which enhances the overall quality of clinical encounters. This innovation fits into a broader pattern of integrating state-of-the-art technology into medical practice, highlighting AI's potential to streamline processes and enhance diagnostic reliability. As the field evolves, addressing ethical and pragmatic concerns associated with adopting these technologies will be instrumental in maximizing their benefits (Alaa et al., 2024).

7.1.3. Integration with Radiology Workflows

The integration of AI and ML into radiology procedures has the potential to improve diagnostic imaging quality and effectiveness. Using complex algorithms, AI systems can assist radiologists in interpreting medical images, enhance diagnostic accuracy, and reduce the risk of human error. One of the primary developments involves the use of convolutional neural networks (CNNs), which excel at processing visual information and identifying complex patterns from radiographs and CT scans. These technologies can prioritize cases, highlighting outliers that require immediate follow-up, which is particularly significant in emergency care. But seamless implementation relies on having smooth integration paths with existing radiology systems, whereby the AI tools augment the workflow and do not add to it. Overcoming these challenges fosters a setting whereby technology can have a significant contribution towards improving patient outcomes and operational efficiency in radiological practice (Bartoszek et al., 2025) (Figure 7.5).

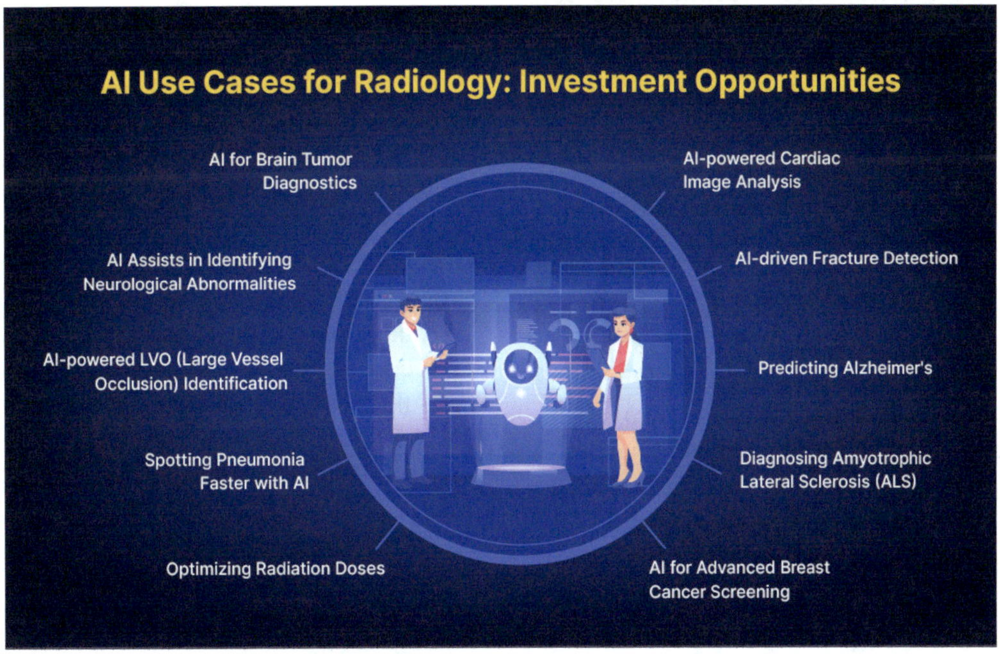

Figure 7.5. AI in radiology helps radiologists with decision-making.

Source: https://assets.bacancytechnology.com/blog/wp-content/uploads/2024/04/09051437/AI-Use-Case-for-Radiology.jpg.

Effective integration of AI into radiology workflows involves addressing issues related to model interpretability and diverse training data. Effective AI systems require robust training datasets that reflect diverse patient populations and span broad pathology coverage to ensure generalizability in practice. Also, practitioners' faith in AI results is essential, where they should feel at ease with the technology's recommendation. Breaking the issue of the black box status of some AI models, where decision-making is not transparent, is paramount to acceptance by healthcare professionals. Additionally, radiologists must be trained not only to implement these new technologies but also to critically examine AI output alongside what they see. This is an interdisciplinary approach that can optimize human and machine interaction to lay the foundations for improved diagnostic processes in radiology (Bartoszek et al., 2025). Other considerations arise when the application of digital tools is involved in enhancing clinical processes beyond traditional imaging protocols. Novel tools such as chatbots and natural language processing (NLP) have shown immense potential to simplify information retrieval and enhance patient engagement. These technologies can support the extraction and categorization of useful medical information, thereby reducing the intellectual load on radiologists and enabling them to focus more on challenging diagnostic tasks. The integration of these technologies does, nonetheless, require undertaking challenges linked to data standardization and possible prejudice within AI systems. The way forward needs rigorous clinical testing and examination of ethical, privacy, and legal considerations to prevent the deployment of AI from undermining patient rights and confidentiality. Through its own digital transformation, radiology lessons can be adopted to provide guidelines, resulting in a more efficient and responsive healthcare system.

7.2. Benefits of AI and ML in Diagnostic Imaging

The incorporation of AI and ML into imaging diagnostics is revolutionizing the health sector by making diagnoses more accurate and more effective. The conventional methods of diagnosis rely heavily on human interpretation, which is subjective and prone to error. By applying AI-driven algorithms that quickly and accurately process vast amounts of medical imaging data, radiologists are today efficient diagnostic instruments for detecting anomalies the naked eye cannot easily discern. Diagnosis can be made earlier with this technology for conditions such as tumors or neurological disorders, improving patient outcomes through timely interventions. ' ability to synthesize data from different sources, such as neuroimaging and electronic health records, underscores their increasing prominence in healthcare environments, showcasing an unmistakable advantage in contemporary diagnostic procedures (Depp et al., 2020).

Beyond enhancing diagnostic accuracy, AI and ML technologies streamline workflows in radiology departments and notably reduce the time required for image analysis. General imaging processes are time-consuming and delay timely reporting of results. Automating routine tests and streamlining priority cases with intelligent algorithms not only enhances process efficiency but also reduces the burden on radiologists. This transition allows physicians to focus on more complex cases and patient consultations, resulting in greater productivity and, ultimately, improved overall quality of care. Second, the decrease in interpretation time can reduce patient anxiety about diagnostic results, thereby improving the overall patient experience (Harwood et al., 2019). Another significant benefit of AI and ML in diagnostic imaging is that they can enable ongoing training and development for healthcare professionals. As AI platforms become more proficient at recognizing patterns and predicting outcomes, they can be used as tools for education, assisting radiologists in sharpening their image interpretation and decision-making skills. AI-based feedback mechanisms will be able to analyze a radiologist's performance and recommend areas for improvement, encouraging the medical community to cultivate a culture of continuous learning. Moreover, novel strategies facilitated by these technologies challenge clinicians to stay abreast of progress in medical imaging and diagnostics. By combining innovation in AI with ongoing clinical education, there is high potential to enhance diagnostic capability on all fronts and have a better-educated and responsive healthcare workforce (Depp et al., 2020) (Figure 7.6).

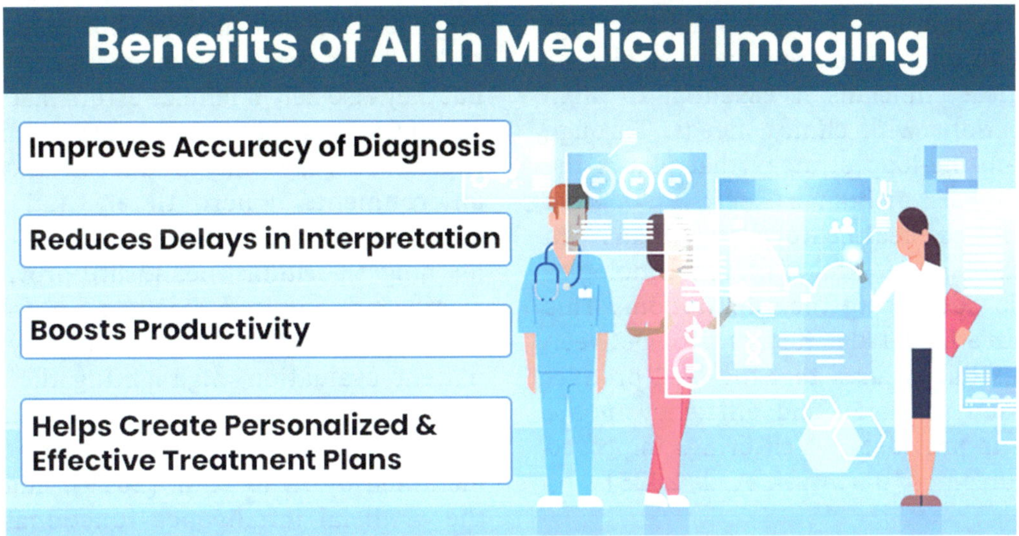

Figure 7.6. Benefits of AI in clinical imaging.

Source: https://cdn.educba.com/academy/wp-content/uploads/2024/03/Benefits-of-AI-in-Diagnostic-Imaging.png.

7.2.1. Increased Accuracy and Efficiency

The intersection of AI and ML in diagnostic imaging has played a significant role in accuracy and efficiency. The most intriguing development is the usage of CNNs for image inspection. The networks are necessary features. Experiments have shown that CNNs outperform traditional diagnostic methods in detecting pulmonary diseases such as pneumonia, tuberculosis, and lung cancer. Greater diagnostic accuracy not only benefits the patient but also relieves radiologists of intensive workloads, allowing them to focus on more complex cases. This then makes the use of AI in diagnostic imaging transform the way health professionals approach the interpretation of medical data, making it a crucial element in improved treatment outcomes (Bartoszek et al., 2025). Additionally, the use of AI in diagnostic imaging improves efficiency for healthcare systems in today's resource-scarce healthcare settings. By automating laborious tasks, AI reduces the time radiologists spend reading medical images, leading to faster and more consistent diagnoses. The application of AI tools supports rapid scanning of large volumes of imaging data, which is especially advantageous in emergency rooms where timely intervention may mean life or death. For instance, AI systems can quickly scan images on short notice, identify severe cases for immediate attention and thus simplify the workflow within very busy health facilities. In addition, the deployment of AI systems enhances diagnostic quality to such an extent that opportunities to miss problems are minimized, thereby enhancing overall patient safety and operational efficiency in medical facilities (Ginley et al., 2018). Although the spectacular advantages of AI in imaging diagnostics are promising, there are still apprehensions about incorporating these technologies in existing medical practices. The explainability of AI techniques and the quality of training data remain areas of concern, which could retard uptake on a mass scale. There is an urgent need for standardized protocols and training solutions to address shortcomings effectively. In addition, coordinating technologists with clinical clinicians is essential to align AI applications with clinical needs. Through a human-in-the-loop strategy that places the utmost emphasis on human expertise alongside AI capabilities, healthcare professionals can harness the full potential of these technologies while also addressing their limitations. This collaborative model also fosters trust between AI systems but ensures that the final product of increased precision and efficiency in the diagnosis is provided, which brings improved patient outcomes (Bartoszek et al., 2025).

7.2.2. Reduction in Human Error

In diagnostic imaging, nevertheless, the conjoining of AI and machine learning prowess is well-placed to eradicate the possibility of human error virtually. The ABCD technique for diagnosing skin cancers, for example, relies very much on subjective assessment and can vary considerably from one clinician to the next. Such traditional methods of diagnosis tend to be unreliable in reliably picking up malignancies and therefore risk misdiagnosis or treatment delays. Thus, there is a growing realization that conventional techniques are insufficient to ensure accurate diagnosis. AI systems, particularly those based on deep learning algorithms, can examine vast amounts of medical imaging at unprecedented speed and accuracy. Through the augmentation of human capability by machine intelligence, diagnostic imaging can be transformed into a discipline that involves greater reliability and fewer mistakes, even further propelling tremendous strides in patient treatment and treatment outcomes, as indicated in Ayub et al. (2019).

Additionally, various deep learning approaches are being researched with the aim of enhancing disease diagnosis and identification in diagnostic imaging. For instance, CNNs have been great tools in the area of medical image analysis, effectively identifying tumors and other anomalies that might escape human eyes. Not only do these technologies accelerate the diagnostic process, but they also help minimize errors that naturally arise from fatigue or complacency among human experts. This capability is handy in risky medical environments, where timely and accurate diagnoses are indispensable. Through machine learning algorithms, healthcare providers can significantly improve diagnostic precision and consistency. This enables more systematic patient evaluation, highlighting the key role of AI in mitigating the inherent limitations of human judgment in diagnostic cases, as identified by Ayub et al. (2019). Additionally, the artificial intelligence functionality goes beyond mere image examination and includes full evaluation metrics to enable improved practitioner decision-making. The inclusion of sophisticated algorithms enables diagnostic performance testing using measures such as sensitivity, specificity, and accuracy. This provides a more detailed understanding of diagnostic effectiveness than traditional methods typically offer. Furthermore, AI developments are making it possible for ongoing learning processes in which algorithms enhance their analysis based on previous outcomes, constantly sharpening their diagnostic skills. In this context, the potential of machine learning's capacity to evolve over time presents a revolutionary opportunity for enhanced diagnostic precision. Ultimately, utilizing these technologies not only minimizes the risk of human error but also establishes a paradigm under which medical clinicians can operate more confidently in their diagnostic assessments, consistent with empirical gains reflected in studies measuring AI deployment in diagnostic imaging, as described.

7.2.3. Enhanced Patient Outcomes and Satisfaction

The application of AI and ML to diagnostic imaging has certainly helped in enhancing patient outcomes and satisfaction. AI machines employ advanced algorithms that process large volumes of data to improve the accuracy and speed of diagnoses, enabling appropriate treatment interventions at the right time. With machines able to identify subtle patterns in imaging information, doctors can detect ailments that would go unnoticed using traditional approaches. This increased diagnostic ability is directly attributable to improved therapeutic decision-making and, in turn, to improved patient health outcomes. Furthermore, with the increasing pace of AI adoption in diagnostic imaging, the potential to reduce unnecessary procedures and optimize workflows comes into consideration, contributing to patient-centered care and satisfaction. Patient satisfaction goes beyond accuracy; it encompasses the overall experience within the health setting. As AI optimizes imaging processes and reduces waiting times, patients are treated faster, creating a nicer experience. AI integration further enables personalized imaging protocols tailored to the specific needs of an individual patient, creating unique pathways to diagnosis. Machine learning, for instance, can be programmed to adjust based on patient history and preference, ensuring that imaging procedures are executed with efficacy and efficiency. Enhanced communication by AI with patients, explained in simpler language and easier-to-read results, builds trust and transparency, which further enhances patient satisfaction and engagement with their healthcare providers. AI is thus leading the revolution in transforming the patient experience in diagnostic imaging. AI and ML's role in diagnostic imaging is more than just improved accuracy and patient satisfaction; they enhance the overall quality of healthcare delivery. The possibility of standardizing treatment and diagnosis through AI-driven insights could introduce an equalized healthcare system. Through precise and standardized diagnostic capabilities, healthcare professionals can provide treatments that better align with clinical guidelines. Automation of monotonous tasks also allows clinicians to manage time more effectively and focus on patient interactions and complex decision-making. As depicted in fields such as oro-facial trauma and prosthodontics, the effective use of AI not only improves clinical outcomes but also fosters a culture of cooperation between patients and healthcare practitioners. Lastly, with the application of AI alongside diagnostic imaging, the path to better patient outcomes and satisfaction is more tangible, thus making AI a cornerstone of the current healthcare revolution.

7.3. Challenges and Limitations

Integration of ML and AI in diagnostic imaging brings along a list of issues and limitations that are increasingly important to examine under a microscope. One fundamental issue is maintaining the completeness and quality of the datasets used to train these algorithms. Datasets that are not adequately diverse or are restricted will lead to mediocre model performance and so-called adversarial biases in diagnostic results. This issue is further compounded in niche fields such as oncology, where samples may not represent subpopulations. Furthermore, the nature of real-world medical data, which is inherently riddled with inconsistencies and discrepancies, makes the issue of algorithmic robustness even more challenging. For instance, the demands of precise data collection and preprocessing are essential to ensure that machine learning techniques can learn appropriately from the nuances of imaging data. Until these inherent dataset limitations are addressed, AI effectiveness for imaging diagnostics is drastically inhibited (Abbas et al., 2024). Besides dataset difficulties, another fundamental issue is that the interpretability of AI models has been a real challenge. The majority of machine learning models, profound learning models, are black boxes, and clinicians cannot untangle the way individual results are generated. Such transparency may be corrosive to trust between healthcare providers and patients, who rely on open explanations to guide their treatment. The demand for explainable AI (XAI) is significant as healthcare providers navigate the intricacies in diagnosis imaging. XAI techniques improve model explainability, enabling clinicians to understand and validate model decisions. Yet developing these interpretive models requires additional resources and expertise, making the incorporation of AI in clinical settings more challenging. Ignoring these interpretability concerns may incite resistance to applying AI technologies to diagnosis (Depp et al., 2020). Lastly, ethical considerations and regulatory frameworks pose significant barriers to the widespread adoption of AI technologies in diagnostic imaging. As AI technology finds more and more applications in clinical practice, the concerns of patient privacy, consent, and data security need to be addressed immediately by regulatory bodies. The potential of AI models to reinforce ingrained bias in healthcare is another pressing ethical concern. Regulatory bodies also need to develop long-term guidelines for evaluating the safety and efficacy of AI interventions. As of now, the pace of AI solution development has remained ahead of regulatory measures, and the landscape is brimming with uncertainty. Therefore, these regulatory and ethical questions must be addressed to establish a space where AI can be used effectively and safely in diagnostic imaging. Failure to solve these complex issues can impede technological advancements and the benefits of AI in clinical diagnostics (Abbas et al., 2024) (Figure 7.7).

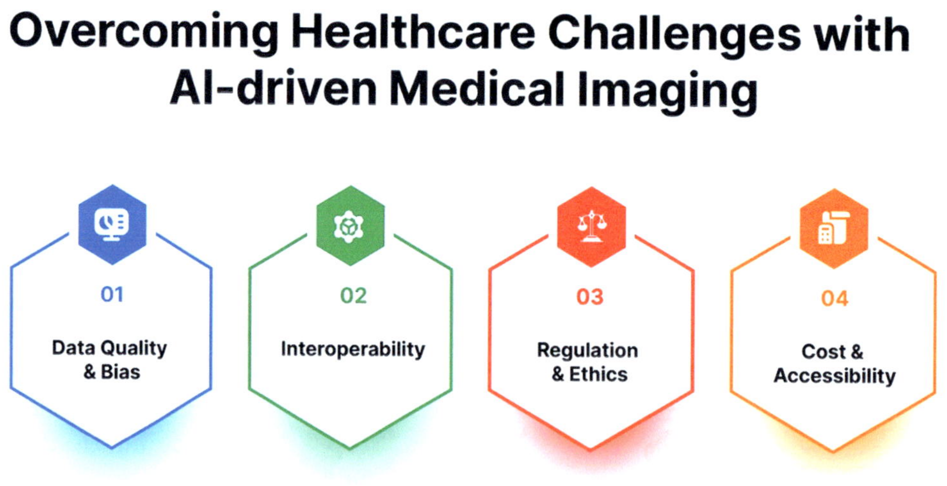

Figure 7.7. Challengers of AI and ML in diagnostics.

Source: https://assets.bacancytechnology.com/blog/wp-content/uploads/2024/05/22120929/Overcoming-Healthcare-Challenges-with-AI-driven-Medical-Imaging.webp.

7.3.1. Data Privacy and Security Concerns

AI and ML application in medical diagnostic imaging poses critical issues of data security and privacy that must be addressed to ensure safe and effective healthcare operations. With increased reliance on AI diagnosis on analysis of patient data, unauthorized access to confidential data is also elevated.

Such confidential information often includes personally identifiable information (PII) and medical histories that, if compromised, can lead to identity theft or abuse. Healthcare providers thus have to use robust security controls, such as encryption and tight access controls, to secure patient information. Without proper protection, patients' and stakeholders' faith in AI-driven healthcare solutions is bound to dwindle, and the innovation and adoption of this crucial industry can be stunted (Farooq et al., 2017). Moreover, the use of federated learning (FL) also complicates the data privacy landscape further in diagnostic imaging. FL facilitates training models across decentralized devices without sharing data, thereby minimizing some privacy risks associated with data sharing. However, the technology is not risk-free either. Unless checked, hackers can exploit vulnerabilities in network communication to snoop on the sensitive information being passed around and breach patient confidentiality. FL's adoption of AI-enabled systems raises fundamental ethical and operational issues regarding data management and compliance with healthcare regulatory requirements. Solutions should not only work to enhance technical specs but also address the ethical environment in which data is used in diagnostic settings. Conquering these hurdles will be essential to developing a secure AI-based healthcare system (Muthuramalingam et al., 2024). Finally, though AI and ML promise tremendous possibilities for diagnostic superiority and convenience, ethical management of patient data remains the cornerstone of their successful implementation. The relationship between technology and ethics is brought into focus when patients are unaware of how their data is utilized to train algorithms or the potential outcomes of the latter. Greater transparency in AI, enabled by XAI methods, is crucial, as it allows clinicians to understand and justify AI-based diagnoses using patient data. Establishing trust is a matter of compliance with ethical standards and regulatory guidelines that focus on data protection in these emerging technologies. Continuous communication among the involved stakeholders—healthcare providers, technologists, and patients—will be essential to addressing privacy and data security issues in AI-ML-driven diagnostic imaging (Muthuramalingam et al., 2024).

7.3.2. Dependence on High-Quality Data

The success of AI and ML in imaging diagnostics is deeply rooted in the quality of data upon which these models are trained. The datasets must be high-quality and diverse, as they are the foundation on which AI algorithms learn to recognize patterns and abnormalities in medical images. When data is incomplete or inaccurate, the output models may exhibit defects or biases in their diagnostic functions. The growth of imaging informatics has therefore put this dependence on robust data in the limelight, with recent research indicating that improvements in diagnostic accuracy are strongly dependent on integrating diverse data types, which corrects biases introduced by homogeneous data sets (Baumgartner et al., 2019). Thus, pushing for high-quality data is paramount to enhancing the generalizability and validity of AI instruments in diagnostic contexts. In addition, ongoing standard development for data reporting and measuring data quality in medical research also remains a major challenge. Dissimilarity in quality across published studies might lead to inconsistencies between findings and the feasibility of applying AI in diagnostic imaging. Several experiments have revealed advanced approaches that increase the replicability and interpretability of AI models, yet no reporting requirements hold back their widespread use (Baumgartner et al., 2019).

This kind of heterogeneity requires researchers and practitioners to collaborate to develop metrics that ensure optimal data quality and transparency. Creating a standard for the evaluation and sharing of datasets can enhance the validity of AI solutions in diagnostic imaging and encourage clinicians' confidence in relying on such innovative technologies for patient management. New technologies such as virtual reality and AI applications are also emerging as beneficial adjuncts in medical imaging. These technologies not only enhance the visual display of information but also provide more immersive, user-friendly experiences for clinicians and patients alike. As an example, the use of AI in the visual arts has shown promise in therapy to improve cognitive capacity and behavior in patients with dementia. These transdisciplinary approaches highlight the requirements for high-quality data beyond standard medical imaging and encourage research that broadens to include fields of creativity and interactive technology. As machine learning in diagnostic imaging advances, upholding data integrity will remain key to developing models capable of driving adaptive clinical applications and enhancing overall health outcomes.

7.3.3. Resistance from Healthcare Professionals

The use of AI and machine learning in diagnostic imaging has not been without opposition among clinicians. There is frequent resistance from healthcare workers because it stems from fear of job loss, with several practitioners worried that the use of AI may render them irrelevant. Even though AIs can increase accuracy and efficiency in diagnostics, clinicians are wary of letting algorithms take over control of patient care.

This is also propagated by misinformation surrounding the capabilities of AI technologies and what they can do. Healthcare workers view AI as a competitor rather than as a means to expand their capabilities, which has led them to reject its adoption. Hence, to address and clarify these problems is essential to facilitate AI adoption in healthcare institutions and ensure that health professionals can effectively collaborate with such advanced technologies to promote better patient outcomes (Cordeiro et al., 2023). Further, resistance is usually due to the absence of experience and training in AI technologies among the health professionals. Studies have shown that the majority of practitioners feel poorly qualified to incorporate AI in practice due to a lack of proper training and education regarding the use of digital health.

This creates an enormous barrier to adoption, as professionals are less likely to use systems they feel they lack full knowledge of or are not comfortable working with. Moreover, there is concern over AI algorithm quality and transparency, i.e., their training data and how they make decisions. In the lack of proper education on these issues, clinicians may be reluctant to believe that AI products are reliable and will improve patient care (Abualigah et al., 2024). Thus, addressing these training and knowledge gaps is critical in developing a more open approach to AI diagnostic imaging. Finally, ethical concerns also play a significant role in the resistance experienced by medical practitioners.

Data privacy, security, and the proper use of AI in clinical environments are most worrying to most practitioners. Issues of consent and algorithmic decision-making bias arise when large volumes of patient data are used to train AI algorithms. Furthermore, clinicians are concerned about the accountability of AI-driven recommendations and diagnoses, as they may contradict current medical guidelines and standards. Inasmuch as trust is part and parcel of the patient-provider relationship, any prospect of a loss of trust arising from AI interventions may further compound resistance. Thus, developing an ethical openness culture and engaging healthcare professionals in discussions regarding AI's role in diagnostic imaging will be crucial to dispelling fears and promoting the uptake of these innovative technologies (Cordeiro et al., 2023).

7.4. Ethical Considerations

With the continued advancement of AI and ML in imaging diagnostics, ethical considerations become increasingly important. Integrating these technologies requires careful examination of data privacy and patient consent. Because AI-based systems are built on large datasets that often contain sensitive health information, confidentiality is important for patients. Health organizations must implement stringent data protection measures against unauthorized access and misuse of personal data. The way informed consent is obtained from patients must also be modified, providing clear explanations about the use of their data in AI diagnostics. Ignorance of these ethical concerns will compromise public trust in healthcare technology, ultimately slowing down its implementation and affecting patient care outcomes in the long term. The concept of accountability also comes up as a leading ethical concern in the use of AI and ML in radiology. As AI systems become more entangled in clinical decision-making, it is harder to decide who is accountable for diagnostic errors. This becomes especially evident where the AI algorithms are black boxes, hiding the decision-making processes behind their outcomes. Without understanding the inner workings of the algorithms, practitioners may not be able to explain using AI-generated diagnoses to stakeholders and patients. This perceived lack of transparency raises questions regarding the ethics of putting decision-making capabilities in the hands of machines and their implications for patient-centered care. It then becomes important to strike a balance between capitalizing on technological advancements and maintaining a commitment to open, transparent medical practices that respect patient autonomy and understanding, as highlighted by the controversy surrounding black-box medicine (Bjerring et al., 2020). Lastly, the intersection of AI in imaging diagnostic work and ethics highlights the importance of equal access to these technologies. Health inequities might limit access to AI technologies in certain populations, exacerbating current disparities in disease detection and treatment outcomes. Furthermore, if an AI system is trained on unrepresentative datasets, it risks reinforcing existing biases, leading to inaccurate diagnoses in underrepresented populations. It is important that policymakers and developers pay attention to inclusivity in the training data as well as in the deployment of the AI tools within healthcare settings. Addressing these ethical issues not only ensures equal treatment for all patients but also enhances the overall validity and reliability of AI-based diagnostic solutions for treating multi-factorial medical conditions, such as various types of cancer (Abbas et al., 2024).

7.4.1. Bias in AI Algorithms

Embedding AI in diagnostic imaging has the potential to revolutionize healthcare by making diagnoses more accurate and efficient. But this comes with the critical challenge of AI algorithmic bias. Algorithmic bias arises when data employed in training AI systems reflects past injustices or the underrepresentation of certain groups. This is particularly problematic in medical applications, where biased algorithms can disproportionately misdiagnose or mistreat certain populations. To illustrate, if training sets consist primarily of images of a single ethnicity, the AI might not accurately interpret scans of underrepresented groups, leading to unequal treatment and outcomes. Therefore, bias elimination is less a matter of technical necessity than of core importance to ensuring fairness in healthcare, especially in high-risk fields like diagnostic imaging, where accuracy and trust are paramount. Beyond that, black-box medicine also complicates the problem of bias in AI systems. As AI algorithms grow more sophisticated, their reasoning processes grow opaque to healthcare practitioners. This transparency can hinder the identification and rectification of biases embedded in the models. Professionals can feel compelled to accept AI suggestions without knowing the reasoning supporting them, which can perpetuate existing biases in patient treatment. This is counter to principles of patient-centered care, which favor informed decision-making and shared deliberation with patients. Therefore, the issue also includes, in addition to detecting bias in AI algorithms, developing a health culture in which practitioners are empowered and willing to critically examine AI output ethically (Bjerring et al., 2020). Secondly, the concern about biased AI algorithms in imaging diagnostics also resonates strongly with broader concerns about healthcare disparities. Studies have shown that machine learning models may vary widely in accuracy across demographic measures, suggesting that such biases might be a factor in an unequal health care access and quality environment (Depp et al., 2020). Early detection and intervention are crucial in the prevention of disease progression, especially with neurocognitive impairment that has significant effects on aging populations. When AI programs repeatedly fail for specific patient groups, they can inadvertently perpetuate widening health disparities, limiting access to early treatment for already at-risk populations. Remediating bias in AI algorithms is thus not only critical to maximizing the technological advantages of diagnostic imaging but also to protecting principles of justice and fairness in health outcomes across diverse patient populations (Figure 7.8).

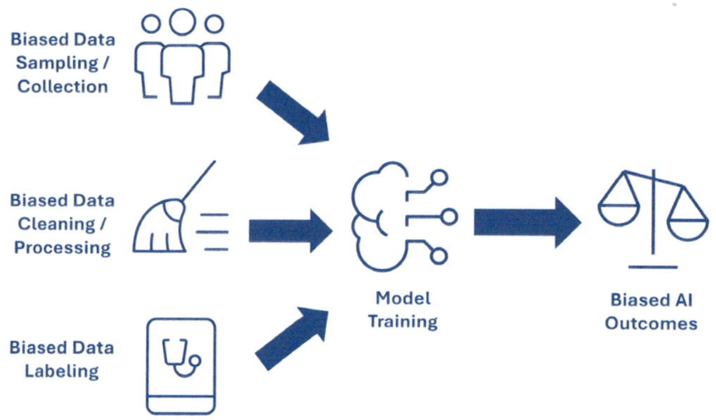

Figure 7.8. Data curation practices to minimize bias in medical AI

Source: https://miro.medium.com/v2/resize:fit:1400/1*_W741xqSPb76MPkQbFffcg.png.

7.4.2. Accountability in Diagnostic Decisions

In diagnostic imaging, applying AI and ML requires profound introspection on responsibility in decision-making. With healthcare providers increasingly reliant on AI-based diagnosis, the framework for responsibility on outcomes delivered through these solutions must remain clearly established. Delegating diagnostic authority to AI presents grave ethical as well as legal challenges, particularly if mistakes lead to misdiagnosis or delayed treatment. Lastly, clinicians must remain actively engaged and watchful while perusing AI-generated outcomes; otherwise, the responsibility is not retained as technology dominates. Such constant scrutiny instills a spirit of working together, fostering the proper use of AI while keeping the intuitive role of human experience central to clinical decision-making. Moreover, the integration of AI in diagnosis also upends conventional assumptions of clinical governance. The stakeholders have to engage in navigating the intricate balance between AI's capabilities and its ethical concerns in applying to patient care. Emphasized in controversies regarding new technologies, such as A.I. neuroprediction in forensic psychiatry, are the far-reaching implications of applications of AI, which need to undergo serious weighing of benefits and harms (Bijlsma et al., 2020) (Figure 7.9).

There is a critical need for a formal system of governance to provide transparency and ethical conduct in clinical settings. This includes creating mechanisms for allocating responsibility among technology developers and healthcare providers. There needs to be collaboration, underpinned by solid ethics, to address concerns about bias, accuracy, and the potential negative impact on patients' trust in health care systems. Further, making AI and ML accountable in imaging diagnostics involves addressing interoperability and standardization issues across healthcare platforms. Healthcare facilities have to adopt stringent standards in AI mechanisms to ensure results consistency and guard against threats to patient well-being (Balaskas et al., 2023). Lack of transparent regulatory processes poses the risk of variability in diagnostic standards, creating inconsistencies in patient care and undermining the welfare these technologies can bring. It is vital that various stakeholders, like clinicians, IT professionals, and regulatory bodies, become involved in formulating policies that address not only technological advancement but also moral accountability. This integrated approach will ultimately make the use of AI-facilitated diagnostics more certain and usher in safer and more effective health care.

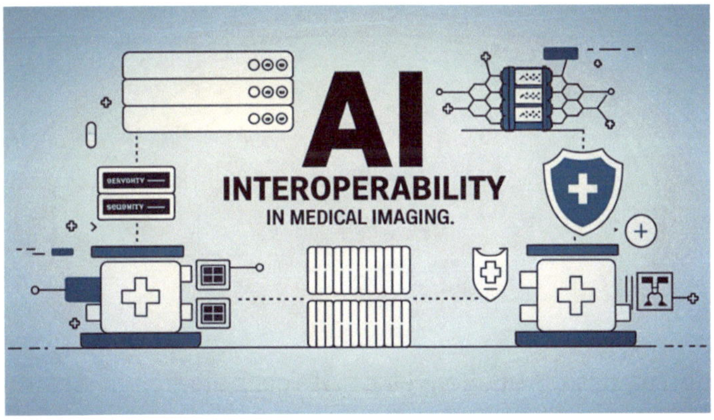

Figure 7.9. AI Interoperability in Medical Imaging: A Roadmap to Improved Patient Outcomes.

Source: https://media.licdn.com/dms/image/v2/D5612AQGPHo_G3ZXPkA/article-cover_image-shrink_600_2000/article-cover_image-shrink_600_2000/0/1730962621789?e=2147483647&v=beta&t=ORu4gT5sU1_5xPeXQFR2ykL6VdXUYySpy3_KCEFAwJc.

7.4.3. Informed Consent and Patient Autonomy

The marriage of AI and machine learning in diagnostic imaging raises key ethical questions regarding patient autonomy and informed consent. As systems become more complex, their functions are increasingly becoming black boxes that healthcare professionals find difficult to decipher or explain. This lack of transparency undermines the core principles of patient-centered care, which is premised on having mutual deliberation between patients and practitioners. Informed consent relies on patients being adequately informed about the technologies impacting their diagnosis and treatment choices. When clinicians do not understand the operation of AI technologies, this undermines the quality of the information communicated to patients, in practical terms, preventing them from making autonomous health choices aligned with their values and preferences (Bjerring et al., 2020). In addition, the difficulties of AI in medicine go beyond technical challenges; they cut across legal and ethical systems that manage patient autonomy. Greater reliance on algorithms for image analysis can indirectly lead to the undervaluing of human judgment in medical practice. As professionals focus more on the recommendations made by AI than on their professional judgment, it may undermine trust within the clinician-patient relationship. Patients must be reassured that AI systems do not solely make their clinical decisions but are still overseen and decision-making, allowing them to apply their autonomy to the maximum. Thus, developing a framework in which patients feel safe enough to ask questions and demand an explanation about AI's role in their treatment becomes imperative (Kanagarajah et al., 2024) (Figure 7.10).

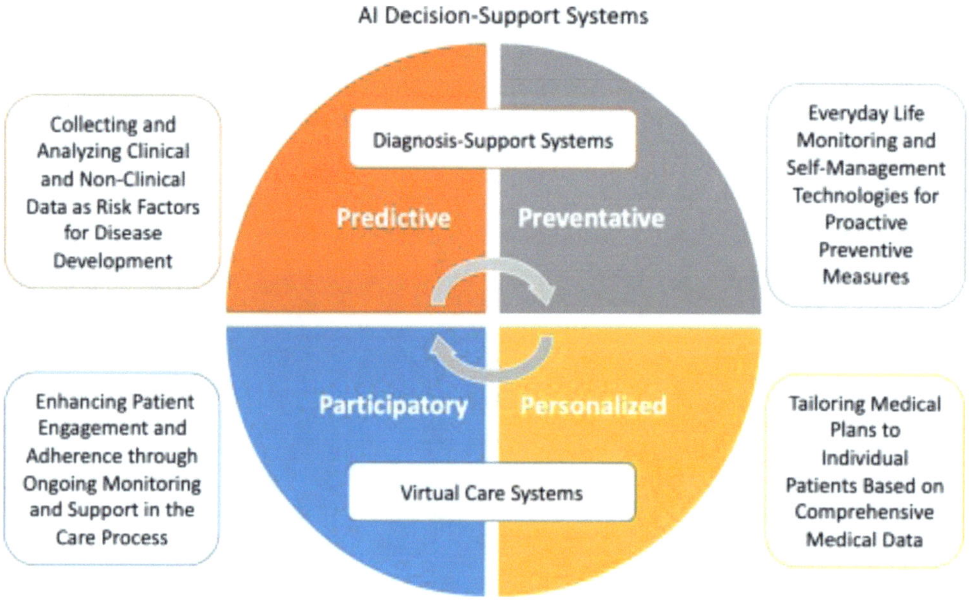

Figure 7.10. Ethical and regulatory challenges of AI technologies in healthcare.

Source: https://ars.els-cdn.com/content/image/1-s2.0-S2405844024023284-gr002.jpg.

To combat these challenges, developing robust frameworks that ensure transparency and promote informed consent in AI and machine learning scenarios is of utmost priority. Healthcare professionals must be properly trained to communicate the consequences of AI-based diagnoses to patients, ensuring they understand the basis for their diagnoses and treatments. Further, regulatory bodies should implement final directives requiring adequate disclosure of the use of AI in the clinical setting. By creating an informed consent model that not only illustrates the power of AI technologies but also their limitations, medical personnel can better ensure patient autonomy values and promote an interactive paradigm of decision-making. As AI technologies become increasingly integral to diagnostic imaging, the healthcare industry must proactively address these ethical concerns to safeguard patients' rights and build trust within the emerging medical technology community (Kanagarajah et al., 2024).

7.5. Future Trends and Innovations

The integration of ML and AI into diagnostic imaging is not only a continuing trend but also an enabler of revolutionary future trends that will redefine healthcare provision. One of the most significant developments is the advent of 5G wireless technology, which offers high-throughput, low-latency connectivity essential for the big data required to run AI algorithms (Figure 7.11). This technological innovation, combined with the commoditization of computing power through cloud computing, enables immediate image analysis, accelerating diagnosis and improving its accuracy. As has been pointed out, the union of AI and 5G enhances the prospects for telemedicine and remote diagnosis, particularly in poor areas where traditional healthcare access is limited. These innovations not only address current gaps in healthcare systems but also complement global efforts, such as the UN Sustainable Development Goals, to ensure equal access to quality healthcare (Farooq et al., 2017).

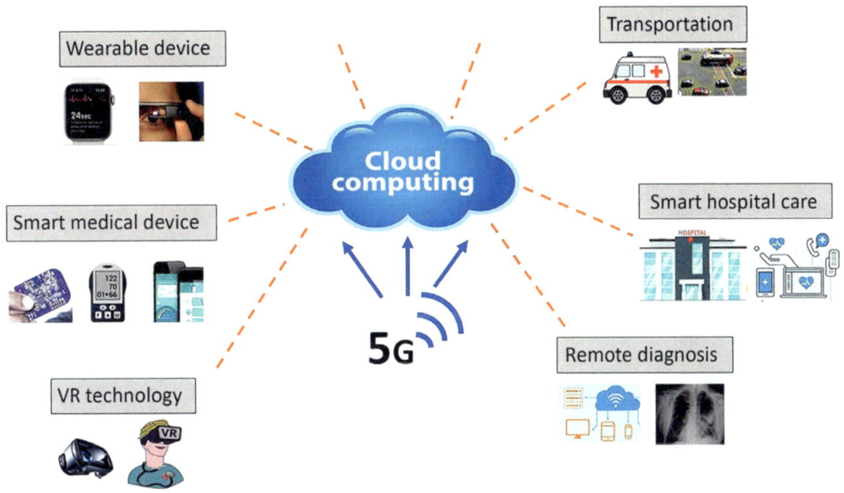

Figure 7.11. Applications of 5G technology in healthcare.

Source: https://www.researchgate.net/profile/Nixon-Amuomo/publication/340447512/figure/fig1/AS:885044566568960@1588022476007/Applications-of-5G-technology-in-healthcare.jpg.

Beyond that, AI utilization in diagnostic imaging is rapidly transforming, influencing all aspects of patient care and clinical practice. Key developments include strides in precision medicine that are introduced by AI-driven diagnostic equipment, which review imaging information with unmatched accuracy. This development encourages personalized treatment protocols since algorithms can predict patient response to various therapies from individual imaging markers. Also, the incorporation of AI in remote monitoring equipment enables constant monitoring of patients, changing healthcare workers' engagement with patients beyond clinical environments. As indicated, the integration of AI capabilities in clinical decision support systems enhances diagnosis accuracy, ultimately improving patient outcomes while avoiding the resource burden on healthcare systems (Adertinto et al., 2024). Despite these promising advances, AI in diagnostic imaging futures are not without challenges. Algorithm accuracy issues, data interoperability issues, and AI tools' incorporation into existing clinical workflows remain challenges. While health systems implement these advanced technologies, it is essential to prioritize the development of robust validation policies and ethical guidelines to ensure maximum patient safety and data security. Moreover, the concurrent existence of AI technologies alongside traditional diagnostic methods necessitates redefining training programs for medical practitioners to enable them to use AI effectively. They will be crucial in unleashing the full potential of AI and ML in diagnostic imaging to build innovations that enhance patient care, operational efficiency, and ultimately reimagine healthcare delivery models (Farooq et al., 2017).

7.5.1. Advancements in Deep Learning Techniques

Advances in deep learning techniques have significantly transformed diagnostic imaging in machine learning and artificial intelligence. Historically, traditional machine learning techniques were not capable of handling complex medical images due to the high dimensionality and intricate features inherent in such data. Deep learning, particularly CNNs, has been a strong alternative for processing such images by effectively analyzing them in terms of hierarchical features. Such networks can automatically learn to recognize patterns and differences in the data without requiring extensive manual feature engineering (Figure 7.12).

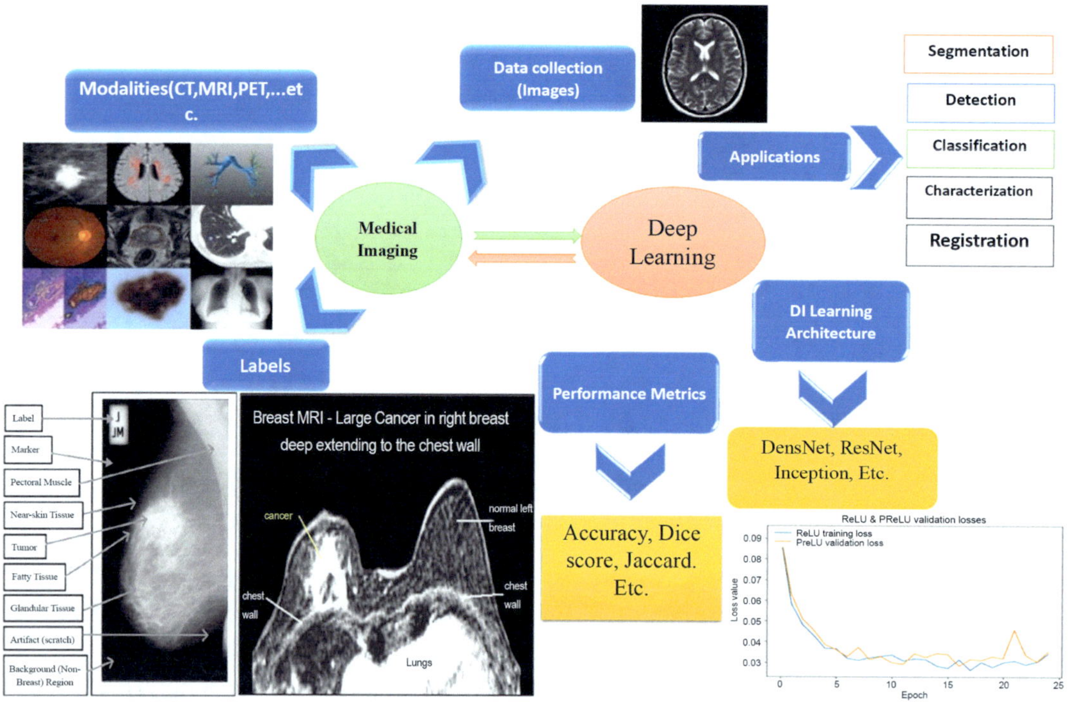

Figure 7.12. A holistic overview of the deep learning approach in medical imaging.

Source: https://media.springernature.com/lw1200/springer-static/image/art%3A10.1007%2Fs00530-021-00884-5/MediaObjects/530_2021_884_Fig1_HTML.png.

The smooth integration of these techniques into imaging diagnostic procedures has enhanced the accuracy and effectiveness of disease diagnosis, thereby maximizing patient outcomes and facilitating timely clinical decision-making. Apart from this, the current trend in deep learning research for diagnostic imaging is heavily focused on large, heterogeneous data sets. Current studies have shown the need for comprehensive data for training deep learning models. Working with large volumes of imaging data, coupled with increased processing power, has consequently propelled advances in this research area. For instance, deep learning models have begun to achieve successful results in several medical disciplines. Oncology and radiology are case in point; machine learning has contributed immensely to tasks such as tumor detection and classification. In addition, the emergence of federated learning approaches supports decentralized model training, which can help address patient privacy challenges by training models on distributed data without revealing sensitive information. With the increasing growth in deep learning techniques, challenges also arise that need to be overcome prior to further integration into clinical practice. Interpretability questions, model stability, and the requirement for validation across diverse populations raise fundamental questions regarding using these models in real-world applications. XAI approaches are central to this as they seek to enhance the transparency of model choices and uncover what happens inside them. Integrating such approaches not only helps describe how models arrive at specific conclusions but also increases clinicians' trust in AI-assisted diagnostics. It is thus essential to conduct research to overcome such challenges while leveraging the revolutionary potential of deep learning to markedly improve diagnostic imaging outcomes, as emphasized in recent reviews (Abbas et al., 2024; Geetu, 2023).

7.5.2. Potential for Personalized Medicine

As diagnostic imaging advances, the combination of machine learning and AI is ushering in a new era of personalized medicine. Both technologies have the potential to analyze vast amounts of data in real time and enable the development of tailored treatment plans that are more effective for each patient. Using powerful algorithms, AI can detect patterns in imaging information that the naked eye cannot perceive, making earlier and more accurate diagnoses. In diseases such as cancer, where early detection dramatically improves patient outcomes, this is particularly valuable. Moreover, the democratization of AI technologies provides assurance that even small healthcare centers can make advanced diagnostic devices affordable, thereby enhancing overall care quality and making personalized medicine available on a wider scale (Farooq et al., 2017) (Figure 7.13).

The capabilities of personalized medicine are also enhanced by the ability of machine learning models to adapt over time. With increased exposure to data, these systems frequently refine the precision of their predictions, which subsequently benefits the patient's care. By correlating imaging findings with a patient's genetic makeup, clinical history, and lifestyle factors, AI-based systems can identify the most suitable treatments tailored to the patient's unique profile. Such a combined approach not only increases the efficiency of the treatment but also diminishes the side effects of standardized one-size-fits-all treatments. The convergence of AI and diagnostics brings us to an age of more patient-centered care, with interventions selected based on a profound understanding of individual characteristics rather than simply according to generalized clinical guidelines (Dethlefs et al., 2019). Secondly, the vision of personalized medicine by AI imaging diagnosis is intrinsically tied to the emergence of preventive healthcare strategies. By examining imaging data alongside advanced patient profiles, AI platforms can predict disease vulnerability and recommend anticipatory interventions to adequately mitigate harm to health. It breaks away from the traditional path of healthcare, where response follows prevention. As AI technologies continue to evolve, they will transform public health programs by detecting population-level trends and high-risk groups, thereby enabling more targeted intervention strategies. Conjoining AI-powered diagnostic features and personalized medicine can redefine healthcare as a proactive rather than reactive system, resulting in improved population health outcomes and better resource allocation (Farooq et al., 2017).

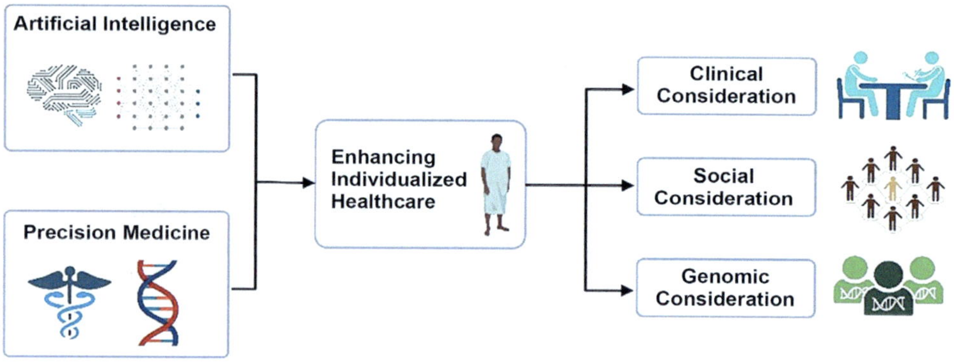

Figure 7.13. The integration of AI and precision medicine enhances individual healthcare by optimizing therapy planning and diagnostic methods.

Source: https://www.researchgate.net/publication/378589955/figure/fig1/AS:11431281238820329@1714073210672/The-integration-of-AI-and-precision-medicine-enhances-individual-healthcare-by-optimizing.tif.

7.5.3. Collaboration Between AI and Human Radiologists

The integration of AI into diagnostic imaging has opened the way for a revolutionary partnership between AI systems and human radiologists.

This is encapsulated under the umbrella of the Bionic Radiologist, where technology supports human ability and leverages it, rather than replacing it. With the rapid growth of radiological exams—over 3.6 billion annually—AI programs can streamline image reading, thereby enhancing diagnostic efficiency and accuracy. By allowing AIs' processing power to handle image review, radiologists can spend more time focusing on crucial decision-making functions. However, the successful deployment of such solutions is contingent on a cautious management of issues like organizational culture and AI suggestion trust, which remain paramount to building an effective collaborative environment, enhancing patient safety and care (Dewey et al., 2019) (Figure 7.14). AI application in diagnostic imaging necessitates a strategy focusing on the interpretability of machine-provided insights, particularly in complex medical cases. As AI technologies continue to advance, issues surrounding their black-box nature have motivated the creation of XAI. This paradigm caters to the need for transparency in AI use, allowing radiologists to see and believe in the AI's suggestions. Through the use of methods that make it clear how AI models come to their decisions, radiologists can better integrate machine-derived insights into their clinical choices.

This combination not only promotes radiologists to make the right decisions but also adds the human touch with patients and a global outlook while providing care, thus further enhancing diagnosis (Parmar et al., 2023). Secondly, with the collaboration of AI, the potential is not just limited to individual-level diagnosis but also includes the ongoing process of learning and adjustment through the continuum of healthcare. Artificial intelligence systems can analyze vast datasets to identify patterns and trends that are not readily apparent to human practitioners. This reservoir of knowledge can inform evidence-based practice and refine imaging testing protocols to a greater degree. As radiologists collaborate with AI tools, they can refine their skills to remain at the forefront of new technologies while driving a culture of continuous improvement. This new alliance not only streamlines diagnostic procedures but also fosters a healthcare culture that promotes personalized, effective patient care, thereby transforming the radiologist's work in the age of AI (Dewey et al., 2019).

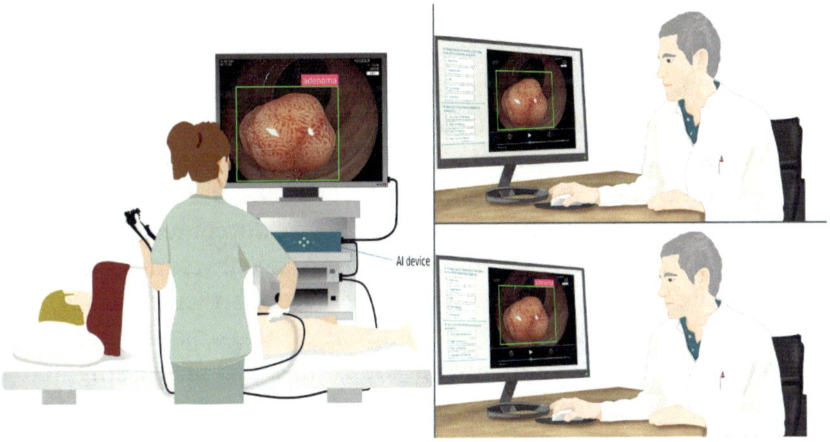

Figure 7.14. Experimental evidence of effective human–AI collaboration in medical decision-making

Source: https://media.springernature.com/lw1200/springer-static/image/art%3A10.1038%2Fs41598-022-18751-2/MediaObjects/41598_2022_18751_Fig1_HTML.png.

SUMMARY

The integration of AI and ML in imaging diagnosis is a paradigm shift in health technology. This revolution is very noticeable when it comes to cancer diagnosis, which entails traditional procedures such as the ABCD method and seven-point detection method, both of which have been proven to be ineffective and not accurate. The shifting horizon of diagnostic means has necessitated seeking better processes, and AI is a viable solution. Deep learning models, particularly CNNs, have been incredible driving forces for image evaluation. With the help of large datasets and high-performance computing techniques, these models improve diagnostic accuracy and speed, thereby benefiting healthcare professionals in making more precise decisions in cancer identification and detection (Ayub et al., 2019). Besides, the role of data mining has become increasingly vital in medical imaging, particularly in the context of vast amounts of medical data generated in contemporary practice. Data mining techniques enable the identification of significant patterns and trends in data, which can be vital for early cancer detection and treatment protocols. Various methodologies, including classification and clustering, have been shown to be successful in dermatology and other branches of medicine. Classification techniques, such as Neural Networks and Genetic Algorithms, have been particularly mentioned for their ability to enhance diagnostic outcomes. They operate by classifying images based on learned features, thereby enhancing more accurate identification of skin diseases and cancer, with clustering assisting in dataset pattern detection (Adibi et al., 2011). The success of ML and AI in diagnostic imaging is heavily dependent on the organization that integrates these technologies. The procedure goes through several steps, like pre-processing, image segmentation, and post-processing, all of which are crucial to achieving the best output. Through these steps, algorithms are fine-tuned to detect and classify different cancer types effectively. The necessity of standardized evaluation metrics, such as the receiver operating characteristic curve and measures of accuracy, cannot be overstated; they are required to quantify model performance. Coupling deep learning architectures with stringent methodological evaluation is conducive to the development of smarter diagnostic devices, thereby complementing the inefficiencies of past approaches and, in the long run, enhancing patient care (Ayub et al., 2019; Adibi et al., 2011).

CLOSER LOOK

THE FUTURE OF AI AND ML IN DIAGNOSTIC IMAGING

The intersection of AI and ML with diagnostic imaging can revolutionize healthcare with highly effective tools for more effective and accurate diagnoses. As these technologies continue to develop, they enable the analysis of large volumes of imaging data to realize the full potential of standard diagnostic techniques. Advances such as advanced imaging technology and computer-aided diagnostic systems greatly improve the visualization and interpretation of complex information. These innovations minimize the reliance on human ability only, increasing diagnostic precision and decreasing the incidence of errors. As proposed through recent studies, novel technology in the form of digital photographic imaging and optical coherence tomography is an illustration of how AI has the capability to boost conventional practice, thereby providing more precise diagnoses while limiting the invasiveness of procedures such as biopsies (Gold et al., 2021). The future diagnostic imaging environment thus promises a radical shift towards AI- and ML-driven practices that will deliver greater safety and care for patients. Although AI and ML promise much in diagnostic imaging, their integration with healthcare systems is not simple. Explainability and transparency in AI, or what is commonly termed black-box medicine, make professional-technology interactions challenging (Bjerring et al., 2020). As AI systems operate with intricate algorithms that are maybe not explainable at all, physicians can become entangled in conflicts on whether to adopt AI-developed conclusions or remain with traditional diagnostic approaches. The complication raises ethical questions about responsibility and informed consentas practitioners would have the burden of making decisions based on AI recommendations which lack, as practitioners would have the burden of making decisions based on AI recommendations that lack an apparent rationale. Thus, it is essential that future research and development focus on enhancing the interpretability of these AI systems, promoting collaboration between healthcare providers and technology to build confidence and improve patient outcomes. Additionally, the advancement of AI and ML in diagnostic imaging demands robust training programs for healthcare providers to empower them to use these advanced tools effectively. As the pace of technological advancement accelerates, practitioners will be expected to engage in continuous learning and professional education to remain competent in a more AI-centric world. Medical school curricula will be forced to increasingly integrate AI literacy, not only training doctors to interact with such systems but also to vet and contextualize their output. Through creating an adaptive workforce, the health care sector can ensure that technological progress is in a position to translate into improving patient care. Ultimately, the destiny of ML and AI in imaging diagnostics lies not in replacing human ability but in optimizing co-work between man and machine to create a smoother, more accurate healthcare environment (Gold et al., 2021).

REFERENCES

1. Abbas, S., Asif, M., Rehman, A., Alharbi, M., Khan, M. A., & Elmitwally, N. (2024). RETRACTED: Emerging research trends in artificial intelligence for cancer diagnostic systems: A comprehensive review. *Heliyon*, *10*(17), e36743. https://doi.org/10.1016/j.heliyon.2024.e36743Abualigah, L., Banu, S. A., Dhama, K., et al. (2024). Unleashing the future: Exploring the transformative prospects of artificial intelligence in veterinary science. https://core.ac.uk/download/620832362.pdf (accessed on 5th August 2025).
2. Adertinto, N., David-Olawade, A. C., David-Olawade, et al. (2024). Advancements and applications of artificial intelligence in cardiology: Current trends and future prospects. https://core.ac.uk/download/603653360.pdf (accessed on 5th August 2025).
3. Adibi, N., Ahmadzadeh, M. R., Barati, E., et al. (2011). A survey on utilization of data mining approaches for dermatological (skin) diseases prediction. https://core.ac.uk/download/1667194.pdf (accessed on 5th August 2025).
4. Ahmed, S., Bajwa, M. N., Braun, S. A., et al. (2020). On interpretability of deep learning-based skin lesion classifiers using concept activation vectors. http://arxiv.org/abs/2005.02000 (accessed on 5th August 2025).
5. Alaa, R., Jawad, A. T., Khalid, M., & Mays, et al. (2024). Advances in artificial intelligence for polyp detection: A comprehensive review. https://core.ac.uk/download/641562679.pdf (accessed on 5th August 2025).
6. António, N., Marreiros, A., Pereira-Macedo, J., et al. (2024). The role of artificial intelligence and machine learning in managing carotid stenosis. https://core.ac.uk/download/621578663.pdf (accessed on 5th August 2025).
7. Arain, Z., Chowdhury, T. T., David, A. L., Iliodromiti, et al. (2023). Machine learning and disease prediction in obstetrics. https://core.ac.uk/download/571216446.pdf (accessed on 5th August 2025).
8. Ayub, A., Elahi, H., Frezza, F., Munir, et al. (2019). Cancer diagnosis using deep learning: A bibliographic review. https://core.ac.uk/download/231746843.pdf (accessed on 5th August 2025).
9. Balaskas, K., Hogg, H. J., Keane, P. A., Taribagil, et al. (2023). Integrating artificial intelligence into an ophthalmologist's workflow: Obstacles and opportunities. https://core.ac.uk/download/554845105.pdf (accessed on 5th August 2025).
10. Bartoszek, L., Kapłan, W., Kaus, M., Klepacz, et al. (2025). Application of artificial intelligence in radiological image analysis for pulmonary disease diagnosis: A review of current methods and challenges. https://core.ac.uk/download/636386127.pdf (accessed on 5th August 2025).
11. Baumgartner, C., Deserno, T., Hsu, W., et al. (2019). Advancing artificial intelligence in sensors, signals, and imaging informatics. https://core.ac.uk/download/323076975.pdf (accessed on 5th August 2025).
12. Bijlsma, J., Ferracuti, S., Meynen, G., Tortora, et al. (2020). Neuroprediction and A.I. in forensic psychiatry and criminal justice: A neurolaw perspective. https://core.ac.uk/download/323191898.pdf (accessed on 5th August 2025).

13. Bjerring, J. C., & Busch, J. (2020). Artificial intelligence and patient-centered decision-making. https://core.ac.uk/download/286027525.pdf (accessed on 5th August 2025).
14. Burczyk, R., Duszyński, K., Michalska, M., et al. (2025). The role of artificial intelligence in detecting breast lesions using ultrasound. https://core.ac.uk/download/636385693.pdf (accessed on 5th August 2025).
15. Cordeiro, J. V., Cunha, A. S., Dias, M. B., Laranjo, et al. (2023). A comprehensive survey of medical doctor's perspectives in Portugal. https://core.ac.uk/download/591215979.pdf (accessed on 5th August 2025).
16. Depp, C. A., Graham, S. A., Jeste, D. V., Kim, et al. (2020). Artificial intelligence approaches to predicting and detecting cognitive decline in older adults: A conceptual review. https://core.ac.uk/download/287623887.pdf (accessed on 5th August 2025).
17. Dethlefs, B. A., Lee, K. L., Li, S. C., et al. (2019). Breathing signature as vitality score index created by exercises of Qigong: Implications of artificial intelligence tools used in traditional Chinese medicine. https://core.ac.uk/download/323075335.pdf (accessed on 5th August 2025).
18. Dewey, M., & Wilkens, U. (2019). The bionic radiologist: Avoiding blurry pictures and providing greater insights. https://core.ac.uk/download/228064788.pdf (accessed on 5th August 2025).
19. Farooq, S., Imran, M. A., Latif, S., Qadir, et al. (2017). How 5G wireless (and concomitant technologies) will revolutionize healthcare? https://core.ac.uk/download/143476480.pdf (accessed on 5th August 2025).
20. Geetu. (2023). The role of artificial intelligence, machine learning, and deep neural networks in medical imaging: Applications, strengths, and challenges. https://core.ac.uk/download/654637202.pdf (accessed on 5th August 2025).
21. Ginley, B., Govind, D., Jain, S., et al. (2018). Iterative annotation to ease neural network training: Specialized machine learning in medical image analysis. https://core.ac.uk/download/573411151.pdf (accessed on 5th August 2025).
22. Gold, M. H., Goldust, M., Grabbe, S., et al. (2021). New diagnostic and imaging technologies in dermatology. https://core.ac.uk/download/621759723.pdf (accessed on 5th August 2025).
23. Harwood, T., Maltby, J., & Mukaetova-Ladinska, E. (2019). Role of artificial intelligence (AI) art in care of ageing society: Focus on dementia. https://core.ac.uk/download/228191193.pdf (accessed on 5th August 2025).
24. Kanagarajah, A. (2024). AI-driven innovation in healthcare product development: Challenges and ethical implications. https://core.ac.uk/download/630299457.pdf (accessed on 5th August 2025).
25. Lastrucci, A., Giansanti, D., Carico, E., & Giarnieri, E. (2024). Revolutionizing cytology and cytopathology with natural language processing and chatbot technologies: A narrative review on current trends and future directions. https://core.ac.uk/download/638802373.pdf (accessed on 5th August 2025).
26. Muthuramalingam, S., & Thiyagarajan, P. (2024). Impact of federated learning and explainable artificial intelligence for medical image diagnosis. https://core.ac.uk/download/642649643.pdf (accessed on 5th August 2025).

27. Parmar, J., Parmar, J., Sahatiya, P., Tulsani, et al. (2023). XAI applications in medical imaging: A survey of methods and challenges. https://core.ac.uk/download/591405083.pdf (accessed on 5th August 2025).

28. Wadhawan, R., Singh, S. D., Tiwari, A. S., Bora, S. P., Khareliya, D. K., & Tamta, V. P. (2024). Beyond scalpel: Artificial intelligence in risk prediction and managing oro-facial trauma. https://core.ac.uk/download/640070294.pdf (accessed on 5th August 2025).

29. Wadhawan, R., Singh, V. D., Roshan, N., Sharma, R., Narayan, Y., & Tamta, V. P. (2024). Artificial intelligence in prosthodontics: Revolutionizing diagnosis, treatment, and prosthetic design. https://core.ac.uk/download/640070377.pdf (accessed on 5th August 2025).

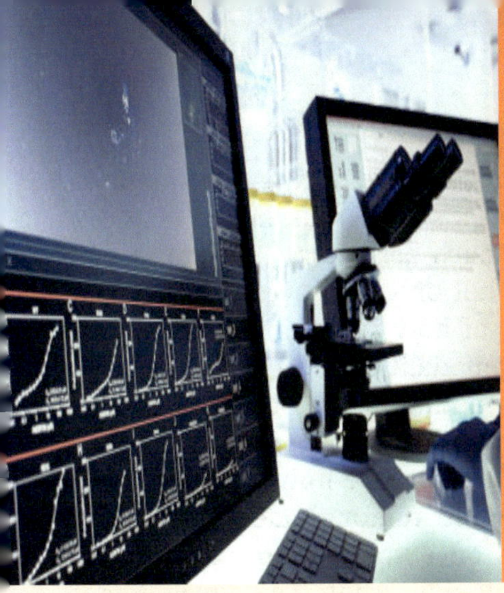

Chapter 8

QUANTITATIVE IMAGING BIOMARKERS AND RADIOMICS

Contents

Introduction

Increasing complexity in cancer management calls for a shift towards individualized care, in which treatment is tailored to the specific characteristics of each patient. The forefront of this transition is the development of quantitative imaging biomarkers that are critical for evaluating tumor heterogeneity and assessing treatment response. Imaging-derived biomarkers contain key information that can inform improved decision-making in oncology. As tumors are biologically heterogeneous, there is a need for incorporating new strategies that facilitate a better understanding of cancer dynamics. For this purpose, radiomics came as a revolutionary tool that utilizes advanced imaging analysis to extract and quantify features from medical images, thus paving the way for more predictive and personalized therapeutic paradigms. Radiomics differs from conventional imaging, with the extraction of vast amounts of data from standard medical scans related to effectively structuring such information into useful patterns that are associated with clinical outcomes. Use of radiomics in lung cancer, for instance, has been embraced owing to its ability to track tumor response and recurrence during treatment. As summarized in recent studies, radiomics can quantitatively associate numerous image features, which enhances predictive capability for various clinical events, such as distant metastasis and radiation-induced damage (Benedict et al., 2018). Such capability not only improves the decision-making of oncologists but also promotes a better understanding of how imaging characteristics reflect underlying biology. The inclusion of these advanced imaging modalities in the clinical setting marks a new era in cancer diagnosis and treatment planning. In addition, the potential uses of radiomics are far-reaching and extend well beyond lung cancer into other oncologic settings, such as breast cancer. By combining multimodality imaging data, researchers are now demonstrating that PET and MRI-derived radiomic features can distinguish between tumor grades and predict disease recurrence (Arasu et al., 2018). This new method relies on extracting specific textural features, which have been statistically shown to be prognostically significant. The development of such technology underscores the promise of quantitative imaging biomarkers in personalizing patient care and maximizing treatment results. As research continues, the incorporation of radiomics into routine clinical practice will likely transform cancer care, enabling us to shift towards more objective, data-driven approaches that maximize prognostication and intervention success.

8.1. Principles of Quantitative Imaging

The foundation for quantitative imaging is the extraction and interpretation of data from medical images to obtain numerical estimates that can be used to understand patient condition and treatment efficacy. Traditional imaging techniques, while helpful, are qualitative and will not show subtle differences detectable by quantitative analysis. This quantitative analysis identifies imaging biomarkers that underlie personalized medicine, enhancing diagnostic accuracy and therapeutic monitoring. Radiomics, specifically the process of extracting high-dimensional data from medical images, applies advanced computational methods to identify features imperceptible to the naked eye. This method is a paradigm shift in imaging since it allows non-invasive detection of important prognostic indicators and therapeutic response in many disorders, especially in cancer therapy, as outlined in Dhermain et al. (2022) (Figure 8.1).

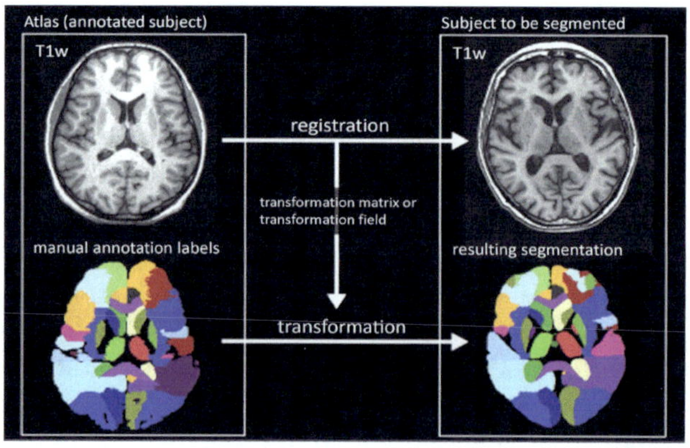

Figure 8.1. Quantitative imaging.

Source: https://ars.els-cdn.com/content/image/1-s2.0-B9780128029732000057-f05-10-9780128029732.jpg.

The integration of quantitative imaging biomarkers into the clinician's practice demands robust methodologies that yield reproducibility and repeatability across imaging modalities. The challenge lies not only in obtaining relevant metrics but also in establishing standardized protocols that can be widely adopted in clinical practice. Current research focuses on harmonizing imaging modalities and establishing guidelines for radiomic analyses to enable an integrated framework that can be used reliably across a range of clinical contexts. A case in point is the potential to automatically extract quantitative biomarkers from patient scans to enhance decision-making in oncology and tailor treatment planning using targeted information rather than general assessment (Dekker et al., 2019). However, reproducibility challenges of these biomarker measurements necessitate ongoing research to develop further improved, more stable, and better-validated methods for clinical applications. The future of radiomics and quantitative imaging is promising but also fraught with challenges that must be solved before its full potential reaches clinical application. Although powerful, quantitative imaging methods remain not fully ingrained in routine clinical practice, primarily due to constraints on applicability and interpretive complexity. With the rising tide of artificial intelligence incorporation in the medical field, a fresh intersection is forming between radiomics and advanced computational approaches, which could enrich the diagnostic value of quantitative imaging. Moreover, the research into Semantic Web and Ontologies here can offer new solutions towards filling the gaps of incorporating quantitative imaging biomarkers in clinical processes, creating a culture of cooperation between healthcare professionals to ensure their maximum potential in treating patients (Dekker et al., 2019). Thus, how these challenges are addressed will be pivotal in unleashing the transformative potential of quantitative imaging in healthcare.

8.1.1. Imaging Modalities Used in Biomarker Analysis

The quest for effective biomarker analysis in oncology has fueled the growth and convergence of imaging modalities, with techniques such as magnetic resonance imaging (MRI) and positron emission tomography (PET) central to this convergence. The imaging modalities are focal instruments in radiomics, through which quantitative imaging biomarkers critical to tumor characterization and response to therapy can be derived. For instance, studies have established that MRI-derived parameters, particularly those dealing with textural patterns, can differentiate between breast cancer subtypes and pre-empt prognosis. Such data are worthwhile, as they allow for personalized therapy to be implemented, thereby informing health care practitioners to make clinical choices regarding their patients' management. The broad applicability of these imaging modalities underscores their role in facilitating personalized medicine and advancing our understanding of cancer heterogeneity. Furthermore, the combination of PET and MRI also illustrates the power of multimodal imaging for biomarker analysis. By combining the complementary advantages of the two modalities, researchers can obtain a richer feature set for analysis. For breast cancer alone, radiomic features from PET and MRI have statistically been shown to be correlated with tumor characteristics and disease prognosis and therefore hold great promise as a prediction tool for recurrence risks.

This fusion improves the clinical imaging prognostic ability by enabling the identification of patients at higher risk of disease progression. There have been recent evaluations that have pointed out the effectiveness of these multi-modality radiomic approaches, showing that they significantly improve the accuracy of prognostic models, thereby informing follow-up treatment protocols and improving patients' quality of life (Arasu et al., 2018). Further, as the field of radiomics continues to advance, addressing the various problems and limitations in terms of imaging modalities used in biomarker analysis is increasingly essential. The power of using sophisticated imaging techniques to reveal hidden patterns in tumor biology is great, yet the standardization of imaging protocols and the need for robust computational methods remain critical problems. Radiomics also relies heavily on accurate extraction and analysis of imaging features from imaging datasets, and this demands advancements in machine learning and artificial intelligence to handle large volumes of imaging data. Additional investigation is also needed to validate and standardize the clinical application of these imaging biomarkers to render them effective in real-world environments. These endeavors will not only enhance the interpretive value of imaging modalities but also anchor them in the paradigm shift of personalized cancer treatment (Benedict et al., 2018).

8.1.2. Quantification Techniques in Imaging

Imaging quantification techniques play a pivotal role in optimizing cancer diagnosis and treatment follow-up, particularly in non-small cell lung cancer (NSCLC). These techniques employ advanced imaging technologies to extract salient information from clinical images and convert it into quantitative values, which are then transformed into usable measurements for clinicians to evaluate tumor characteristics and response to treatment. Radiomics, the most prominent among them, involves quantitative feature extraction from images of numerous parameters. By analyzing patterns not normally perceptible to the naked eye, radiomics is a key tool to identify tumor heterogeneity and the risk of recurrence following treatment. This approach not only enables customized surveillance strategies but also underscores the need for ongoing research into the predictive validity of these imaging biomarkers, reflecting their pivotal role in contemporary oncology practice (Benedict et al., 2018) (Figure 8.2).

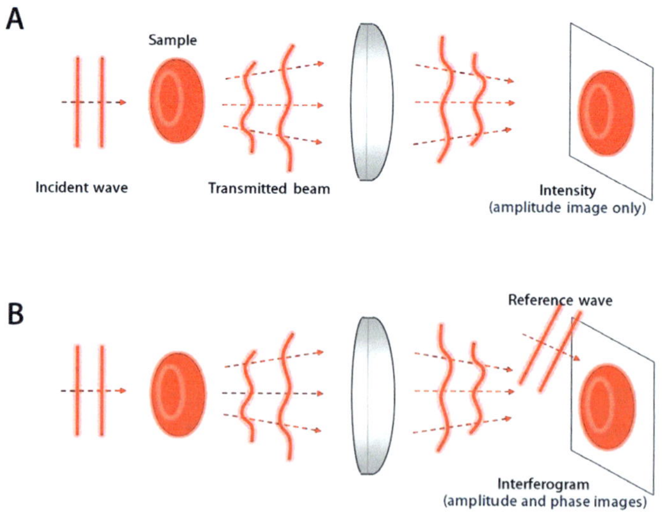

Figure 8.2. Quantitative phase imaging techniques for the study of cell pathophysiology.

Source: https://www.mdpi.com/sensors/sensors-13-04170/article_deploy/html/images/sensors-13-04170f1.png.

The increased density and complexity of information provided by imaging modalities necessitate novel, advanced quantification techniques that do not sacrifice valuable information. Radiomics is particularly well-positioned to meet this challenge by applying data mining and machine learning algorithms to process large datasets, extracting relevant correlations among image features and clinical outcomes. Such capability is most applicable in NSCLC, wherein variations in tumor features can dramatically influence treatment outcome. As noted in recent literature, radiomics has attracted considerable attention because it holds the potential to predict tumor response and quantify treatment response across modalities, including chemotherapy and radiotherapy. With the large volumes of data now available, integrating robust quantitative techniques into clinical models has become imperative to optimize predictive models and achieve optimal treatment personalization. Further, the use of imaging biomarkers extends beyond the diagnostic domain, providing a real-time interface for monitoring therapeutic response and outcomes. Imaging-based quantification of tumor parameter changes enables clinicians to adjust therapeutic regimens in a timely manner. As research in radiomics is ongoing, imaging procedures such as region-of-interest segmentation and feature classification are intrinsic to the effective use of imaging data. The ongoing development of standardized image acquisition methods, analysis techniques, and interpretation rules will increasingly affirm the role of quantitative imaging biomarkers in daily clinical applications, highlighting the revolutionary impact of quantitative methods on oncology advancement (Benedict et al., 2018).

8.1.3. Role of Artificial Intelligence in Imaging Analysis

The integration of artificial intelligence (AI) into imaging analysis has transformed the quantitative imaging biomarkers and radiomics domain tremendously. AI algorithms, namely machine learning and deep learning algorithms, have enhanced the effectiveness and accuracy of image interpretation, which is critical in medical diagnosis. For instance, with the introduction of multiparametric MRI (mpMRI), tumors can now be evaluated more closely to better differentiate between muscle-invasive and non-muscle-invasive bladder cancer.

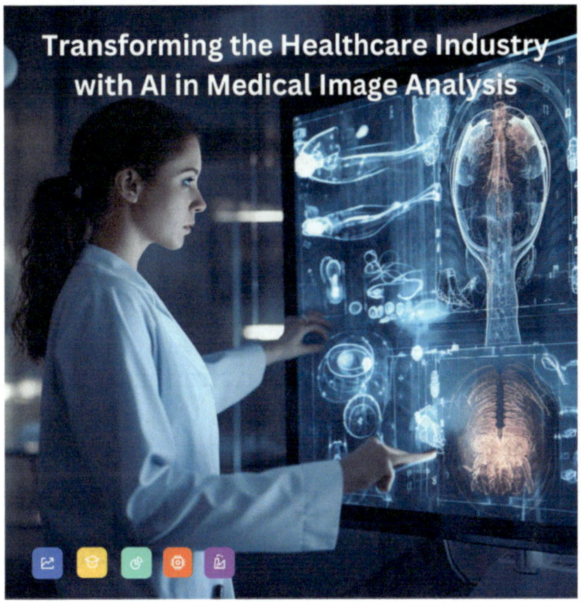

Figure 8.3. Transforming the healthcare industry with AI in medical image analysis.

Source: https://encrypted-tbn0.gstatic.com/images?q=tbn:ANd9GcT-r6dHK3IQz894fVidjrrwLvjNzwLd4HIEBQ&s.

AI enhances the sensitivity to detect minute changes in imaging features that may signal a response to therapy or disease recurrence, thereby enabling prompt decision-making by doctors. These developments are not mere theories; they have practical applications for patients, in the sense that applying AI in image analysis has the potential to result in more focused and better treatment plans, particularly in complex conditions like bladder cancer, where precise evaluation plays a significant role in patient management (Akin et al., 2025).

Radiomics also benefits immensely from AI, enabling it to extract high-dimensional features from medical images. By converting imaging characteristics into quantitative parameters, AI serves as a bridge between traditional imaging techniques and advanced quantitative analysis. To illustrate, the application of machine learning techniques enables the derivation of numerous quantitative imaging biomarkers that quantify different aspects of a tumor, paving the way for even more comprehensive assessments of prostate cancer (Figure 8.3). This process not only improves the information content of existing imaging data but also enables the development of predictive models that utilize both imaging and clinical data. This dual application is key to personalizing patient management approaches, as it can improve risk stratification, make treatment regimens more individualized to each patient's profile, and hence enhance the overall quality of prostate cancer management (Barone et al., 2021). Further, the intersection of imaging analysis and AI holds potential for significant breakthroughs in monitoring response and treatment assessment. Delta-radiomics, or the measurement of changes in imaging characteristics over time, illustrates the potential of AI to better track therapy response compared with conventional methods. By analyzing quantitative differences in imaging biomarkers, AI can potentially provide earlier alerts on treatment efficacy, allowing treating physicians to revise treatment plans proactively. Such technologies are particularly relevant in bladder cancer, where the morphology of treated tissue can make evaluation challenging. AI-based solutions are expected to simplify such analyses, minimizing ambiguities inherent in conventional methods of interpretation. With ongoing research and verification, the complementary application of AI in imaging evaluation marks a new era, maximizing clinical processes and improving patient outcomes in the arena of quantitative imaging biomarkers and radiomics (Akin et al., 2025).

8.2. Applications in Oncology

In oncology, the advent of quantitative imaging biomarkers and radiomics is a quantum leap to personalized management of cancer. Radiomics involves extracting quantitative features from medical images, ranging from tumor morphology to texture analysis. This method is particularly robust for assessing intratumoral heterogeneity—variability that strongly affects treatment response. Through algorithms that identify and quantify such features, oncologists can improve diagnostic accuracy and tailor treatment modalities for patients based on unique tumor features. Merging radiomic data with clinical variables is invaluable for predicting treatment responses, thereby maximizing the likelihood of optimizing treatment efficacy while minimizing side effects (Benedict et al., 2018) (Figure 8.4).

Radiomics is not only applicable to cancers; its predictive potential has been thoroughly tested across various cancers. For instance, in non-small cell lung cancer, radiomics has been employed to analyze pre-treatment imaging data to assess the likelihood of tumor response to radiotherapy or chemotherapy. Through intensive imaging characteristic analysis, researchers have even identified possible tumor recurrence and metastasis signs that are crucial in monitoring the evolution of the disease. It is especially critical given the limitations of standard imaging techniques, which are incapable of noticing subtle changes in the tumor during treatment. As envisaged in modern research, predictive validity of the aforementioned imaging biomarkers enhances oncologists' ability to perform timely interventions and possibly improve patients' survival rates (Benedict et al., 2018). Furthermore, the breathtaking diversity of radiomics' prospective applications can be encapsulated in its applicability to constructing robust predictive models to address locoregional recurrences and distant metastases. In head-and-neck cancer research, the incorporation of radiomics and clinical factors has led to models that demonstrate outstanding prognostic performance. By applying advanced machine learning algorithms such as random forests, researchers have developed predictive models with area under the curve (AUC) values that reflect their performance in assessing treatment response. These advances underscore the clinical utility of radiomic features, which can stratify patients into clinically relevant risk classes. Not only does this stratification facilitate more individualized chemotherapy and radiotherapy, but it also guides clinical decision-making based on a response tailored to individual risk profiles (Aerts et al., 2017).

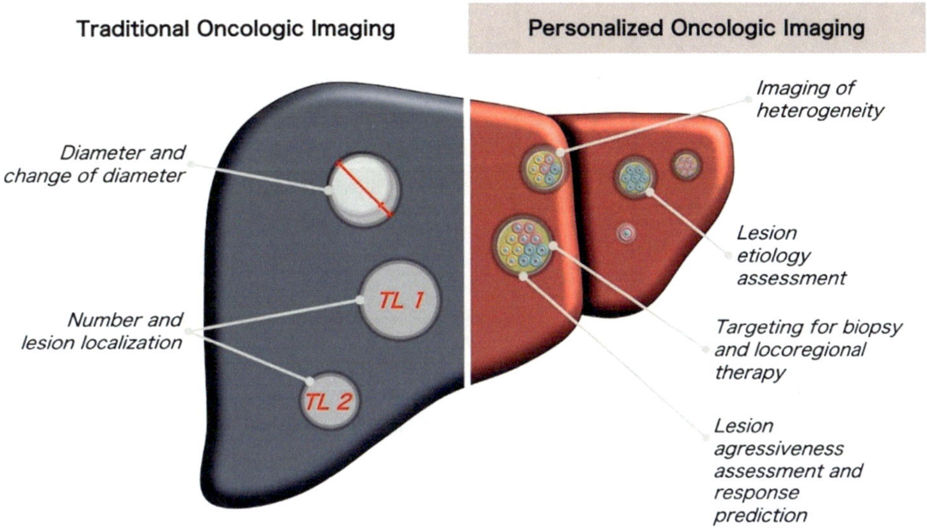

Figure 8.4. The potential and emerging role of quantitative imaging biomarkers for cancer characterization.

Source: https://www.mdpi.com/cancers/cancers-14-03349/article_deploy/html/images/cancers-14-03349-g001.png.

8.2.1. Tumor Characterization and Classification

Within the context of tumor classification and characterization, the application of quantitative imaging biomarkers has become increasingly prominent, notably through radiomics.

This novel method enables researchers to derive a large number of imaging features from clinical scans, thereby permitting the discovery of previously unseen patterns and correlations. For instance, it has been established in studies that multimodal data fusion between modalities such as PET and MRI greatly enhances prognostic prediction for breast cancer patients. Through unsupervised clustering analyses of radiomic features derived from these images, it is possible to distinguish tumor subgroups and identify correlations with tumor grade, overall stage, and recurrence risk. These findings underscore the ability of radiomic analysis not merely to improve diagnostic precision but to inform personalized treatment choices in oncology (Arasu et al., 2018) (Figure 8.5).

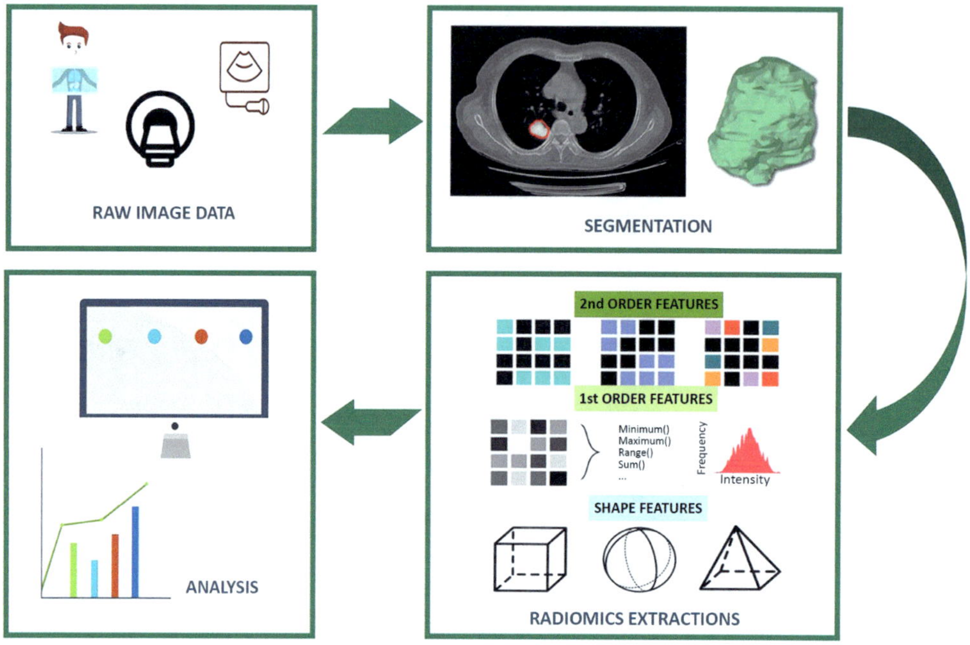

Figure 8.5. The role of radiomics in lung cancer: from screening to treatment and follow-up.

Source: https://www.frontiersin.org/files/Articles/603595/fonc-11-603595-HTML-r1/image_m/fonc-11-603595-g001.jpg.

The combination of radiomics with clinical practice also addresses the inherent heterogeneity of tumors, particularly in complex cancers such as NSCLC. Informative as they are, traditional evaluation methods are often inadequate to fully describe tumor behavior and treatment response. Radiomics enables the recovery of quantitative data from longitudinal imaging, thereby matching imaging features to clinical outcomes, enhancing the predictive validity of treatment responses. Pretreatment imaging biomarker studies have shown promise in predicting tumor behavior, recurrence, and metastasis. Subsequently, clinicians can employ more tailored surveillance methods tailored to the unique characteristics of each tumor in the patient, resulting in improved management and prognosis in cancer care (Benedict et al., 2018). In conclusion, as radiomics expands, it offers rich information about tumor characterization and classification, which is important in contemporary cancer care. The ability to analyze large image datasets using advanced computational methods is a paradigm shift in tumor understanding and treatment. With the help of robust feature extraction algorithms and multi-modal imaging data, radiomics has the potential to change the face of oncology, enabling more evidence-based decision-making regarding treatment regimens and follow-up. The integration of quantitative imaging biomarkers into routine clinical practice could not only enhance tumor characterization but also redefine personalized oncology (Arasu et al., 2018; Benedict et al., 2018).

8.2.2. Treatment Response Assessment

Assessment of response to treatment in cancer therapy is critical in optimizing patient outcomes and constructing personalized treatment protocols. Traditional strategies have primarily relied on anatomical imaging techniques and standard criteria, such as the Response Evaluation Criteria in Solid Tumors (RECIST). These techniques are typically hampered by the inability to accurately represent the dynamic tumor biology that could provide more detailed insight into response to therapy (Figure 8.6).

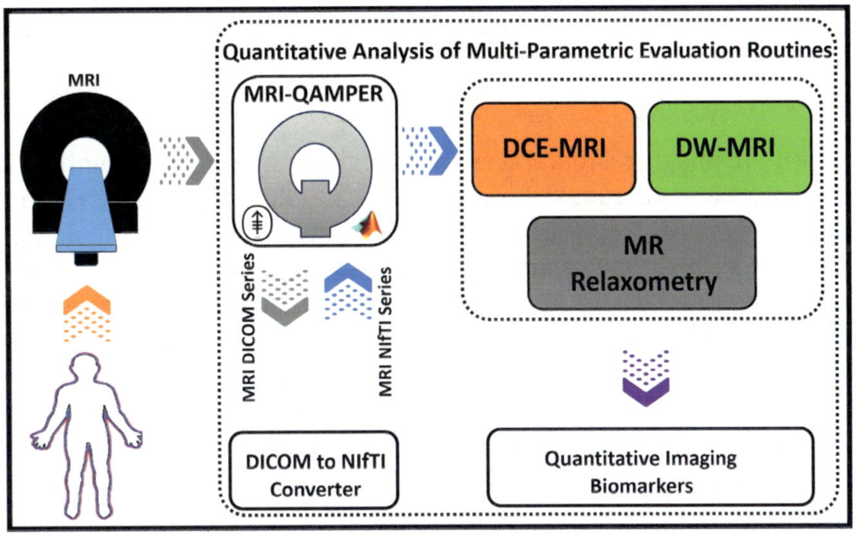

Figure 8.6. Imaging biomarkers in clinical oncology.

Source: https://pub.mdpi-res.com/tomography/tomography-09-00161/article_deploy/html/images/tomography-09-00161-ag-550.jpg?1704961866.

Inclusion of quantitative imaging biomarkers (QIBs) has also been proposed as a solution, using cutting-edge imaging modalities such as multiparametric MRI to provide deeper insight into the tumor microenvironment. Biomarker-based measurements enable early detection of therapy-induced changes, ultimately leading to improved prognostic estimates and therapeutic adjustments. Their growingly leading position in clinical practice underscores the continuing utility of investigation and verification of such new approaches across diverse oncological contexts, from bladder cancers and beyond (Akin et al., 2025). Radiomics, an emerging technology that analyzes complex patterns in medical imaging data, has shown tremendous promise in enhancing the assessment of treatment response. By extracting a broad range of quantitative imaging features from pre-treatment and follow-up images, radiomics enables a more comprehensive evaluation of tumor characteristics that may affect therapeutic outcomes. Radiomic features are matched with clinical outcomes through this data-driven approach, encouraging personalized medicine. Recent studies have demonstrated the potential of radiomics to detect treatment responses earlier than conventional imaging modalities, particularly in therapies such as radiotherapy and chemotherapy for heterogeneously responding tumors. The fusion of radiomics and artificial intelligence elevates this process to include high-level feature extraction and classification, thereby improving the accuracy of treatment predictions from assessments (Benedict et al., 2018). In addition, emphasis on robust validation through multicenter trials is important for the clinical application of QIBs and radiomics for monitoring treatment response. While the conceptual basis and initial results are promising, their translation into routine clinical practice requires an agreed-upon process and unambiguous criteria for use. The establishment of reliable protocols will aid in overcoming challenges related to interobserver variability and tumor heterogeneity. In addition, integration of these emerging imaging modalities into existing clinical routines is ready to address the growing need for patient-specific surveillance approaches, particularly in cancer, with broad variability in patterns of recurrence and responsiveness. With continued advances in the field, the interconnection among clinicians, researchers, and AI professionals will be the determinant in realizing the ultimate potential of radiomics and quantitative imaging biomarkers in making evidence-based treatment decisions (Akin et al., 2025).

8.2.3. Prognostic Value of Imaging Biomarkers

The predictive power of imaging biomarkers has received significant attention in recent years, especially in oncology. Because tumor heterogeneity is challenging to treat and monitor, the need for personalized treatment options has become extremely important. Imaging biomarkers, particularly radiomic quantifications, enable clinicians to obtain information about tumor features that were previously inaccessible. By quantifying features such as texture, shape, and intensity in medical images, these biomarkers enable more precise assessments of tumor behavior and potential treatment responses. This advance in imaging paradigms marks a departure from the past and provides more integrated information to guide clinical practice and, ultimately, improve patient outcomes, particularly in today's fast-changing landscape of cancer care. Radiomics, with its use of machine learning and data mining techniques to analyze imaging data, is a crucial tool in the prognostic evaluation of cancer. For example, research has found that some radiomic features correlate strongly with clinical endpoints, such as tumor recurrence and metastasis (Figure 8.7).

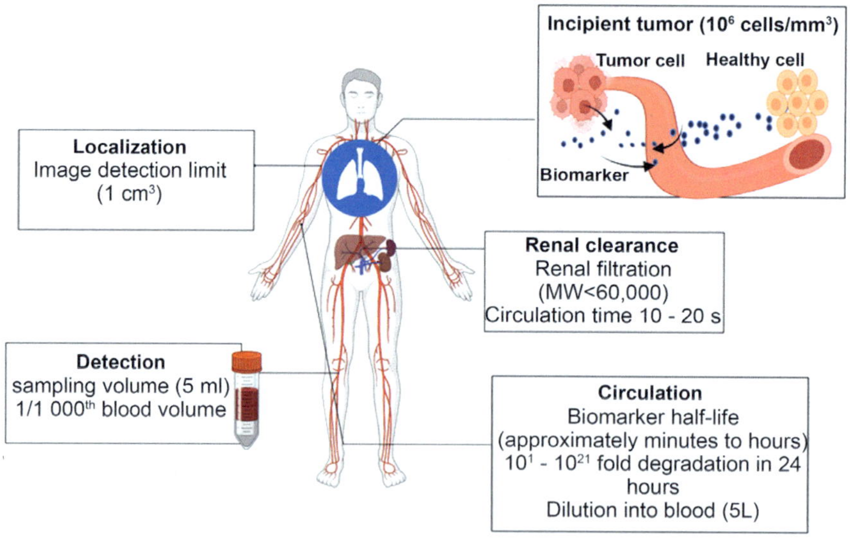

Figure 8.7. Biomarkers in cancer detection, diagnosis, and prognosis.

Source: https://www.mdpi.com/sensors/sensors-24-00037/article_deploy/html/images/sensors-24-00037-g001.png.

With a comprehensive analysis including 1615 pre-treatment FDG-PET and head-and-neck cancer patients' CT scan radiomic features, models integrating both radiomics and clinical data showed robust predictive performance. These models achieved an area under the curve (AUC) of 0.69 for locoregional recurrences and 0.86 for distant metastasis, revealing the robustness of radiomics in classifying patient risk levels (Aerts et al., 2017). These predictive accuracies pave the way for more detailed therapeutic interventions, ultimately maximizing the effectiveness of treatment protocols. Furthermore, integration of imaging biomarkers into clinical protocols has significant implications on the management of patients with multifocal cancer manifestations. As highlighted in recent studies, not only do radiomics predict therapy response, but also possible side effects, e.g., radiation-induced lung damage. Notably, advanced radiomic assessment can detect early signs of therapeutic response, enabling appropriate intervention in time and maximizing patient benefit. Ongoing research on radiomics in assessing non-small cell lung cancer is what underscores the potential of this emerging field. By correlating volumetric imaging data with patient outcomes, doctors are now more able to inform decision-making, address tumor heterogeneity, and individualize monitoring measures more effectively (Benedict et al., 2018). Thus, the prognostic role of imaging biomarkers is a revolutionary phase for oncology, ushering in a new era of personalized cancer treatment.

8.3. Applications in Neurology

Quantitative imaging biomarkers have contributed significantly to the field of neurology, particularly in the diagnosis and management of complex neurological disorders. The integration of multimodal image data, including MRI, PET, and clinical biomarkers, has improved diagnostic sensitivity and enabled individualized treatment plans. Through the complementarity of information from various image sources, health care providers can form a comprehensive understanding of neurological diseases (Figure 8.8). Multimodal data fusion processing accounts for key challenges in working with heterogeneous medical data, including dimensionality reduction and biomarker relevance extraction. Such processing enables the determination of patient-specific disease mechanisms and progression patterns, thereby improving the overall efficiency of neurological interventions (Xin et al., 2021). As a result, the application of quantitative imaging biomarkers in neurology goes beyond simple diagnosis, impacting treatment considerably and prognostic evaluation. In the case of gliomas, notorious for their infiltrative behavior, conventional structural MRI is often not up to the task of providing precise information on tumor genotype and behavior. This limitation underscores the importance of employing advanced imaging modalities, such as magnetic resonance spectroscopy (MRS) and chemical exchange saturation transfer (CEST), which yield more useful data on tumor biology. The GliMR COST action underscores the imperative to raise awareness and to translate advanced MRI modalities for enhanced preoperative assessment of gliomas (Arzanforoosh et al., 2023). As these methods become more widely accepted, they are incorporated into standard protocols, hence revolutionizing the field of neurological imaging. In time, these advances promise improved delineation of diffuse gliomas, potentially with more effective surgical planning and improved patient care. The future of neurology quantitative imaging is intrinsically linked to the integration of AI and machine learning algorithms, which fortify the analysis of imaging data. These technologies enable the exploration of minor imaging features and clinical outcomes, broadening the boundaries of prevailing diagnosis. With the application of AI, researchers aim to develop algorithms that automatically detect and characterize neurological diseases to help clinicians make timely and informed decisions. In addition, continuous radiomics optimization—quantitatively assessing large volumes of imaging data—identifies new biomarkers related to disease extent and treatment response. This combination of quantitative imaging, AI, and clinical practice not only has tremendous potential to improve diagnostic processes but also offers a path for visionary innovations that can transform the neurology discipline (Xin et al., 2021).

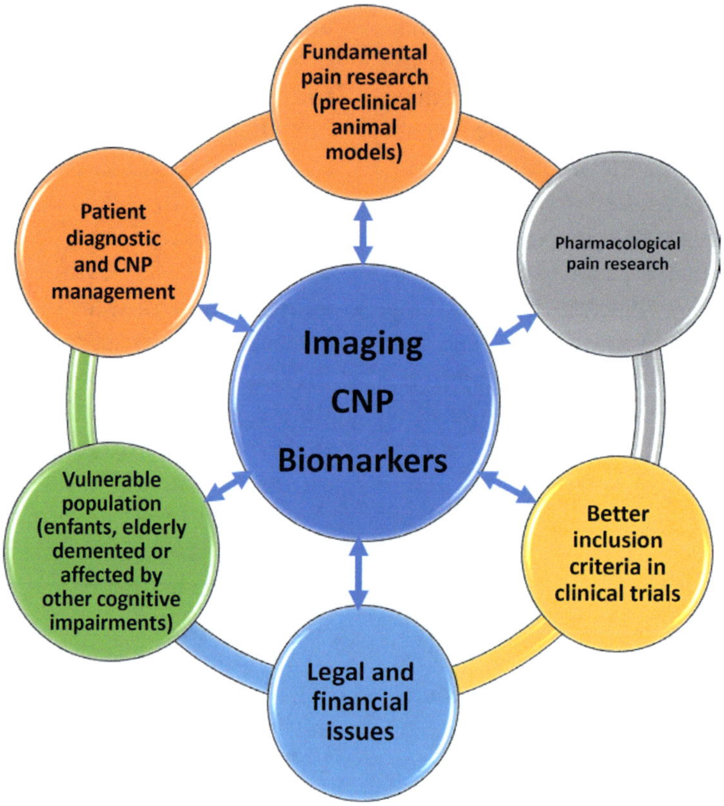

Figure 8.8. The roles of imaging biomarkers in the management of chronic neuropathic pain.

Source: https://pub.mdpi-res.com/ijms/ijms-23-13038/article_deploy/html/images/ijms-23-13038-g002.png?1666919443.

8.3.1. Imaging Biomarkers in Neurodegenerative Diseases

The identification of imaging biomarkers for neurodegenerative diseases has advanced significantly due to technological and methodological advances. Neurodegenerative disease, such as Alzheimer's and Parkinson's diseases, is characterized by progressive impairment and loss of neurons in specific areas of the brain. Therefore detection and quantification of these changes are critical for early diagnosis and treatment. New imaging modalities, particularly MRI, have proven invaluable in identifying the structural alterations that are linked to such disorders. However, conventional MRI approaches do not always have the capacity to provide comprehensive insight into the biochemical and functional alterations in the brain, hence the necessity of complementing them with sophisticated analytical techniques like Radiomics, which employs quantitative values produced from scanning images for enhanced diagnostic accuracy and therapy protocols (Carvalho et al., 2021). The application of Radiomics in neurodegenerative disease research is particularly promising as it involves the extraction of a wide array of quantitative features from radiological images. Such features encompass a wide variety of characteristics, such as texture, shape, and intensity, which can be harnessed as potential biomarkers indicative of disease progression (Figure 8.9).

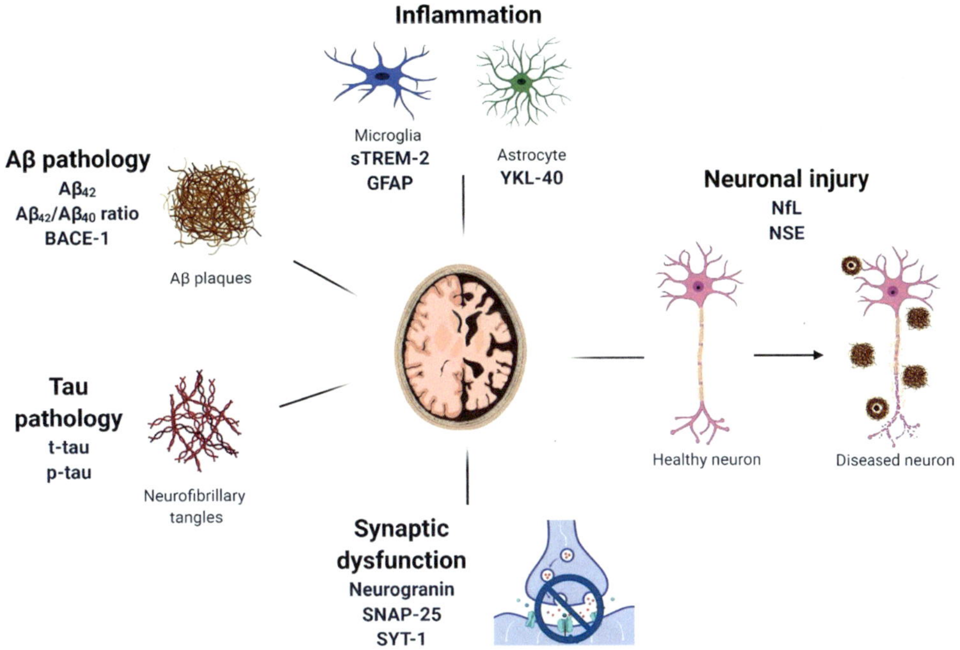

Figure 8.9. Main pathological mechanisms occurring in Alzheimer's disease and their associated fluid biomarkers.

Source: https://www.mdpi.com/jpm/jpm-10-00061/article_deploy/html/images/jpm-10-00061-g001-550.jpg.

With the application of machine learning algorithms, researchers can now study these features to develop patterns associated with specific neurodegenerative diseases. Not only do such analyses lay the groundwork for improved disease classification and differentiation, such as Parkinson's disease classifications based on SPECT imaging, but they also pave the way for personalized medicine, wherein treatment protocols can be formulated around an individual patient's imaging profile (Spanu et al., 2020). Thus, the union of imaging biomarkers and advanced computational algorithms has certainly the potential to transform the treatment of neurodegenerative disorders. Also, ongoing development of bioinformatics tools is required to standardize and facilitate the use of Radiomics in clinical practice. Tools such as PyRadiomics, as open-source software, enable the extraction and analysis of imaging features from MRI information and offer a solid platform for collaboration between researchers and clinicians. This multicentric collaboration is paramount in enhancing reproducibility and quality of imaging biomarker studies toward the generation of normative databases that can contribute to decision-making in the clinic. As advances are made, there is also a need to integrate these imaging biomarkers with other diagnostic methods, such as biochemical tests, to formulate an integrated approach that incorporates both structural and functional assessment of neurodegenerative disorders. Finally, the possible contribution of imaging biomarkers to enhancing our understanding and management of such diseases underscores the value in adopting a multidisciplinary approach to addressing one of the most significant challenges facing contemporary medicine (Carvalho et al., 2021).

8.3.2. Role in Stroke Assessment

Stroke assessment by quantitative imaging biomarkers and radiomics is significant for enhancing clinical decision-making and patient outcomes. Radiological imaging techniques such as CT and MRI are key for the timely detection of ischemic strokes, allowing clinicians to evaluate the extent of brain damage and determine the best therapeutic interventions. By using advanced imaging modalities, physicians can gain extensive knowledge of brain structure and disease, thereby enhancing the determination of stroke subtype and risk factors. Significantly, the use of quantitative imaging biomarkers enables the identification of subtle cerebral microstructural alterations that cannot be detected with conventional imaging modalities (Figure 8.10).

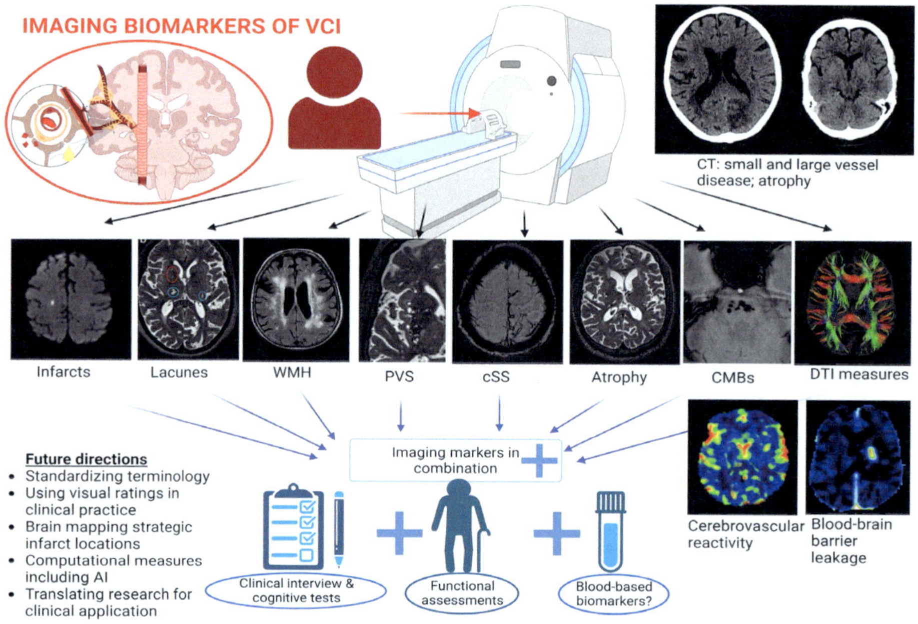

Figure 8.10. Imaging biomarkers of VCI.

Source: https://www.frontiersin.org/files/Articles/619721/fneur-12-619721-HTML/image_m/fneur-12-619721-g001.jpg.

Subsequently, this allows for early intervention measures that could make a dramatic difference in patient outcomes, further highlighting the necessity for continued investigation into the application of radiomics in stroke evaluation (Dewey et al., 2019). In addition, the new paradigm of precision medicine is increasingly image biomarker-dependent to customize treatment plans for patients suffering from strokes. Radiomics, the extraction of a large number of quantitative features from radiological images, enables lesion characterization beyond visual rating. It is a new technique that can reveal unique biological and pathological profiles associated with some stroke mechanisms and be helpful for prognostication. Advanced imaging analysis has been shown to predict outcomes such as the potential for recovery and the risk of recurrent events, based on studies. For instance, imaging characteristics indicating carotid artery disease have been associated with an increased risk of ischemic strokes, thus providing actionable information for preventive treatment. Lastly, the use of radiomics in stroke assessment improves risk stratification, promoting more effective and targeted care (Aluigi et al., 2022). Further, success in the use of radiomics for stroke assessment will depend on addressing existing flaws in the application of such advanced imaging techniques in the clinical setting. The concept of the Bionic Radiologist reflects the imperative to bridge the gap between technology and expertise to achieve optimal patient outcomes. Though transforming imaging data into usable insights holds great potential, challenges such as variation in imaging protocols, the need for standardized data interpretation, and healthcare professionals' inertia toward dropping traditional methods must be addressed. New models emphasizing shared decision-making and continuous learning can trigger such change by promoting a culture of innovation and collaboration among healthcare professionals. By bridging these gaps, the full potential of quantitative imaging biomarkers and radiomics for stroke evaluation can be realized, ultimately culminating in improved patient outcomes and a reduction in the burden of stroke as an underlying cause of morbidity and mortality (Dewey et al., 2019).

8.3.3. Predictive Modeling for Neurological Disorders

The advent of predictive modeling in neurologic disorders has significantly enhanced our ability to predict treatment outcomes and tailor therapeutic interventions. This approach employs quantitative imaging biomarkers from advanced neuroimaging technologies, such as MRI and functional MRI (fMRI). Recent studies underscore the deficiency of traditional radiomics, which often focus on localized lesion characteristics and detect inherent heterogeneity in such radiological features among patients. As a new paradigm, prediction based on brain connectomics exploits large-scale brain network dynamics rather than relying solely on local tumor morphology, offering a more comprehensive representation of disease progression and prognosis.

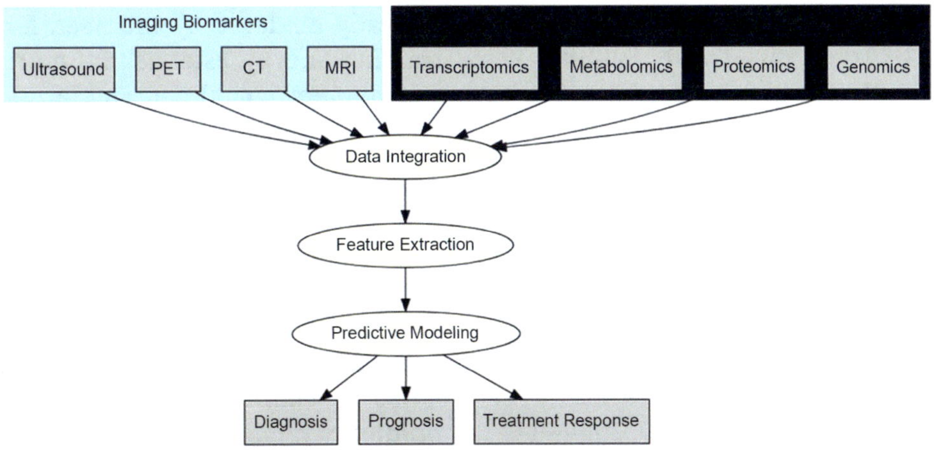

Figure 8.11. Predictive modeling for neurological disorders.

Source: https://www.researchgate.net/publication/386219130/figure/fig4/AS:11431281293858497@1732892222146/Predictive-modeling-using-imaging-biomarkers-and-molecular-profiling.png.

For instance, by integrating heterogeneous neural connection patterns, researchers have demonstrated an impressive predictive rate for global survival in high-grade glioma patients, showcasing how predictive modeling can transform patient outcomes and tailored treatment regimens (Aibaidula et al., 2018). Furthermore, integrating multimodal data is important for enhancing predictive model accuracy and validity, particularly in neurological disorders. Neurological disorders are usually complex and multifactorial, requiring data-driven strategies that integrate imaging and non-imaging biomarkers (Figure 8.11). Recent advances in multimodal data integration address the challenges posed by medical data heterogeneity and complexity, as the literature presents.

By integrating complementary information from diverse sources—e.g., imaging results from PET or CT scans with electronic medical records—researchers can train models that provide a more comprehensive view of disease processes. The prospects for use in predictive modeling are vast, leading to improved diagnostic accuracy, better prognostic prediction, and more personalized medical care tailored to each individual's profile (Xin et al., 2021). In the future of predictive modeling, the solution to feature-level, information-level, and knowledge-level fusion will be key. Multimodal datasets typically have high dimensionality and may include redundant or irrelevant features, which can mask significant predictors of disease outcome.

Hence, new frameworks that can effectively mine multimodal biomarkers while being understandable are most crucial. The development of integrated models by combining deep learning and canonical correlation analysis enables the analysis of disparate data types to identify cross-modal associations that may underpin pathophysiological processes. By employing topological analyses of interconnected multi-focus areas, scientists can better describe the intricate dynamics underlying neurological conditions and thus enhance the biological relevance and medical utility of their forecasting models (Aibaidula et al., 2018; Xin et al., 2021).

8.4. Challenges and Limitations

Its use in clinical medicine poses several significant challenges and limitations. Chief among these is the imminent absence of standardization of imaging protocols and imaging techniques across institutions. Differences in these can have a dramatic effect on reproducibility and validity of radiomic features since differences in even one imaging parameter can lead to differences in images of tumor characteristics. Also, integration of radiomics into existing clinical practice remains a problem, where doctors have to balance the demands of traditional diagnosis against the need for sophisticated analytical techniques. Despite the potential for more accurate prediction and personalized therapy, the transition towards the inclusion of radiomics in everyday practice is typically hindered by the need for specialized training and by establishing multidisciplinary collaboration among data specialists, oncologists, and radiologists (Figure 8.12).

Additionally, critical limitations arise from the sheer size of data generated by radiomic analyses. The isolation of hundreds of features extracted from imaging data may generate vast amounts of potentially useful information, but separating clinically relevant features from noise is challenging. Therefore, overfitting predictive models is more likely, and they may generate results that are not generalizable to heterogeneous patient groups. Robust statistical methods are required to resolve these issues; however, the literature has been heterogenous in feature extraction and validation methods.

As evidenced from a more recent study, radiomics has shown some potential for describing tumor heterogeneity and potential treatment responses. Still, without unifying methods, the clinical use of these biomarkers remains uncertain (Benedict et al., 2018). In addition, patient-focused and ethical considerations should also be taken into account when listing the disadvantages of adopting radiomics in cancer treatment. The reliance on advanced imaging strategies and algorithms means serious attention to patient confidentiality and how sensitive health information is handled. Also, interpretability in advanced models based on imaging data raises concerns on clinician trust and patient understanding. If clinicians cannot effectively explain the basis for radiomic prediction, it may erode patient acceptance and engagement in novel treatment strategies. Furthermore, there are ethical issues related to the suggestion of variability in access to next-generation technology that could inadvertently exacerbate healthcare disparities. Therefore, although radiomics holds promise for revolutionary advances in personalized medicine, addressing these deficits and challenges is crucial to its successful integration into clinical practice (Arasu et al., 2018).

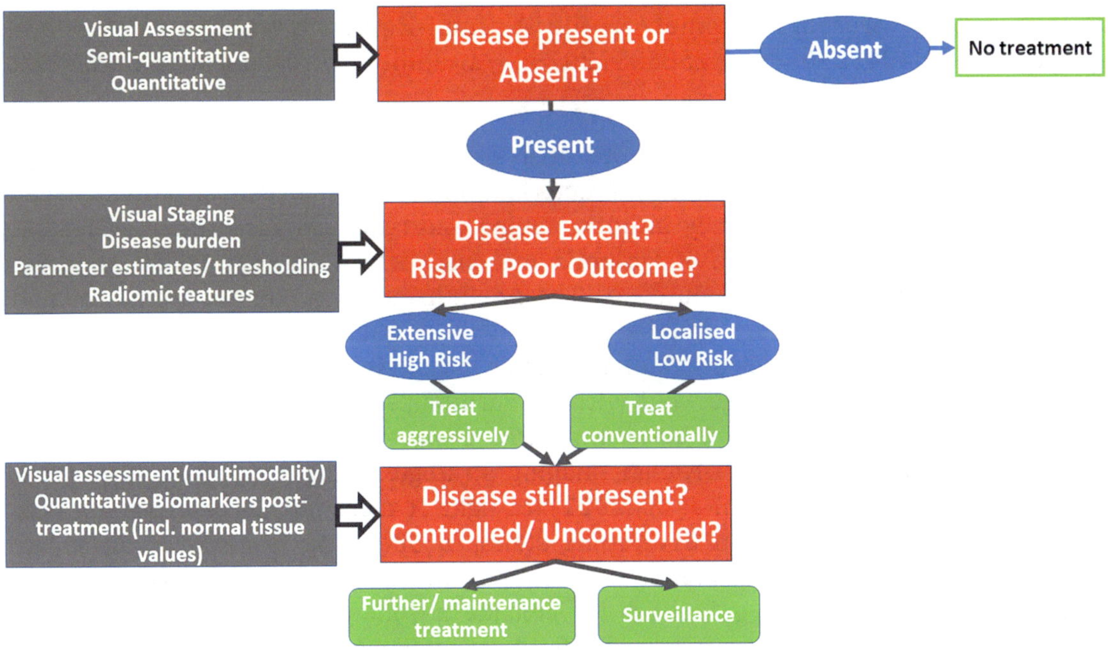

Figure 8.12. Validated imaging biomarkers as decision-making tools in clinical trials and routine practice.

Source: https://media.springernature.com/lw685/springer-static/image/art%3A10.1186%2Fs13244-019-0764-0/MediaObjects/13244_2019_764_Fig1_HTML.png.

8.4.1. Variability in Imaging Protocols

Heterogeneity of imaging protocols has been among the biggest challenges in quantitative imaging biomarkers and radiomics. The heterogeneity could be attributed to various factors, including machine calibration variations, imaging settings, and patient positioning. These inconsistencies will lead to variability in image quality and feature extraction, which are central to developing reliable biomarkers for use in diagnosis. As this heterogeneity may affect the generalizability and reproducibility of radiomic models, standardization of imaging protocols is required to enable different research teams to validate and compare their findings effectively. Standardization should cover not only technical parameters but also data preprocessing and segmentation methods, since these steps play significant roles in subsequent analysis (Brunetti et al., 2022). Solving these issues is crucial to progressing the integration of radiomics into practice (Figure 8.13).

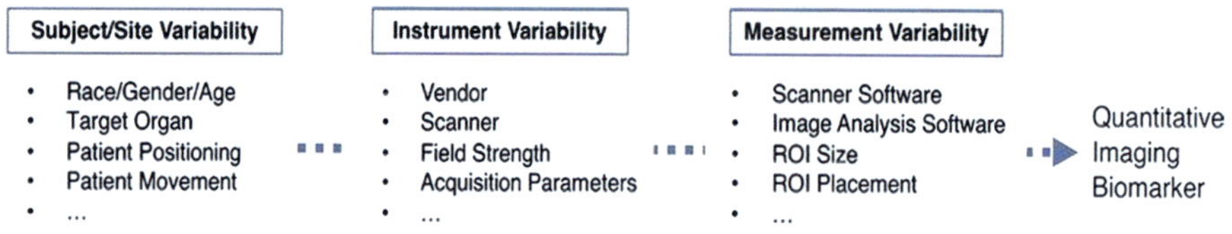

Figure 8.13. Variability sources of quantitative imaging biomarkers.

Source: https://www.researchgate.net/profile/Akifumi-Hagiwara/publication/340237657/figure/fig1/AS:873840452308993@1585351207952/ariability-sources-of-quantitative-imaging-biomarkers.jpg.

The significance of variability in imaging protocols is also heightened in specialty oncology, where accuracy is critical. By way of illustration, characterization of tumors in cancer patients treated for rectal cancer must have high accuracy in both staging and response assessment. Variability can significantly impact the performance of radiomic analysis, particularly assessment of response to therapy or the prediction of patient outcome. The breakthroughs in computational methods and imaging analysis software can help overcome some of these issues; however, the underlying data have to be harmonized and trustworthy. Radiomics aims to exploit sophisticated algorithms to derive quantitative data from clinical images, but without harmonized imaging protocols, the predictive value of such algorithms will remain undermined. As seen, the transition towards personalized medicine is based on consolidating robust imaging strategies that are universally transferable across varied clinical settings (Laghi et al., 2021). In light of these challenges, ongoing radiomics research programs should focus on developing standard operating procedures for all imaging modalities. Collaboration among academic institutions, clinical centers, and regulatory bodies is needed to create comprehensive guidelines for considering imaging variability complexities. By developing harmonized imaging protocols, the field can enhance the reproducibility of research studies and provide a stronger foundation for translating radiomic results into clinical applications. This focus on standardization will not only increase quantitative imaging biomarker accuracy but also facilitate the innovation to fit more seamlessly into routine clinical practice as well. With the advancement of the field, overcoming inconsistencies in imaging protocols and the consequent hurdles will be part of realizing the full promise of radiomics to revolutionize patient management and outcomes (Brunetti et al., 2022).

8.4.2. Data Standardization Issues

The emerging field of quantitative imaging biomarkers and radiomics is primarily threatened by data standardization problems, which are crucial to facilitating the reliability and reproducibility of the study findings. Heterogeneity in image acquisition protocols, processing algorithms, and analysis pipelines can introduce inconsistencies that undermine the validity of biomarker measurements.

For instance, differences in imaging modalities, such as MRI versus CT, can yield different radiomic features, making it hard to draw generalizable conclusions. As noted in recent reviews, these methodological differences pose a challenge to the use of radiomics in everyday clinical practice, as they make results difficult to compare across studies or to incorporate into decision-support systems tailored to individual patients (Brunetti et al., 2022). Addressing these problems of standardization is therefore critical for the onward march of quantitative imaging biomarkers in oncology and optimizing personalized medicine strategies. Solving data standardization issues entails developing standardized methods for image acquisition and preprocessing. This involves institutionalizing consensus guidelines that specify how medical images are acquired, processed, and analyzed uniformly across different research environments. Furthermore, using techniques that are suitable to the broad range of imaging equipment utilized in clinical environments is crucial. Applying automation and machine learning techniques may enhance the reproducibility of image processing through minimized human error and bias. The challenges regarding the reliability of image-derived biomarkers must be addressed to build trust in quantitative imaging applications and encourage their inclusion in clinical decision-making frameworks (Traverso et al., 2021). A systematic standardization methodology not only enhances the quality of radiomic analysis but also aligns with the overarching aim of establishing credible, actionable biomarkers in clinical settings. Furthermore, the data standardization challenge also extends to validating the radiomic model, which is critical for its adoption in clinical settings. Validations must consist of external validation sets from diverse populations as well as imaging protocols so that models do not become overfit to one dataset. This demands the use of robust statistical methods to assess the models' prognostic capability. By data standardization across multiple nodes along the pathway—from image acquisition to analysis and validation—researchers can establish a strong foundation for applying quantitative imaging biomarkers to personalized cancer therapy. Without moving forward with standardization practices, the potential of capitalizing on radiomics in oncology will remain unfulfilled, limiting strides towards individualized treatment strategies that are tailored to the specific characteristics of each patient's malignancy (Traverso et al., 2021; Brunetti et al., 2022).

8.4.3. Ethical Considerations in Biomarker Research

In the realm of biomarker research, and particularly quantitative imaging biomarker development, ethics are paramount. Researchers must operate in an arena with multiple layers, where scientific innovation and patient advantage are factors. The need for precise biomarkers as an aid in diagnosis in the detection of conditions such as ovarian cancer is evident through the challenge of diagnosing earlier, especially when alone laboratory tests are not sufficient. Ethical concerns necessitate that researchers ensure that any biomarker derived from imaging or biological specimens adheres to the principles of beneficence and non-maleficence. This commitment of concern for the well-being and safety of patients is not only crucial for establishing public trust but also for ensuring that the advancement in imaging modalities is utilized responsibly and prudently, thus potentially saving lives and enhancing treatment outcomes as stipulated in the broader mission of ongoing research activities in the field (Bacalbasa et al., 2024). Besides, informed consent is a critical element of ethical biomarker research, particularly where personal sensitive information is being used. Researchers have an obligation to adequately inform patients regarding how their information will be utilized and what it could mean if they are involved in research. This becomes more complex with the use of artificial intelligence and machine learning in biomarker research because it involves complex interpretations and data-driven outcomes. The intricacies of imaging algorithms, researched within the ambit of radiomics, need to be made transparent and comprehensible in terms of the computation of the results and how they affect patient treatment options (Figure 8.14).

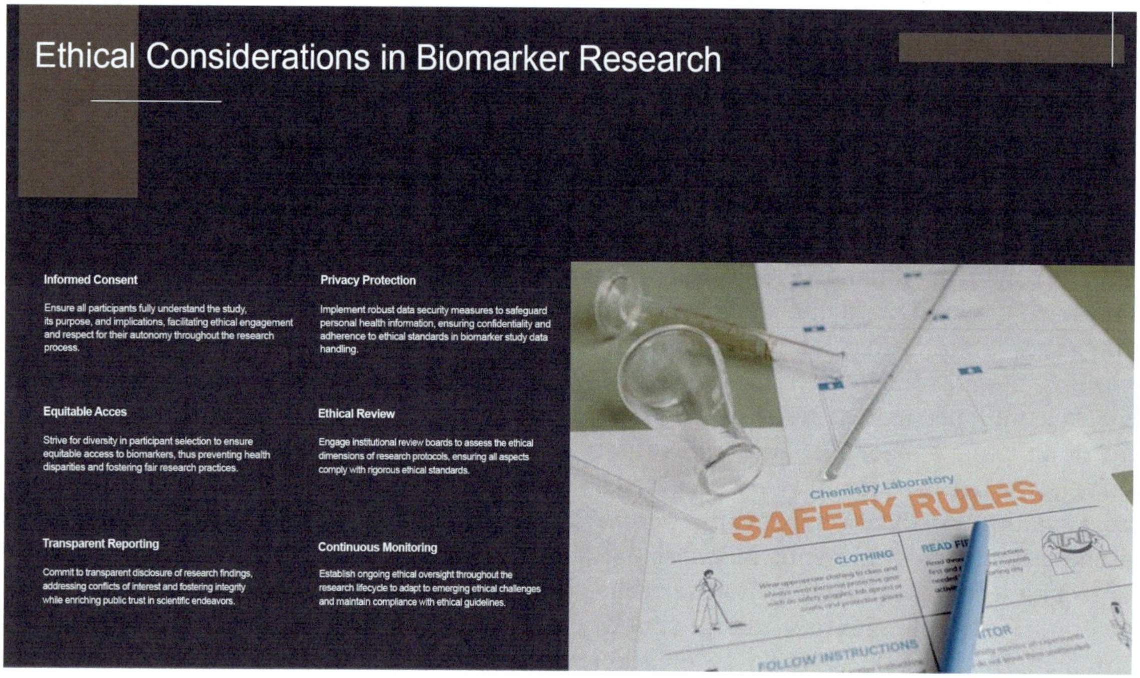

Figure 8.14. Ethical considerations in biomarker research.

Source: https://www.slideteam.net/media/catalog/product/cache/1280x720/e/t/ethical_considerations_in_biomarker_research_cancer_antigen_ppt_summary_st_ai_ss_slide01.jpg.

These ethical obligations are crucial in establishing research environments that respect patient autonomy and promote ethical integrity in science (Budach et al., 2017). Finally, issues of equity and access in biomarker development complicate ethical concerns. With the progress of quantitative imaging technologies, the benefits of these advances may not be available to all patients, particularly those in resource-poor settings. Disparities in access could perpetuate current health inequalities and pose ethical questions for researchers and clinicians. It is thus the responsibility of the scientific community to speak out and advocate policies that guarantee equal access to research results on biomarkers and clinical applications. By outlining these values, researchers can ensure that progress in quantitative imaging biomarkers and radiomics not only equates to improved diagnostic and prognostic tools but also preserves the inherent values of justice and fairness in healthcare delivery (Bacalbasa et al., 2024; Budach et al., 2017).

8.5. Future Directions

The potential of quantitative imaging biomarkers and radiomics in the future is to revolutionize the management and treatment of cancer fully. As efforts continue to be actualized, the combination of advanced machine learning models and artificial intelligence will raise the power of radiomic analysis in precisely predicting patient outcomes, such as never before. These emerging strategies will enable progressively more advanced data sets from imaging modalities to be delineated, facilitating the development of patient-specific treatment plans based on a patient's unique tumor characteristics. These developments have the potential to improve the predictive accuracy of existing models, thereby facilitating a paradigm shift in oncologists' diagnostic and treatment approaches across a wide variety of cancers, ultimately resulting in better patient care. Further research also emphasizes the importance of validated radiomic features in prognostic models. Radiomic data extracted from magnetic resonance imaging were shown to reveal survival correlations in a study of soft tissue sarcomas, underscoring their clinical utility (Ball et al., 2019). Future endeavors will likely focus on developing and expanding validated databases and multicenter trials to confirm the reproducibility of results across different cancer types and treatments. This emphasis on reproducibility will enhance the reliability of radiomics as a fundamental component of oncological assessment, thereby integrating imaging sciences into clinical decision-making. Ultimately, these efforts will propel further evolution of radiomics into a key component of precision medicine. Finally, future directions for quantitative imaging biomarkers and radiomics must also address ethical concerns and the need for regulatory guidelines. With increasingly expanding healthcare uses of artificial intelligence, it will be critical that the utilization of these technologies is guaranteed in a responsible manner. The creation of patient safety guidelines, protection of data, and disclosure regarding algorithms will be crucial in building patient and practitioner trust. Moreover, continued multidisciplinary engagement among radiologists, oncologists, data scientists, and ethicists will be critical in addressing these challenges. Such cooperation will ensure that quantitative imaging biomarkers and radiomics evolve not only to enhance clinical benefits but also to be ethically aligned with precision medicine practices and principles (Aerts et al., 2017).

8.5.1. Integration of Multi-Omics Data

The use of multi-omics data is a game-changing approach in radiomics and quantitative imaging biomarkers. The approach integrates various forms of biological data—genomics, transcriptomics, proteomics, and metabolomics—into a single platform that provides deeper insight into complex disease mechanisms, particularly cancer. By combining imaging biomarkers with multi-omics data, researchers and doctors can gain a clearer view of tumor biology. This integrative strategy enables the detection of subtle phenotypic variations between tumors, enabling an indistinct sort and may subsequently lead to stronger personalized treatment strategies for patients. The multi-omics method, therefore, not only improves tumor heterogeneity understanding but also promotes predictive model design based on both imaging and biological data, thereby optimizing patient therapy. New AI-driven advances have significantly enhanced the analysis of multi-omics data. AI-driven methods leverage machine learning algorithms that can efficiently process and integrate vast amounts of data, revealing intricate patterns that are hard to detect with conventional statistical methods alone (Figure 8.15).

These technologies have been particularly promising in oncology, where accurate stratification of patients based on their unique molecular profiles is central to improving therapeutic outcomes. Specifically, AI techniques for analyzing multi-omics data can improve prognostic predictions and guide clinicians in the prevention, diagnosis, and treatment of complex cancers, such as Non-Small Cell Lung Cancer (NSCLC) (Darvish et al., 2024). Thus, the integration of multi-omics data by AI enables a shift towards more targeted and personalized therapeutic regimens. Studies on integrated models that incorporate imaging and multi-omics data have made significant advances in disease risk stratification. For example, in the diagnosis of clear cell renal cell carcinoma (ccRCC), a study demonstrated the effective use of PET/MRI-based radiomics, combined with multi-omics datasets, to achieve an excellent accuracy of 95.65% in differentiating between molecular subtypes (Brooks et al., 2018). This underlines the potential prospects in leveraging complementary information from different omics layers in enhancing diagnostic accuracy and treatment recommendations. Evolution of these integrative approaches represents a paradigm shift in the application of large-scale data by clinicians to improve patient management, an important milestone towards addressing the complexities of cancer treatment. As the field evolves, continued research into the integration of quantitative imaging and multi-omics shall be pivotal to optimise the therapeutic model in oncology further.

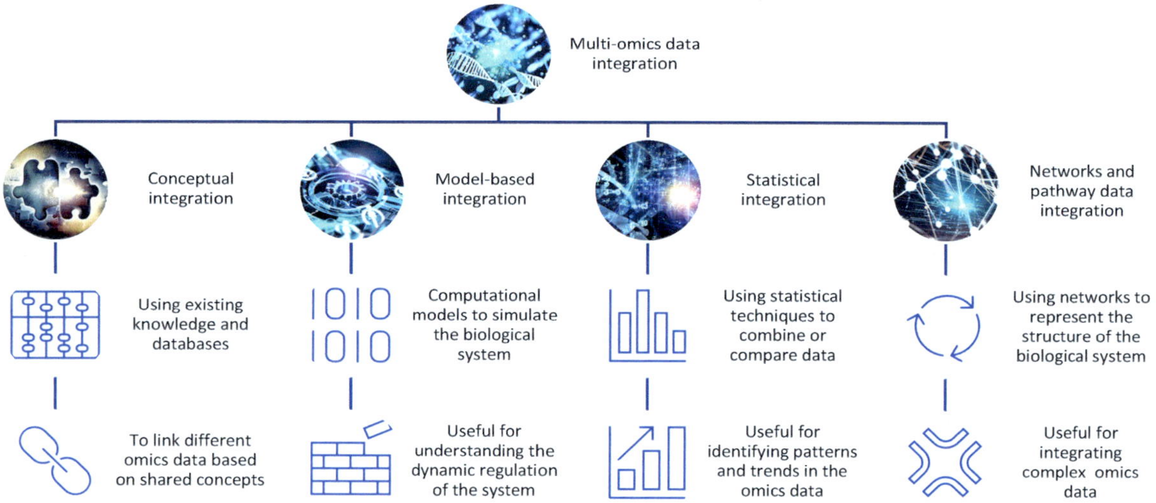

Figure 8.15. Multi-omics integration for the design of novel therapies and the identification of novel biomarkers.

Source: https://pub.mdpi-res.com/proteomes/proteomes-11-00034/article_deploy/html/images/proteomes-11-00034-g001.png?1697795846.

8.5.2. Advances in Machine Learning Techniques

The integration of machine learning techniques into medical imaging is a groundbreaking step in the field, particularly for quantitative extraction of imaging biomarkers. These techniques enable clinicians to analyze vast amounts of data based on modern imaging modalities, which have transformed considerably over the past decades. The increasing number and complexity of medical images need not only to enhance diagnostic correctness but also to aid more efficient workflows in oncology. Computerized technology developed for this purpose uses deep learning techniques and radiomics to semi-automatically or automatically assess imaging data, thereby serving as a vital support system for clinicians who may be bogged down by the volume of scans that need careful analysis (Astaraki et al., 2022) (Figure 8.16).

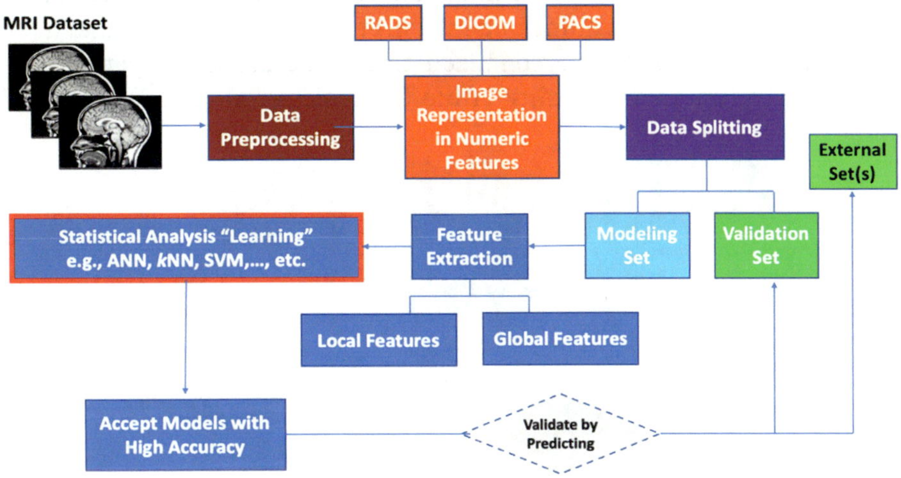

Figure 8.16. Identification of tumor-specific MRI biomarkers using machine learning (ML).

Source: https://www.mdpi.com/diagnostics/diagnostics-11-00742/article_deploy/html/images/diagnostics-11-00742-g001.png.

Among the areas of significant progress in machine learning, the design of sophisticated deep learning models for tumor segmentation and classification has been a major focus. Research has shown that the use of prior knowledge in deep learning can significantly increase segmentation accuracy, improving the identification of tumor characteristics across various cancers, such as lung and head-and-neck tumors. For instance, some studies propose new unsupervised segmentation methods to alleviate the drawback of small labeled datasets, ultimately demonstrating substantial improvements in segmentation accuracy (Astaraki et al., 2022). Moreover, the fusion of traditional radiomics with learned deep features is a fascinating new field, with the potential for creating more effective quantitative biomarkers that are capable of informing the treatment decision and prognostic evaluation more effectively in oncology. Furthermore, the implementation of artificial intelligence methods, notably survival prognosis for brain tumor patients, underscores the profound impact of machine learning on patient management. By employing quantitative imaging data from MRI and other modalities, researchers have developed models that achieve high classification accuracy. These machine learning algorithms enable a nuanced understanding of survival times and the stratification of patients into well-defined groups based on predicted survival. Quantification of individual survival times remains challenging, but progressive advances in machine learning algorithms hold promise for enhanced predictive models that will eventually provide more personalized treatment prognoses and improved clinical decision-making in oncology.

8.5.3. Potential for Personalized Medicine

The vision of personalized medicine, in the context of quantitative imaging biomarkers and radiomics, is currently redrawing the landscape of cancer diagnosis and treatment at a breakneck pace. Employing sophisticated imaging technology, radiomics aims to extract from medical images large quantities of quantitative data that enable clinicians to draw relevant correlations between imaging features and patient outcomes. This noninvasive technology is particularly pertinent in the case of lung cancer, with non-small cell lung cancer (NSCLC) being a leading cancer-related mortality worldwide. The ability to examine and interpret advanced imaging data not only enhances diagnostic accuracy but also enables personalized treatment based on patient-specific profiles, thereby increasing survival rates and quality of life (Benedict et al., 2018) (Figure 8.17).

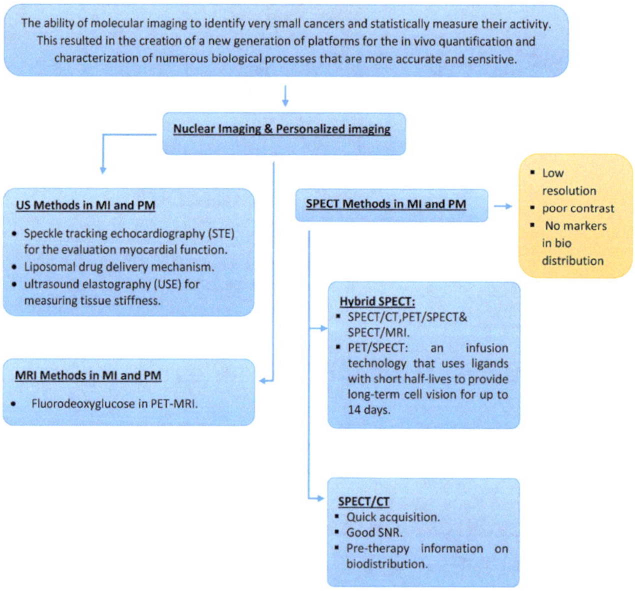

Figure 8.17. Role of biomarkers in personalized medicine.

Source: https://media.springernature.com/lw685/springer-static/image/chp%3A10.1007%2F978-981-16-5759-7_10/MediaObjects/508041_1_En_10_Fig4_HTML.png.

With the evolution of personalized medicine, the convergence of machine learning and deep learning approaches is likely to enhance the performance of radiomics further. These algorithmic processes data and clinical variables, and have the potential to revolutionize clinicians' capacity to predict outcomes and personalize interventions. For instance, pre-treatment imaging-derived radiomic features can provide critical insights into tumor heterogeneity and treatment response, thereby informing therapeutic decisions. The new oncology paradigm emphasizes the need for predictive models that, in addition to assessing disease status, can forecast future progression, recurrence, and treatment response for the disease and the patient. To this end, quantitative imaging biomarkers may substantially enhance the level of predictability to enable personalized treatment protocols (Darvish et al., 2024). Lastly, the adaptability and precision offered by precision medicine, through the use of radiomics and quantitative imaging biomarkers, represent a paradigm-shifting development in oncology. By focusing on every patient's and his or her cancer's unique characteristics, caregivers can create treatment plans that reduce much trial-and-error thinking commonly associated with cancer therapies. Such personalized care enables not only improved clinical outcomes, but enhanced usage of health resources as well. With ongoing research revealing the secrets of the underlying biological processes of radiomic information, the medical fraternity is poised for a revolutionary phase in which personalized treatment will take center stage in improving cancer therapy and patient survival (Benedict et al., 2018; Darvish et al., 2024).

SUMMARY

The combination of quantitative imaging biomarkers and radiomics has thus far gained immense understanding of cancer characterization, but predominantly for breast cancer. Multi-modality radiomics data derived from combined PET and MRI analysis show how sophisticated imaging can be used to improve tumor phenotype and prognosis. Notably, the study established clearly delineated subgroups of breast cancer patients using unsupervised clustering techniques on 84 extracted features. These subgroups demonstrated strong statistical correlations with significant clinical parameters, including tumor grade, stage at diagnosis, and recurrence status, indicating the potential of radiomics to inform personalized treatment options and enhance patient outcomes (Arasu et al., 2018). Besides, the transferability of some texture features from PET and MRI images to prognostic modeling was evident.

The first-order statistics and gray level co-occurrence matrix (GLCM) features not only had a significant effect on predictive model performance, where the area under the receiver operating characteristic curve (AUC) was 0.76 for tumor grade differentiation, but were also capable of predicting recurrence-free survival, pointing to their application in clinical settings. The research emphasizes the importance of multimodal imaging in developing strong, non-invasive biomarkers that can precisely guide treatment decisions and improve prognostic estimates for breast cancer patients (Arasu et al., 2018).

For non-small cell lung cancer (NSCLC), the application of radiomics has revolutionized the evaluation of treatment response and recurrence significantly. Because the disease tends to be highly heterogeneous, traditional approaches are likely to miss key subtleties in patient management. Radiomics, which can quantify many features from medical images, is instrumental in identifying early signs of tumor response and recurrence. Recent reviews have emphasized the importance of employing sophisticated image analysis tools for correlating pre-treatment image features with treatment response. This approach not only enhances the accuracy of prediction of treatment outcome but also serves as an effective tool for individualized follow-up after treatment, addressing the long-standing need for personalized therapy in the management of NSCLC.

The growing body of evidence on quantitative imaging biomarkers and radiomics has several implications for future research, particularly for the enhancement of methods to assess cancer risk. As demonstrated by research, radiomic features can enhance prognostic models and patient grouping (e.g., 1615 radiomic features from FDG-PET and CT scans were shown to predict locoregional recurrences in head-and-neck cancer) (Aerts et al., 2017).

This raises a critical area for future research: the need for standardized methodologies for analysis and feature extraction. Having a common framework would be helpful in order to enable reproducibility and broader applicability of results across different populations. Discussion about these methodologies continues to be refined, and better prediction models will improve patient outcomes by enabling more tailored treatment protocols. Furthermore, the explosive growth in published radiomics literature, particularly for lung cancer, necessitates a critical evaluation of the clinical applications of radiomic signatures. Future research must deal with the integration of such imaging biomarkers into clinical applications, both for therapy and diagnosis. This will include, in addition to the identification of radiomic features predictive of tumor response, the exploration of their application to staging and prognosis. Multidisciplinary partnerships among oncologists, radiologists, and data scientists will be essential to address challenges posed by the rapid evolution of radiomics. Emphasis on interdisciplinary research can significantly contribute to the development of practical clinical guidelines that leverage radiomic information to improve patient management. Lastly, as radiomics develops as a field of study, overcoming technical issues about imaging techniques will be on the agenda. Future research in the past should have addressed studies on machine learning and AI software, as these pertain to improving the accuracy of radiomics analysis. As image technology advances, understanding how technical advancements, e.g., higher-resolution images and new feature-extraction metrics, affect radiomics will be key. These developments will have the potential to enhance our ability to detect minute variations in tumor biology, ultimately culminating in better stratification of treatment approaches. Activities geared towards harmonizing data across various imaging modalities will prove invaluable in enabling the discipline to stay adaptable and responsive to the ever-evolving profile of cancer treatment.

CLOSER LOOK

ROLE OF RADIOMICS IN HEALTHCARE

The evolving health landscape increasingly recognizes the potential of radiomics as a novelty in patient care and treatment customization. Through the extraction and quantification of imaging data, radiomics enables more advanced understanding of tumor characteristics and behavior. The shift to data-driven approaches makes it possible for clinicians to provide improved cancer risks and intratumoral heterogeneity estimates, thereby improving prognostic capability. As illustrated by recent studies, integrating radiomic features with clinical variables has been promising for predicting conditions such as locoregional recurrences and distant metastases, indicating a clear direction towards individualized treatment protocols. Such advancements in predictive modeling not only enhance patient prognosis but also align with the general goals of precision medicine, where treatments are aimed at being individually customized to each patient's unique biological profile. The Bionic Radiologist concept further reflects the integration of radiomics into practice, noting the intersection of technological advancement and human ability in radiology. The application of artificial intelligence techniques to support radiological decision-making fosters a collaborative team environment in which data access is aligned with improved patient care. As indicated, the overcoming of challenges to implementation, such as resistance to shifting from entrenched practices and ongoing physician education, remains relevant. It is interesting that shared decision-making initiatives and early quantification of uncertainty can engender trust and buy-in among medical professionals. Ultimately, the Bionic Radiologist aims to improve the quality of care being delivered, and therefore, radiomics adoption is not only a technological leap but also an imperative towards more empathetic and personalized medical practice (Dewey et al., 2019). Institutionalizing radiomics in the healthcare sector will require overcoming technical as well as cultural barriers throughout health systems. This entails facilitating enhanced interoperability of image data, standardizing radiomic feature extraction protocols for radiology, and establishing an organizational culture that fosters continued learning and shared decision-making. The ability to incorporate radiomics as part of a whole clinical practice has vast potential, particularly in oncology, as it can lead to improved prognostication accuracy and treatment individualization. Studies supporting the use of radiomic features to predict tumor outcomes also further establish their clinical relevance in the treatment of conditions such as head-and-neck cancer (Aerts et al., 2017). As the medical community is more and more adopting this innovative approach, the future of radiomics is poised to significantly improve the patient experience and simplify treatment protocols in different oncological settings.

REFERENCES

1. Liu, L., Zhang, H., Wu, J., Yu, Z., Chen, X., Rekik, I., Wang, Q., Lu, J., & Shen, D. (2018). Overall survival time prediction for high-grade glioma patients based on large-scale brain functional networks. *Brain Imaging and Behavior, 13*(5), 1333–1351. https://doi.org/10.1007/s11682-018-9949-2Aerts, H. J. W. L., Furstoss, C., Kay-Rivest, E., Khaouam, N., et al. (2017). Radiomics strategies for risk assessment of tumor failure in head-and-neck cancer. http://arxiv.org/abs/1703.08516 (accessed on 5th August 2025).
2. Akin, O., Arita, Y., Edo, H., Kwee, T., et al. (2025). Multiparametric MRI and artificial intelligence in predicting and monitoring treatment response in bladder cancer. https://core.ac.uk/download/653308070.pdf (accessed on 5th August 2025).
3. Aluigi, L., Antignani, P. L., Avgerinos, E. D., Balu, R., et al. (2022). International Union of Angiology (IUA) consensus paper on imaging strategies in atherosclerotic carotid artery imaging: From basic strategies to advanced approaches. https://core.ac.uk/download/534390786.pdf (accessed on 5th August 2025).
4. Laghi, A., Defeudis, A., Cattabriga, A., Caruso, D., Regge, D., Neri, E., Coppola, F., et al. (2021). Radiomics and magnetic resonance imaging of rectal cancer: From engineering to clinical practice. https://core.ac.uk/download/542627265.pdf (accessed on 5th August 2025).
5. Spanu, A., Palumbo, B., Bianconi, F., Fravolini, M. L., & Nuvoli, S. (2020). Artificial intelligence techniques support nuclear medicine modalities to improve the diagnosis of Parkinson's disease and Parkinsonian syndromes. https://core.ac.uk/download/589947997.pdf (accessed on 5th August 2025).
6. Arasu, V. A., Behr, S. C., Copeland, T. P., Esserman, L., et al. (2018). Exploration of PET and MRI radiomic features for decoding breast cancer phenotypes and prognosis. https://core.ac.uk/download/323073101.pdf (accessed on 5th August 2025).
7. Arzanforoosh, F., Barkhof, F., Booth, T., Calvo-Ímirizaldu, M., et al. (2023). Advanced MR techniques for preoperative glioma characterization: Part 2. https://core.ac.uk/download/586994301.pdf (accessed on 5th August 2025).
8. Astaraki, M. (2022). Advanced machine learning methods for oncological image analysis. https://core.ac.uk/download/541039877.pdf (accessed on 5th August 2025).
9. Bacalbasa, N., Balalau, C., Balescu, I., Bucur, M., et al. (2024). Artificial intelligence in ovarian cancers—from diagnosis to treatment: A literature review. https://core.ac.uk/download/624145776.pdf (accessed on 5th August 2025).
10. Bak, S. H., Park, H., Lee, G., & Lee, H. Y. (2020). Radiomics in lung cancer from basic to advanced: Current status and future directions. https://core.ac.uk/download/336856588.pdf (accessed on 5th August 2025).
11. Ball, K. C., Chapman, T. R., Combs, S. E., Hippe, D., et al. (2019). MRI radiomic features are independently associated with overall survival in soft tissue sarcoma. https://core.ac.uk/download/212868561.pdf (accessed on 5th August 2025).
12. Barone, B., Busetto, G. M., Carrieri, G., Cormio, L., Crocetto, F., de Cobelli, O., Del Giudice, F., et al. (2021). Prostate cancer radiogenomics—from imaging to molecular characterization. https://core.ac.uk/download/541678203.pdf (accessed on 5th August 2025).

13. Benedict, S., He, Y., Qiu, J., Rong, Y., et al. (2018). Radiomics for response and outcome assessment for non-small cell lung cancer. https://core.ac.uk/download/323070464.pdf (accessed on 5th August 2025).
14. Bernard, S., Cao, H., Heutte, L., Sabourin, R., et al. (2018). Dissimilarity-based representation for radiomics applications. http://arxiv.org/abs/1803.04460 (accessed on 5th August 2025).
15. Brooks, S. A., Fielding, J. R., Hung, S. C., Khandani, A., et al. (2018). Integrative radiomics expression predicts molecular subtypes of primary clear cell renal cell carcinoma. https://core.ac.uk/download/619688870.pdf (accessed on 5th August 2025).
16. Brunetti, A., Cuocolo, R., Maurea, S., Romeo, V., et al. (2022). Oncologic imaging and radiomics: A walkthrough review of methodological challenges. https://core.ac.uk/download/541161781.pdf (accessed on 5th August 2025).
17. Budach, V., Kotzerke, J., Leger, S., Linge, P., et al. (2017). A comparative study of machine learning methods for time-to-event survival data for radiomics risk modelling. https://core.ac.uk/download/199429272.pdf (accessed on 5th August 2025).
18. Carvalho, S. M. G. de. (2021). Classification of dementias based on brain radiomics features. https://core.ac.uk/download/556218236.pdf (accessed on 5th August 2025).
19. Castelli, M., Di Noia, C., Fabozzi, M., Grist, J., et al. (2022). Current state-of-the-art of AI methods applied to MRI. https://core.ac.uk/download/533756684.pdf (accessed on 5th August 2025).
20. Darvish, M., Hershman, M., Khansari, M., Ren, Y., et al. (2024). AI-enabled lung cancer prognosis. http://arxiv.org/abs/2402.09476 (accessed on 5th August 2025).
21. Dekker, A., Shi, Z., Traverso, A., Wee, L., et al. (2019). FAIR quantitative imaging in oncology: How Semantic Web and ontologies will support reproducible science. https://core.ac.uk/download/593035608.pdf (accessed on 5th August 2025).
22. Dewey, M., & Wilkens, U. (2019). The Bionic Radiologist: Avoiding blurry pictures and providing greater insights. https://core.ac.uk/download/228064788.pdf (accessed on 5th August 2025).
23. Dhermain, F., Franceschi, E., Galldiks, N., Lohmann, P., et al. (2022). Radiomics in neuro-oncological clinical trials. https://www.zora.uzh.ch/id/eprint/221053/1/PIIS2589750022001443.pdf (accessed on 5th August 2025).
24. Traverso, A. (2021). Quantitative imaging in radiation oncology. https://core.ac.uk/download/395380680.pdf (accessed on 5th August 2025).
25. Xin, B. (2021). Multimodal data fusion and quantitative analysis for medical applications. https://core.ac.uk/download/479568823.pdf (accessed on 5th August 2025).

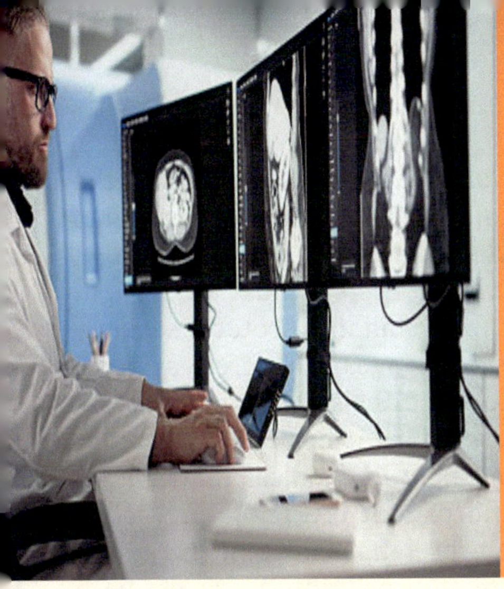

Chapter 9

TELERADIOLOGY: WORKFLOW AND QUALITY ASSURANCE

Contents

Introduction

The advent of teleradiology is a revolutionary shift in medical imaging, facilitating rapid transmission and interpretation of radiological data over long distances. Through teleradiology, physicians can communicate vital patient images and information in real time, thereby augmenting diagnostic capabilities and improving patient care. Teleradiology has evolved into a vital tool in modern-day healthcare, especially in areas where access to specialized radiological expertise is lacking. But with such development come problems, particularly regarding the efficiency of work processes and quality control within the system. To address these issues, there must be a deep understanding of operational workflows, integration protocols, and quality management, especially as legal concepts and interoperability standards evolve. The interfacing of different health information systems, such as those based on DICOM and HL7 protocols, and their implementation will be of significant importance in achieving effective and secure operation of teleradiology systems. These protocols already specify how patient information may be transferred, which is a matter of great concern regarding the confidentiality, integrity, and availability of sensitive data. Radiology information departments must be confident that their systems will talk to each other, most commonly by wading through the intricacies of interoperability problems. Each radiology information system must be brought in with great care to ensure unimpeded workflow, which requires understanding protocol security and its broader context of patient safety and quality of care. The challenges of discrete systems underscore the necessity for extreme quality assurance. Legal considerations also play an important role in the practice of teleradiology, particularly within the European Union. As healthcare becomes increasingly digital, regulatory tools have emerged to govern the flow of medical information between organizations, ensuring that legal obligations are met and patient privacy is protected. Nevertheless, the sheer volume of legal documents complicates the interpretation and implementation of these directives across member states. The varying degrees of interoperability issues, both technical and semantic, create significant legal uncertainties, underscoring the need for intense coordination and collaboration among radiologists, healthcare administrators, and policymakers to address these challenges. It is important to plan strategically to align technological upgrades with legal frameworks and to support the ongoing development of teleradiology by improving quality assurance and overall healthcare delivery.

9.1. Historical Background of Teleradiology

The history of development of teleradiology down the years traces its roots back to the 1960s, a decade that witnessed technological breakthroughs in medical imaging machinery and telecommunication. Telecommunication networks were interconnected with analog imaging devices during this time to transmit radiological images over long distances. Initial efforts focused on remote consultations, in which specialists could interpret pictures remotely. The rapid development of computer technologies and the advent of digital imaging later on triggered a new phase in teleradiology, where images of higher resolution could be handled faster and with greater security (Figure 9.1).

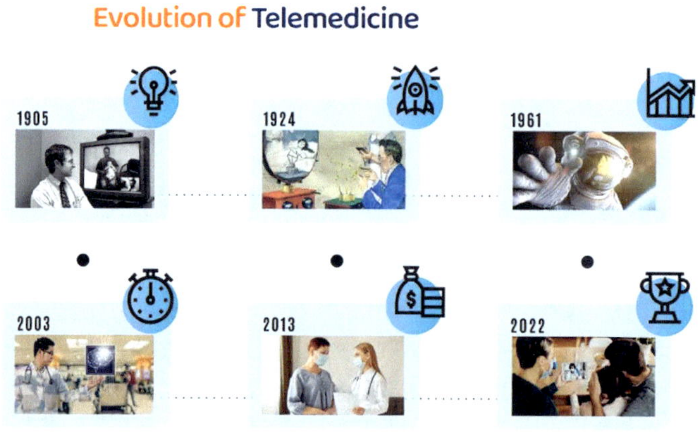

Figure 9.1. Evolution of telemedicine.

Source: https://www.bigscal.com/wp-content/uploads/2023/09/Evolution-of-Telemedicine.webp.

This development made way for a practice that facilitates real-time access to diagnostic expertise across geographical regions and improves patient care, particularly for rural communities. The late 20th century was a defining era for teleradiology, particularly with the arrival of industry standards such as the Digital Imaging and Communications in Medicine (DICOM) and Health Level 7 (HL7). These protocols are necessary to ensure interoperability among various systems and provide assurance regarding the quality of care delivered through teleradiology. DICOM advocated an international standard for sharing images in file format, while HL7 advocated data exchange guidelines across various healthcare systems. As Clark et al. (2018) mandate, harmonizing these protocols is of utmost criticality for ensuring the CIA triad of confidentiality, integrity, and availability of medical imaging. The evolution of Picture Archiving and Communication Systems (PACS) later transformed the industry by enabling centralized storage and rapid image retrieval, significantly streamlining radiological workflows, and increasing the efficiency of diagnostic facilities. When analyzing the contemporary teleradiology scenario, it is imperative to consider the impact of digitalization on the healthcare infrastructure. According to Hristova et al. (2020), the integration of infrastructures like PACS, DICOM, and HL7 has not only changed workflows but also reshaped the labor dynamics of health professionals. Advances in digital technologies have enabled complex supply chains that enhance collaboration among radiologists, data engineers, and other stakeholders. However, with such advancements come pitfalls that require stringent quality assurance strategies to enable reliable, precise diagnoses. As teleradiology continues to expand, adherence to standard protocols and implementation of quality control programs are crucial to taking advantage of the waves of medical imaging change and to earning the trust of patients and clinicians as well.

9.1.1. Evolution of Radiology Practices

Radiology practice has been significantly shaped by technological advances, which have transformed medical imaging. Beginning with Wilhelm Roentgen's announcement of the discovery of X-rays in 1895, radiology rapidly progressed from incorporating emerging technologies to being solidified through digital imaging. The transition from film radiography to digital radiography not only improved the quality and accessibility of imaging but also laid the ground for technologies such as teleradiology. The new paradigm allowed radiologists to interpret images remotely, both accelerating and simplifying diagnostic processes. Therefore, the spatial brick-and-mortar boundaries of radiology units were minimized, enabling healthcare systems to increase patient care substantially. With these advancements, the processes of radiology groups also began to change, prompting new standards and protocols to ensure quality assurance in the sharing and interpretation of images. As teleradiology advanced, several issues arose regarding interoperability and the legal frameworks under which such technologies operated. The digitization of healthcare information enabled image sharing and workflows between medical professionals and patients, but also had complex challenges. Utilizing shared workflows for images highlighted technical and semantic interoperability amid the differences in image sharing across organizations, healthcare organizations, or even nationally (Pohjonen et al., 2011). To add, the legal context regarding teleradiology has become more complex, particularly given the various EU directives that regulate its use. Despite immense efforts to enhance eHealth solutions, Member States remain responsible for planning, supplying, and paying for health care, which implies that successful implementation of teleradiology requires coordination among radiologists, health administrators, and relevant authorities. The evidence supporting the effectiveness of teleradiology continues to pile up, as evidenced by a systematic review of the literature in recent years. Findings consistently demonstrate that teleradiology is equal to conventional radiology in diagnostic accuracy and reliability, and it is essential for substantiating its use in clinical practice (Bashshur et al., 2016). Most significant among the benefits attributed to teleradiology are reductions in patient transfers, rehospitalizations, and overall lengths of stay, all of which contribute directly to better patient outcomes and healthcare system efficiencies. As radiology continues to advance with new technology, it is increasingly important to create and optimize workflows that support high-quality imaging interpretation. Thus, the application of teleradiology is a prime example of the dynamic evolution of radiological practice, which most clearly illustrates how innovation can be integrated into improved healthcare provision at the cost of constraints inherent in traditional imaging processes (Figure 9.2).

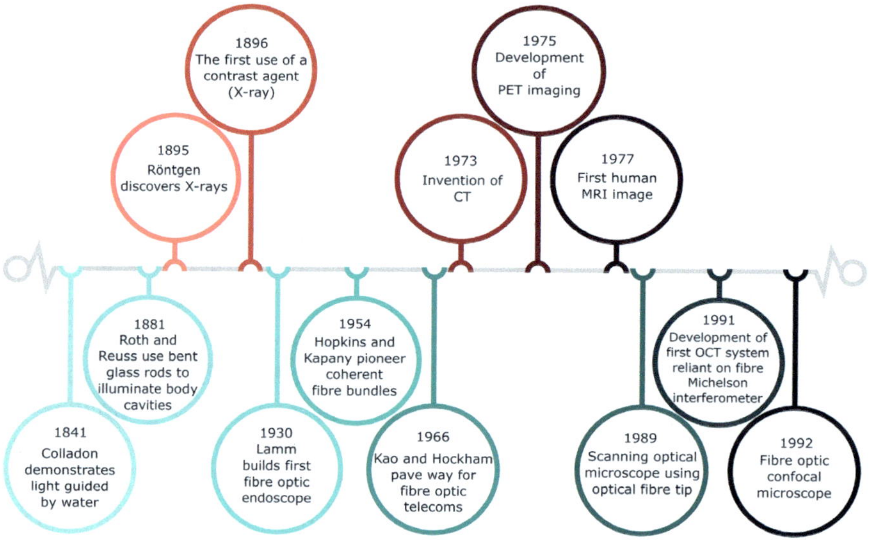

Figure 9.2. Timeline of medical imaging developments. (Top) A brief overview of developments in medical imaging, such as CT (computed tomography), PET (positron-emission tomography), MRI (magnetic resonance imaging), and OCT (optical coherence tomography). (bottom) Timeline of the development of optical fibers and some applications in medical imaging.

Source: https://www.researchgate.net/publication/338553673/figure/fig1/AS:11431281390660138@1745286998721/Timeline-of-medical-imaging-developments-Top-Brief-overview-of-developments-in-medical.tif.

9.1.2. Technological Advancements

In the rapidly evolving medical imaging landscape, technology is the answer to enhancing the efficiency and effectiveness of teleradiology. Cloud computing, more specifically, is a revolutionary technology that enables faster, more convenient imaging data storage and retrieval than ever before. This revolution offers a significant advantage over traditional Picture Archiving and Communication Systems (PACS), which are generally restrictive in scalability and interoperability. The evolution of mobile applications and online programs further accelerates such developments, with radiological images readily available to medical professionals anywhere. According to findings in recent research, such innovations are crucial to improving workflows as well as reducing time for diagnostic evaluations, hence resulting in better patient care and timely clinical decisions, as noted in the literature documenting trends in the radiology practice (Archer et al., 2014). In addition, the development of diagnostic imaging repositories represents a major leap forward in teleradiology's information management. These repositories allow patient imaging reports to be centrally stored, making data sharing convenient across different platforms and institutions. It enhances collaborative care and preserves the continuity of diagnosis and treatment planning by overcoming challenges in managing distributed imaging datasets. These centers offer access to external examination management systems, which further reflect the growth in sophistication of teleradiology solutions, wherein a comprehensive approach that optimizes workflow between radiologists and referring physicians is adopted. From the literature reviewed, it is apparent that these advancements not only improve processes but also enable healthcare providers to focus on delivering quality care without being distracted by administrative stress (Bashshur et al., 2016). The advances in teleradiology are not merely technical developments; they represent a paradigm shift toward a networked, adaptive health care system. Diagnostic quality and reliability have significantly improved through continued research and development in the area, resulting in high concordance between teleradiology and conventional radiology. In addition, the increasing use of electronic health records (EHR) and telemedicine solutions in teleradiology enables radiologists to make expert opinions from remote locations, overcoming geographical limitations that historically prevented patients from accessing quality diagnostic services. This strategic use of technology not only allows for diagnosis and treatment of illness but also improves patient outcomes through decreased need for unnecessary transfers and hospitalizations, highlighting the inalienable significance of technological innovation in shaping the future of healthcare delivery (Archer et al., 2014; Bashshur et al., 2016) (Figure 9.3).

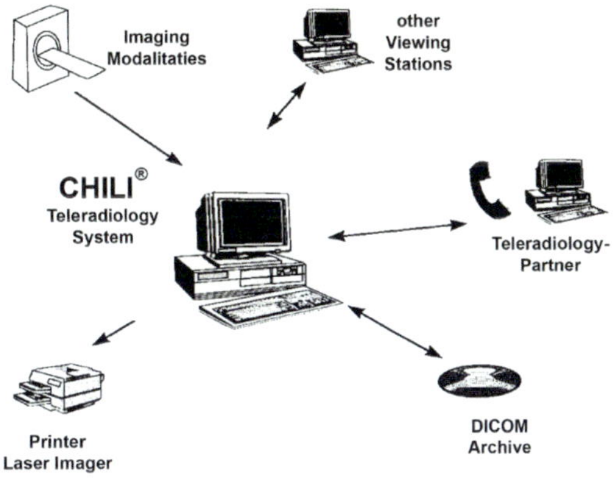

Figure 9.3. Second-generation teleradiology system CHILI in the context of radiology.

Source: https://www.researchgate.net/profile/Henning-Mueller-3/publication/12595424/figure/fig2/AS:667652989153285@1536192285932/Second-generation-teleradiology-system-CHILI-in-the-context-of-radiology.png.

9.1.3. Regulatory Changes Impacting Teleradiology

The legal landscape within which teleradiology has come to function has transformed radically in recent years, mirroring the rapid technological advancements and the increasing incorporation of telehealth services into the conventional healthcare system. As hospitals and other healthcare facilities adopt teleradiology solutions, policymakers have issued guidelines to facilitate the safe and efficient use of the modality and to maintain patient confidentiality and data security. For instance, enforcing stringent regulations on patient authorization and the handling of electronic health records (EHR) is necessary to offset the threat of data breaches. Compliance with the Health Insurance Portability and Accountability Act (HIPAA) remains the paramount mandate, with teleradiology providers compelled to invest in secure communication channels and sophisticated encryption methods to protect sensitive patient information. These changes not only highlight the importance of patient trust but also facilitate more efficient workflows because healthcare professionals can operate confidently within a healthy regulatory framework focused on quality assurance and patient safety. Furthermore, the intersection of teleradiology and regional health policies illustrates how regulatory reforms can influence the workflow efficiencies and the quality of radiologic services.

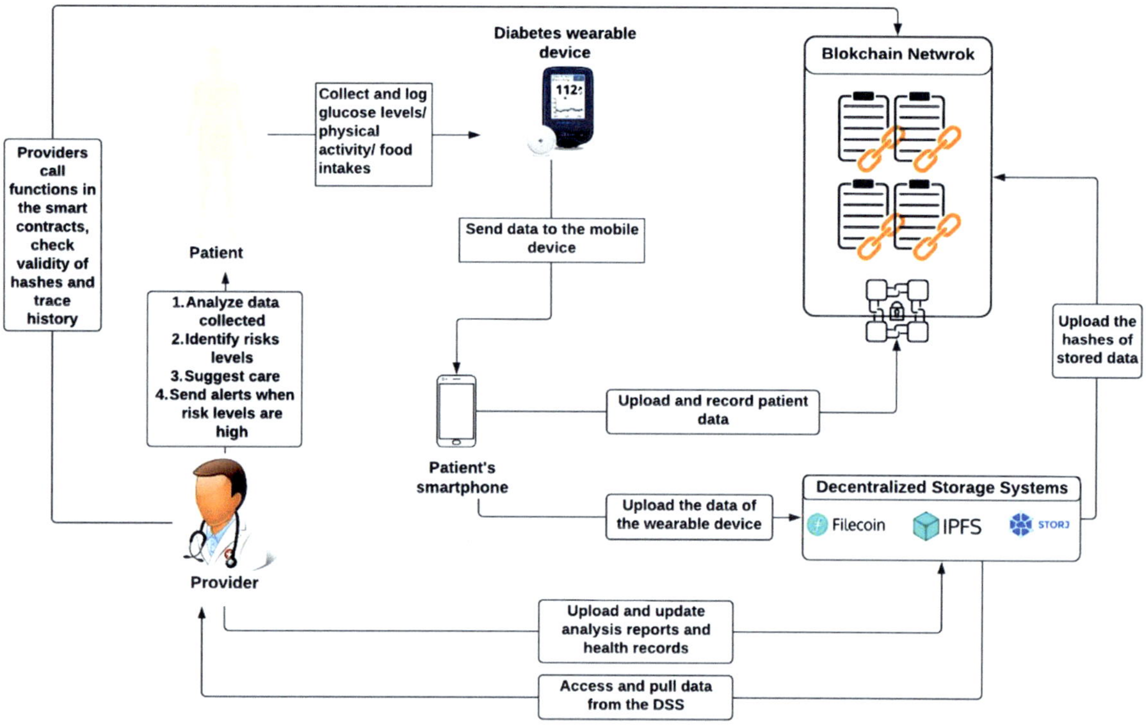

Figure 9.4. A Blockchain-Based Regulatory Framework for mHealth.

Source: https://www.mdpi.com/data/data-07-00177/article_deploy/html/images/data-07-00177-g001.png.

As described by the pre-implementation phase case study of a teleradiology project in rural Thailand, a systematic approach based on Patient Care Pathways can improve service delivery outcomes substantially. Through an identification of the interdependence of systems in health care and an overcoming of probable obstacles before implementation, stakeholders can create a teleradiology service that is less susceptible to policy changes. This proactive strategy enables process optimization and streamlining of clinical and administrative processes, which are essential in rural settings where specialized service access may be limited. Responsive rules that encourage such planning are most likely to lead to enhanced clinical practice and ultimately improved patient outcomes for teleradiology initiatives (Jones et al., 2009). As telehealth expands, the regulatory environment will need to keep pace with the new technologies revolutionizing healthcare provision.

New Hampshire, for instance, demonstrates how a higher EHR utilization rate, in conjunction with an existing telecommunications infrastructure, sets teleradiology and mHealth up for expansion. When these technologies are recognized, policymakers can streamline regulations to allow remote diagnostic services to be easily incorporated. This entails developing open payment and licensure procedures to facilitate teleradiology across state borders and improve patient access in underserved areas. Effective management of these policy reforms can significantly enhance the quality of care provided through teleradiology, ensuring that patients receive timely and accurate diagnoses, even when face-to-face consultation is not feasible (Arnault et al., 2017) (Figure 9.4).

9.2. Teleradiology Workflow

The teleradiology workflow is a dynamic, complex process of transmitting medical images from one site to another, typically by a healthcare institution to radiologists who read the images remotely. This workflow begins with acquiring images, which include such diagnostic imaging devices as X-ray, CT scan, and MRI, and creating digital files. After acquisition, images must be compressed and encrypted to ensure safe transmission over networks. Effective transmission protocols are crucial in avoiding data loss and ensuring images arrive in good condition and on time for interpretation. The first process within this workflow emphasizes the importance of technological advancements in digital imaging and telecommunications to enable effective image sharing across platforms, thereby facilitating timely radiological evaluation essential to patient care. Once images have been sent, the next critical phase is interpretation, in which radiologists examine the images and generate reports. This phase is not only about ensuring that the quality of the images has been evaluated but also about rapidly accessing prior studies and patient histories to enhance diagnostic accuracy (Figure 9.5).

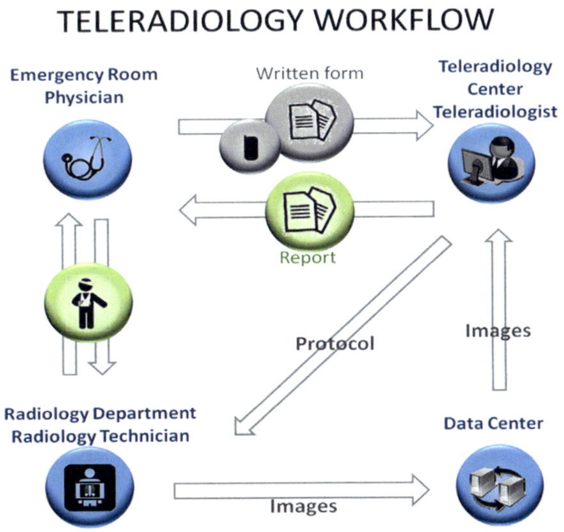

Figure 9.5. Teleradiology workflow using RADSpa.

Source: https://epos.myesr.org/posterimage/esr/ecr2012/112460/media/411792.

Integrating advanced software applications simplifies the radiologist's workflow by introducing highlight features to identify abnormalities and annotate images. Transparency is essential in the communication between the patient, referring doctors, and radiologists at this stage. The reports must be conveyed in explicit detail, particularly tailored for individual providers to enable them to make rational clinical decisions. Introduction of the standard reporting formats, coupled with adherence to the pre-established guidelines, results in the maximum workflow efficiency and is a significant contributor to quality assurance of teleradiology. Successful workflows in teleradiology are based on overcoming interoperability and regulatory problems that are likely to affect quality assurance of healthcare environments. The legal and technical complexities of sharing medical images, particularly across nations, underscore the need for comprehensive frameworks and coordination among stakeholders. As noted in recent literature, disparities in interoperability issues, whether technical or semantic in type, make a need for having an aggregated effort to produce seamless communication networks (Pohjonen et al., 2011). In addition to basic technology, the adoption of a systems analysis model is advantageous for the design and implementation of teleradiology services, enabling improved understanding of patient care trajectories and information exchange (Jones et al., 2009). Therefore, the encouragement of cooperation among radiologists, healthcare administrators, and policymakers remains at the forefront of addressing these challenges, ensuring that teleradiology is taken to its optimal level to improve healthcare delivery.

9.2.1. Image Acquisition and Transmission

Image capture in the teleradiology process is important in ensuring that diagnostic interpretations become effective and precise. It is the process by which quality images are captured via numerous modalities, such as X-rays, CT scans, and MRIs, which play a critical role in providing comprehensive information about a patient's condition. Modern imaging technologies employ sophisticated digital techniques to enhance image sharpness and resolution, thereby increasing diagnostic accuracy. However, the images captured need to follow specific protocols and standards, such as Digital Communications in Medicine (DICOM), in order to be made compatible with diverse systems (Figure 9.6).

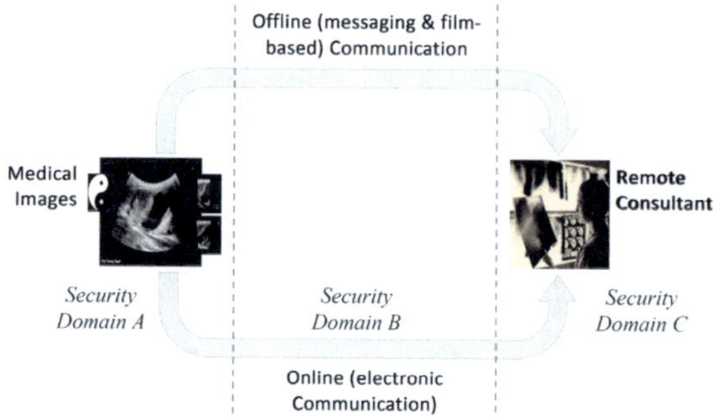

Figure 9.6. Process of image acquisition in teleradiology.

Source: https://www.researchgate.net/profile/Hussain-Nyeem/publication/230849286/figure/fig1/AS:300449581289472@1448644170037/Teleradiology-model.png.

This coupling is essential to maintaining the structured flow of information required for reliable diagnosis and to fulfilling the underlying pillars of confidentiality, integrity, and availability, as identified in recent texts (Clark et al., 2018). Once images have been acquired, the second important step in the teleradiology process is their transmission. Safe transmission of large files, including high-resolution images, relies on robust information systems and new communications technologies. Safe networks must be used to protect patient information when it is sent, in accordance with

HIPAA standards that place privacy within the context of healthcare. Besides, standards such as Health Level 7 (HL7) facilitate seamless data sharing between various healthcare systems, making it not only easy but also ensuring that what is shared is correct and up-to-date. It is important that communication lines of this nature are reliable because any interference can delay treatment and diagnosis, undermining patient outcomes and the quality of care in general (Clark et al., 2018). Integrating teleradiology into the overall healthcare system is both promising and challenging, particularly with respect to ensuring image quality and diagnostic validity. Large-scale studies have established that a high degree of conformity with conventional diagnoses has been confirmed as effective. Care should be taken to maintain the workflow at optimal levels and ensure quality standards. Regular quality imaging audits, constant education of radiologists, and adherence to regulatory guidelines are essential to optimize both the acquisition and transmission processes. With high standards in these processes, healthcare professionals can reap the and most significant advantages of teleradiology, avoid unnecessary patient transfer, and ultimately enhance patient care in terms of timely and accurate diagnoses.

9.2.2. Interpretation by Radiologists

The radiologist's core function in teleradiology is to interpret diagnostic images, a crucial process that significantly impacts patient care.

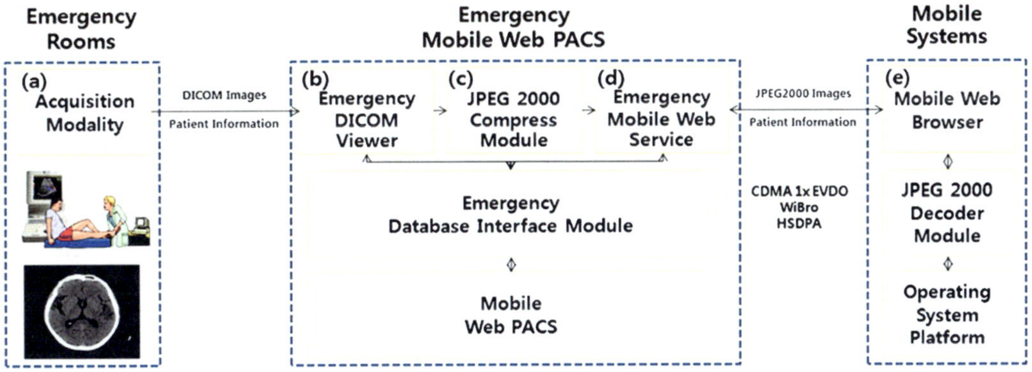

Figure 9.7. The configuration of a mobile tele-radiology imaging system composed of an emergency mobile Web PACS and mobile system with five components: a acquisition modality, b emergency DICOM viewer, c JPEG2000 compression module, d emergency mobile Web service, and e mobile browser as end-user mobile devices.

Source: https://www.researchgate.net/profile/Dongkeun-Kim/publication/46171005/figure/fig1/AS:277223979405330@1443106755820/The-configuration-of-a-mobile-tele-radiology-imaging-system-composed-of-an-emergency.png.

The job involves evaluating various imaging modalities, such as X-rays, CT scans, and MRIs, to identify abnormalities ranging from fractures to tumors. With the application of digital imaging and teleradiology, radiologists now face new challenges: images are communicated across networks to remote locations, requiring them not only to possess clinical competence but also digital system competence. Accurate interpretation under these circumstances is crucial, as it enables timely treatment and diagnosis and bridges geographical distances between specialists and patients.

Therefore, bringing together efficient tools for communication and secure systems for information is most important for sustaining quality assurance throughout the teleradiology workflow (Clark et al., 2018). Additionally, the quality of interpretation plays a central role in guaranteeing that diagnostic findings are reliable and correct. Studies have shown that concordance rates between teleradiology and conventional radiology are equally high, indicating that telemedicine interpretations are equivalent to in-person inspection (Bashshur et al., 2016) (Figure 9.7). This reliability is not only based on technological development but also on extensive training and ongoing education of radiologists in understanding advanced imaging techniques and interpretation methods. Guaranteeing that radiologists can use digital resources and have an adequate understanding of the procedures involved fosters a culture of trust within the clinic. Therefore, continuing professional development is essential for radiologists who practice teleradiology, as it directly impacts patient outcomes. In addition to clinical expertise, teleradiology interpretation requires a robust workflow and high-quality assurance processes. Effective integration of digital communications supports smooth data transfer and is important in ensuring patient data privacy and integrity, adhering to standards like DICOM and HL7 (Clark et al., 2018). These protocols enable radiologists to focus on their core activity—accurate interpretation—without increasing the likelihood of errors caused by technical setbacks or mishandling of data. Performance metrics and auditing also become part of the quality assurance process. They provide data that can be applied to practice improvement, enabling radiologists to continually improve interpretation and remain excellent at patient diagnosis. Thus, the relationship among workflow efficiency, technology, and quality assurance is the crux of quality radiologist interpretation in teleradiology.

9.2.3. Reporting and Communication of Results

Result reporting and result communication in the teleradiology sector are paramount process that determines the effectiveness of patient treatment. Radiologists employ advanced imaging procedures, such as Digital Communications in Medicine (DICOM) and Health Level 7 (HL7), to transmit significant patient information among different information systems. These standards enable not just the sharing of medical images but also the reports through which clinicians get information about findings and diagnoses. Integration of such systems is essential to ensure that healthcare professionals will be able to access accurate and timely information, hence resulting in better decision-making. However, organizing such communication smoothly poses significant challenges, particularly ensuring the confidentiality, integrity, and availability of data in the workflow, which is central to patient information protection and trust among healthcare practitioners. In addition, the complexity of the legal framework in teleradiology means that ensuring compliance with proper knowledge of regulatory implications when sharing imaging results becomes vital. As highlighted by recent publications, there is possible legal ambiguity, particularly while crossing national boundaries, based on the varied EU directive interpretations and legal rules applicable to teleradiology (Pohjonen et al., 2011). This creates a multifaceted environment for radiologists and health administrators to navigate not only technological obstacles but also legislative requirements. Interoperability problems typically play out in both technical and semantic domains, affecting how information is exchanged between organizations, underscoring the need for cross-disciplinary teamwork. Effective handling of these legal challenges requires teamwork between radiologists, administrators, and clinicians to ensure that reporting and communication quality is not sacrificed in the presence of the regulatory landscape. Furthermore, challenges encountered at the various image and workflow sharing levels significantly affect the reporting mechanisms used in teleradiology. The evolution to digital has brought on the rise of new paradigms of communication that enable the sharing of data in real time between healthcare providers. However, these advancements must be accompanied by rigorous security protocols to ensure the level of care expected in medical imaging (Clark et al., 2018). The integration of disparate healthcare systems demands a common approach to mitigate potential vulnerabilities, ensuring patient safety in the workflow. By fostering common communication among stakeholders such as radiologists and IT professionals, healthcare organizations can ensure the quality assurance mechanisms that underpin effective reporting and the overall patient experience in teleradiology.

9.3. Technology in Teleradiology

The interfolding of technology in teleradiology is profoundly transformative, enabling instant communication of medical imaging across diverse geographic boundaries. By digitizing medical information, medical doctors can instantly exchange images and workflows, thereby encouraging greater collaboration among radiologists, general physicians, and specialists. The revolution of technology not only accelerates diagnosis but also responds to the growing demand for efficiency in healthcare delivery. However, implementing such cooperative workflows is challenging, particularly regarding interoperability and legal certainty. The complexities of running image sharing across various levels—organization, country, or among caregivers and patients—pose technical and semantic challenges. These challenges need to be overcome to derive the maximum benefits of teleradiology, thereby enabling smooth integration and improved patient outcomes and operational workflows (Pohjonen et al., 2011). Also, successful technology implementation in teleradiology is contingent on establishing a broad framework for its realization, as revealed by current studies. For instance, using an adapted Patient Care Pathway provides a structured process for assessing and optimizing e-health programs. In addition to considering the patient's journey through the healthcare system, this pathway follows the course of information essential to the teleradiology service. Case study of a teleradiology project in rural Thailand underscores the criticality of applying a systems analysis methodology. By identifying key points in the healthcare system and forecasting clinical practice changes, the methodology assists stakeholders in addressing technology integration complexities. In response, systematic planning and change management enhance the potential success of teleradiology programs, rendering them operational and sustainable across different healthcare environments (Jones et al., 2009). Furthermore, as technology in teleradiology continues to improve, the necessity for robust quality assurance mechanisms becomes increasingly apparent. Technology is critical to maintaining consistent image quality, accurate interpretation, and secure data. Through the application of state-of-the-art imaging technology, coupled with rigorous quality control measures, the dependability of diagnostics is not only improved but also patient trust in remote radiological services is reinforced. Furthermore, the interfacing of teleradiology with EHRs and cloud-based platforms creates an environment where information is readily accessible and editable, thereby improving the quality assurance process. With coordinated effort to bridge interoperability gaps and standardize procedures, the field of teleradiology can maximize technology's potential to offer better quality healthcare services while at the same time overcoming the hurdles in an increasingly digitized medical setting (Jones et al., 2009; Pohjonen et al., 2011) (Figure 9.8).

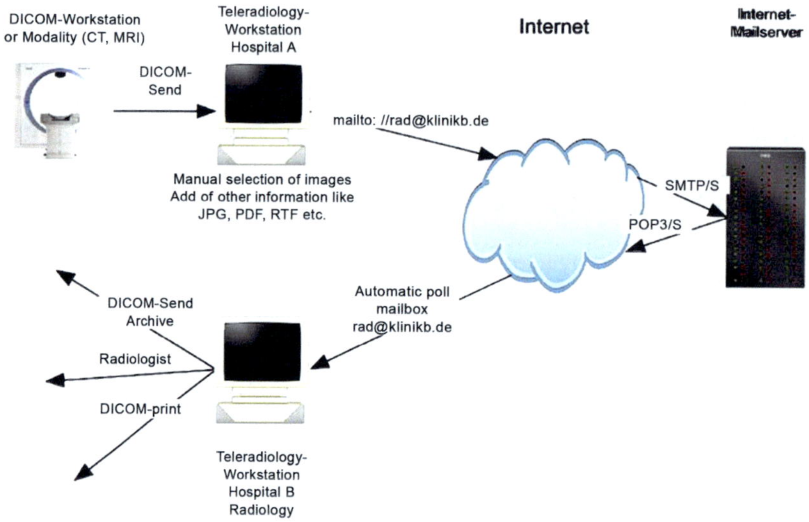

Figure 9.8. Integration of a DICOM- e-mail teleradiology workstation.

Source: https://www.researchgate.net/profile/Uwe-Engelmann/publication/6764633/figure/fig1/AS:277768832077830@1443236658338/ntegration-of-a-DICOM-e-mail-teleradiology-workstation.png.

9.3.1. Imaging Modalities Used

The evolution of imaging modalities has also significantly impacted teleradiology practice by enhancing the diagnostic and management potential of diseases at a distance. Modalities such as CT, MRI, and standard X-rays are all fundamental components of this evolving environment. Each modality offers a distinct advantage; for instance, CT scans enable rapid imaging of internal structures, and MRI provides superior soft-tissue contrast. The widespread adoption of these modalities has improved clinical workflows, enabling radiologists to interpret images from remote locations. With advances in teleradiology, the advantages of these imaging modalities are continually improving, leading to more accurate diagnoses and faster decision-making in patient care. Generally, the integration of advanced imaging modalities into teleradiology represents a significant shift in how healthcare workers handle imaging data. Flexibility of the imaging modality in teleradiology requires stringent QA processes to provide diagnostic quality and ensure patient safety (Figure 9.9).

Since different imaging modalities provide different information, maintaining the highest standards is essential. This includes strict adherence to established standards, such as Digital Communications in Medicine (DICOM) and Health Level 7 (HL7), that enable secure data exchanges (Clark et al., 2018). Consistency in image quality is also essential because differences in image resolution can significantly affect diagnosis and treatment guidelines. The QA measures taken should extend beyond technical calibration of imaging devices to include extensive training for radiologists and imaging technologists in the interpretation of teleradiographic data. Such QA measures ensure the integrity and reliability of imaging modalities in a teleradiology environment. The historical background of teleradiology provides the track record of imaging modalities and their applications in real-world settings. Initially established in the 1940s, teleradiology has undergone radical change, primarily driven by technological advancements (Bashshur et al., 2016). The initial focus was on the transmission of basic radiographic images, but today's applications range to advanced imaging techniques such as digital angiography and therapeutic ultrasound. Such growth demonstrates a growing reliance on multi-modal imaging in clinical practice, which can deliver a comprehensive assessment of patient status. The convergence of sophisticated imaging technologies and robust teleradiology platforms not only optimizes patient results but also simplifies traditional barriers, such as geography and access to specialized care. Hence, the development of teleradiology testifies to how computer advancements continually enhance medical practice today.

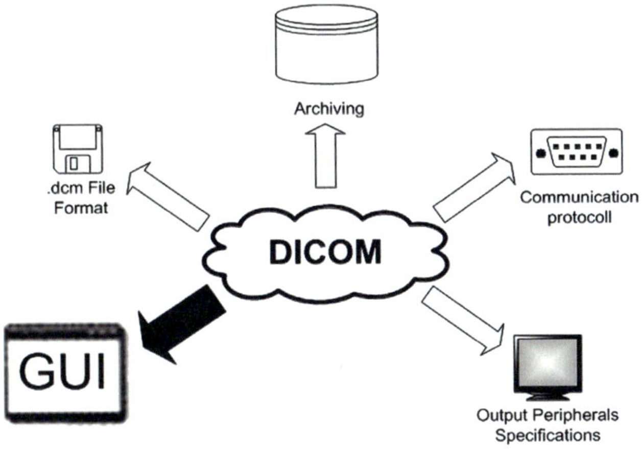

Figure 9.9. The DICOM standard involves various aspects of the medical software standardization except the GUI structure.

Source: https://www.researchgate.net/profile/Roberto-Pirrone/publication/221328281/figure/fig1/AS:393937433972741@1470933411450/The-DICOM-standard-involves-various-aspects-of-the-medical-software-standardization.png.

9.3.2. Software and Platforms for Teleradiology

In teleradiology, the software and platforms used play a significant role in ensuring optimal workflow and quality assurance. They assist in the transfer of medical images and associated information between various healthcare centers so that radiologists can provide timely diagnosis, irrespective of geographical location. Among the technological upgrades needed are robust image-sharing protocols, such as Digital Imaging and Communications in Medicine (DICOM) and Health Level 7 (HL7), which are essential for the seamless sharing of life-saving information. By adhering to them, healthcare institutions can offer interoperability, which is required for effective communication between different systems and improving patient outcomes. The difficulties in using these technologies primarily concern maintaining the smooth integration of dissimilar systems, for which well-designed workflows must be put in place to preserve the confidentiality, integrity, and availability of patient data (Pohjonen et al., 2011). Further, teleradiology software must enable several legal and regulatory matters, particularly about cross-border data exchange. The complexity of interoperability is not only technical; semantic complexity, in the form of language differences and variations in national laws, is also involved. For instance, the European Union legal law on teleradiology comprises several directives that ensure safe and effective image-sharing procedures. Recent EU reports indicate that these directives call for coordination among radiologists, healthcare managers, and policymakers to optimize the use of eHealth solutions (Figure 9.10).

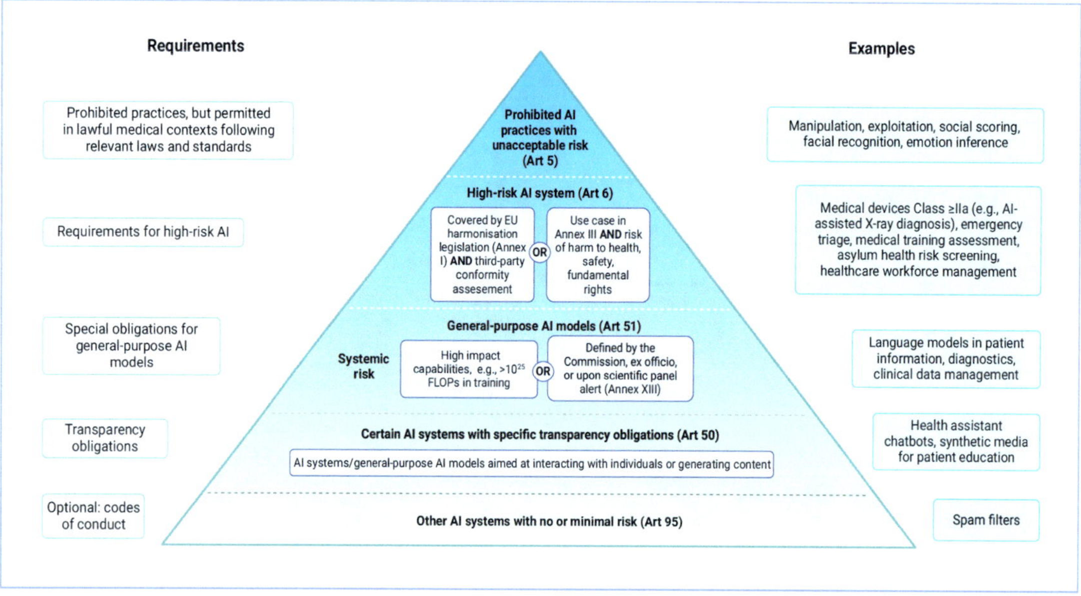

Figure 9.10. Navigating the European union artificial intelligence act for healthcare.

Source: https://media.springernature.com/full/springer-static/image/art%3A10.1038%2Fs41746-024-01213-6/MediaObjects/41746_2024_1213_Fig1_HTML.png.

Given the complex legal landscape, the deployment of teleradiology systems must navigate these nuances carefully, and data-sharing procedures must comply with existing regulations while promoting innovation in remote diagnosis (Pohjonen et al., 2011). The effectiveness of teleradiology systems also depends on user experience and clinical workflows provided by chosen software platforms. Those platforms must be designed from a user-centric approach so radiologists can easily access and analyze images and minimize potential mistakes. More advanced features, such as automated reporting and clinical decision support tools embedded within, can significantly enhance workflow effectiveness and diagnostic quality. In addition, there is a mandatory overarching quality assurance system necessary for monitoring teleradiology system performance, ensuring diagnostic-quality images, and providing timely reports. By leveraging advanced software options that balance functionality and compliance, healthcare organizations can enhance the reliability of teleradiology services, ultimately improving patient care and outcomes (Clark et al., 2018).

9.3.3. Security Measures for Data Protection

In the context of teleradiology, strong security measures for data protection are essential to safeguard sensitive patient information. The electronic form of medical information enables greater connectivity among healthcare professionals, patients, and institutions, but at the same time creates vulnerabilities open to misuse by malicious forces. The implications of common workflows call for a multi-directional approach to address interoperability challenges and the legal complexities associated with data sharing. As health care infrastructure increasingly relies on online platforms, a structured process combining technical and legal considerations is essential to ensure that patient confidentiality and data integrity are maintained (Pohjonen et al., 2011). Adequate security practices not only protect patients' information but also enhance the quality and reliability of teleradiology services, thereby building public trust in electronic health infrastructure. Strict compliance with well-established protocols such as DICOM and Health Level 7 (HL7) is a prerequisite in the transfer of medical imaging data and associated patient data. The protocols aim at allowing various healthcare systems to interoperate, allowing critical data to be sent promptly and accurately. However, the integration of multiple information systems most of the time poses mammoth challenges, particularly with regard to security for data being moved (Figure 9.11).

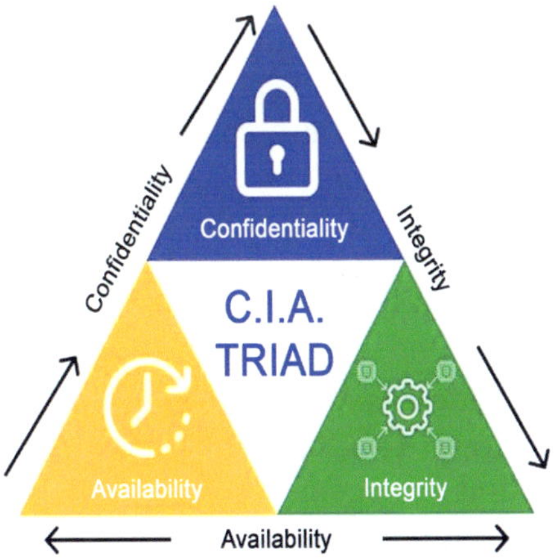

Figure 9.11. Shows the CIA triad.

Source: https://cdn.prod.website-files.com/5ff66329429d880392f6cba2/66a372b4a3d814c4fc284041_63fdd44daa2d3e1f527b40e7_CIA%2520Triad.jpeg.

The CIA triad of confidentiality, integrity, and availability is a global framework for assessing and enhancing the security of such protocols (Clark et al., 2018). While emphasizing these considerations, healthcare providers can prevent possible vulnerabilities so that sensitive information is kept safe and maximize the effectiveness of teleradiology operations. Moreover, the dynamic nature of regulatory environments and compliance measures implies ongoing vigilance in data protection for teleradiology. As foreseen in most EU directives, defining legal standards for data sharing can be complex, particularly when transnational activities are involved. This complexity increases the need for cooperation among stakeholders, such as radiologists, healthcare administrators, and control authorities, to establish standard procedures that adhere to technical and legal standards (Pohjonen et al., 2011). Through developing a culture of compliance and collaboration, healthcare organizations can develop suitable strategies that enhance both the security of patient data and the quality assurance of teleradiology services, which will enable best practices within the industry.

9.4. Quality Assurance in Teleradiology

Quality assurance in teleradiology is necessary to ensure diagnostic accuracy and patient safety. Rapid growth in digital technology has facilitated the sharing of radiological images and patient information across various platforms by medical practitioners. However, the trend poses challenges for maintaining image integrity and consistency during transmission. There must be functional quality assurance procedures to address potential discrepancies arising from technical and semantic interoperability issues. These become more complicated, particularly for a teleradiology context where services might be offered across borders, thereby subjecting the practice to diverse regulating bodies and bodies of law. Solving these issues is paramount in building trust between medical professionals and patients and ensuring the integrity of diagnostic outcomes in a business that relies on precise image interpretation and analysis (Pohjonen et al., 2011). Effective implementation of rigorous quality assurance protocols also needs a good grasp of the workflow that governs teleradiology services. These precautions must include regular assessment of equipment, continuous training for radiologists, and implementation of standardized image acquisition and interpretation protocols. Emphasizing structured workflows enables in-depth consideration of the patient care pathway, which is vital for identifying and controlling risks inherent in teleradiology services. For instance, a tailored Patient Care Pathway can prove to be a critical element in planning and implementing e-health efforts, including teleradiology services. The stepwise approach enables healthcare systems to have a clearer view of the patient experience and information flow, thereby facilitating the provision of real-time interventions and adjustments to improve quality (Jones et al., 2009). By providing an exact schematic representation of relevant processes, healthcare professionals can more comfortably address the consequences of alterations introduced by new technologies. Second, quality assurance in teleradiology demands cooperation among participants, including stakeholders within the healthcare setting. Strong cooperation among radiologists, healthcare managers, and policymakers is essential for developing effective teleradiology solutions. As outlined in various strategic publications from the European Union, establishing clear lines of duty and responsibility can help ensure the legal certainty required in teleradiology processes. This is particularly important given the myriad regulatory directives that govern cross-border healthcare supply. By encouraging inter-professional communication and compliance among health professionals, the efficiency of teleradiology can be significantly improved, leading to better patient outcomes. Under this dynamic setup, continuous assessment and enhancement of quality assurance procedures will eventually enable teleradiology services to reach the highest levels of clinical excellence (Pohjonen et al., 2011).

9.4.1. Standards and Guidelines

Standards and guidelines are also significant to the efficiency and reliability of teleradiology, standardizing processes across platforms and regions. With medical data becoming digital, image and workflow exchange between caregivers has become more complicated. This is because interoperability and legal clarity are needed when data is being exchanged between organizations or nations.

The European Union has enacted various directives for the regulation of teleradiology, which are consistent with the different challenges in its implementation. The regulations provide guidelines that can affect healthcare professionals, while also directing them to cooperate with radiologists, healthcare administrators, and policymakers. As such, the acceptance of standards improves workflow efficiency and conformity with legal requirements set by bodies such as the EU (Pohjonen et al., 2011). In essence, standards application in teleradiology is not merely a matter of compliance but encompasses the entire workflow management system. Systems analysis models, such as the modified Patient Care Pathway, contribute to the strength of planning and management of e-health programs, such as teleradiology services. An application of a complete systems approach guarantees stakeholders fully understand patient pathways and information flows through the health system. Such a model allows the identification of the key factors that may influence clinical practice upon implementation. Such forethought is essential for creating a smoother integration of teleradiology services into existing healthcare setups, thereby ensuring quality assurance programs and placing patients' welfare above technological advancements (Jones et al., 2009). The establishment of standard guidelines and protocols also facilitates the training and education of radiology professionals, emphasizing the need for standardized methods in image acquisition, interpretation, and reporting. By applying pre-programmed protocols, variability and errors in teleradiology can be minimized, thereby increasing diagnostic precision and patient treatment. Furthermore, these guidelines should be reviewed and revised regularly as technology advances, so that the standards remain up to date and beneficial. An interagency team composed of healthcare practitioners, professional organizations, and regulatory bodies will be tasked with developing guidelines responding to acute needs and long-term issues to the practice of teleradiology. The group's conformity to these standards will ensure an environment that values quality assurance, ultimately enhancing the overall integrity of radiological care (Pohjonen et al., 2011).

9.4.2. Role of Accreditation Bodies

Accreditation agencies play a significant role in guaranteeing that services offered in teleradiology are of good quality and reliable. Through formulating strict standards and guidelines, these agencies provide a framework for evaluating the performance of infrastructure and processes employed in teleradiology. This supervision is important because teleradiology is a complex systems that integrate various elements, such as Picture Archiving and Communication Systems (PACS) and protocols such as DICOM and HL7, which allow for unrestricted transfer of medical imaging information from one area to another. Effective accreditation can enhance trust among health workers and patients by ensuring that such systems meet established quality standards, thereby minimizing the scope for human error and enhancing the overall quality of patient care. Such accredited teleradiology, therefore, can be crucial in improving healthcare outcomes, particularly in rural or underserved areas where radiology experts might not be readily available. The impact of accreditation extends beyond compliance to the workflow efficiency in teleradiology networks. By adhering to accreditation organizations' best practices, teleradiology services can streamline operations, reduce diagnostic delays, and improve turnaround times for imaging exams. For instance, the application of systems engineering principles, as presented in a case study of a teleradiology project in rural Thailand, addresses the need for a systematic process for implementing e-health solutions [^31]. This procedure serves as a model for organizations to rationalize patient care pathways, not only improving the quality of care delivered but also enhancing operational effectiveness across all service delivery levels.

Hence, accreditation plays a vital role in ensuring that clinics and hospitals successfully and safely implement technology-driven solutions. Accreditation agencies also serve as the link between technological advancements and human resource training in teleradiology. The complexities introduced by various technologies necessitate continuous education and adaptation among radiologists and administrative personnel. Accreditation programs usually include performance checks and ongoing education to keep health professionals abreast of evolving standards and practices in teleradiology [^32]. This focus on education not only prepares staff to operate new systems, but also enables collaboration among interprofessional teams providing patient care. Accreditation organizations here not only uphold standards but also foster a culture of constant improvement and quality assurance. Ensuring practitioners possess the necessary skills and knowledge ultimately leads to a stronger teleradiology infrastructure capable of delivering high-quality diagnostic services efficiently.

9.4.3. Continuous Quality Improvement Processes

Initiating continuous quality improvement (CQI) processes in the domain of teleradiology is important for enhancing workflow efficiency and quality assurance. CQI is an orderly process that works towards improving healthcare services by continuous review and workflow improvement. In the case of teleradiology, this can involve the creation of some benchmarks for the interpretation of imaging studies to evaluate the efficacy of technological tools and clinicians' skills. By developing a feedback loop between information from referring physicians and radiologists, healthcare systems can identify areas for improvement and provide a quick, accurate assessment for patients. In doing this, not only does this promote an organizational culture of ongoing learning and adjustment among healthcare workers, but it also drives service innovations based on evolving clinical standards and patient needs. A component of CQI in teleradiology is the integration of a systems analysis model that considers the interdependencies among healthcare complexities. According to previous research, healthcare systems fail to integrate total change management when implementing e-health programs, leading to inefficiency and care fragmentation. With an applied Patient Care Pathway model, teleradiology schemes can create a clearer picture of patient pathways, information flows, and potential risks that may arise during diagnosis. With planning of these pathways, healthcare providers are in a position to detect challenges and prepare staff and technology accordingly. This vision not only enhances the quality of care delivered but also demonstrates the organization's commitment to continuous improvement processes, which are essential for achieving long-term success in teleradiology services (Jones et al., 2009). Furthermore, the empirical support for teleradiology highlights its value in improving diagnostic accuracy and operational efficiency. Evidence demonstrates that teleradiology is not only feasible but also provides results equal to those of traditional radiology practice, notably in diagnostic accuracy and overall impact on patient management (Bashshur et al., 2016). Adoption of CQI processes in this system can facilitate regular reviews of both diagnostic practices and technology enhancements. To illustrate, a continuous audit of teleradiology activities allows organizations to analyze diagnostic concordance and turnaround time data and verify that any results that do not meet pre-specified benchmarks are addressed immediately. This continuous monitoring and realignment eventually streamline patient care pathways, reduce unnecessary transfers, enhance the patient experience, and, by implication, align with the inherent aspects of CQI in healthcare settings.

9.5. Challenges in Teleradiology

The integration of teleradiology into healthcare settings is facing a range of challenges that have broader implications for workflow and quality assurance. One of the key challenges is the heterogeneity of radiology information systems, which are often designed to support distinct imaging protocols, such as Digital Communications in Medicine (DICOM) and Health Level 7 (HL7) (Figure 9.12). These protocols are also critical for patient data transmission. Still, their integration between platforms needs to be done with great care to preserve the CIA triad of confidentiality, integrity, and availability. Failure to achieve proper integration may result in life-threatening delays in diagnosis and treatment, thereby compromising patient safety and healthcare delivery efficiency. Therefore, addressing such systemic issues is essential to advancing teleradiology practices and harnessing its full potential to provide timely medical care. The second significant challenge confronting teleradiology is the effective management of change in its deployment process in healthcare organizations. Most e-health initiatives do not take into account the interdependencies and complexities of healthcare processes, and hence, they cannot develop appropriate change management processes. This gap is particularly problematic in teleradiology, where radiologic evaluations need to be intuitively woven into the composite patient care processes. Through adopting a systems analysis model, as proposed by recent research, healthcare organizations can better equip themselves for such changes by mapping the patient care process and identifying critical points within the system. Such a method aids in improved understanding of how teleradiology services can re-engineer clinical practice without causing disruptions usually associated with new technology adoption (Jones et al., 2009). Quality assurance in teleradiology is also problematic, particularly in ensuring diagnostic accuracy and the integrity of transferred images. Alterations in clinical practice require healthcare practitioners to adhere to high image-quality and interpretation standards, and these standards may vary considerably across radiology practices. Ensuring conformity with standards by all stakeholders is important because differences can lead to misdiagnosis and poor-quality care. Furthermore, the heterogeneous technology environment complicates the task further because variations in equipment and transmission methods can lead to discrepancies. Overcoming these challenges demands ongoing training and education for technicians and radiologists, as well as the implementation of effective quality control processes that adapt to the evolving face of teleradiology (Clark et al., 2018).

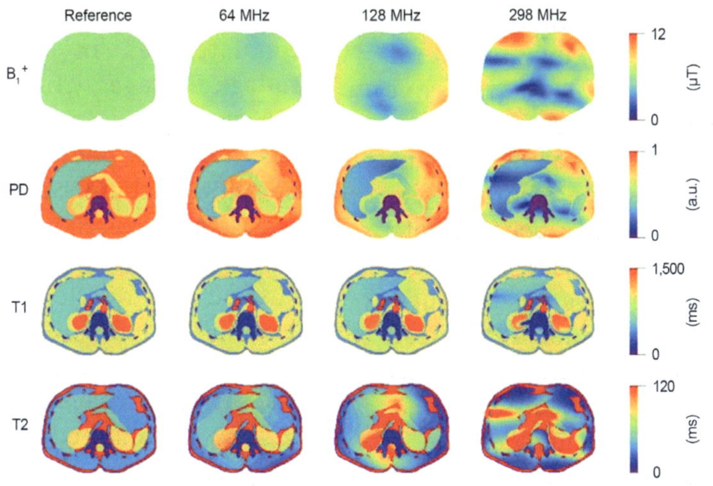

Figure 9.12. Multiparametric imaging with heterogeneous radiofrequency fields.

Source: https://media.springernature.com/m685/springer-static/image/art%3A10.1038%2Fncomms12445/MediaObjects/41467_2016_Article_BFncomms12445_Fig1_HTML.jpg.

9.5.1. Technical Issues and Limitations

In line with the expansion of teleradiology, several technical challenges and limitations can impede its effective implementation. Interoperability of systems is one of the significant challenges that leads to inefficiencies and miscommunication among healthcare providers. Various technological standards and protocols can pose hindrances in relation to sharing data among institutions or even within an organization. Without free flow of information, the possible advantages of teleradiology, such as prompt diagnosis and improved patient care, are subverted. Moreover, legal intricacies in image sharing complicate the development of integrated systems. As has been stressed in current research, such complexities are further amplified when planning for interoperability involves more than one party and environments that are differently governed, further weighing on healthcare professionals required to move between these complex environments (Pohjonen et al., 2011). The teleradiology infrastructure also must face bandwidth and data transfer rate limitations inherent to it. Strong internet connections are required for high-resolution images to allow timely transfer without compromising image quality for diagnostic images. Rural or underserved areas with slow internet connectivity often delay transmission of critical imaging results, potentially impacting patient outcomes. Moreover, reliance on technology is a fault, as system crashes, cyberattacks, or data leakage can disrupt workflows and negatively impact the quality of patient care. These sound measures for quality assurance should therefore include elaborate plans to prevent such risks through redundancy and highly secure schemes. The implementation of new technologies should not only aim to maximize capabilities but also anticipate potential disruptions and develop strategies to address such issues as they arise (Jones et al., 2009). Finally, addressing the human aspects of teleradiology is important for successfully overcoming technical issues. Remote working among radiologists, health care administrators, and IT professionals is critical to the success of teleradiology, with workflows appropriately synchronized. Delays in developing change management plans may lead to resistance among healthcare staff, who may be disappointed by the introduction of new processes and technologies. A systems analysis model can encourage a more integrated understanding of these interdependencies and establish the integration of teleradiology with current healthcare systems. By mapping the process of patient care, stakeholders can identify critical points in the system where additional support or training may be required, thereby designing an environment conducive to embracing technology without disrupting patient care (Jones et al., 2009).

9.5.2. Variability in Image Quality

In teleradiology, inconsistent image quality poses a serious threat, undermining diagnostic accuracy and patient outcomes. Inconsistency results from variations in image acquisition modalities, processing algorithms, and transmission modalities across various health care facilities. It has the potential to introduce inconsistencies in the interpretation of radiological images, which is crucial for ensuring accurate diagnosis and treatment planning. As highlighted by peer-reviewed publications, maintaining a standard level of image quality is essential, as research has repeatedly reaffirmed that improved imaging quality correlates with improved diagnostic concordance between teleradiology and conventional radiology practices (Bashshur et al., 2016). Modulating these variations becomes essential to get the workflow streamlined and foster a culture of quality assurance in teleradiology. Another source of complexity in maintaining image quality arises from interactions between technological advances and clinical work practices. While imaging technologies have advanced as much as they have in enhancing resolution and reducing noise, the successful integration of these technologies into existing workflows remains a problem. Protocol changes, for instance, the standardization of processes for reporting images, are generally met with skepticism because they disrupt workflows. Structured reporting, for instance, has been proposed as a means of increasing the organization and readability of radiological reports, but its adoption has been delayed by concerns about productivity and clinician workflow (Kong et al., 2009). While health organizations strive to improve service delivery, most significant importance must be given to extremely careful consideration of how emerging technology can be adapted into current processes without compromising image quality. Quality assurance activities play a role in curbing variability in image quality in teleradiology. Roll-out of comprehensive training programs for radiologists in image interpretation can enhance their ability to identify and make up for differences in quality. Periodic audit and feedback arrangements can further facilitate ongoing improvement and adherence to best practices in imaging. The data accumulated through these quality assurance processes can thus guide equipment maintenance policies, standard imaging protocol development, and better communication between radiologists and referring physicians. By establishing a systemic quality assurance process in teleradiology, health organizations effectively minimize risks related to variable image quality, ultimately leading to better diagnostic competence and patient care outcomes (Bashshur et al., 2016).

9.5.3. Legal and Ethical Considerations

The advent of teleradiology has raised a range of legal and ethical questions that require careful consideration, particularly regarding the security and privacy of patient information. Through remote transmission of radiological images and patient data, medical practitioners must negotiate a complicated maze of regulations designed to maintain patient confidentiality. The American Health Insurance Portability and Accountability Act (HIPAA) mandates robust safeguards for the protection of confidential health information and requires that teleradiology systems use encryption and secure transmission mechanisms. Violation thereof could lead not only to legal proceedings but also to loss of patient confidence, which could lead to disastrous repercussions to the provision of care. As teleradiology continues to integrate more deeply into the world's healthcare practices, it is crucial to understand and comply with these legal systems to protect patients and promote a culture of ethical responsibility within the profession. Furthermore, ethical principles go beyond legal requirements, addressing the issues of consent, equity, and access to care. In an ever-changing industry, informed consent poses special challenges in teleradiology, especially when images are sent across international boundaries. The patients must be adequately informed about what will be done with their information, to whom it will be disclosed, and about the potential consequences of disclosing their medical information, particularly in regions where regulatory requirements may vary significantly. Practitioners must also address ethical concerns about equal access as teleradiology services reach underserved communities. Provision of such technological advancements to marginalized communities so that they may be provided with a just share ensures concerted efforts to address differences in healthcare delivery systems and infrastructure, enabling an inclusive practice of teleradiology. The dynamic nature of technology also means that debates about the ethical implications of artificial intelligence and machine learning continually arise in the practice of teleradiology. With advanced AI capabilities augmenting diagnostic processes, strong concerns are raised about accountability and the role of human observation in clinical decision-making. Radiologists must weigh the convenience and speed afforded by automated processes against the ethical obligation to deliver appropriate and compassionate care. AI-guided decisions should supplement, not supplant, licensed practitioners' experience, underscoring the importance of maintaining a patient-focused approach amid advancing technology. These are most vital in ensuring teleradiology not just enhances workflow and quality control but also upholds the highest ethical standards of medical practice, reaffirming patient care in an increasingly digitalizing health care setting (Chatterjee et al., 2008; Reponen et al., 2010).

9.6. Future Trends in Teleradiology

With the changing landscape of healthcare, technology innovations are likely to redefine the future of teleradiology profoundly. One of the primary trends is the implementation of AI and machine learning algorithms that have the potential to enhance image evaluation and diagnostic quality. By processing vast amounts of data, these technologies can identify patterns and anomalies that human radiologists may not detect. These technologies not only accelerate workflows but also improve quality control in diagnostic imaging. The introduction of AI-driven platforms that automatically notify radiologists of high-risk findings allows the prioritization of such cases, enabling timely intervention and improved patient outcomes. With AI-enhanced instruments, their incorporation into teleradiology procedures is bound to introduce greater efficiency and reliability in diagnostic workflows, aligning with the evolving demands of healthcare providers and patients alike (Archer et al., 2014). Moreover, cloud technology and mobile applications are transforming how radiologists obtain and read imaging tests. As reliance on mobile technology increases, medical professionals can now perform remote consultations, enabling on-time discussion of patient cases regardless of physical distance. Apart from encouraging coordination among specialists, this mobile link also enables continuity of care, particularly during emergencies. This is combined with the development of zero-footprint image viewers that can be used in web browsers without excessive software installation, making them easy to integrate with current workflows. These advancements align with a broader trend towards flexibility and adaptability in healthcare technology, in line with the very principles of teleradiology that emphasize improved workflow and quality control (Reponen et al., 2010). Last but not least, the future of teleradiology will be shaped by a greater focus on regulatory affairs and data protection as telehealth services expand. As patient information is increasingly digitized and shifted across platforms, protecting the confidentiality and integrity of sensitive information is crucial. New regulatory frameworks can require strong data transmission and storage standards, affecting the design and implementation of teleradiology services. Additionally, sustaining strict quality assurance controls will not only be crucial for such regulations but also vital to establishing confidence among patients and healthcare providers. Lastly, these emerging trends point towards the imperative to balance innovation with responsible governance in teleradiology, the future of enhanced patient care and outcome assurance in the healthcare system (Archer et al., 2014).

9.6.1. Integration of Artificial Intelligence

The use of AI in teleradiology is a paradigm change in the precision and speed of radiology workflows. As computing power and data processing develop exponentially, AI algorithms are becoming increasingly skilled at assisting radiologists in interpreting challenging imaging studies. It not only enhances diagnostic precision but also speeds up workflow so that radiologists can process an increased number of cases without any dip in quality. The COVID-19 pandemic further emphasized the need to incorporate teleradiology services, making AI an essential component that enables quick and precise diagnosis in remote areas. Through optimized workflows and resource utilization, the incorporation of AI appears as a critical driver for enhanced patient outcomes and maintaining continuity of care, furthering the continued transformation of radiology as a field inextricably linked to technology (Agrawal, 2023). Moreover, the contribution of AI to teleradiology is more than mere efficiency; it encompasses broader areas, including improving quality assurance and standardizing care. Through machine learning algorithms, healthcare systems can analyze vast amounts of imaging data to identify patterns and abnormalities that are not readily apparent to the naked eye. These innovations have the potential to enhance diagnostic quality by minimizing human error and providing real-time feedback to radiologists. In addition, AI-driven tools can standardize report preparation processes so that diagnostic assessments adhere to set guidelines and frameworks. This structured approach not only boosts confidence in radiological conclusions but also supports a culture conducive to team practice. The ongoing evolution of regulatory and ethical standards for AI integration will be instrumental in addressing future challenges, ensuring that these technologies are aligned with patient safety and quality-of-care standards (N/A, 2022). Finally, the journey to establish a fully integrated AI architecture in teleradiology is not without challenges. While the final benefit is excellent, challenges such as data privacy, integration costs, and investment in long-term radiologist training are likely to delay. The dependency on sophisticated algorithms demands in-depth expertise in AI technologies with a commitment to continuous learning and fine-tuning. Moreover, the different perspectives within the radiology community on the use of AI underscore the need for communication and collaboration among professionals. As the combined experience of biomedicine, technology, and bioethics comes together, it is evident that the adoption of AI in teleradiology needs to be carefully managed. By overcoming these hurdles, healthcare facilities can leverage the full potential of AI, ensuring its effective integration into the workflow and maintaining high standards of quality assurance (N/A, 2022; Agrawal, 2023).

9.6.2. Expansion of Telehealth Services

Telehealth services have emerged as a crucial characteristic of modern health care delivery, particularly within teleradiology. With healthcare facilities facing increased patient volumes and fiscal constraints, telehealth is seen as an effective means to improve access to quality care. For instance, video-based technologies that are part of daily life can be effectively applied in clinical settings to facilitate virtual consultations and remote diagnosis. The integration of telehealth into existing infrastructure allows healthcare providers to expand their coverage to underserved populations, particularly in remote areas where specialists are difficult to reach. The interface of technology and healthcare delivery not only enhances operational effectiveness but also ensures a more robust patient experience, thus illustrating how telehealth enhances overall healthcare objectives (Arnault et al., 2017). In addition, the central role of ICT in the expansion of telehealth cannot be overstated. Unequal access to care is a common global phenomenon due to numerous systemic barriers, including cost and workforce shortages. However, as underscored by the existing literature, the application of ICT in healthcare systems can help bridge gaps. For instance, health facilities that adopt ICT devices have demonstrated increased efficiency in service delivery and increased the accessibility of patients, an argument reflected by the findings indicating a high linkage rate of ICT adoption to better healthcare outcomes. Therefore, when the teleradiology sector adopts these technologies, health care providers should prioritize end-user training and assistance to maximize benefits (Gabonewe et al., 2017). Lastly, the expansion of telehealth services, such as teleradiology, is a healthcare provision revolution that boosts traditional methods with technology utilization. As telehealth continues to evolve, more and more healthcare units will need to integrate these services into existing activities wisely. Moreover, as health policymakers underscore the value of remote access to care, professional education, and successful ICT implementation, these will be critical to realizing the potential of telehealth. By fostering a culture of technological uptake and expertise, health care practitioners can ensure improved quality, effectiveness, and accuracy in the provision of services, which ultimately results in improved patient outcomes in a dynamic health care system (Arnault et al., 2017; Gabonewe et al., 2017).

9.6.3. Potential for Global Collaboration

The teleradiology environment provides immense scope for worldwide collaboration among medical professionals to share information and resources across national borders. Advances in communications technology have enabled radiologists to transmit reports and images within moments, transcending geographical limitations that had restricted access to expert treatment. Collaboration is extremely vital, especially in regions with a shortage of radiology specialists. With teleradiology, low-resource facilities can access specialist opinions from centers of excellence worldwide, instilling a culture of collective knowledge and collaborative problem-solving. Furthermore, the sharing of best practices and standard guidelines can enhance diagnostic accuracy and overall patient care and illustrate how collaboration not only improves individual cases but also makes broader, systemic improvements possible in the delivery of healthcare. Incorporating teleradiology into global healthcare raises significant workflow and quality-assurance issues that are critical to maintaining high standards of patient care. Practical communication standards, such as DICOM and Health Level 7 (HL7), are central to ensuring secure transmission of confidential patient data. These standards promote a synergistic environment in which radiologists can collaborate within a single system, thus providing the CIA triad of confidentiality, integrity, and availability of patient information (Clark et al., 2018). With secure processes in teleradiology, healthcare providers can utilize international collaborations, thus enabling accelerated diagnoses and timely treatments. When radiology centers adopt such new-generation technologies, they can ensure consistency in quality assurance processes, thereby promoting a patient-safety- and effective-communication-focused culture within collaborative networks. In addition, the potential for global cooperation in teleradiology extends beyond practice to research and innovation, accelerating developments in medical imaging and diagnostic techniques. Pooling of expertise and resources from different regions of the globe enables it to perform large-scale studies that will eventually lead to the development of improved imaging technologies and techniques. Based on the available literature, the feasibility of teleradiology has been sufficiently established, with studies revealing equivalent performance between teleradiology and conventional radiology (Bashshur et al., 2016). This empirical foundation is the starting point for collaborative research studies, enabling institutions to share findings and contribute to the ongoing evolution of radiological practice. Collaboration among clinicians and researchers enables them to tackle key global health problems, opening the door for new solutions that will positively impact patients worldwide. Such synergies not only enhance clinical outcomes but also advance the understanding of teleradiology's role in today's healthcare, further cementing teleradiology as a vital part of the global healthcare landscape.

SUMMARY

Looking at the workflow in teleradiology, several pertinent points can be observed that define its contribution to today's healthcare. Teleradiology optimizes for the possibility of remote diagnosis, and radiologists are able to interpret images from any geographical location remotely, which is particularly significant for rural or underserved regions. Pre-implementation planning takes center stage, as working with an adapted Patient Care Pathway provides an organized way of creating and implementing teleradiology projects. This framework not only explains the patient pathway but also incorporates the necessary information flow to provide continuity of care. By analyzing these pathways, health professionals can identify critical points that warrant additional emphasis, thereby enhancing overall service delivery and clinical outcomes in radiology settings. Planning in this holistic context lays the foundation for the successful deployment of teleradiology systems (Jones et al., 2009). Moreover, the integration of specialist protocols into teleradiology is pivotal to workflow efficiency and quality assurance. Protocols such as DICOM and Health Level 7 (HL7) are important to guarantee safe and smooth transmission of medical images as well as patient information. The protocols ensure interoperability among different healthcare systems to support minimal data compromise or loss. As reaffirmed, achieving the CIA triad—availability, integrity, and confidentiality—is crucial for safeguarding sensitive patient information, particularly given the potential risks involved in integrating heterogeneous healthcare radiology information systems. An understanding of these protocols and how they operate is necessary for radiology departments to ensure maximum utilization of teleradiology benefits while maintaining the highest standards of care (Clark et al., 2018). Finally, quality assurance measures are key to the successful application of teleradiology services. The establishment of standardized protocols during the process of integration can significantly constrain the variability of image quality and interpretation. Regular audits and feedback systems help remove deviations from established standards in a timely manner, thereby fostering a culture of ongoing improvement. Besides, training and support for health practitioners involved in teleradiology are critical to maintaining high-quality interpretation in the long term. By implementing effective quality assurance mechanisms, healthcare organizations can better manage potential risks and enhance patient trust in remote diagnostic services. Ultimately, emphasis on quality assurance benefits not only the organizations but also directly impacts patient outcomes and levels of satisfaction, thereby improving the role of teleradiology in modern healthcare delivery (Jones et al., 2009).

CLOSER LOOK

IMPORTANCE OF ONGOING QUALITY ASSURANCE

The need for continuous QA of teleradiology cannot be overemphasized, especially given the complexities of digital workflows in remote diagnostic settings. As healthcare increasingly relies on digital technologies for diagnostics and medical images, it becomes imperative to introduce a stringent quality assurance process to ensure the validity of results. The use of technology such as Picture Archiving and Communication Systems (PACS) and standards such as DICOM and HL7 is a case in point of how technology can assist in driving the overall quality of care provided. These are advanced technologies that rely heavily on accurate data transfer and storage; therefore, quality assurance is central to avoiding diagnostic errors that can have critical consequences for patient outcomes (Hristova et al., 2020). Regular audits and reviews not only help in the identification of discrepancies in the workflow but also help in creating guidelines to ensure quality medical imaging. Continuous quality assurance also helps in enhancing the efficiency of the teleradiology workflow. Through regular training and support for healthcare providers using such technological platforms, centers can ensure that personnel can effectively manage the complexity of digital imaging. Research has proven that the application of quality assurance practices can have the impact of enhancing efficiency in healthcare delivery, particularly in teleradiology departments whose turnaround time is typically of most significant concern (Gabonewe et al., 2017). As a case in point, when organizations embrace simplified guidelines for image acquisition and interpretation, variation in results can be minimized to enhance the speed and accuracy of diagnosis. This practice not only fosters a culture of continuous improvement but also helps address challenges arising from an evolving healthcare environment driven by increased technology dependence. Further, continuous quality assurance serves as a primary regulatory compliance mechanism and a mechanism for enhancing patients' and stakeholders' trust in healthcare. Because teleradiology involves complex interdependencies between various healthcare providers, any decline in quality compromises the integrity of the service. Regular quality assurance mechanisms ensure that care delivery adheres to prescribed standards, which are vital for accreditation and for pleasing regulatory bodies and patients. With such a thin margin for error in an industry, systems monitoring can help minimize risk associated with misinterpretation or technology failure. Therefore, incorporating quality assurance into the very roots of teleradiology practice not only enhances diagnostic accuracy but also fosters an open culture that ensures patient safety and high-quality care across all levels of the healthcare system (Hristova et al., 2020).

REFERENCES

1. Agrawal, A. (2023). Digital transformation of career landscapes in radiology: personal and professional implications. *Frontiers in Radiology, 3*, 1180699. https://doi.org/10.3389/fradi.2023.1180699Archer, N. P., McClung, A., McKibbon, A., & McMaster eBusiness Research Centre (MeRC). (2014). Novel eHealth trends in the field of radiology: A scoping review. https://core.ac.uk/download/639169329.pdf (accessed on 5th August 2025).
2. Arnault, S., Bartels, S. J., Blount, A., Cameron, D., et al. (2017). Telehealth and mobile health applied to integrated behavioral care: Opportunities for progress in New Hampshire. https://core.ac.uk/download/215540990.pdf (accessed on 5th August 2025).
3. Bashshur, N., Bashshur, R. L., Krupinski, E. A., Thrall, J. H., et al. (2016). The empirical foundations of teleradiology and related applications: A review of the evidence. http://deepblue.lib.umich.edu/bitstream/2027.42/140295/1/tmj.2016.0149.pdf (accessed on 5th August 2025).
4. Chatterjee, S., Murthy, S., Obal, L., Tulu, B., et al. (2008). Stakeholder analysis framework for IT-enabled healthcare outsourcing: Critical success factors. https://core.ac.uk/download/301347796.pdf (accessed on 5th August 2025).
5. Clark, S. A. (2018). Secure integration of information systems in radiology. https://core.ac.uk/download/217361887.pdf (accessed on 5th August 2025).
6. Gabonewe, K. S. (2017). The impact of information and communication technology (ICT) on the efficiency of healthcare delivery at Radiology Department of Inkosi Albert Luthuli Hospital. https://core.ac.uk/download/288926087.pdf (accessed on 5th August 2025).
7. Hristova, T. (2020). Data infrastructures and digital labor: The case of teleradiology. https://core.ac.uk/download/426937685.pdf (accessed on 5th August 2025).
8. Jones, K. (2009). The remodelling of patient care pathway for e-health. https://core.ac.uk/download/336465.pdf (accessed on 5th August 2025).
9. Kong, A., Plumb, A. A., Reiner, B. I., Sundaram, B., Mozumdar, B. C., Reiner, B. I., et al. (2009). The challenges, opportunities, and imperative of structured reporting in medical imaging. https://core.ac.uk/download/pdf/8352572.pdf (accessed on 5th August 2025).
10. N/A. (2022). The artificial intelligence in digital pathology and digital radiology: Where are we? https://core.ac.uk/download/534899615.pdf (accessed on 5th August 2025).
11. Pohjonen, H., & Ross, P. (2011). Images crossing borders: Image and workflow sharing on multiple levels. https://core.ac.uk/download/pdf/8670905.pdf (accessed on 5th August 2025).
12. Reponen, J. (2010). Teleradiology—Changing radiological service processes from local to regional, international and mobile environment. https://core.ac.uk/download/628862722.pdf (accessed on 5th August 2025).

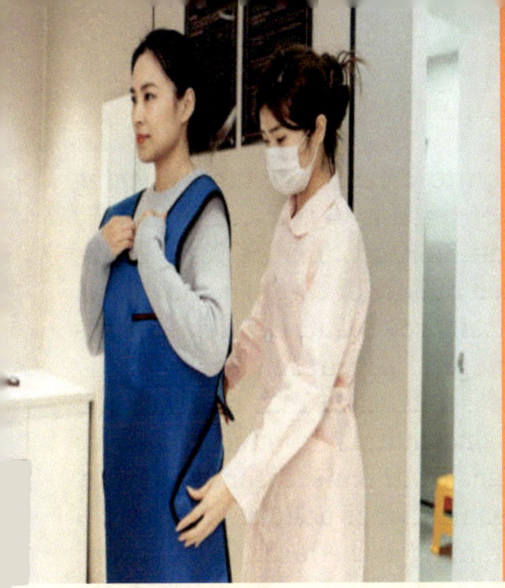

Chapter 10

RADIATION PROTECTION REGULATIONS AND ACCREDITATION IN MEDICAL IMAGING

Contents

Introduction

Radiation protection is a significant consideration in the medical imaging world, an industry that relies more and more on state-of-the-art technologies to detect and treat all forms of medical conditions. As radiation use in interventions for diagnosis and therapy continues to expand, there is an expanding necessity to balance the benefits of these medical technologies with the imperative to ensure that these technologies do not injure patients and medical practitioners. This challenge demands the institution of strict regulations and standards governing the safe use of radiation within a clinical setting. Most important are the functions of regulatory bodies, professional associations, and accrediting organizations, which develop guidelines intended to safeguard health while maintaining the effectiveness of imaging modalities. There is an orchestrated collaboration that follows from this synergistic effort, necessitating the maintenance of high standards of medical practice involving radiation. Accreditation is a formal recognition of an institution's commitment to assuring compliance with established safety standards and best practices for radiation usage. In addition to bringing medical imaging facilities into compliance with mandated regulations, accreditation instills a perpetual striving for excellence in practice. In the case of medical imaging, accreditation compliance to rigorous requirements can result in improved patient outcomes and enhanced quality of care. The American Association of Physicists in Medicine (AAPM), for instance, periodically revises its Medical Physics Practice Guidelines to incorporate the latest practices and technological advancements following a thorough consensus process (Seibert et al., 2018). The guidelines recognize that the safe and effective provision of diagnostic and therapeutic radiation depends on a suitably trained workforce with advanced skills and techniques to protect patients and clinicians from unnecessary exposure. Further, the integration of radiation protection guidelines into organizational policies enhances a safety and vigilance culture in healthcare organizations. Ongoing training and education programs are important in ensuring the employees are well informed about the existing safety procedures and regulatory requirements. Likewise, teamwork among healthcare workers is core to a proper understanding of radiation hazards and to developing strategies to mitigate them. Moreover, community action cannot be overlooked in the context of radiation safety, as it makes the patient an active participant in healthcare decisions. By fostering a co-responsibility culture for radiation safety, the medical imaging community can not only advance clinical practice but also uphold its ethical responsibility to promote patient wellness (Barr et al., 2016).

10.1. Current Radiation Protection Regulations

The success of radiation protection regulations in medical imaging is imperative to safeguard both patients and medical professionals from the potential hazards of ionizing radiation. In the United States, regulatory procedures, for instance, those of the American Association of Physicists in Medicine (AAPM), require medical physicists to follow strict guidelines and implement safe imaging protocols. Such guidelines not only emphasize the quality of specialized training and expertise among professionals but also encourage systematic patient care through the implementation of quality standards. Adhering to reviewing and revising such guidelines enables developments aligned with evolving medical technologies, allowing health institutions to improve the quality of service while remaining compliant with regulatory requirements. Compliance with these guidelines constitutes an important component of avoiding risks of exposure to radiation and patient safety as well as the proper use of imaging (Seibert et al., 2018) (Figure 10.1).

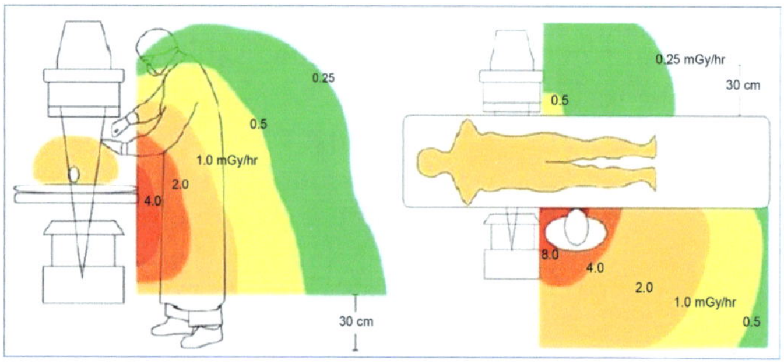

Figure 10.1. Radiation protection.

Source: https://radiologykey.com/wp-content/uploads/2023/04/C21-FF4.gif.

The creation of quality standards most often requires interdisciplinary collaboration among stakeholders within the medical imaging community. Radiotherapy, for instance, has also seen an enhancement in its interdisciplinary approach, as it entails complex planning and monitoring at every level of treatment delivery. Guided by legislative law and professional practice, as defined by groups such as the AAPM and other global organizations, quality assurance practice intersects with various areas, including organizational, clinical, and technical matters. The impact of the standards is only as long-lasting as the continued focus on their review and enhancement. Institutions are encouraged to scrutinize their practices regularly, thereby promoting a culture of responsibility and quality in the profession. As regulations are continually updated to align with existing scientific knowledge, the need for strict adherence becomes more pressing to improve patient care outcomes (Bogusz-Czerniewicz et al., 2012). Beyond their direct impact on patient protection, the existing radiation protection directives also help improve public confidence in medical imaging procedures. Certainty in adherence to guidelines set gives patients and medical practitioners alike the confidence that they are cared for according to the highest standards. Accreditation procedures often demand facilities to demonstrate compliance with radiation safety practices, thus further cementing their credibility and image in the medical profession. Moreover, regular education and training programs are essential for staying abreast of the latest regulations and laws, ensuring that all personnel working in imaging departments have up-to-date information and skills. As medical imaging's face evolves with advancing technology and in response to changing regulations, commitment to prudent radiation protection continues as an ethical base of good medical practice, ensuring quality outcomes for all concerned in the imaging process (Seibert et al., 2018).

10.1.1. Overview of National Regulations (e.g., NRC, FDA)

The regulation of radiation protection in medical imaging is characterized by a framework comprising a series of important national agencies, each performing a particular function in public health protection. The Nuclear Regulatory Commission (NRC) primarily oversees the use of radioactive materials, with the aim of ensuring that their use in diagnostic imaging is consistent with safety standards. NRC regulations govern the licensing, operation, and decommissioning of facilities that use radioactive materials. It is this lack of oversight that is considered necessary, particularly to ensure that procedures under nuclear medicine and radiologic technologies do not have the unintended consequence of increasing the radiation burden on patients and healthcare workers. The NRC also works in close collaboration with state governments and other government agencies, thereby maintaining a multi-level mechanism for regulating and enforcing compliance in the medical imaging sector, and building a robust regulatory framework to minimize the inherent risks of radiation use. In addition to the NRC, the Food and Drug Administration (FDA) is crucial for enforcing regulations on medical equipment such as X-ray machines and MRI systems (Figure 10.2). The task of the FDA is the evaluation of the safety and efficacy of imaging equipment for preventing misuse or improper complications due to incorrect use. The company also establishes performance standards that ensure products possess the required safety features before they are released into the market. Above all else, the FDA's regulation is not just confined to pre-market inspection. Still, it extends to labeling and post-market surveillance, which safeguard patients and operators from the negative consequences of radiation exposure. The other role played by the FDA in imaging center accreditation also helps maintain stringent quality assurance practices and, therefore, enhances the safety of medical imaging practice in the clinical setting overall. Coordination of national regulations, such as those of the NRC and FDA, forms a general system to ensure the intricacies of radiation protection in medical imaging. In addition to applying direct safety attributes, they facilitate educational programs under which best practices and current risks of radiation exposure are learned by medical experts. For instance, both agencies aid in the release of guidelines that specify proper patient evaluation and monitoring, which is most crucial in determining cases of overexposure, particularly among vulnerable populations, such as children, who are most likely to display heightened sensitivity to radiation effect (as observed from the past regarding I-131 exposure) (Agency US for Substances T and Registry D. Division of Toxicology and Medicine E.). Not only do efforts of this nature enhance the efficacy of regulatory actions, but they also serve as preventive measures against potential long-term health implications, thereby ensuring that patient safety is never compromised in the delivery of medical imaging services (Davies et al., 2025).

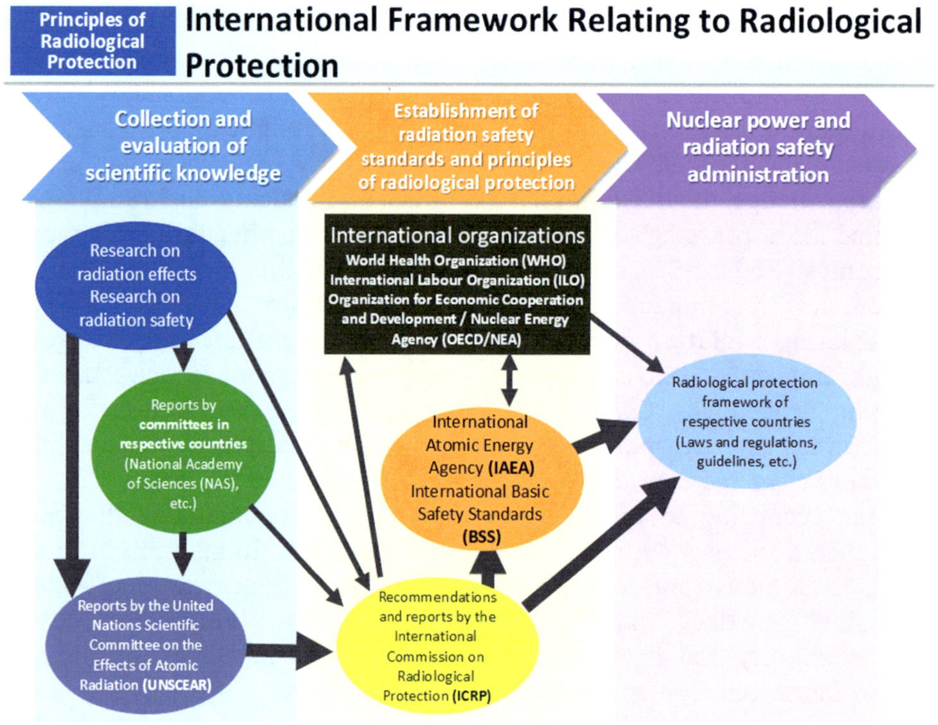

Figure 10.2. International framework relating to radiological protection (MOE).

Source: https://www.env.go.jp/en/chemi/rhm/basic-info/1st/img/img-04-01-01.png.

10.1.2. International Guidelines (e.g., ICRP, WHO)

International guidelines from organizations such as the International Commission on Radiological Protection (ICRP) and the World Health Organization (WHO) dictate radiation protection legislation in medical imaging (Figure 10.3). These guidelines are intended to provide a benchmark for the restriction of exposure of patients and members of staff to radiation, so that the benefits of medical imaging are more than the harm caused. The ICRP, for instance, puts particular stress on the principle of justification such that any radiological examination is justified in terms of its benefit in relation to the risk. These guideline recommendations are not only meant to protect individuals from unwarranted exposure but also to inspire medical practitioners to carefully consider the necessity of imaging examinations. Implementation of the above practices is essential in developing a culture of safety in the healthcare system as outlined in the best practice promotion papers for radiation protection. Furthermore, the application of the guidelines is essential in securing accreditation for medical imaging facilities. The accrediting agencies occasionally require compliance with their standards to qualify health care institutions to offer imaging services that are safe and effective. For example, guidelines from the ICRP and WHO set crucial standards for educating healthcare professionals, including continuing education on radiation protection. This includes an understanding of radiological risk and optimal techniques for optimizing image quality while limiting exposure. Such institutions adopting these international standards reflect a commitment to patient care and professional excellence. Hence, effective governance and adherence to such guidelines are key to formulating a sustainable accreditation model that not only enhances operating efficiency but also enhances public trust in medical imaging practice. In addition, the importance of stakeholder engagement is underscored in the international guideline environment. A thorough examination of training in radiation protection indicates the need for a unified effort across healthcare workers, including collaboration among European societies to establish training needs and develop best practices (Alves et al., 2022). By addressing the strengths and weaknesses of current educational systems, stakeholders can work together to effectively integrate the principles of radiation protection into daily medical practice. The absence of adequate training and sensitization is a significant hindrance to the efficient enforcement of radiation protection rules, and it demands national and international levels of amendment. The inclusion of multiple professional groups ensures that radiation safety information flows increasingly, ultimately providing quality care offered under medical imaging as well as fostering an environment of collective responsibility to safeguard patients.

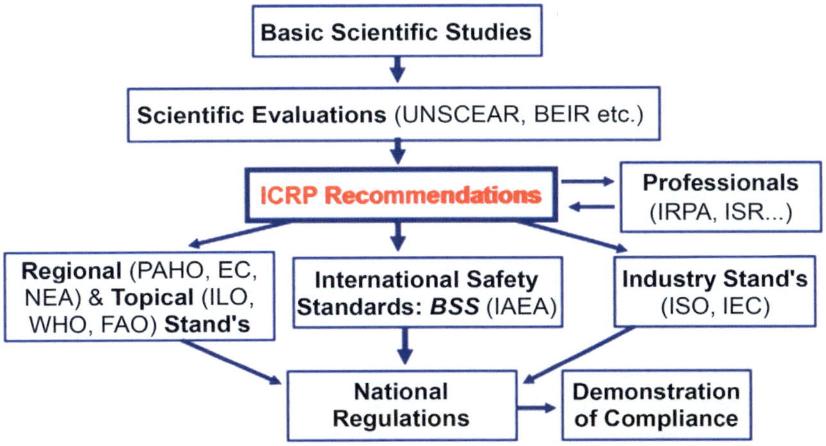

Figure 10.3. The basis for and use of ICRP recommendations on radiological protection policy (Clarke and Valentin, 2009, p. 102).

Source: https://www.researchgate.net/profile/Mariano-David/publication/332473865/figure/fig1/AS:748889229508608@1555560514086/The-basis-for-and-use-of-ICRP-recommendations-on-radiological-protection-policy-Clarke.png.

10.1.3. Role of State Regulations in Medical Imaging

State legislation plays a pivotal role in the medical imaging sector, serving as the basis for regulations that determine the use and safety of radiation. Laws guarantee that medical units adhere to norms of practice to protect patients and doctors from potential harm arising from exposure to radiation. Through the development of specific guidelines and protocols, state law instills a culture of safety and accountability in medical imaging practice. Regulatory bodies, with the help of agencies such as the American Association of Physicists in Medicine (AAPM), work tirelessly to develop and revise medical physics practice guidelines. These guidelines are the standards of quality necessary for successful practice in the profession and give topmost consideration to patient welfare, thereby enhancing the quality of medical imaging services offered in any healthcare facility (Seibert et al., 2018). Beyond compliance, the importance of state regulations extends to making medical imaging facilities eligible for accreditation. Accreditation plays the central role of ensuring that patients, as well as the service providers, know that the diagnostic imaging services provided are of quality. In this regard, state laws help make it easier to meet accreditation standards by simplifying regulatory requirements, while ensuring facilities maintain desired performance standards by conducting regular audits, inspections, and evaluations that encourage conformity with best practices and improvements in the provision of imaging services. The general agreement among stakeholders tends to emphasize the imperative of comprehensive radioprotection training, a point underscored by a recent review that delineates strengths and weaknesses in education and training among medical professionals (Alves et al., 2022). Under such conditions, state regulation becomes critical to promoting professionalism and a culture of safety in the medical imaging industry. Finally, as state laws evolve, they must keep up with the rapidly changing world of medical technology and the increasing complexity of imaging modalities. The melding of sophisticated imaging modalities necessitates regulations that keep pace with evolving technology and altering best practices. For instance, the move towards sophisticated imaging modalities such as MRI and CT scans poses new challenges for radiation safety and patient care. It is important that state legislation be re-evaluated and brought up to date to reflect these developments. The regulatory agencies take the opinions of medical professionals and industry experts to ensure that regulations are viable and implementable, which is critical for developing a robust framework capable of fostering innovative practices without undermining safety standards. Ultimately, state regulations must strike a balance between protecting public health and advancing developments in medical imaging technology.

10.2. Accreditation Bodies in Medical Imaging

The role of accreditation bodies in medical imaging is paramount in ensuring that there is compliance with radiation protection regulations and imaging service quality. The bodies are involved in a multi-role that includes practice guideline development, compliance monitoring, and application of quality assurance. For instance, the AAPM makes a notable contribution by sometimes implementing practice guidelines that advance medical physics and benefit patient care. By ensuring that specific training and capabilities are required for those working with diagnostic and therapeutic radiation, agencies such as the AAPM move toward a unified measure of expertise in the discipline (Figure 10.4).

Figure 10.4. American Association of physicists in medicine.

Source: https://history.aip.org/phn/Photos/aapm_logo.jpg.

The use of these guidelines enhances public trust and overall security of medical imaging practice with the long-term goal of lowering patient radiation exposure while maximizing diagnostic efficacy. Furthermore, the coordinated efforts of various accredited bodies underscore the significance of harmonization in education and training on radiation protection. The recent survey conducted across professional organizations in Europe shows widespread consensus on the need for a harmonized training strategy in radiation protection. The research established four themes, including the creation of models for training needs assessment and the importance of funding support to enable effective,adequate governance arrangements. These collaborations not only raise the educational levels of healthcare professionals but also refer to the collaborative effort that goes into implementing better radiation safety protocols. By providing professionals with appropriate training and equipment, accreditation bodies play an important role by offering a single set of standards that prioritize radiation protection across different medical imaging modalities. Lastly, the inclusion of accrediting processes within the healthcare system supports enhanced total quality and safety in medical imaging. Recognizing accrediting bodies encourages a culture of continuous improvement and accountability, compelling facilities to continually evaluate their practices. The emphasis on guideline compliance, such as those developed by the AAPM, provides a means to achieve successful radiation protection. Moreover, as there are still problems with awareness and prioritization of radiation protection at both national and international levels, the function of accreditation becomes increasingly important. These organizations not only ensure improved practice standards, as seen through the collaborative efforts and infrastructural investments under programs such as the European Radiation Protection education framework, but also promote change to improve safety and efficacy in medical imaging practices (Seibert et al., 2018; Alves et al., 2022).

10.2.1. Overview of Major Accreditation Organizations (e.g., ACR, JCAHO)

The American College of Radiology (ACR) is pivotal in medical imaging accreditation, particularly in establishing standards to guarantee the safety and efficacy of imaging practice. As a reputable professional association, ACR seeks to raise the quality of radiology services by promoting stringent guidelines that practitioners must follow. Its accreditation programs, in MRI and other imaging modalities, address not only technical standards but also ethical standards regarding patient care and safety. By promoting the appropriate use of imaging technologies, ACR promotes radiation protection protocols, thereby contributing to the overall well-being of patients. Furthermore, the organization's commitment to continued education keeps medical professionals abreast of the latest innovations and safety procedures regarding radiation protection, solidifying its position as a pioneer in maximizing medical imaging practice. Except the ACR, the Joint Commission on Accreditation of Healthcare

Organizations (JCAHO) is also a large accrediting organization for healthcare organizations, including those involved in medical imaging (Figure 10.5).

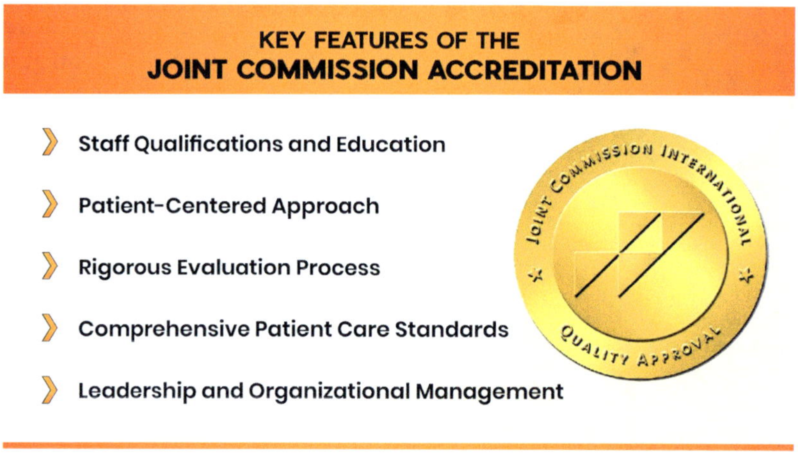

Figure 10.5. Key features of JCAHO.

Source: https://www.strategiquepartners.com/wp-content/uploads/2024/07/SP-25.jpg.

JCAHO's guidelines aim to ensure that health care organizations provide safe, effective, and high-quality care to patients. The organization's holistic initiative covers most aspects of health care provision, including safety standards that must be implemented in imaging departments. JCAHO accreditation is applied as a measure of quality that indicates an organization's compliance with national standards, which subsequently results in better patient safety practices. Furthermore, JCAHO's focus on implementing risk management techniques fosters an improvement culture within medical imaging facilities, making it an essential partner in promoting radiation safety and delivering the best patient care. Accreditation by organizations such as ACR and JCAHO not only provides a template for safety and quality but also has more widespread implications for public health. With increased awareness in medicine of potential imaging-related risks, particularly in modalities like MRI, accreditation is an important factor in mitigating such risks through sound safety practices. For instance, mounting evidence indicates that healthcare providers without an MRI connection also require additional training in MRI safety guidelines to prevent risks arising from strong magnetic fields and other hazards. This demand emphasizes the importance of accreditation programs, which can encourage improved training and education for all medical imaging personnel. By providing employees with sufficient education and training in safety protocols, accredited institutions ensure that a culture exists in which patient protection is prioritized, as evidenced by research indicating healthcare providers' knowledge and satisfaction levels when handling MRI (Downie et al., 2007; Houser et al., 2019).

10.2.2. Accreditation Process and Requirements

Medical imaging accreditation is an essential process for ensuring high standards of radiation safety and effectiveness. Accreditation involves a thorough evaluation against set standards and guidelines developed by such notable bodies. The institutions need to submit comprehensive documentation demonstrating compliance with regulatory requirements, including safety protocols, staff training, and quality assurance procedures. For example, the American Association of Physicists in Medicine (AAPM) emphasizes the importance of ongoing education and practice guidelines that require special training in medical physics, making adherence to these guidelines essential for accreditation. Therefore, successful accreditation not only enhances the institution's reputation but also ensures uninterrupted quality in patient care, thereby safeguarding public health in medical imaging. Accreditation requirements can vary widely by accrediting agency, but they typically share fundamental commonalities. In the normal course of events, medical imaging facilities must undergo rigorous inspections that assess technical and operational standards. Establishing standards of quality is very important, as studies highlight the necessity of classifying standards in terms of organizational, physical, and clinical dimensions, which are essential to guaranteeing high service quality in imaging practice. The data submitted in the course of accreditation assessment is reviewed to ensure that the appropriate procedures are used for protection against radiation, like compliance with national and international standards, like those of the International Atomic Energy Agency (IAEA). Having high-quality accreditation requirements helps uphold a culture of responsibility and safety in the medical imaging industry. Furthermore, continuous accreditation is equally vital as initial accreditation. Institutions must undergo continuous cycles of quality improvement, including regular audits, performance assessments, and updates to procedural documents to keep pace with regulatory changes. Accreditation agencies can require re-assessment at regular intervals and adherence to current practice guidelines to keep the facilities up to date with technological advancements and safety protocols. Quality assurance procedures, as prescribed by the AAPM and complemented by international standards such as ISO 9001:2008, are necessary to ensure compliance monitoring and to implement improvements where required. The process of accreditation is thus no mere checklist, but a dynamic process that compels institutions to continually uphold radiation safety and imaging service quality and ultimately enhance patient care in the healthcare system.

10.2.3. Importance of Accreditation for Healthcare Facilities

Accreditation plays a vital role in enhancing the quality and safety of medical facilities, particularly in medical imaging (Figure 10.6). By maintaining compliance with established standards issued by accrediting agencies, medical facilities demonstrate their commitment to providing operational excellence and patient safety. Because the medical imaging profession often involves complex procedures involving radiation, the need for accreditation is compounded. The accredited facilities must systematically examine their processes to reduce risks to patients and employees from radiation exposure. Moreover, accrediting agencies will typically check for compliance with standards governing the use of radiation in a way that best practices are applied uniformly. These protections not only improve patient care but also build confidence in the general healthcare system, as part of a broader drive to prioritize safety and enhance service quality (Belcher and Watson). Accreditation not only improves safety standards but also confers significant advantages to healthcare organizations in terms of operating efficiency. Accreditation organizations typically undergo a thorough review that identifies areas for improvement, thereby encouraging practices that boost clinical outcomes. This ongoing process of quality improvement affects how facilities manage resources, address waste production, and adopt sustainable measures, particularly regarding medical waste and radiation emissions. The drive to attain and sustain accreditation prompts healthcare facilities to adopt cutting-edge technologies and protocols that minimize radiation-related risks. Additionally, with developments in healthcare regulations, accredited organizations are better positioned to respond to changes, thereby preparing them to address new compliance challenges. Therefore, accreditation is not only a regulatory instrument but also a driver of change in medical imaging practices (Moore et al., 2020). The impacts of accreditation go beyond the immediate benefits to health facilities and engender a culture of transparency and accountability in the medical imaging industry. Health care providers are compelled to address radiation safety with intent, hence building a safety culture that is of overriding importance over patient care. This is long overdue, given it is in the company of the intricate interdependence of various variables that propel radiation safety behavior, viz., leadership, teamwork, and organizational learning. With all parties, from technologists to administrative staff, having to meet accredited standards, an integrated approach to radiation protection is established. This, in turn, enhances decision-making processes to produce high-quality imaging services that meet stringent safety standards. Ultimately, the accreditation of health facilities not only enhances patient confidence but also paves the way for a robust healthcare system committed to continuous improvement and radiation protection (Moore et al., 2020).

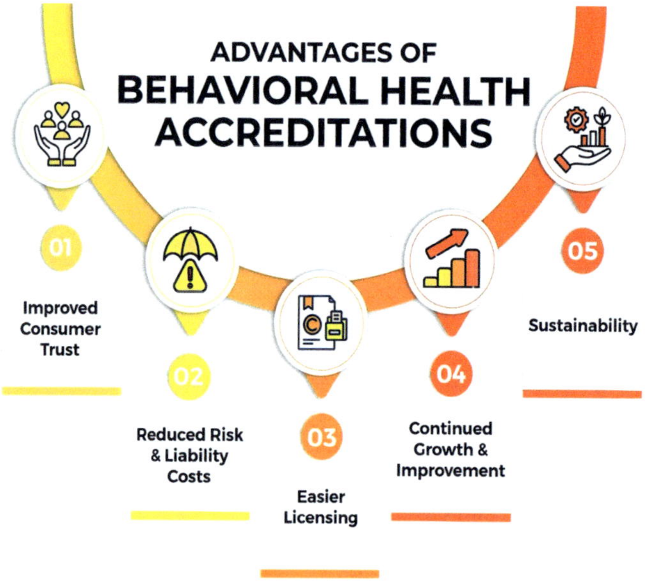

Figure 10.6. The benefits of accreditations in the healthcare business.

Source: https://www.strategiquepartners.com/wp-content/uploads/2024/08/blog-1.jpg.webp.

10.3. Impact of Regulations on Medical Imaging Practices

The regulatory influence of medical imaging activities is extensive, extending not only to safety procedures but also to quality assurance practices that underlie the delivery of patient care. In the United States, institutions such as the AAPM play a significant role in shaping those regulations. By developing Medical Physics Practice Guidelines (MPPGs), the AAPM establishes standards to ensure the safe application of diagnostic and therapeutic radiation. These guidelines undergo rigorous consensus processes to incorporate stakeholder input, and their fulfillment is critical to regulatory and accrediting body requirements. Ultimately, these efforts result in a safer environment for patients, reducing the risk of radiation exposure while enhancing the overall quality of medical imaging services (Seibert et al., 2018). Apart from guaranteeing safe procedures, regulations encourage ongoing education and self-assessment on the profession (Figure 10.7).

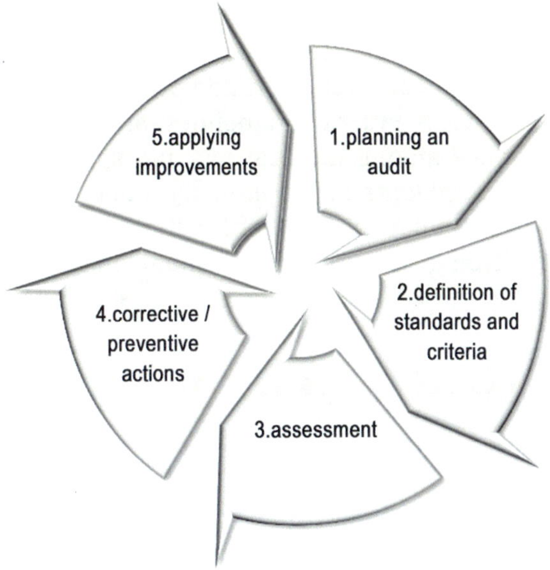

Figure 10.7. QUANUM 3.0, an updated tool for nuclear medicine audits.

Source: https://encrypted-tbn0.gstatic.com/images?q=tbn:ANd9GcTYPCDZb7jSEZwOqvLXv-lSTE2FKmff5c6i_Q&s.

The use of comprehensive quality management programs, such as the Quality Management Audits in Nuclear Medicine (QUANUM) developed by the IAEA, is one of these commitments to improvement. QUANUM not just imposes strict quality standards but also stimulates a systematic and patient-centered auditing culture. Audits are key to enabling medical centers to evaluate how well they are following established protocols, thereby identifying areas where they can do better. The beneficial effects of such audits validate the efficacy of regulatory frameworks in nudging health care institutions to improve conformance levels, which, in turn, contribute to patient outcomes in nuclear medicine (Delaloye et al., 2018). The interface between regulations and medical imaging practices is also evident from visible changes after compliance audits in centers. Data from participating centers in the QUANUM program show a large-scale improvement in global standard conformity. For instance, among the participating centers that underwent internal audits after external evaluations, a high percentage showed improved compliance scores across several quality assurance areas. Such data highlight how adopting and adhering to regulatory standards can lead to systemic improvements in diagnostic performance and patient safety. These results not only support the demand for regulation but also underscore the more significant role of accreditation in impacting the quality of medical imaging service, proving that compliance is not merely a process but a pathway to improved patient care and protection in medical imaging service (Delaloye et al., 2018).

10.3.1. Changes in Imaging Technology and Techniques

Technological innovations in imaging affect the landscape of radiation protection law and medical imaging accreditation. Computed tomography (CT), magnetic resonance imaging (MRI), and digital radiography are significant developments that have revolutionized the diagnostic imaging landscape. These developments not only enhance image quality but also reduce radiation exposure to patients. For instance, advanced algorithms employed in digital imaging enable decreased dose applications with the same diagnostic impact. This evolving technological environment necessitates periodic updating of radiation protection standards to ensure ongoing patient safety and keep pace with new knowledge. Organizations tasked with setting standards, including the American Association of Physicists in Medicine, must develop and revise practice guidelines to reflect these developments, thereby necessitating continuing education and training for medical physicists (Seibert et al., 2018). The introduction of artificial intelligence (AI) and machine learning to imaging modalities is a paradigm shift for medical imaging. The technologies assist in automating image interpretation, thereby speeding up diagnosis and eliminating the possibility of human error. As AI platforms operate on large datasets to identify patterns, the accuracy and speed of interpretation can be enhanced, which is pivotal for timely patient treatment. But with these advancements come questions regarding liability, ethics, and the requirement for sound training among practitioners. Accrediting bodies need to integrate these evolving methodologies into standards so imaging professionals can use AI optimally while maintaining stringent radiation protection guidelines. As these technologies change, there needs to be ongoing review of prevailing regulations to reduce related risks while optimizing patient benefits (N/A, 1991). Furthermore, the transition from analog to digital systems necessitates rigid quality control measures to ensure image standards. Digital technology demands strict calibration and performance monitoring to minimize risks of overexposure and improper imaging procedures. Regulations governing such transitions need to take such shifts into consideration, imposing stricter operating parameters and operator training. Adoption of the most recent medical physics practice guidelines, as promoted by bodies such as the AAPM, fosters a spirit of compliance among medical imaging specialists, keeping them up to date with best practices and new developments in the industry. Coordination among technology developers, educational facilities, and regulatory authorities is necessary to develop inclusive frameworks that ensure patient safety through ongoing improvements in imaging methodologies and technologies (Seibert et al., 2018).

10.3.2. Training and Certification Requirements for Professionals

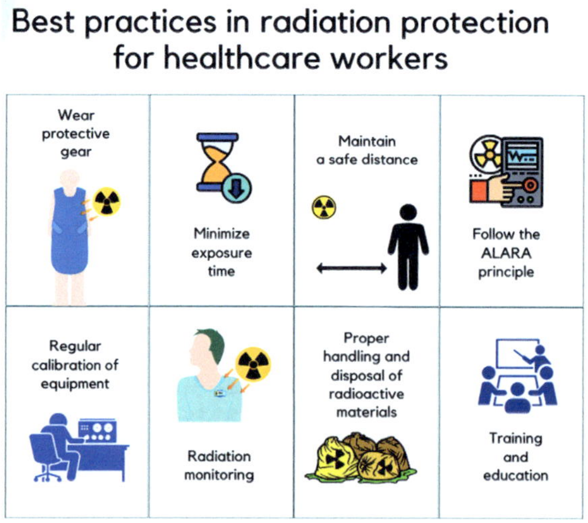

Figure 10.8. Best practices in radiation protection for healthcare workers.

Source: https://www.dhaalindia.com/wp-content/uploads/2024/03/15-1.png.

The training and certification requirements for professionals engaged in radiation protection, especially in the health imaging practice, are crucial to ensuring patient safety and the appropriate application of radiological procedures (Figure 10.8). The medical physicists, for example, have the mandate to enhance the utilization of ionizing radiation in clinics, which necessitates rigorous education and specialized training. According to recent European reference documents like the European Union Council Directive 2013/59/EURATOM, the medical physics professional is at the center, with a focus on ensuring higher qualifications that integrate theoretical and practical competence. The need to establish comprehensive qualification frameworks that enable clinical specialization and certification is increasingly acknowledged by institutions, highlighting the significance of educational standards within the health profession. All these measures not only meet regulatory requirements but also enhance the overall quality of medical care for practitioners and patients and radiation protection (Lopes et al., 2016).

Beyond professional education, professional renewal and development, and recertification are critical to achieving high-quality radiation protection. Various accrediting agencies offer certification programs that require professionals to demonstrate proficiency in radiological safety protocols and imaging procedures. These courses, in most instances, have continuing education requirements that keep professionals up to date with evolving technologies and methods in medical imaging. For example, the International Atomic Energy Agency prescribes formal training and continuing education as part of its guidelines, suggesting periodic testing and recertification as a means of guaranteeing a professional's capability in upholding safe practice. By enforcing rigorous certification requirements, governmental agencies can successfully limit the risks associated with ionizing radiation, ultimately generating a safety culture and a sense of responsibility within the healthcare environment (Davies et al., 2025). Further, harmonization of training and certification processes has far-reaching consequences beyond immediate occupational safety; it also influences public confidence and outcomes of medical imaging practice. If workers are well-trained and certified in radiation protection, patients cannot help but be assured of the safety of ionizing radiation diagnostic tests. The evident provision of guidelines and educational standards operates to standardize the quality of proficiency among professionals, which could translate into improved patient care and reduced instances of radiation-induced health complications. Also, regulatory bodies have an ethical and legal duty to encourage these training procedures so that they are applied uniformly across healthcare systems. This is a declaration of commitment to maintaining public health while developing professional excellence in medical imaging, thereby aligning with international efforts to protect radiation in healthcare (Lopes et al., 2016).

10.3.3. Patient Safety and Risk Management Strategies

Patient safety in medical imaging demands efficient risk management, particularly regarding radiation exposure. To avoid potential injury from diagnostic and interventional procedures, healthcare facilities must make staff training in equipment use and optimization techniques their top priority.

Training shortfalls can lead to extreme overexposures, as documented at an International Atomic Energy Agency Technical Meeting, where accidents resulted in critical doses that caused tissue reactions during examinations such as computed tomography. The use of checklists and time-outs before operations is a preventive measure that guarantees all the safety protocols are in place. Moreover, the installation of dose alerts that trigger when thresholds are reached can significantly enhance safety and reduce the likelihood of unwanted effects during imaging.

Beyond procedural and training protections, clearly documented policy guidelines must be in place to ensure appropriate risk management (Figure 10.9).

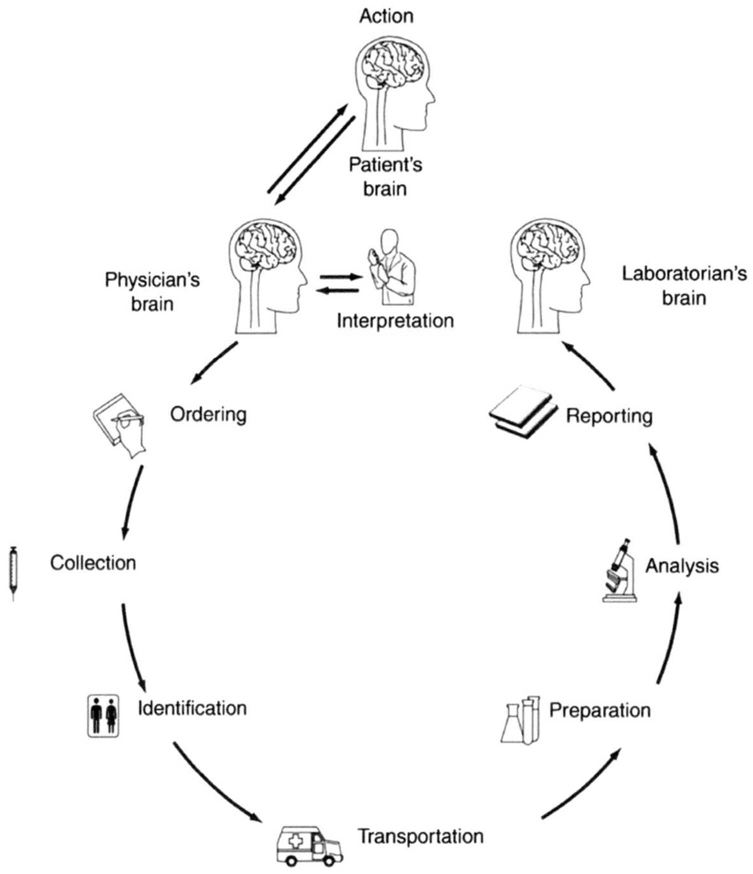

Figure 10.9. Patient safety in laboratory medicine.

Source: https://media.springernature.com/lw685/springer-static/image/chp%3A10.1007%2F978-3-030-59403-9_24/MediaObjects/480571_1_En_24_Fig1_HTML.png.

Responsibilities for radiation overexposure must be delineated in formal written policies, with accountability imposed on personnel to investigate and prevent such incidents. The orders further underscore the importance of root cause identification and rectification at the time of incident occurrence, in line with the learning culture in healthcare facilities. Through comprehensive investigations, facilities are able to examine the situation of overexposures and introduce improved protocols and practices. Furthermore, when overexposures occur, it is necessary to estimate doses accurately to assess their impact on patients and act accordingly. The explanation of risks from stochastic effects in nonmathematical terms, rather than in mathematical terms, minimizes misunderstandings about personal risk and enhances communication about safety measures and results. Finally, environmental implications come into perspective as an aspect of planning for risk management in healthcare. The health care sector is not only tasked with the provision of patient safety utilizing radiation protection, but also faces broader environmental effects as a result of its activities. An evaluation of the health service sector identifies that various routine healthcare processes, such as waste disposal and hospital hygiene, may have a significant environmental effect. Such processes need serious attention and management to restrict pollution and enhance the sustainability of medical imaging activities. Moreover, healthcare sector suppliers wield immense influence over products used within medical imaging; thus, managing risks associated with toxic materials, including mercury and plastics, is essential. Through strict management practices, the healthcare sector can promote patient safety and environmental stewardship, ultimately improving the quality of care in medical imaging (Damilakis et al., 2017; Davies et al., 2025).

10.4. Challenges in Compliance with Regulations

In medical imaging, compliance with radiation protection regulations presents a significant challenge to healthcare institutions. One of the significant challenges is compliance with quality assurance standards, which are important for patient safety and equipment efficacy. For instance, levels of compliance in computed tomography centers in Kenya stood at only 50±3% nationwide, while individual image quality and quality assurance were 61±3% and 37±3% respectively. These results reveal a deficiency in meeting internationally recognized standards set by the AAPM and other equivalent regulatory bodies. Although facilities strive to improve compliance, they are often constrained by resource limitations, inadequate training, and a poor understanding of regulatory requirements, all of which compromise their capacity to maintain the required quality levels for medical imaging procedures (Korir et al., 2012). The impact of changing regulatory environments further complicates compliance activity in medical imaging. Regulatory reforms, while intended to improve safety and efficiency, may pose unexpected hurdles to healthcare professionals and institutions. These are especially significant in settings with strict or dynamically changing regulations. As a case in point in healthcare technology, certain regulatory shifts have unintentionally put smaller companies at a disadvantage, leaving them struggling to keep up and compete. This is also reflected in the medical imaging sector, where compliance with new regulations may require significant investment in technology and training upgrades. As such, while regulatory reforms are aimed at enhancing innovation and patient safety, the actual implications could conflict with existing operating infrastructure and thus inhibit potential improvements in imaging methods (Mkwashi et al., 2020). Moreover, sustaining accreditation in medical imaging entails rigorous, often burdensome compliance that tests resources and institutional focus. Accreditation not only demands compliance with established regulations but also involves a constant effort towards quality enhancement, which can prove overwhelming for facilities already facing workforce shortages and economic challenges. During the accreditation process, variations in compliance scores can provide insight into more ingrained issues in quality management systems, such as outdated equipment or poorly trained employees. Such problems can contribute to a culture of non-compliance in which facilities lack the capability to change. Hence, as the medical imaging profession evolves, overcoming these compliance issues will be essential to ensuring patient safety and fostering an optimal environment for high-quality care (Korir et al., 2012; Mkwashi et al., 2020).

10.4.1. Financial Implications for Healthcare Facilities

The financial implications of radiation protection standards and accreditation in medical imaging extend far beyond healthcare facilities. With changing regulations aimed at enhancing patient safety, institutions must invest significant funds to keep pace with new standards. The cost of implementing stronger radiation protection controls—such as purchasing new technologies, training personnel, and conducting routine compliance audits—can be overwhelming. For most health centers, especially small ones, this expense will be a pinch to their existing budgets, thereby diverting funds from other sectors of patient care that are similarly critical. Compliance with such laws not only requires short-term financial resources but could also lead to higher operating expenses in the long run, making strategic financial planning in healthcare units that deal with imaging diagnostics all the more critical. Accreditation processes also complicate the financial situation because health institutions need to spend additional funds to achieve and maintain accreditation status. Ongoing education and updated training sessions to meet radiation protection regulations can place financial strain on organizations. The training sessions are critical to ensuring staff members are adequately informed about the ethical and pragmatic aspects of radiation safety, thereby improving patient care. Additionally, accredited institutions often have to invest in more advanced technology to meet strict accreditation standards, which can be reflected in higher operational costs. The interaction between accreditation and viability is found to correlate directly: the drive for increased standards brings innovative change within the healthcare sector, while, at other times, the financial cost poses a deterrent to operational effectiveness. Secondly, the threat of monetary fines enters the picture when medical facilities are not compliant with radiation protection guidelines by regulatory authorities. Non-compliance could lead not only to monetary fines but also to damage to their reputations, which could seriously impact patient trust and facility profitability. Hospitals and imaging centers, therefore, have to invest in compliance initiatives to circumvent these risks. Compliance investment can yield long-term financial benefits, including lower liability insurance costs and increased operational efficiency. Every facility faces a different challenge in balancing the costs of regulatory compliance and accreditation against the requirements to deliver high-quality patient care and maintain operational viability. Finally, understanding and interpreting the financial implications of such regulations are critical for healthcare administrators who wish to make sense of the complex medical imaging environment in an impactful way, as highlighted in research by Cimasi et al. (2015).

10.4.2. Variability in Adherence Among Different Institutions

Regulation of radiation protection laws among medical imaging centers often reveals substantial heterogeneity in compliance levels. Heterogeneity can result from a variety of different factors, including institutional policy frameworks, levels of resources, and the degree of training and education of employees. For instance, certain facilities may have more detailed guidelines and higher levels of compliance intensity due to efficient governance and control, thereby raising adherence to radiation protection controls. On the other hand, less resourced or informal administrative arrangements may lack the capacity to implement and enforce necessary regulations. Moreover, the lack of in inconsistent implementation of best practices across institutions, thereby compromising patient safety and overall quality of care. When radiation protection regulations are examined in the context of compliance, the role of accreditation comes to the forefront. Accredited facilities usually face frequent inspections that ensure adherence to accepted safety standards, which can serve as inspiration to sustain high levels of adherence. Variation tends to remain, though, due to the various accrediting organizations and their respective demands. Certain facilities can meet the minimum accreditation requirements, leading to superficial adherence rather than actual devotion to patient safety. Conversely, compliance-promise institutions might make long-term investments in ongoing training, quality assurance, and risk management practices that foster safety culture. Pre-emptive measures such as these can indeed optimize rates of compliance and ultimately protect patients from unnecessary radiation exposure, which demonstrates that safety commitment need not be limited to regulatory compliance at times. Lastly, most recent research underscores that institutional culture must be a decisive factor in determining adherence to radiation protection behaviors. A safety-conscious and accountability-oriented culture is likely to promote higher levels of staff compliance, since employees are empowered to place patients' health foremost. Conversely, institutions lacking a strong commitment to radiation safety are likely to promote non-compliance, as staff develop complacency about the hazards of radiation exposure. Importantly, evidence has indicated that staff teamwork, leadership support, and communication of best practices can increase adherence considerably. Given the constant growth in the medical imaging industry, it will be crucial to have an understanding and management of the subtleties of compliance across institutions in order to improve safety measures, further significant impacts on policy development and practice at the institutional level in radiation protection legislation (Kitsiou et al., 2013; Valjakova et al., 2015).

10.4.3. Technological Advancements Outpacing Regulations

The rapid development of imaging technologies has challenged existing radiation protection legislation. With technologies such as photon-counting CT and ultra-high-field MRI, greater diagnostic capability can be achieved with lower radiation exposure (Seibert et al., 2018). The regulatory landscape that will cover such technologies usually trails their implementation. Even though some organizations, such as the AAPM, try to develop practice guidelines and adapt to the evolving landscape of medical physics, such efforts may be insufficient to address the complexities introduced by emerging technologies (Seibert et al., 2018). Consequently, professionals in the field are often required to function within a regulatory environment not inherently well-suited to consider the connotations of advanced imaging technology, thereby creating uneven patient safety and quality care. In addition, the incorporation of AI into medical imaging makes compliance with existing regulations even more challenging. AI has the potential to enhance image interpretation, automate processes, and personalize patient protocols to individual requirements, thereby reducing unnecessary radiation exposure (Adadzi et al., 2024). However, with the rapid adoption of AI technologies into clinical practice comes the challenge of how to regulate them. The regulatory bodies in place now may not know or may not have the set-up to assess these innovations adequately, which results in applications of AI in imaging being poorly regulated. This can lead to future risks since healthcare professionals find themselves relying on equipment that has not undergone rigorous testing. Accordingly, a proactive regulatory approach that keeps pace with emerging technology is necessary to mitigate potential risks associated with the application of AI in medical imaging. To address these issues, regulatory agencies and professional organizations need to participate actively with technology developers to establish an increasingly responsive regulatory framework. This entails not only updating existing guidelines but also anticipating future industry trends (Seibert et al., 2018). By maintaining ongoing engagement with industry players, regulatory bodies can establish an environment that promotes innovation while ensuring that patient safety takes precedence. Moreover, addressing the economic considerations involved in implementing high-end imaging technology is critical to preventing disparate access to healthcare (Adadzi et al., 2024). With advances in medical imaging, the dynamic relationship between innovation and regulation will be at the forefront in determining the quality and accessibility of imaging services, with far-reaching consequences for patient outcomes in the health system.

10.5. Future Directions in Radiation Protection

The future of radiation protection in medical imaging is promising, as it is driven by technological innovation and evolving regulatory paradigms. With the medical profession increasingly digitalized and employing more advanced imaging technologies, deep capabilities such as AI are rising to prominence as key assets for advancing radiation safety. AI techniques can be used to maximize image protocols to minimize radiation doses to the lowest reasonably achievable (ALARA), in keeping with best practice in patient protection. Also, ongoing advances in imaging equipment will require updated regulations to address new safety concerns, and practitioners who employ such advanced technology will be required to abide by them. The incorporation of newer technologies into present frameworks of regulations will make way for an effective, more responsive and flexible response to radiation protection in clinical settings, contributing to a safer environment overall for patients and caregivers and solving shifting issues associated with radiation exposure (South Carolina Department of Health and Environmental Control, 2021). As healthcare workers continue to perform interventional procedures, the need for ongoing training and education in radiation protection is even greater. Research has shown an evident link between the amount of training completed by medical staff and adherence to radiation protection best practices. For instance, studies have shown that staff trained in radiation protection are more likely to use protective devices and implement safety measures during fluoroscopic procedures (Alahmari et al., 2015). Therefore, future projects should prioritize systematic training programs that foster the development of knowledge and competence in radiation safety among medical staff. Such prioritization entails that workers are not only equipped with applicable skills but also have the confidence to make protection possible. When connecting training schemes with the accreditation standards, medical facilities will not only improve patient outcomes but also assist in instilling a culture of safety within their work environments. Moreover, coordination among regulatory bodies, medical associations, and technology firms provides the platform for the updating of radiation protection standards. Joint ventures can result in the evolution of inclusive guidelines that integrate the best practices from various areas of medical imaging. For instance, contributions from frontline healthcare workers can result in practical ideas that inform regulations, enabling them to look back on contemporary practice. Further. This cooperative diagnostic plan can result in harmonizing accreditation processes that really reflect diagnostic changes in medical imaging technologies. It should be proactive in applying new regulations and diagnostic measures and avoid being reactive in order to prevent risks beforehand. Through engaging in cooperative activities, stakeholders can collectively work towards building the system of radiation protection regulation, promoting a safer future in medical imaging, and ultimately building public trust in healthcare systems (South Carolina Department of Health and Environmental Control, 2021).

10.5.1. Emerging Technologies and Their Implications

The introduction of advanced technologies in medical imaging has introduced new portals to improved diagnostic performance and patient safety. Technologies such as AI and advanced imaging modalities, such as CBCT and MRI, are transforming fundamental practices in medical imaging. These advancements improve disease detection and treatment planning accuracy, which in turn demands strict radiation shielding policies. Organizations like the AAPM are spearheading the development of practice guidelines to ensure these technologies are used safely. With mature guidelines evolving in accordance with the latest scientific facts and technological innovation, strong professional education and standards compliance become critical in minimizing risks from radiation exposure and optimizing patient care in a progressively complex field (Seibert et al., 2018). The shift towards non-ionizing radiation technologies such as MRI and ultrasound is a sign of an impressive change in the medical imaging sector, with the aim of reducing patient exposure to ionizing radiation. The International Commission on Non-Ionizing Radiation Protection (ICNIRP) has emphasized the application of established guidelines for the use of non-ionizing radiation (NIR) in diagnostic imaging. With the advancement of newer non-invasive technologies, there is a need for the regulatory environment to adapt to different NIR devices. Recent research has questioned existing safety guidelines, particularly regarding potential health risks to both patients and healthcare workers. Evidence continues to emerge, particularly for specific groups, such as fetuses in the first trimester (Alfirevic et al., 2017). Existing policies should therefore grant comprehensive assessments of health risks posed by NIR exposure to ensure that the growing trend in the application of cutting-edge technologies does not come at the expense of safety. Further, accreditation processes in medical imaging must also keep pace with the accelerating pace of technological development. As newer technologies become integrated into medical imaging facilities, the regulatory agencies are required to conduct conformity checks against new safety standards and guidelines. The shift from conventional imaging technologies to intelligent solutions, such as AI-based diagnostic imaging, calls for medical professionals to learn and updatekeep up to date continually. Accreditation programs must incorporate such advances into their assessment processes so that practitioners become accustomed to new technologies and their roles in protection against radiation. In this way, these programs can provide high standards of care and promote an innovative culture in medical imaging. No significance should be given to accreditation's contribution to patient health protection, as it is a critical checkpoint in the deployment of new technologies (Seibert et al., 2018).

10.5.2. Potential Updates to Existing Regulations

The changing environment of medical imaging necessitates the reevaluation and perhaps revision of the present radiation protection regulations. As technology continues to improve, the modalities and techniques used in medical imaging become increasingly sophisticated, hence the need for regulation that is reasonable with modern practices and understands new safety issues. It is the responsibility of organizations such as the AAPM to set these standards. The AAPM revises its medical physics practice guidelines at regular intervals in order to stay current with the latest scientific evidence and regulatory criteria, and ensure that its standards promote not only safe practice but also continuing improvement in service delivery in the context of medical imaging facilities (Seibert et al., 2018). Incorporating stakeholders' input, the revisions could benefit most importantly practitioners and patients, ultimately having the greatest overall public health impact. In addition to guideline review, special attention has to be paid to implementing quality assurance (QA) procedures in medical imaging services. There should be careful QA protocols established to manage radiation exposure risks. When creating effective QA systems, organizations match regulatory frameworks with international standards to create benchmarks that are comparable in different countries (Bogusz-Czerniewicz et al., 2012). would impose certain QA processes to ensure the consistency and effectiveness of imaging modalities. Besides, the requirements need to focus not just on compliance but also on a safety culture that includes continuous monitoring and improvement as a standard expectation. This will not only enhance the quality of services offered to patients but also ensure the integrity of healthcare centers involved in medical imaging. Finally, amendments to regulations to ensure training and competency requirements for staff operating imaging machines cannot be overstated. With ongoing advances in imaging technology, it is important that staff are trained and experienced in best practices to minimize radiation exposure risks. Regulatory bodies could specify stricter standards for certification and continuing education of medical imaging staff. Incentivizing multidisciplinary collaboration, as outlined in a number of guidelines, is also beneficial. For instance, convening the expertise of different professional groups can inform the creation of new regulations that balance safety with technical and clinical factors in medical imaging (Seibert et al., 2018). By developing an appropriately trained workforce with up-to-date knowledge, healthcare professionals can effectively improve patient outcomes while ensuring the highest possible levels of radiation protection.

10.5.3. The Role of Education and Training in Future Compliance

The relevance of training and education in future compliance with the practice of legislation in the area of radiation protection cannot be overstated. As technology in medical imaging improves, so does the training of professionals. Proper training ensures that radiologic technologists, medical physicists, and other professionals possess the skills needed to use imaging devices safely and properly. Furthermore, adherence to regulatory standards, such as those set by the American Association of Physicists in Medicine, relies on continuously developing educational practices. These guidelines underscore the importance of practitioners engaging in ongoing professional education to ensure imaging quality and patient safety. With more advanced medical treatments involving radiation, effective educational programming will enable future healthcare workers to handle the intricacies of compliance more effectively and ultimately provide improved patient care and outcomes. Furthermore, the enforcement of effective training programs that are in compliance with regulatory standards further solidifies a safety culture within health centers. By emphasizing the importance of radiation protection guidelines, educational institutions can build an employee base that values compliance and ethical performance. The training programs need to include not only the technical aspects of imaging but also the core principles that underpin good practice, so that future professionals are provided with adequate knowledge of the legal and ethical issues associated with their profession. Those institutions offering such educational courses will have to update and rework their curricula periodically to reflect recent technological advancements as well as regulatory changes, as required by bodies regulating the practice of medical imaging. Anticipatory changes ensure an industry workforce not only in compliance with existing regulations but also responsive to new practices and standards as they emerge. In the coming years, the future prospects for compliance in radiation protection will be dominated by collaboration among regulatory bodies, schools of education, and medical caregivers. Joint action among these parties can lead to new training programs that equip practitioners with the skills needed to meet evolving standards. Such feedback loops among these parties can also inform the development of educational products to address the issues that practitioners face in medical imaging. With regulations such as those outlined by the AAPM that point to the need for independent training in the safe use of therapeutic and diagnostic radiation, it becomes important that education programs meet these requirements (Seibert et al., 2018). The commitment to strict educational frameworks and continuous professional improvement will not only ensure compliance but also build a strong healthcare environment capable of meeting the challenges of modern medical imaging (South Carolina Department of Health and Environmental Control, 2021).

SUMMARY

In reviewing the context of radiation protection rules and accreditation in medical imaging, one should focus on the most significant conclusions drawn from recent surveys of training and education in this field. A review stated a commonality among various stakeholders, including professional bodies and healthcare providers, on the current strengths and potential in RP training. The identified strengths included developed training models and the need for an in-depth analysis of RP training requirements, reflecting a model with a systemized approach to education and training, ensuring safety in medical imaging procedures. Besides, areas for improvement were identified, with an emphasis on the harmonization and accreditation of RP education to enhance the quality of training for medical professionals and, ultimately, patient safety (Alves et al., 2022). The review also gave major insights into the strengths and limitations of radiation protection training in medical imaging. Notably, there has been a gap in emphasizing the importance of radiation safety at national, international, practitioner group, and research levels. Lack of attention to RP principles in practice has led to uneven application of safety provisions, jeopardizing patient and practitioner health. To address such issues and enable the proper implementation of radiation protection measures, stakeholders must plan strategically at European, national, and regional levels. Harmonization in such efforts can lead to a robust training network that efficiently enhances the quality and scope of RP education in medical imaging (Alves et al., 2022). In addition, the role of regulatory reforms in medical imaging technology and in companies' capacity in the sector cannot be overemphasized. Recent studies indicate that while regulatory reforms can promote innovation and forge cooperative relationships between firms, they can also impose tight conditions on such firms, whose effects fall most heavily on small firms in the healthcare sector. The evidence suggests that regulatory systems must be selective and enabling, upholding the technological capability of the firms to achieve their desired outcomes effectively. Through a platform that promotes innovation while avoiding unnecessary market entry barriers, the medical device industry can efficiently address affordable healthcare technology issues, ensuring equal access to safe imaging procedures for all.

CLOSER LOOK

IMPROVED PRACTICES IN MEDICAL IMAGING

In recent years, the radiological community has been subject to growing criticism regarding radiation safety and the quality of care. There is a critical need to enhance practices implemented under the radiation protection legislation. One solution proposed through international standards is to apply holistic quality management systems, such as those of the International Atomic Energy Agency. Such initiatives as QUANUM not only provide clear guidelines but also foster a culture of continuous quality improvement in nuclear medicine practice. By continuously auditing compliance with these standards, facilities can identify areas of noncompliance and make the necessary adjustments, supporting patient well-being and improving imaging methods. Practical application of QUANUM has been proven to enhance levels of conformance significantly, and this underscores the value of routine internal audits and external inspections in the validation of high practice standards in medical imaging (Delaloye et al., 2018). An indispensable element towards enhancing medical imaging practices is the creation of an effective radiation safety culture among imaging practitioners. An awareness that safety culture is shaped by many factors—interpersonal relationships, organizational policy, and community attitudes—can lead to more effective radiation practice. New research shows that leadership behavior, teamwork, and organizational learning are key to increasing radiologic technologists' perception of radiation safety. Organizations can create a supportive environment that prioritizes safety and reduces patient exposure to unnecessary radiation by addressing these determinants. Secondly, implementing targeted training programs based on these findings can equip professionals to take action in the workplace, thereby optimizing overall safety protocols in healthcare settings. Continued efforts to drive improvement must be grounded in such research to make medical imaging safe and effective, fostering patient and healthcare provider confidence (Moore et al., 2020). To bring about true change, stakeholders at every level of the medical imaging chain must unite and drive for heightened regulatory conformity and accreditation standards. This is not just an appeal by radiologic technologists but encompasses clinical leaders, policymakers, and educational institutions. Collaborative efforts must focus on establishing effective channels of communication to facilitate the exchange of best practices and lessons learned among institutions. Furthermore, inclusion of these findings in curricula for educational institutions can ensure that future professionals prioritize radiation safety right from the beginning of their careers. The process of having a harmonized approach toward radiation protection legislation and accreditation, aside from enhancing patient outcomes, will strengthen the medical imaging professional. By reinforcing a common commitment to enhanced practices, the industry can easily eliminate risks and deliver top-quality imaging care to each patient (Delaloye et al., 2018; Moore et al., 2020).

REFERENCES

1. Kerna, N. A., Ngwu, D. C., Kadivi, K., Carsrud, N. V., Pruitt, K. D., Flores, J. V., Holets, H. M., Jomsky, B. M., Chawla, S., Azi, C. I., McKee, D., Nwokorie, U., Anderson II, J., Dugeri, J. L., Hammam, H. S. H., Chiedozie, O. B., Nnake, I., David, C. O., & Adadzi, J. (2024). Transformative Advancements in Diagnostic Imaging: Reducing Risks, Enhancing Accuracy, and Promoting Sustainability. *European Journal of Medical and Health Research*, *2*(5), 153-172. https://doi.org/10.59324/ejmhr.2024.2(5).16Alahmari, M. A. S. (2015). Awareness and knowledge of radiation protection in interventional laboratory: A comparative study between Australian and Saudi Arabian hospitals. https://core.ac.uk/download/195631630.pdf (accessed on 5th August 2025).
2. Alfirevic, Z., Bause, L., Bouyssi-Kobar, M., Bucher, C., De Santis, M., Fatemi, M., Fiechter, M., et al. (2017). ICNIRP statement on diagnostic devices using non-ionizing radiation: Existing regulations and potential health risks. https://core.ac.uk/download/76975622.pdf (accessed on 5th August 2025).
3. Alves, F., Andersson, J., Bacher, K., Damilakis, J., et al. (2022). Education and training in radiation protection in Europe: An analysis from the EURAMED rock-n-roll project. https://core.ac.uk/download/541044065.pdf (accessed on 5th August 2025).
4. Bajraktarova Valjakova, E., Gigovski, N., Korunoska Stevkovska, V., Mijoska, A., et al. (2015). Implant-prosthetic therapy failure in smoker and nonsmoker patients. https://core.ac.uk/download/35343836.pdf (accessed on 5th August 2025).
5. Barr, H., Blanco, S. A. A., Butler, P., Craig, P., et al. (2016). Mammography services quality assurance: Baseline standards for Latin America and the Caribbean. https://core.ac.uk/download/343666765.pdf (accessed on 5th August 2025).
6. Bogusz-Czerniewicz, M., & Kaźmierczak, D. (2012). Organizational, technical, physical and clinical quality standards for radiotherapy. https://core.ac.uk/download/pdf/81975775.pdf (accessed on 5th August 2025).
7. Cimasi, R. J., & Zigrang, T. A. (2015). *Adviser's Guide to Health Care, Volume 1: An Era of Reform—The Four Pillars*. https://core.ac.uk/download/551513560.pdf (accessed on 5th August 2025).
8. Cimasi, R. J., & Zigrang, T. A. (2015). *Adviser's Guide to Health Care, Volume 2: Consulting Services*. https://core.ac.uk/download/551513559.pdf (accessed on 5th August 2025).
9. Damilakis, J., Ebdon-Jackson, S., Frush, D. P., Loose, R., et al. (2017). Unintended and accidental medical radiation exposures in radiology: Guidelines on investigation and prevention. https://core.ac.uk/download/96883276.pdf (accessed on 5th August 2025).
10. Davies, J. C., & Lowe, A. (2025). Environmental implications of the health care service sector. https://core.ac.uk/download/pdf/9307987.pdf (accessed on 5th August 2025).
11. Delaloye, A. B., Dondi, M., Giammarile, F., Lobato, R., et al. (2018). Implementation of quality systems in nuclear medicine: Why it matters. An outcome analysis (Quality management audits in nuclear medicine part III). https://core.ac.uk/download/156955537.pdf (accessed on 5th August 2025).
12. do Carmo Lopes, M., Casar, B., Drljević, A., Gershkevitsh, E., et al. (2016). Medical physics in Europe following recommendations of the International Atomic Energy Agency. https://core.ac.uk/download/604617660.pdf (accessed on 5th August 2025).

13. Downie, J., Malisza, K., Marshall, J., Martin, L., et al. (2007). A comprehensive analysis of MRI research risks: In support of full disclosure. https://core.ac.uk/download/478607605.pdf (accessed on 5th August 2025).

14. Esler, J., Harrison, K., Jeffrey, R., Kirby, J., et al. (2007). Oocyte cryopreservation as an adjunct to the assisted reproductive technologies. https://core.ac.uk/download/12759048.pdf (accessed on 5th August 2025).

15. Houser, T. (2019). Assessment of magnetic resonance imaging safety: Allied health professional clinical competence. https://core.ac.uk/download/214094399.pdf (accessed on 5th August 2025).

16. Kitsiou, A. L. P., Caforio, A., Porta-Sanchez, A., Vahanian, A., Iung, B., Carrera, C., Szymanski, C., et al. (2013). ESC core curriculum for the general cardiologist (2013). https://core.ac.uk/download/55756305.pdf (accessed on 5th August 2025).

17. Korir, G. K., Korir, I. K., Ochieng, B. O., Wambani, S., et al. (2012). Establishing the quality management baseline in the use of computed tomography machines in Kenya. https://core.ac.uk/download/47254975.pdf (accessed on 5th August 2025).

18. Mkwashi, A. S. (2020). Medical device regulations, industrial capabilities, and affordable healthcare technology development: Case studies from the United Kingdom and South Africa. https://core.ac.uk/download/323055215.pdf (accessed on 5th August 2025).

19. Moore, Q. T. (2020). Radiation actions and dimensions of radiation safety among U.S. radiologic technologists. https://core.ac.uk/download/643706003.pdf (accessed on 5th August 2025).

20. N/A. (1991). *Focal Spot, Spring 1991*. https://core.ac.uk/download/129069286.pdf (accessed on 5th August 2025).

21. Seibert, A. J., Baird, C. T., Clements, J. B., de Boer, S. F., et al. (2018). AAPM medical physics practice guideline 10.a.: Scope of practice for clinical medical physics. https://core.ac.uk/download/286729023.pdf (accessed on 5th August 2025).

22. South Carolina Department of Health and Environmental Control. (2021). Regulation 61–64 X-rays (Title B). https://core.ac.uk/download/588861585.pdf (accessed on 5th August 2025).

23. United States Agency for Toxic Substances and Disease Registry. Division of Toxicology and Environmental Medicine. (2025). Radiation exposure from iodine-131. https://core.ac.uk/download/144200170.pdf (accessed on 5th August 2025).

INDEX

D

E

F

G

H

I

L

M

N

O

P

R

S

T

U

V

W

X

ABOUT THE AUTHOR

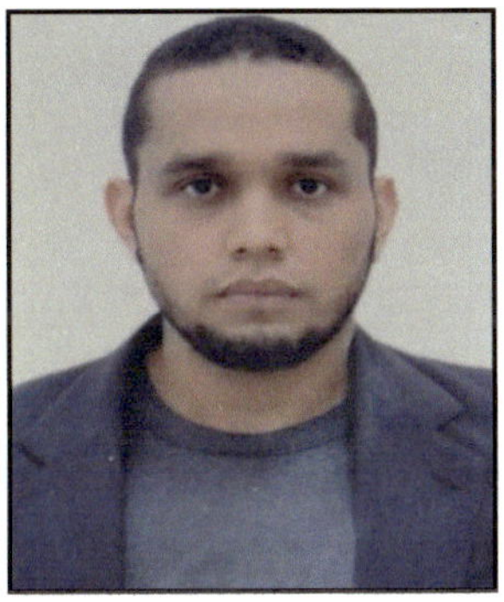

Dr. José Abraham Amaya Duarte is a radiologist with extensive clinical and academic experience in diagnostic imaging, advanced image interpretation, and image-guided procedures. His expertise includes ultrasound, computed tomography (CT), magnetic resonance imaging (MRI), and radiography across a broad range of clinical applications.

He earned his Doctor of Medicine and Surgery degree from the Universidad Nacional Autónoma de Nicaragua (UNAN-León) and completed his specialization in Diagnostic Imaging at the Universidad de Defensa de Nicaragua (UDENIC). To further enhance his expertise, Dr. Amaya pursued advanced subspecialty training in musculoskeletal, neuro, and women's imaging, and is currently completing a Master's degree in Obstetric and Gynecologic Ultrasound.

Dr. Amaya currently serves as a Radiology and Imaging Specialist at Sugar City Medical Center in Belize, where he provides comprehensive diagnostic evaluations and supports multidisciplinary clinical teams. His professional background also includes academic instruction, pediatric medicine, and international teleradiology services for hospitals and clinics worldwide.

A dedicated educator and researcher, Dr. Amaya's professional focus lies in improving diagnostic accuracy, clinical workflow, and imaging quality through continuous education and collaboration. His commitment to excellence and his contributions to clinical radiology continue to advance the field across Latin America and beyond.

Brief Table of Contents

Detailed Table of Contents

CHAPTER 7

Gastrointestinal Tract Imaging: CT, MRI, and Fluoroscopy 181

CHAPTER 8

Genitourinary Imaging: Kidneys, Bladder, and Prostate 213

CHAPTER 9

Musculoskeletal Imaging: Bone and Soft Tissue 245

CHAPTER 10

Pediatric Diagnostic Imaging Principles 273

CHAPTER 11

Emergency and Trauma Imaging Protocols 303

LIST OF FIGURES

PREFACE

Diagnostic imaging has transformed medical practice by giving clinicians an instantaneous glimpse into the human body. Over the past decades, advances in X-ray technology and cross-sectional imaging have made it possible for practitioners to identify disease processes at an earlier stage, better target therapeutic measures, and assess success while on or following therapy with greater confidence. From acute trauma examination to assessment of chronic disorder, imaging is currently a central tool that assists in diagnosis, directs patient management, and improves prognostic capability.

With evolving technology, the workload for radiologists and referring physicians becomes more complex. The clinicians should be familiar with principles of all modalities, should understand the merits and limitations of different approaches, and integrate imaging findings with clinical and laboratory data. Interpretation of images and communication of diagnostic impressions are most important in patient care, and education in new technologies is imperative for all healthcare professionals dealing with imaging.

Handbook of Diagnostic Imaging: Volume 2 offers an in-depth review of modern imaging methods in a variety of anatomic locations and settings. It expands fundamental principles by covering extensive discussions of technique, application, and the future direction. With input from prominent neuroradiologists, head and neck, thoracic, and cardiovascular imagers, as well as breast, abdomen, genitourinary, musculoskeletal, pediatric, and emergency imagers, the book serves as a deserving reference for both trainees and practitioners.

Chapter 1 provides an introduction to neuroimaging, discussing principles and realities of central nervous system computed tomography (CT) and magnetic resonance imaging (MRI). It begins with a concise overview of the fundamentals of neuroimaging techniques and modalities, and subsequently explains CT physics, clinical use, and hazards. The session then shifts to MRI technology, discussing sequence choice, advantages in contrast for soft tissues, and safety. Clinical uses, including CT for trauma, tumor imaging, and stroke evaluation, are followed by MRI sections on multiple sclerosis, brain tumors, and neurodegenerative diseases. The chapter concludes about emerging technologies, such as advanced imaging equipment and the use of artificial intelligence to provide personalized care.

Chapter 2 prioritizes head and neck imaging, beginning with ultrasound for evaluation of the thyroid gland and salivary tissue. The ultrasound section presents transducer selection, image optimization, pitfalls, and limitations. The following section discusses positron emission tomography (PET) and radiotracer mechanisms, as well as its oncologic use in head and neck cancers. The chapter proceeds to discuss contrast agents, their types, and safety profiles, followed by applications in the clinic, such as tumor detection, trauma assessment, and measurement of response to therapy. Future research directions, like advances in technology or computer intelligence in the interpretation of images, conclude the chapter.

Chapter 3 addresses thoracic imaging of the lung and mediastinum. It starts with a review of thoracic anatomy, merges chest X-ray interpretation basics, and builds up to CT and MRI techniques used in lung assessment. Representative pathologies such as pneumonia, lung cancer, and interstitial lung disease are described based on their imaging features. The mediastinal chapter covers CT, ultrasound, and MRI uses, addresses mediastinal tumors, lymphadenopathy, and detection of an aortic aneurysm. It emphasizes recent advances and the increasing application of machine learning in thoracic radiology.

Chapter 4 discusses cardiovascular imaging with CT angiography and MRI. The chapter introduces the principles of CT angiography, the aspects of contrast media, and the indications for assessing coronary and vascular disease. It then discusses cardiovascular MRI, its relevant sequences, functional assessment techniques, and clinical applications. Relative discussions cover procedural time, image resolution, soft-tissue characterization, radiation dose, and patient comfort. The chapter concludes by noting the limitations of each modality and offering advice on modality selection in clinical situations.

Chapter 5 discusses breast imaging from classic mammography to ultrasound and then MRI. It covers screening versus diagnostic mammography, procedure details, and advantages and limitations. The ultrasound section covers indications for adjunctive imaging and its sensitivity compared to mammography. MRI use for breast cancer detection and high-risk screening comes next, including patient preparation and interpretation criteria. A final comparison of sensitivity, specificity, cost, and patient experience rounds out the chapter, with comments on future directions and tailored screening approaches.

Chapter 6 discusses abdominal imaging of liver, biliary, and pancreatic disease. The chapter begins with liver anatomy and physiology and then goes on to describe ultrasound, CT, and MRI techniques, including elastography for the measurement of fibrosis. Liver diseases—hepatitis, cirrhosis, and tumors—are outlined by their radiographic features. The biliary section discusses cholangiographic methods, ultrasound evaluation, and cross-sectional imaging of the bile ducts, as well as imaging characteristics of cholelithiasis, obstruction, and cholangiocarcinoma. Key developments and novel emerging imaging methods conclude the subject.

Chapter 7 summarizes imaging of the gastrointestinal tract using CT, MRI, and fluoroscopy. It starts with gastrointestinal anatomy and clinical reasons for imaging. CT protocols and their advantages for obstruction, inflammation, and neoplasia are delineated, followed by MRI techniques for soft-tissue contrast and motion-sensitive sequences. Uses of fluoroscopy—barium studies and dynamic swallow assessments—are covered next. The chapter compares modalities, assesses patient safety issues, and looks ahead to image-guided interventions and adaptive imaging protocols.

Chapter 8 is a description of genitourinary imaging of the kidneys, bladder, and prostate. The anatomy chapter leads to ultrasound, CT, and MRI evaluation of renal parenchyma and collecting systems of the urinary tract. Modalities for bladder imaging, including cystography and cross-sectional studies, come next. The use of transrectal ultrasound, MRI, and PET scanning for evaluating the prostate follows. Disorders that are frequent on all levels—stones, infection, tumors, and benign hypertrophy—are characterized by their imaging appearance. The chapter concludes with the designation of new imaging technologies and the increasing use of computer-aided diagnosis.

Chapter 9 discusses musculoskeletal imaging of bone and soft tissues. It reviews standard radiography for fracture assessment, describes CT's role in assessing complex bony injuries, and details MRI's advantages for soft tissue and marrow evaluation. Common conditions—fractures, tumors, inflammatory disorders—are outlined with corresponding imaging findings. The chapter also presents case studies in sports injuries, arthritis, and trauma to illustrate practical applications. Recent technological enhancements and AI-driven interpretation tools are featured in the closing section.

Chapter 10 outlines principles of pediatric imaging with attention to patient safety and developmental considerations. Methods for reducing dose, recommendations for contrast agents, and age-based protocols are discussed. The psychological impact of imaging examinations on children and parental involvement strategies is covered. The unique interpretation difficulty in the pediatric patient is discussed, along with emerging technologies designed to maximize diagnostic yield while reducing risk. Ethical and legal issues of pediatric imaging bring the chapter to a conclusion.

Chapter 11 summarizes imaging protocols in the trauma and emergency settings. Chapter 11 covers indications of head, chest, and abdominal imaging in acute trauma, such as specific protocols and guidelines for administration of contrast. Time constraints, radiation exposure, and institutional differences are among the issues discussed. The chapter also names triage setting rapid imaging, point-of-care, and portable technology development, as well as the potential of artificial intelligence, as factors to simplify emergency workflows.

This text is aimed at radiologists, fellows, residents, and clinicians who are reliant on diagnostic imaging in daily practice. It is both background information and a guide to practical recommendations, and hence equally helpful to trainees as to experienced clinicians in need of an accessible but authoritative reference.

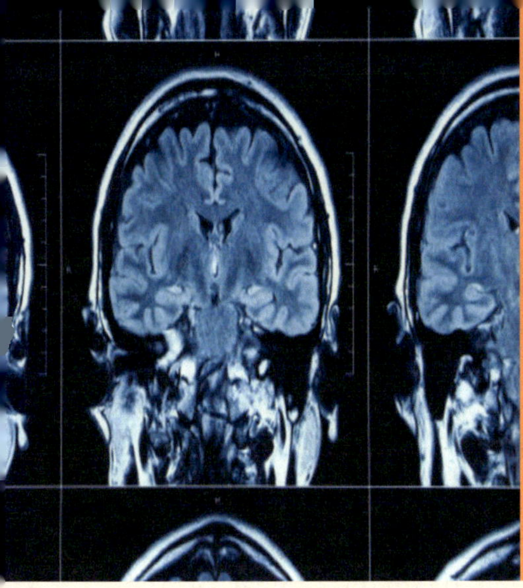

Chapter 1

NEUROIMAGING: CT AND MRI OF THE CENTRAL NERVOUS SYSTEM

Contents

Introduction

The emergence of neuroimaging devices has revolutionized medical diagnostic techniques, particularly of the Central Nervous System (CNS). Two primary modalities for advancing anatomical and functional knowledge of brain disease are Computed Tomography (CT) and Magnetic Resonance Imaging (MRI). With the application of various imaging methods, clinicians and researchers are able to identify neuroanatomical disorders, monitor disease status, and assess treatment response. The development of high-resolution imaging has enabled the visualization of brain structures more precisely, ultimately creating a greater understanding of many neurological diseases. Such increased imaging capability has therefore restored interest in brain-gut interactions and how these influence general health, particularly as far as chronic pain syndromes where dysregulation can be found (Aziz et al., 2019).

CT and MRI fundamentally differ in their functions and applications. CT scans use X-rays to generate cross-sectional images of the brain, making them particularly helpful for detecting acute hemorrhage, fractures, and other structural defects. MRI, however, employs powerful magnetic fields and radio waves to visualize soft tissues in vivid detail. The reason is that MRI can detect subtle structural alterations and functional variations that may go undetected by CT scans. Furthermore, advancements in neuroimaging over the last decade have moved beyond conventional imaging, with functional and metabolic measurements integrated to provide a more comprehensive understanding of brain function. As researchers continue to explore these modalities, significant progress is being made toward identifying the underlying mechanisms and biomarkers for many central nervous system disorders (Basu et al., 2018).

Clinical uses of CT and MRI have repercussions extending beyond mere diagnostics. Brain connectivity and its relationship to behavioral and physiological states are new areas of study. Although tremendous progress has been made in imaging modalities and data analysis, problems still exist regarding standardization and interpretation of imaging data across populations. For instance, the integration of multisite datasets may enhance generalizability but requires collective effort within the scientific community to develop harmonized protocols and datasets. Creation of complete, standardized repositories and consortia will be key in overcoming such impediments, thus enhancing our understanding of the CNS and its intricate web of interactions (Aziz et al., 2019). As we explore these new imaging techniques, hope for revolutionary gains in neurobiology and clinical practice remains optimistic.

1.1. Basics of Neuroimaging

Neuroimaging encompasses a range of techniques essential for diagnosing and understanding numerous Central Nervous System (CNS) disorders. Of these techniques, Computed Tomography (CT) and Magnetic Resonance Imaging (MRI) are the most frequently used because they offer specific advantages. CT scans use X-rays to generate high-resolution cross-sectional views of the brain. They are thus instrumental in emergencies where rapid evaluation is critical, such as for stroke or traumatic brain injury. The immediate assessment made possible by the rapidity and availability of CT scans can be the difference between life and death in clinical settings. In addition, the technology of CT has been improving image quality and reducing radiation doses, hence overall improving its effectiveness as a diagnostic tool. Although CT is effective in identifying acute hemorrhagic strokes, it may not be as sensitive in the identification of early ischemic changes as MRI is. On the other hand, MRI offers superb contrast in soft tissues and is well-suited for imaging of brain anatomy and diagnosing a wide variety of disorders, from tumors to demyelinating diseases. Using strong magnetic fields and radio waves, MRI generates high-quality images without exposing the patient to ionizing radiation. Specifically, the application of T1- and T2-weighted imaging sequences with MRI enables delicate demarcation of various cerebral structures, which is vital for assessing diseases such as Alzheimer's and multiple sclerosis. In addition, MRI modalities such as diffusion-weighted imaging inform us about the integrity of white matter tracts, which aids in illuminating neurodegenerative processes. The global context offered by MRI, along with its ability to image physiological changes in real time, emphasizes its importance in clinical and research settings. The addition of neuroimaging to healthcare has revolutionized the treatment of neurological disorders, allowing for early diagnosis and guiding therapeutic interventions. For example, understanding the BBB permeability dynamics of ischemic stroke through imaging techniques is crucial. As has been pointed out in recent research, BBB disruption occurs in a multiphasic pattern, and it can have direct consequences for drug treatment and patient prognosis (Bernardo-Castro et al., 2020). Moreover, studies that have explored ventricular morphology via neuroimaging have established that age influences cerebral ventricle size and type, and that differences between groups need to be determined (Blanco et al., 2003). By optimizing the use of CT and MRI, clinicians can maximize patient selection for therapeutic interventions and improve delivery protocols, ultimately improving clinical outcomes in neurosciences and neurorehabilitation research. (Figure 1.1).

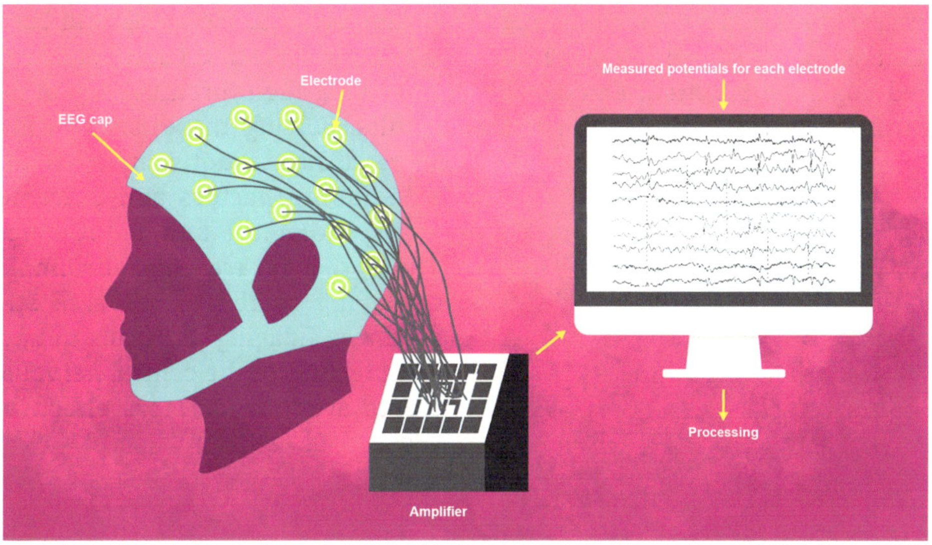

Figure 1.1. Diagram illustrating the physics of MRI: how hydrogen protons behave in a magnetic field. (A) All living tissues have water molecules, two hydrogen nuclei, and one oxygen nucleus. Each hydrogen nucleus consists of a single positive charge, that is, a proton spinning on its axis, which works as a minute magnet. (B) As the person steps into the MRI scanner, the with the direction of the main static magnetic field, B0. Some of the protons will orient "up" or parallel, and some will orient "down" or antiparallel, but still rotating around their axis like a top. (C) When the same frequency RF wave/pulse as that of the precessional frequency of the proton is turned on, the protons oriented upwards flip off from the B0 field and dissipate RF energy.

Source: https://cdn.technologynetworks.com/tn/images/body/neuroimaging-seo-article-fig-11_resized1657187466884.jpg.

1.1.1. Definition of Neuroimaging Methods

Neuroimaging has revolutionized our understanding of the central nervous system, significantly enhancing clinical diagnostics and research capabilities. Two primary modalities—Computed Tomography (CT) and Magnetic Resonance Imaging (MRI)—serve as fundamental tools in neuroimaging. CT utilizes X-ray technology to create cross-sectional images of the brain, making it effective for identifying acute hemorrhages, brain tumors, and other structural abnormalities. It offers rapid imaging, which is crucial in emergency settings. On the other hand, MRI employs strong magnetic fields and radio waves to produce high-resolution images and to provide precise visualization of brain tissue. MRI finds particular utility in assessing soft-tissue differences, i.e., contrast between normal and pathological status, as it provides greater contrast resolution. The choice between CT and MRI may depend on clinical situations in which each is best suited. The development of neuroimaging technology improved diagnostic precision and enabled the exploration of subtle brain structure and function. Novel MRI technologies, including functional MRI (fMRI), help researchers and clinicians to image brain activity by observing changes in blood flow after neural activity. This has illuminated cognitive function, emotional states, and neurotransmission disorders (Figure 1.2).

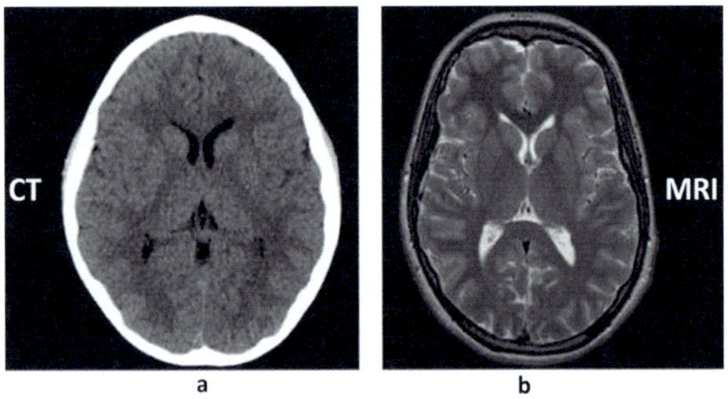

Figure 1.2. Diagram comparing CT and MRI signal contrasts.

Source: https://www.researchgate.net/publication/339429935/figure/fig2/AS:946416839032833@1602654766981/Difference-between-a-MRI-scan-and-a-CT-scan.ppm.

At the same time, diffusion tensor imaging (DTI), an MRI technique, enables white matter tractography, indicating the integrity of neural pathways. The union of these modalities expands our insight on a range of conditions, such as chronic pain syndromes, where deranged brain-bodily interactions can inform therapeutic interventions. Increasing numbers of studies are still using neuroimaging to investigate how structural alterations interact with functional outcomes in the brain, leading to promising treatment and prevention outcomes. Advances as such notwithstanding, there are still challenges in the field of neuroimaging, particularly problems with standardizing procedures and interpreting multifaceted data. As noted, there has been remarkable growth in the development of imaging techniques that quantify structural, functional, and metabolic brain characteristics (Aziz et al., 2019). Nevertheless, harmonization of findings from diverse imaging research is yet to be achieved due to variability in acquisition protocols. Collaborative research, such as the organization of consortia and standardization efforts, is vital to creating stable datasets and improving the reproducibility of neuroimaging results. Solving these issues will allow for a more accurate determination of preclinical vulnerability factors and outcome predictors in psychological and neurological diseases. Thus, the future of neuroimaging lies in deploying combined research strategies and advanced imaging protocols to understand the complexities of the central nervous system and create avenues for more effective treatments (Basu et al., 2018).

1.1.2. Comparison of Imaging Modalities

The advent of several neuroimaging modalities has transformed central nervous system diagnostics to a great extent, particularly with computed tomography (CT) and magnetic resonance imaging (MRI). CT scanning uses X-rays to produce cross-sectional images of the brain, enabling rapid assessment of acute neurological syndromes such as hemorrhages and fractures. This non-invasive technique allows clinicians to visualize bone structures well and is commonly applied in emergency cases due to its rapidity and availability. CT's disadvantage is, however, that there is poorer soft tissue contrast and, as it is ionizing radiation, potential exposure to ionizing radiation, which raises concerns about repeated use in vulnerable groups. On the other hand, MRI uses radio waves and magnetic fields to produce high-resolution images of soft tissues; thus, it is the modality of preference for the diagnosis of disorders such as tumors, multiple sclerosis, and vascular abnormalities (Basu et al., 2018) (Figure 1.3).

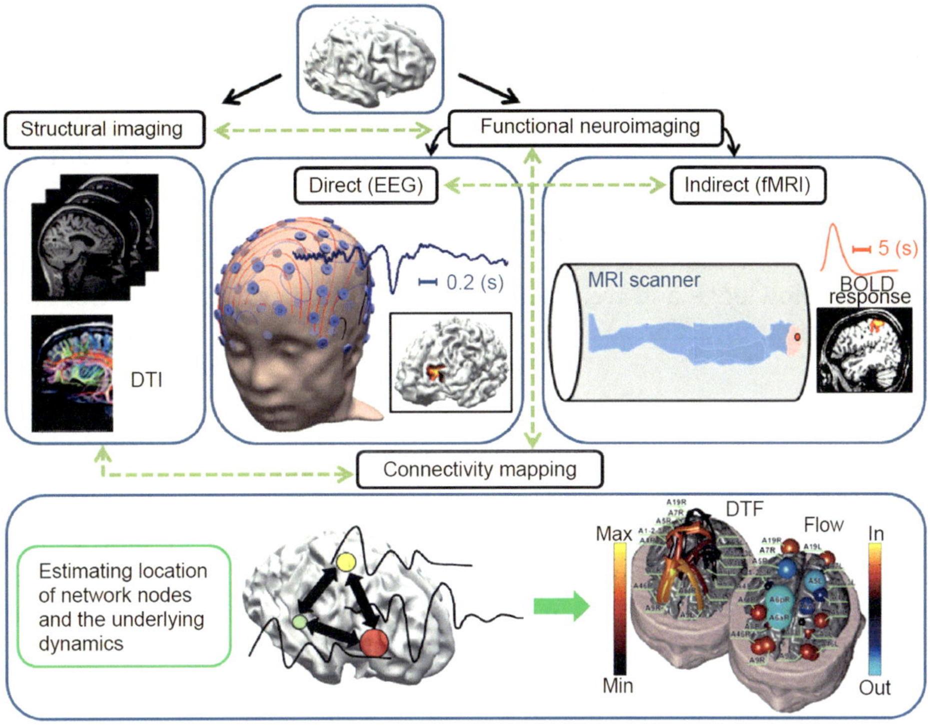

Figure 1.3. Features of major neuroimaging modalities.

Source: https://www.researchgate.net/publication/283753260/figure/fig1/AS:613949510783015@1523388378589/Neuroimaging-at-a-glance-Different-neuroimaging-modalities-interact-with-each-other-to.png.

The differences in the strengths and limitations of these imaging devices underscore the need for proper selection based on clinical scenarios. Clinicians are often faced with challenges in interpreting neuroimaging studies, particularly in considering the minor variation in sensitivity and specificity of CT and MRI. CT imaging is an effective tool for detecting acute hemorrhage, but becomes less useful when it comes to detecting subtle changes in the brain parenchyma. MRI with increased soft tissue contrast is superior to CT for imaging brain anatomy and pathology but perhaps less convenient in the acute environment with longer scan times and susceptibility to motion artifact. Furthermore, certain conditions, such as autoimmune vasculitis, present special challenges to differential diagnosis. Evidence indicates that, although traditional imaging methods are likely to struggle to provide unambiguous diagnoses, newer modalities, such as perfusion brain SPECT, can be helpful in monitoring therapy and evaluating patient responsiveness (Maffione et al., 2015). The strengths and limitations of knowledge can thus help practitioners choose the most appropriate imaging technique for specific cases. In making a comparative analysis of CT and MRI, consideration should be taken of the technological advances as well as the evolving nature of neuroimaging protocols. Advances in MRI technology, such as functional MRI (fMRI) and diffusion tensor imaging (DTI), have broadened its use from purely structural imaging to functional and tractography studies, offering information regarding brain connectivity and activity. Conversely, the rapid development of CT techniques, including dual-energy CT and CT perfusion, aims to enhance diagnostic efficiency while reducing radiation dose. In the emerging future, multimodality imaging approaches may become routine, combining the rapid evaluation potential of CT with the detailed anatomical and functional definition of MRI. This hybridization not only enhances diagnostic precision but also portends greater customized treatment pathways, ultimately leading to better patient outcomes (Basu et al., 2018). Ongoing innovation in imaging modalities will continue to revolutionize our knowledge and treatment of central nervous system disorders.

1.2. Computed Tomography (CT)

Computed Tomography (CT) is the key to neuroimaging diagnosis for diagnosing a wide range of central nervous system pathologies. In this, CT uses X-ray attenuation to produce cross-sectional anatomical images, enabling detailed visualization of brain structures and enabling clinicians to identify abnormalities with great accuracy. Its rapid image acquisition rate makes CT particularly favorable in acute situations, such as the detection of hemorrhagic stroke or traumatic brain injury. Despite advancements in imaging modalities, CT remains a workhorse due to the availability and ease of use, often the first imaging modality before investigation by more advanced methods like MRI. The swift assessment of conditions such as glioblastomas, with an annual incidence of approximately 5.26 cases per 100,000 population, underscores CT's pivotal role in the acute medical environment, rendering it indispensable for immediate clinical management (Omuro, 2013). CT effectiveness in neuroimaging also emerges when its applications in monitoring treatment response for any form of brain tumor and ischemic conditions are considered. For instance, following intervention for glioblastomas, CT can be used to monitor tumor size and complications such as edema or secondary hemorrhage. The CT features of glioblastomas tend to be hyperdense, which is useful for their distinction from other lesions. Although MRI excels in soft-tissue contrast and resolution, CT's ability to provide rapid feedback on tumor response to therapy—especially when paired with contrast agents—demonstrates its enduring value in clinical practice. Recommendations for acute ischemic stroke management also point to the value of CT in initial evaluations because it delineates infarcted areas and better directs treatment protocols (Edward et al., 2013). Additionally, even though CT possesses extreme acute diagnostic power, it is not without some limitations, primarily long-term repercussions regarding radiation exposure. Because of its reliance on ionizing radiation, there has been criticism over the cumulative effects of frequent repetition of CT scans in patients, and the most vulnerable patients are children, who are naturally more susceptible to radiation's adverse effects. As research continues into optimizing imaging techniques and reducing radiation doses, diagnostic efficacy against patient safety becomes more and more a balancing act. In the end, while CT is a staple of neuroimaging, future protocols will depend on continued development and adjunct use with other modalities, for example, MRI, particularly in complex cases such as malignant gliomas, which require multiple specialties for optimal treatment (Omuro, 2013).

1.2.1. Principles of CT Imaging

The fundamental concepts of computed tomography (CT) imaging form the foundation for its application in neuroimaging, particularly in neuroimaging of the central nervous system. CT uses X-ray technology to obtain detailed cross-sectional images of the brain, enabling visualization of anatomical structures and potential pathologies. The process employs a rotating X-ray tube emitting radiation as the patient is placed on a movable table, collecting slices of high-definition pictures. These are reconstructed into a complete view of cranial and spinal anatomy, allowing clinicians to diagnose conditions such as tumors, hemorrhage, and structural defects. The rapid image acquisition also makes CT a valuable tool in emergency settings, where decision speed can make or break patient treatment. One of the advantages of CT imaging is that it can rapidly detect a broad spectrum of conditions. Due to its speed and efficiency, CT is the imaging method of choice in the acute setting, particularly for the diagnosis of stroke or traumatic brain injury. The technology can distinguish between different tissues based on their X-ray attenuation coefficients, which is essential for diagnosing diverse intracranial disease states. Moreover, CT imaging may be supplemented by contrast agents to augment the delineation of tumors or vascular structures. The possibility of doing this is most useful for surgical planning and measuring response to treatment. As an example, studies have proven that the strategic use of high-resolution computed tomography (HRCT) is able to highlight neuroanatomical anomalies that are clinically relevant, especially in patient populations that already have complicating factors, that is, those who require cochlear implants (Aimoni et al., 2015). CT imaging has no limitations at all in its broad spectrum of applications, particularly with respect to radiation exposure. While technological advances have reduced the dose of ionizing radiation applied in scans, there are lingering risks, particularly for vulnerable groups such as children or those requiring repeated imaging tests. CT is also less capable than MRI in creating accurate images of soft tissues, such as central nervous system organs, such as the spinal cord or cranial nerves, and is therefore not suited to certain conditions involving these structures. To this end, integrating CT with other imaging modalities, such as MRI, can yield a more comprehensive evaluation of neuroanatomical structures. Utilizing the modalities in combination enables clinicians to make precise diagnoses and develop treatment plans tailored to the intricacies of each patient's condition, thereby improving patient care overall (Ali et al., 2016) (Figure 1.4).

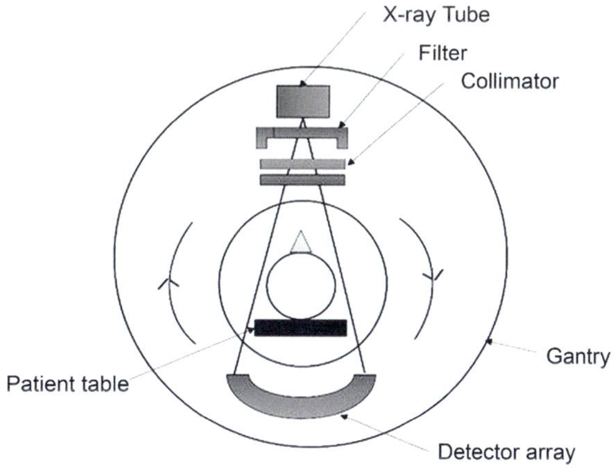

Figure 1.4. Schematic showing CT scanner gantry and rotating X-ray source.

Source: https://cdnintech.com/media/chapter/80151/1512345123/media/F6.png.

1.2.2. Advantages of CT in Clinical Practice

Among imaging approaches in clinical practice, computed tomography (CT) stands out for its rapid acquisition and broad accessibility. The other principal advantage of CT is that it can provide a timely evaluation of acute neurological conditions, especially in emergency cases. For instance, a CT scan plays a crucial role in acute stroke presentations, where it enables the expedited assessment of intracranial hemorrhage and other ischemic insults. Unlike magnetic resonance imaging (MRI), which may be slower and less universally available in every clinical case, CT scans provide clinicians with the ability to make quick decisions regarding patient care and treatment. Expediency of this kind can significantly alter patient outcomes, particularly in cases like stroke, where minutes count in re-establishing blood flow to the damaged brain tissues. Another important advantage of CT is its cost-effectiveness, particularly compared to MRI. The costs of running and equipment for CT tend to be lower, which makes it more appropriate for various healthcare centers, especially in low-budget areas. As illustrated during the period from 1999 to 2008, while MRI utilization increased immensely, CT remained consistently high with negligible fluctuations (92% in 1999 to 95% in 2008) in acute stroke diagnosis utilization (Adams et al., 2012). This cost-effectiveness ensures CT's role as a vital part of diagnostic imaging, allowing many patients access to critical care without the deterrent of prohibitive costs associated with innovative imaging techniques. This aspect of CT is beneficial to healthcare organizations that aim to maximize utilization of resources while not compromising patient care. Also, CT has the flexibility to be used clinically outside neuroimaging, encompassing a wide variety of medical examinations. In trauma, tumor, or infection, the ability of CT to produce sharp, high-resolution cross-sectional images of the brain and its immediate surrounding structures is of immense value. Also, when used with more advanced modalities like CT angiography, it can yield important information about vascular disease, such as aneurysms and vascular malformations. Its inclusion in routine clinical practice enables acomplete evaluation for treatment planning and patient management. With advances in neuroimaging technology, the adjunctive role of CT relative to MRI remains to fulfill the unique needs of diverse patient populations, making it an invaluable modality in modern medicine (Arunogiri et al., 2019) (Figure 1.5).

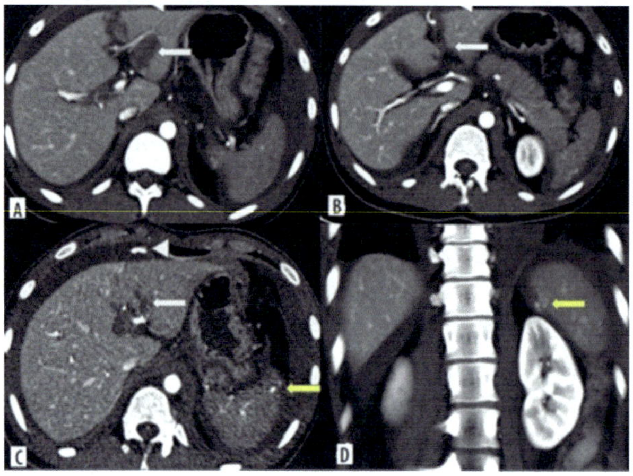

Figure 1.5. CT scan image demonstrating rapid acquisition in trauma.

Source: https://www.polradiol.com/f/pictures/200756_28b34_o.jpg.

1.2.3. Limitations and Risks Associated with CT

Computed tomography (CT) has emerged as a ubiquitous imaging modality in the field of neuroimaging, but its use is not without severe limitations and risks. Perhaps one of the most important disadvantages of CT scanning is the radiation exposure, which may lead to long-term harmful health effects, including an increased risk of cancer. Although technological advancements in CT have endeavored to reduce doses of radiation, cumulative exposure for patients who undergo repeated scans over time can amount to troubling levels. Furthermore, when patients present with overlapping symptoms or disorders, misinterpretation of results is more likely. Such misdiagnoses not only cause delays in treatment but also lead to undue anxiety for patients and their families. As such, a thoughtful risk-benefit assessment is required in determining whether or not to obtain a CT scan, especially among such vulnerable groups as children and those who require repeated imaging. Another significant limitation of CT imaging is its relatively low sensitivity for detecting certain central nervous system disorders compared with MRI. While CT scans provide rapid assessments of acute injuries, they may not detect subtle lesions, particularly inflammatory or infectious lesions in the brain. In central nervous system lymphoma, for instance, CT may yield non-specific findings that undermine proper diagnosis. On the other hand, MRI provides superior soft-tissue contrast, facilitating the visualization of abnormalities such as demyelination or tumor invasion. As the case of Doolittle et al. (2013) illustrates, alternative imaging techniques, such as ultrasound or MRI with contrast agents, for example ultrasmall superparamagnetic iron oxide nanoparticles, may increase diagnostic specificity in some conditions but may not be readily available to all clinics. Limited use of CT in this scenario necessitates careful interpretation and, in some cases, the need to supplement data with other imaging modalities. Additionally, the logistics used in CT scanning also limit it. These scans are often used for time-critical decision-making in emergency care that requires rapid output. Nevertheless, the application of ordinary contrast agents in CT imaging can harm particular groups of patients, including patients with renal insufficiency who are highly susceptible to nephrogenic systemic fibrosis. This condition puts focus on assessing the suitability of patients for CT scans because the risk of reaction to contrast media can lead to further complications. Coordination of neuroimaging protocols with specific patient needs also calls for extensive assessment measures, according to Arunogiri et al. (2019), research integrating neuroscience-informed approaches into clinical practice when addressing addiction. Finally, a greater understanding of patients' medical histories and potential contraindications would be paramount to enhancing the maximum safety and effectiveness of CT scanning in central nervous system disorder diagnosis (Figure 1.6).

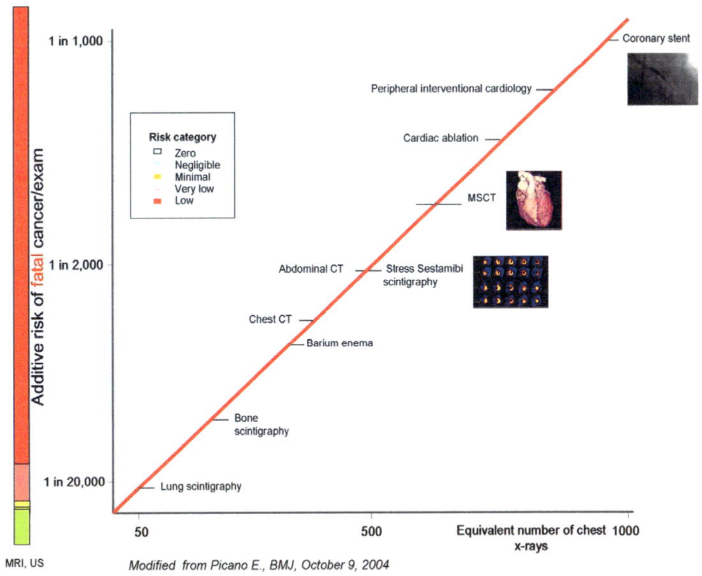

Figure 1.6. Graphic representation of radiation exposure risks from CT.

Source: WHO.int.

1.3. Magnetic Resonance Imaging (MRI)

Magnetic Resonance Imaging (MRI) has revolutionized neuroimaging, yielding images unrivaled in their representation of CNS anatomy and pathology. Unlike computed tomography (CT), which provides only structural information with ionizing radiation, MRI uses powerful magnetic fields and radiofrequency pulses to image soft tissues with high resolution. Being non-invasive, it is also far superior for visualizing complex brain structures and detecting subtle alterations associated with various neurological illnesses. MRI is particularly beneficial for evaluating conditions such as tumors, strokes, and neurodegenerative diseases, facilitating early diagnosis and effective treatment strategies. Furthermore, the ability of MRI to generate multiplanar images enhances its utility in clinical practice and research, positioning it as an essential tool for both neurologists and radiologists in understanding the intricacies of CNS diseases. Advancing MRI technology with the development of ultra-high-field MRI systems has significantly hastened its application in neuroscience. The discovery of 7-Tesla (7T) MRI has become a cutting-edge machine capable of showing cortical details unseen before, even at lower levels of magnetic field strength. According to the North American Imaging in MS Cooperative (NAIMS), the use of 7T MRI is now central to the detection and quantification of pathological features in multiple sclerosis, such as grey matter lesions and central vein sign. The new imaging is not only set to improve diagnostics but also therapeutic follow-up in clinical trials and routine practice. Thus, these technological advances underscore the potential of MRI to facilitate a more sophisticated understanding of CNS illness, which, in turn, will inform individualized treatment modalities and improve patient outcomes (Bagnato et al., 2024).

With the encouraging advances in MRI, however, there are challenges in translating neuroimaging findings into practice. With the gap between neuroscientific inquiry and clinical usefulness still to be bridged, there is a need to develop valid and ecologically valid neuroimaging protocols that translate findings into clinically useful applications. The integration of cognitive tests with neuroimaging, as conceptualized by the studies within the International Society of Addiction Medicine (ISAM), focuses attention on an n-dimensional approach to treating substance use disorders and other cognitive impairments. By enabling collaboration between clinicians and researchers, neuroscience-based interventions can be made more effective and possibly improved assessment and treatment protocols for patients with CNS disorders. It is this collaboration that will enable the full potential of the MRI technology to be used in clinics and provide a platform for ongoing refinement of neuroimaging as a mainstay of modern medicine (Arunogiri et al., 2019).

1.3.1. Principles of MRI technology

MRI technology relies on the inherent properties of atomic nuclei, particularly those of hydrogen, in body tissues due to their high water content. MRI relies on the principle that a strong magnetic field can align the spins of hydrogen nuclei, which are then disrupted by radiofrequency pulses. When the radiofrequency pulse is turned off, the hydrogen nuclei relax back slowly to their original orientation, generating signals that are recorded by the MRI scanner. This creates high-resolution images of structures and tissues in the central nervous system, including tissue differentiation based on their relaxation times—T1 and T2—leading to contrasting effects on the resultant image (Figure 1.7).

One of the most significant aspects of MRI technology is its ability to provide non-invasive observations of the physiological and biochemical conditions of the brain and spinal cord. More advanced MRI techniques, such as quantitative Magnetic Resonance Imaging (qMRI), allow accurate information beyond normal morphological imaging to be recovered. For instance, qMRI can generate quantitative maps that define multiple tissue types, estimate volumes of brain structures, and classify pathology over time. This type of analysis makes it easier for researchers and clinicians to understand complex neurological disorders and track disease development, offering improved diagnosis and prognosis capabilities, particularly with respect to such disorders as spinal cord injury, in which soft-tissue evaluation is so critical (Afshari et al., 2015).

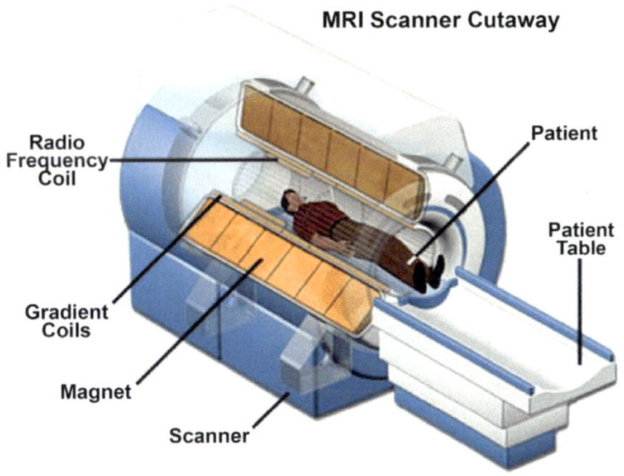

Figure 1.7. MRI machine with labeled components showing superconducting magnet.

Source: https://i.pinimg.com/736x/7a/a4/04/7aa4045c11c9965b90f936218c57ac3e.jpg.

In addition, the application of qMRI has opened up doors to examining subtle changes in brain anatomy that are present in many disorders. By incorporating advanced image processing techniques, clinicians can segment brain tissues and measure volumes, providing an improved description of brain morphology. It has been discovered that an abnormality in structure, such as the deep grey matter, which acts as a relay of brain signals, has been associated with different neurological diseases. These results can assist in advancing our understanding of conditions like Fetal Alcohol Spectrum Disorders (FASD), for instance, by capturing changes in the volume of specific brain areas with age (Yu et al., 2016). Furthermore, the concepts behind MRI technology not only enhance our imaging abilities but also advance neurobiological investigation by rendering intricate brain structure transparent and unlocking insights into the character of disease and health.

1.3.2. MRI Versus CT Advantages

Magnetic Resonance Imaging (MRI) has superior advantages over Computed Tomography (CT) in the assessment of soft tissues of the central nervous system. One of the principal benefits of MRI is its superior tissue differentiation, enabled by its high contrast resolution. MRI, for instance, excels at imaging the brain, spinal cord, and other soft tissues by taking close-up pictures that can detect structural malformations, lesions, and tumors that are not as well detectable on CT scans. This capability is particularly valuable in the diagnosis of conditions such as multiple sclerosis or brain tumors, in which soft tissue characterization can directly affect treatment choices and outcomes. MRI also does not utilize ionizing radiation, another benefit in patient safety terms, and allows repeated imaging without the hazards of radiation exposure that comes with it, and so is a preferable option in children and pregnant patients (Figure 1.8).

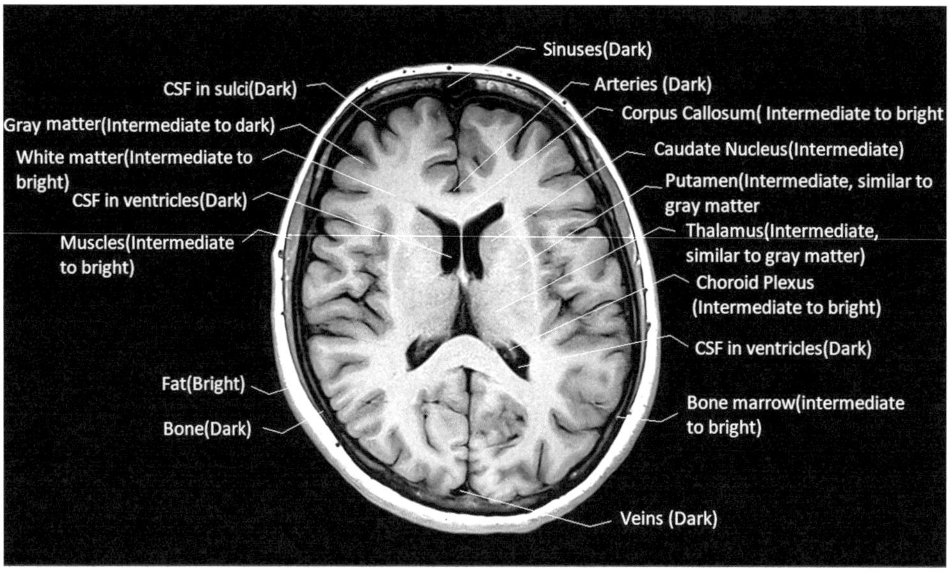

Figure 1.8. Brain MRI image highlighting high contrast of soft tissues.

Source: https://mrimaster.com/wp-content/uploads/2023/09/T1-MRI-appearance-of-various-tissues-in-the-brain-1024x591.jpg.

In addition to tissue differentiation, MRI also possesses outstanding functional imaging capability that provides critical information regarding brain activity and connectivity. Functional MRI (fMRI) is one of the methods that allows researchers and clinicians to investigate real-time changes in blood flow and neural activity and, therefore, measure cognitive and motor function without invasion. This fMRI characteristic is particularly valuable in clinical and research settings, providing a better understanding of psychiatric disease and neurodegenerative illness. Through measurement of activity in the brain for varying states or tasks, fMRI can reveal abnormalities in brain function that are potentially linked to observable behavioral symptoms. Furthermore, the combination of structural and functional imaging provides detailed information that enhances the diagnostic accuracy of various neurological disorders, which is not always possible with CT (Aziz et al., 2019). Furthermore, MRI's ability to obtain multi-parametric data provides a broader level of information that is important in the understanding of complex neuroanatomical structures. A technology breakthrough in MRI, diffusion tensor imaging (DTI), enables neurologists to trace white matter tracts, which could be instrumental in determining connectivity and routes in the brain. This level of specificity is important, especially in cases of traumatic brain injury or stroke, when the integrity of neural pathways would directly correlate with outcomes as well as rehabilitation strategies. Furthermore, the development of standard imaging protocols and computational approaches significantly enhances the interpretation of MRI data to facilitate large-scale studies that determine network attributes and potential biomarkers (Welch et al., 2012). With further advancement of neuroimaging and neuroinformatics technology, the superior advantage of MRI over CT will undoubtedly become central to advancing our understanding of the central nervous system.

1.3.3. Limitations and Risks Associated with MRI

The use of Magnetic Resonance Imaging (MRI) in neuroimaging has revolutionized the understanding of central nervous system illnesses. However, it is essential to determine the limitations and dangers of the imaging method. Among the most significant challenges is that of therapeutic misconception among patients and their parents, particularly children. Parents generally seek the newest technology in the expectation of direct therapeutic benefit for their children, and this can introduce a skewed perception of the research objective.

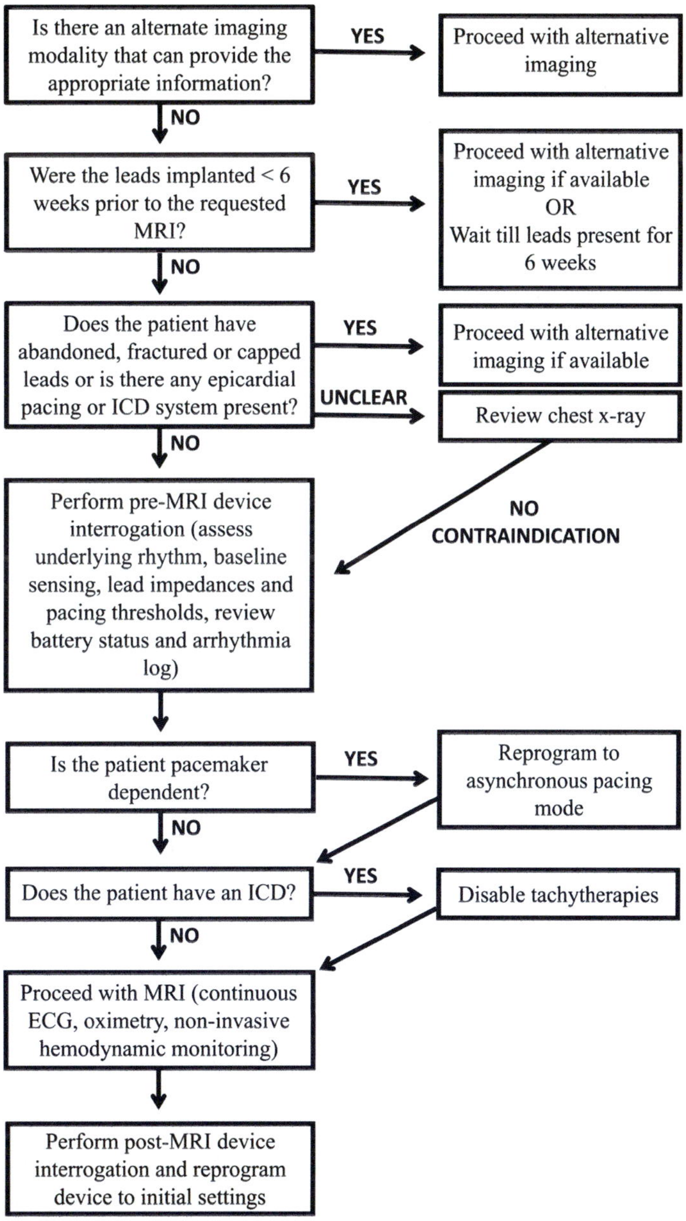

Figure 1.9. Infographic listing MRI contraindications such as pacemakers.

Source: https://www.ajnr.org/content/ajnr/38/12/2222/F2.large.jpg.

Misconception compromises the informed consent process, particularly when enrolling healthy controls or patients with developmental conditions in the expectation of optimistically influencing results in emerging neuroimaging studies. Such circumstances can ultimately undermine the ethical integrity of research and mislead stakeholders about the actual effects of MRI findings (D\u27Arcy et al., 2008). Aside from ethics, the physical constraints of MRI must be taken into account. The procedure is not danger-free, especially to the patient's well-being. The presence of metal implants, such as pacemakers, poses a serious risk when powerful magnetic fields used in MRI scanning are present. Claustrophobia also hinders patient compliance, making it difficult to obtain satisfactory-quality images. Motion artifacts can make MRI ineffective because small movements while the imaging is being done will produce images that are distorted and make diagnosis more difficult. This limitation is especially significant in the pediatric group, where movement is more likely, so in some instances sedation becomes necessary, though with associated risk (Bradford et al., 2018).

Further, interpreting MRI data can be challenging, as anatomical variation and the presence of incidental findings complicate clinical decision-making. Radiologists may be confronted with numerous indeterminate findings that are not immediately correlated to clinical symptoms, leading subsequently to unjustified patient or family distress. The problem is further compounded by the fact that the interpretation of MRI images is operator-dependent and subject to the skill and experience of the radiologists. Hence, even though MRI is a very useful neuroimaging machine, the in-built constraints and risks of its use must be measured accurately in both its application within healthcare settings and its input within research schemes (D'Arcy et al., 2008) (Figure 1.9).

1.4. Clinical Applications of CT

The applications of computed tomography (CT) in neuroimaging have now revolutionized the diagnosis, treatment, and management of numerous central nervous system disorders. CT scans are particularly valuable in the acute environment since they allow for prompt evaluation of such conditions as intracranial hemorrhage, ischemic stroke, and traumatic brain injury. The speed at which CT imaging can be performed makes it a valuable emergency medicine tool, providing clinicians with instant access to information about potentially life-threatening pathologies. The ability to image bone structures also assists in the detection of fractures or abnormalities and complicates neurological examination. Evidence has shown that early CT imaging is significantly associated with improved patient outcomes, especially in stroke care, where every minute counts in restoring cerebral perfusion (Ali et al., 2016).

Aside from emergency settings, CT plays a vital role in the postoperative evaluation of neurosurgical patients. Its ability to produce high-resolution images of brain anatomy enables it to evaluate the integrity of surgical fields and diagnose early complications, such as hematomas or infections. The application of CT angiography enhances its value for cerebrovascular evaluation, aiding in the diagnosis of vascular malformations and guiding therapeutic interventions. As a non-invasive modality, CT puts patients at low risk while acquiring necessary information for effective treatment planning. The integration of CT scans in routine postoperative care best explains its worth in ongoing monitoring of patient recovery, thus treating potential complications before they develop into serious issues (Ali et al., 2016). Furthermore, CT imaging is increasingly being supplemented by technological advances, such as the expansion of dual-energy CT and computer algorithms to enhance image quality and diagnostic sensitivity. These emerging technologies allow for improved differentiation between tissues and the identification of subtle pathologies that would be overlooked on conventional CT scans. Integration of newer algorithms facilitates improved lesion quantification and segmentation, thereby enhancing decision-making at the therapeutic level. With rising strokes still being documented globally, CT's imaging function in prevention and management becomes even more critical. Integration of stroke management concepts with imaging technology can have a crucial impact on patient care, particularly in preventive strategies and risk-factor control.

1.4.1. Use of CT in Acute Trauma Settings

Computed tomography (CT) has revolutionized the assessment of acute trauma patients, particularly in emergency settings where the clock needs to be worked fast. CT scan is preferred because it is able to produce high-quality images of the brain within a matter of a few minutes, allowing rapid assessment of potential intracranial lesions such as hemorrhages, fractures, and contusions. The immediacy of CT scans is imperative in trauma settings where time is a consideration that determines the patient's outcome. CT has been shown to identify life-threatening conditions that may require urgent surgical treatment, enabling clinicians to make optimal treatment decisions. This tool is highlighted by the increasing evidence supporting the use of CT imaging as a routine protocol in the management of trauma, so that clinicians may properly diagnose the severity of neurological injury shortly after the accident has happened, ultimately enhancing survival and recovery patterns of patients who have suffered acute traumatic incidents (Figure 1.10).

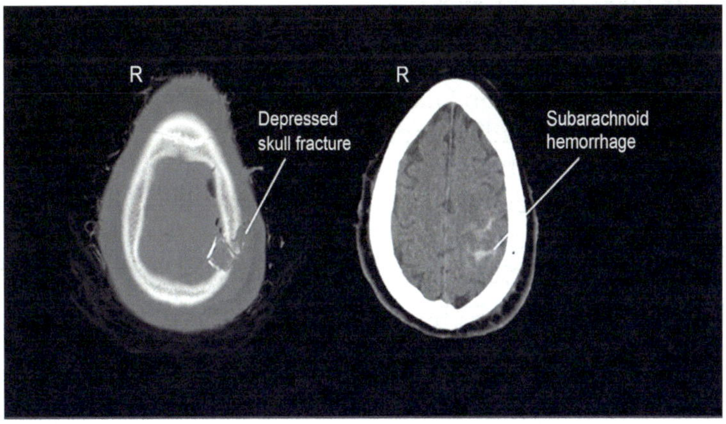

Figure 1.10. Axial CT scan of head trauma showing skull fracture and hemorrhage.

Source: https://d25iein5sonfaj.cloudfront.net/v1/public-drupal-medmastery-assets-production/migrated-images/depressed-skull-fracture-subarachnoid-hemorrhage.png?cfg=eyJ3aWR0aCI6NjAwLCJoZWlnaHQiOjQwMCwib3V0cHV0Ijoid2VicCJ9.

Other than its efficacy and speed, the use of CT in acute trauma also demonstrates to create significant effects on patient management strategies. Other than acute intracranial hemorrhage, CT scanning is a primary diagnostic tool in diagnosing other conditions of immediate threat to life, including spinal trauma and facial fractures, which can be compounded with head trauma. The comprehensive evaluation offered by CT enables an integrated trauma evaluation process, ensuring that every conceivable injury is considered and treated accordingly. Moreover, advances in CT technology have improved image quality while reducing radiation exposure, addressing earlier concerns about safety in imaging trauma. This development is particularly pertinent given the vulnerable condition of trauma patients, some of whom may find themselves spending weeks in the hospital recuperating from their injuries. As such, CT's application in acute trauma keeps advancing and has become a cornerstone of modern emergency healthcare. While CT imaging is prevalent during the initial diagnostic workup of acute trauma patients, its judicious use remains essential. The advantages of CT must be considered against the risk of too much radiation to young or repeatedly scanned patients. Guidelines of the European Resuscitation Council highlight an evidence-based approach to resuscitation and trauma care that includes an adequate imaging strategy (Gavin et al., 2021). This includes not only the use of CT as the primary diagnostic modality but also its integration with clinical assessment and patient history to determine its necessity. Furthermore, in this era of progressive neuroimaging, ongoing research on other modalities, such as advanced MRI technology, can supplement or take over the role of CT in trauma patients. Understanding the intricate dynamics among these technologies will ultimately lead to optimized patient care results in the rapidly evolving field of trauma medicine.

1.4.2. Role of CT in Detecting Tumors

The role of computed tomography (CT) in diagnosing central nervous system (CNS) tumors is integral, as it can provide immediate, accurate imaging. CT scanning uses ionizing radiation to produce cross-sectional images that allow clinicians to visualize structural abnormalities of the brain and spine. CT scanning is particularly useful in emergency settings when time is of the essence, enabling rapid diagnosis and therapy. Studies have proven that CT can detect a variety of tumors ranging from primary malignancies to metastatic lesions as hypo- or hyperdense collections within the brain parenchyma. Additionally, the capability of CT to provide information for biopsies enhances its value in tissue sampling for histological examination, hence considerably influencing management decisions and therapeutic strategies. While CT is an essential first-line tumor detection method, it also finds application in treatment monitoring and detecting tumor recurrence. Enhanced tumor visibility with contrast material enables differentiation between tumors and normal tissue. The latest technology in CT, such as multi-detector CT and perfusion imaging, has significantly improved tumor detection sensitivity and specificity. These developments help radiologists characterize lesions, an essential part of determining appropriate treatment options (Figure 1.11).

Also, the growing convergence of CT with other imaging modalities like MRI provides precise data on tumor behavior, thus maximizing the diagnostic accuracy and therapeutic outcomes. As a result, the overlap between CT imaging and clinical decision-making shifts continuously in CNS tumor treatment. Although there are advantages, CT imaging has limitations that must be appreciated, primarily in soft tissue resolution compared with MRI. Concern regarding CT's exposure to ionizing radiation exists, especially in children or in patients in whom repeated follow-up scans might be necessary. This underlines the need to reserve the use of CT and complement it with MRI, which has improved soft tissue contrast and multi-planar imaging. As technology continues to advance in neuroimaging, new methodologies, such as functional imaging and advanced CT algorithms, will most likely continue to enhance the detection and characterization of tumors. Studies continue to add to the understanding of CNS tumor molecular and biological behavior, observed through findings of atypical presentation, such as with right hemispheric tumors giving rise to new language deficits (Anand et al., 2017) and virus infection giving rise to malignancy (Mailles et al., 2010). Interaction among imaging modalities and clinical data is most crucial in improving patient outcomes in neuro-oncology.

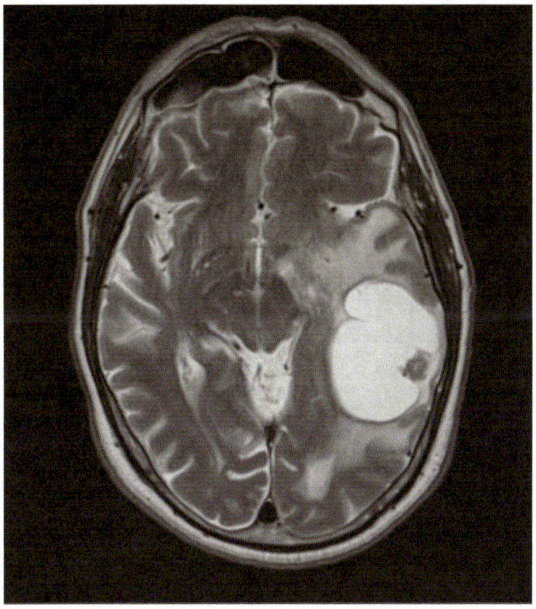

Figure 1.11. Contrast-enhanced CT showing a large frontal brain tumor.

Source: https://prod-images-static.radiopaedia.org/images/24664057/c226c124771bb525888ce739ce4bed_gallery.jpeg.

1.4.3. CT in Evaluating Stroke and Hemorrhage

For the assessment of cerebrovascular insults like hemorrhage and stroke, computed tomography (CT) is a critical tool. The rapidity of imaging of brain structures by CT enables the early diagnosis of acute ischemic strokes and separation from hemorrhagic strokes. The utility of CT is partly because of its velocity, availability, and absence of ionizing radiation in acute settings, and it is now the imaging modality of choice in the majority of hospitals as the first-line imaging. It is this rate, however, that is the major factor, since early treatment can significantly limit the neurological damage of strokes. CT's assistance in emergency neuroimaging has rendered it priceless, where split-second decisions must be made because treatment time is tantamount to determining patient outcome. By establishing the presence or absence of hemorrhage, CT not only guides acute management strategies but also informs patients and families about the nature of the neurological injury. While CT imaging has some advantages, some limitations can affect the diagnostic evaluation in the assessment of strokes. The CT sensitivity for detecting early ischemic changes is much lower than that of magnetic resonance imaging (MRI), particularly in the first few hours after symptom onset. Thus, non-hemorrhagic strokes may go undetected initially and, as a result, there may be potential delays in treatment (Figure 1.12).

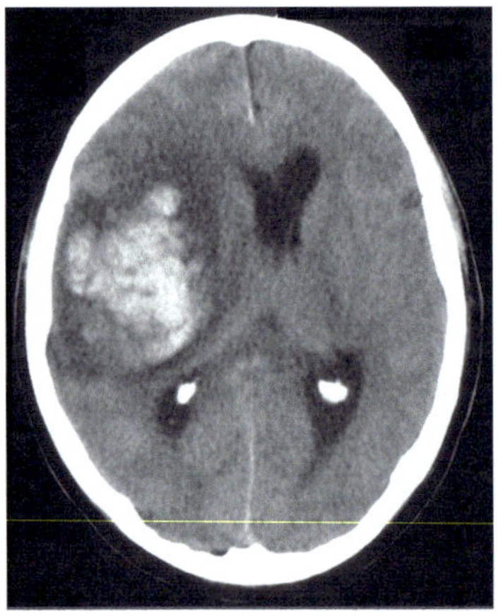

Figure 1.12. CT image illustrating ischemic stroke and hemorrhagic conversion.

Source: https://assets.medlink.com/content/article-media/hcipt3.jpg.

However, the early diagnosis of hemorrhagic strokes is a significant advantage in the sense that it provides vital information for surgical control, as well as surgery if needed. Further, Happonen et al. (2025) suggest that some clinical conditions, such as age and symptoms, can be employed to pre-predict significant findings so that health professionals can establish which patients are most important for further imaging. Thus, while CT has certain strengths, integration with other imaging modalities would be needed for a complete assessment of the patient. Dual imaging of CT and MRI can prove to be advantageous in acute clinical practice for enhancing diagnosis in stroke management. In indeterminate symptoms or when the initial CT is indeterminate, additional MRI may be employed to make the diagnosis or identify complications such as cerebral venous sinus thrombosis, which may not be apparent on CT. MRI's ability to define brain tissue well enables improved comprehension of pathophysiology, especially in ischemic strokes that may develop over time. Also, the significance of keeping in mind the patient's clinical presentation compared to imaging results cannot be overstated; recognition of potential complications, such as those with hematologic malignancies, can enhance the diagnostic workup and treatment plan, according to Annibali et al. (2023). Therefore, the dual-modality application of CT and MRI provides an all-encompassing diagnostic protocol essential for optimizing patient outcomes in stroke and hemorrhage assessment.

1.5. Clinical Applications of MRI

The medical applications of Magnetic Resonance Imaging (MRI) have significantly advanced the neuroimaging discipline, enabling more effective diagnosis and treatment planning of various neurological diseases. MRI offers greater contrast resolution than Computed Tomography (CT) and can identify subtle abnormalities in soft tissues, such as the brain and spinal cord. One of its numerous uses, MRI is a critical diagnostic imaging modality for assessing conditions such as tumors, multiple sclerosis, and stroke. By employing MRI sequences specific to distinct pathologies, doctors can obtain accurate information about anatomical structures and physiologic alterations. For instance, diffusion-weighted imaging (DWI) can swiftly detect acute ischemic stroke, thereby enabling timely intervention. Similarly, MRI is not merely a diagnostic technique but also a tool to follow disease evolution and reaction to therapy, highlighting its central position in the modern neurological practice. Last but not least, functional MRI (fMRI) has transformed our comprehension of brain dynamics and provided insights beyond simple anatomical imaging. fMRI is used to measure brain activity by observing associated changes in blood flow, creating charts of functional areas of the brain responsible for specific cognitive tasks or motor functions. The technology is most valuable in the pre-surgical treatment of tumor or epilepsy patients since it can identify critical areas that must be spared throughout the surgery. The integration of fMRI findings with standard anatomical MRI enhances the ability to see how the various structures of the brain engage and cooperate as an integrated system. Consequently, clinicians can make well-informed decisions that minimize neurological deficits following surgery. The growing visibility of fMRI in clinical environments is a reflection of the continuous evolution of MRI technology and its overarching control over neuroimaging and neurological treatment. In addition to diagnostic and functional applications, MRI is of paramount importance in the intraoperative setting, namely through neurophysiological monitoring modalities. Multimodal real-time intraoperative neurophysiological monitoring (IONM) has proven successful across a wide range of neurosurgeries and has been shown to preserve function and protect against iatrogenic injury to the central and peripheral nervous systems. Monitoring tools such as somatosensory evoked potentials (SSEPs) and electromyography (EMG) provide critical feedback regarding neuronal function during surgery, to allow immediate interventions in case of neurological compromise. The use of IONM, as outlined in clinical findings, reflected that no significant warnings resulted in reversal in operations, which emphasizes its relevance in ensuring patient safety. Hence, clinical applications of MRI far exceed the traditional domains of diagnosis, such as dynamic intraoperative monitoring, which is indispensable for maximizing patient outcomes (Ali et al., 2016). Such broad applications illustrate the critical role of MRI in modern neurology, rendering it a cornerstone of effective patient management (Farooq et al., 2016).

1.5.1. MRI in Diagnosing Multiple Sclerosis

Magnetic Resonance Imaging (MRI) is now the foundation of diagnosing multiple sclerosis (MS), a disease that is chronic in nature and is immune-mediated damage to the central nervous system. The capability of MRI to show detailed images of structures in the brain and spinal cord allows researchers to detect lesions and tissue damage that are characteristic of MS. MRI has traditionally detected hyperintense lesions on T2-weighted images and gadolinium-enhanced lesions, indicating active inflammation. The extreme sensitivity of MRI to alterations in brain tissue enables not only the diagnosis of MS but also the observation of disease progression and the assessment of treatment response.

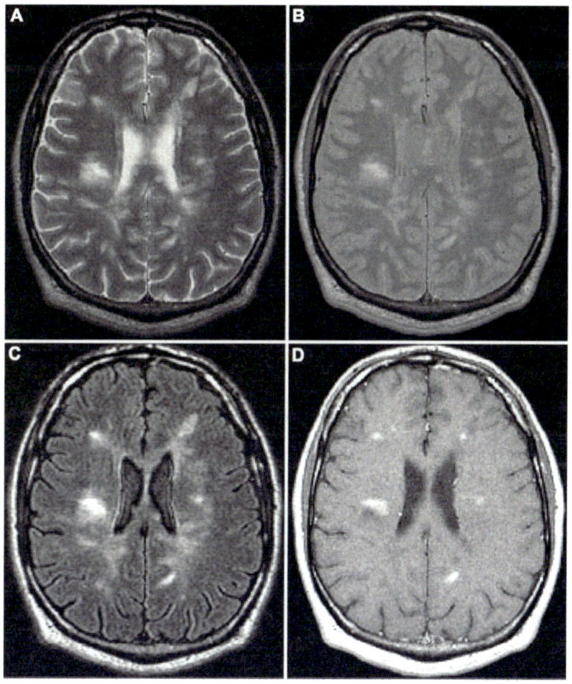

Figure 1.13. T2-weighted MRI showing plaques in multiple sclerosis.

Source: https://jnnp.bmj.com/content/jnnp/76/suppl_3/iii11/F1.large.jpg.

In the face of ongoing technological advancements in MRI, clinicians are increasingly well placed to evaluate the sophistication of MS, enhancing their diagnostic skills and developing patient-tailored management plans to maximize benefits. Aside from detecting active lesions, more advanced MRI techniques, such as quantitative MRI, are becoming increasingly important in the imaging of MS. These include diffusion tensor imaging (DTI) and magnetization transfer imaging (MTI), which provide information on white matter tract integrity and demyelination. Such quantitative measurements have the ability to transcend normal interpretation in the clarification of the disease, such as subtle changes in brain structure before clinical onset (Figure 1.13). Additionally, the use of more advanced MRI distinguishes MS from other neurodegenerative diseases. Visualization of microstructural alterations that occur in neuropsychiatric diseases is very important for proper diagnosis and treatment. Thus, such new techniques accentuate the evolving role of MRI in the comprehensive evaluation of MS patients in the clinical setting. Overall, the use of MRI in the diagnostic workup of multiple sclerosis is a paradigm for neurological medicine. As clinicians embrace the technical advances in MRI, the ramifications for early diagnosis and therapy are all the more profound. The capability to accurately detect and follow MS lesions can not only influence therapeutic intervention but also the quality of the patient's life. Due to the chronicity of MS, interventions at this juncture can lead to better long-term outcomes and adherence to therapeutic regimens. Further research into MRI applications in MS can also enhance diagnostic criteria and predictive models and steer patients toward appropriate treatment in a timely manner. With advances in medical science further elucidating the intricacies of MS, the role of MRI as a monitoring and diagnostic procedure remains key to developing innovative patient care approaches (Bargalló Alabart et al., 2017; Ciesielski et al., 2010).

1.5.2. MRI Application to Brain Tumors

In the past decade, magnetic resonance imaging (MRI) has emerged as the gold standard for the evaluation and follow-up of brain tumors. It is not invasive, with better soft tissue contrast, which allows for accurate visualization of intra- and extra-axial lesions. MRI is most helpful in characterizing the types of tumors since it can highlight certain features, such as edema, necrosis, and enhancement patterns, that are commonly associated with specific types of tumors. This subtle radiological characteristic assists clinicians in developing appropriate treatment plans. MRI also enables observation of the response of tumors to therapy on a temporal scale, which is an extremely important consideration in the management of malignant lesions (Figure 1.14).

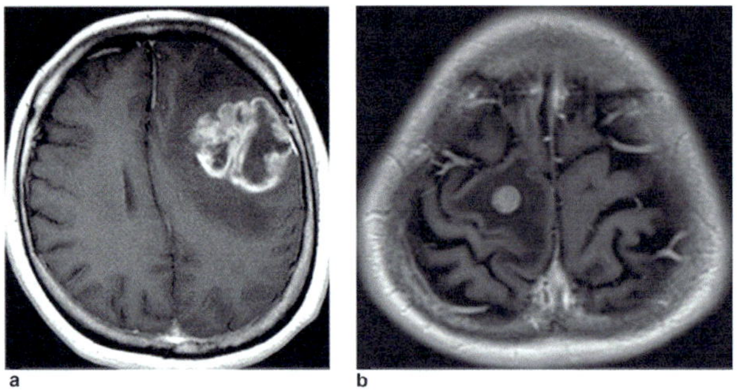

Figure 1.14. MRI scan with contrast showing irregular glioblastoma margins.

Source: https://www.i-mri.org/ArticleImage/1040IMRI/imri-25-23-g001-l.jpg.

The ability to perform dynamic imaging studies, like functional MRI and diffusion tensor imaging, provides additional dimensions of information critical to neurosurgical planning and intervention and renders MRI an invaluable resource to contemporary neuro-oncology. One of the most important advantages of MRI with brain tumor imaging is its ability to follow progression and response to treatment without exposing patients to ionizing radiation. This is particularly vital for patients who may require repeated imaging scans during the course of their treatment. For instance, pediatric patients are more susceptible to the delayed effects of ionizing radiation, and MRI is a more appropriate choice than CT scans. Furthermore, advances in MRI technology, such as MR spectroscopy and perfusion imaging, provide better insight into brain tumors, providing information on metabolic activity and vascularity. Such capabilities facilitate healthcare professionals to make more informed judgments regarding the timing of surgery and adjuvant therapy. In this manner, not only is MRI application enhanced in terms of diagnostic sensitivity, but it also becomes a key factor in the optimization of patient management plans within the context of neuro-oncology. In addition, familiarity with the genetic origin of certain brain tumors, such as those seen in Neurofibromatosis Type 1 (NF1), is crucial for adequate care of patients. MRI can detect incidental findings in patients with this genetic disorder, like minimal pontine lesions that do not always appear with severe symptoms. These are the types of findings as observed in familial NF1, where MRI has demonstrated differences in phenotype, which highlight the necessity for certain methods in managing brain tumors. Also, ongoing research into the genetic mutation in NF1 underscores the need for multidisciplinary collaboration among radiologists, oncologists, and geneticists. Through this collaborative effort, the evolving landscape of genetics and neuroimaging will continue to illuminate the area of brain tumors and treatment, ultimately leading to improved patient outcomes. This integrated approach ensures that neuroimaging remains the central contribution to the diagnosis and treatment of diseases of the central nervous system, as well as for complicated disorders such as those with (Bozzao et al., 2013) and (Ali et al., 2016).

1.5.3. MRI Assessment in Neurodegenerative Diseases

Magnetic Resonance Imaging (MRI) is critical for assessing neurodegenerative diseases, as it is a non-invasive imaging test that provides superior information on structural and functional alterations in the brain. Neurodegenerative illnesses like Alzheimer's and Parkinson's disease often present early in the form of tiny morphological alterations that can be detected on MRI. Early alterations often consist of atrophy of some brain regions, particularly the hippocampus in the case of Alzheimer's. Such changes may not yet be detectable clinically, but MRI gives an enormously valuable technique of making the diagnosis early and starting treatment. By expanding the ability to envision such changes, MRI enables clearer understanding of disease progression, thereby enabling early intervention and improved patient outcomes (Figure 1.15).

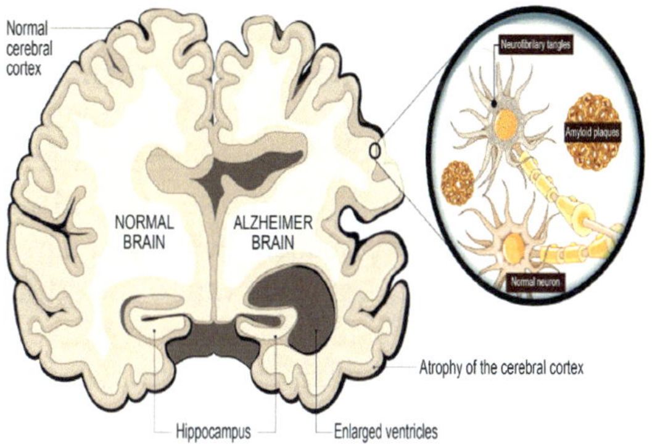

Figure 1.15. MRI images comparing a normal brain with a Alzheimer's-affected brain.

Source: Alzheimer's association.

In neurodegenerative disorders, MRI is unique not only in its structural imaging but also in its ability to assess functional changes with advanced modalities such as diffusion tensor imaging (DTI) and functional MRI (fMRI). These modalities define white matter integrity and local brain activity, which underpin the pathophysiology of dementia and cognitive impairment. For instance, DTI can detect microstructural changes in white matter tracts that correlate with cognitive impairment and other clinical symptoms. In contrast, resting-state fMRI is increasingly being used to examine functional connectivity between brain regions, enabling researchers and clinicians to identify patterns associated with a range of neurodegenerative disorders. All this sophisticated imaging provides greater insight into the nature of these diseases in the brain, more than structural atrophy alone. The integration of MRI findings with clinical evaluation enhances discrimination between various neurodegenerative conditions and, hence, treatment plans in focus. With dementia on the rise, an accurate Alzheimer's disease diagnosis, as compared to other forms of dementia, has direct care and management implications. In research, it is feasible to correlate patterns of atrophy and functional connectivity with various neurodegenerative diseases to enhance diagnosis. It has been found that shrinkage in specific regions of the brain, such as the temporal lobe in Alzheimer's and substantia nigra in Parkinson's, might lead to more intricate understandings of the course and clinical progression of each disease. With advancements in MRI technology, its application to the study of the complexities of neurodegenerative diseases will enhance clinical practice and knowledge of these complex disorders (Ciesielski et al., 2010; Eberling et al., 1995).

1.6. Future Directions in Neuroimaging

The future of neuroimaging looks set for great leaps, specifically with advances from developments in diffusion-weighted MRI (DW-MRI). This technique is gaining favor for its ability to visualize and analyze the structure of white matter in the brain. Using fiber tracking algorithms, physicians can model white matter tract paths, enabling better definition of tumor margins during resections for tumors such as gliomas. The combination of DW-MRI with treatment planning tools allows researchers to create maps of white matter path length, personalized to predict the migration patterns of cancer cells. This technology is important because it can make radiation therapy more efficient by minimizing exposure to healthy tissues and maximizing treatment of migrating tumor cells. These advancements depict the potential of neuroimaging technologies to revolutionize treatment protocols, significantly enhancing patient outcomes, as noted in (Amirbekian et al., 2019). Moreover, research into the implications of neuroimaging extends beyond tumor therapy to become an exploration of uncovering complex disorders associated with obesity and reward circuitry in the brain. Recent studies have indicated alterations in the structural and functional connectivity of regions that are part of reward systems, particularly in individuals with higher body mass indices (BMI). Findings have indicated that individuals with higher BMI have remarkable alterations in the structure in regions such as the nucleus accumbens (NAcc) compared to their non-obese counterparts.

Such individuals also exhibit distinct patterns of functional connectivity, which indicate involvement of the NAcc in aberrant food consumption behaviors. As researchers attempt to further delineate such associations, neuroimaging is increasingly becoming a valuable asset both for diagnosis and for determining the intricate relationships among structure, function, and behavioral outcomes (Ashe-McNalley et al., 2015). Future research integrating neuroimaging modalities such as CT and MRI with advanced computational techniques remains an exciting prospect. Integration of machine learning models into neuroimaging analysis has the potential to enhance diagnostic precision and interpretation of brain pathology.

This cross-disciplinary area can be translated into real-time imaging and automated interpretation of findings, leading to more individualized medicine strategies. The ability to integrate neuroimaging findings with genetic and clinical data can provide insights into specific neurobiological mechanisms underlying various neurological disorders. As the discipline progresses, interdisciplinary collaboration among neuroimaging experts, clinicians, and computational scientists will be essential to building our understanding of the central nervous system and to optimizing therapeutic opportunities for patients afflicted with a broad range of diseases.

1.6.1. Advances in Imaging Technology

The rapid advancement in imaging technology, particularly in magnetic resonance imaging (MRI) and computed tomography (CT), has revolutionized the field of neuroimaging, enabling clearer insight into the central nervous system. These modalities provide high-resolution, detailed images of the brain's structures that assist in the diagnosis and treatment of neurological conditions. CT scans utilize X-rays to build cross-sectional pictures of the brain to identify acute hemorrhages, tumors, and other structural abnormalities.

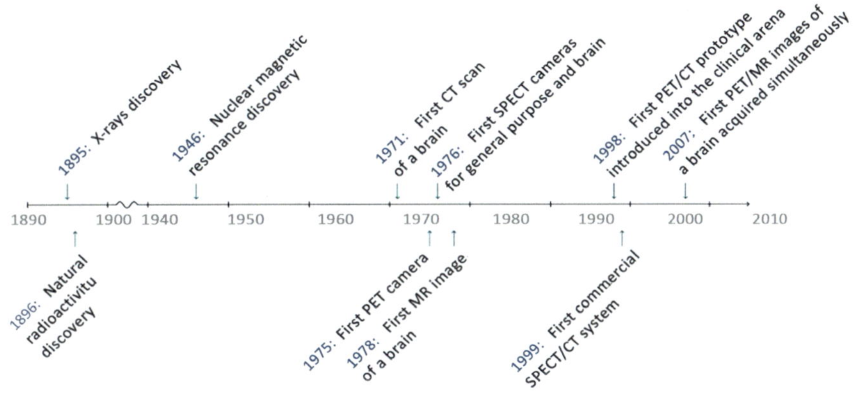

Figure 1.16. Timeline chart showing the evolution of neuroimaging hardware.

Source: https://www.ncbi.nlm.nih.gov/books/NBK597488/bin/515045_1_En_8_Fig1_HTML.jpg.

MRI uses strong magnetic forces and radio waves to create detailed images without ionizing radiation and is particularly suitable for imaging soft tissues and minor neurological changes. The development of advanced techniques such as functional MRI (fMRI) and diffusion tensor imaging (DTI) further increases the capability of MRI to examine brain activity and neural pathway integrity. Beyond enhancing the potential of diagnosis, progress in imaging technologies has significantly impacted treatment planning and monitoring of patients with neurological disorders. For instance, neuroimaging is critical in pre-surgical assessments, allowing clinicians to image important brain regions so that the risk of injury to functional areas during surgery is reduced. In addition, ongoing research into integrating artificial intelligence and machine learning with imaging modalities may simplify image analysis, accelerate diagnosis, and personalize treatment planning (Figure 1.16). These innovations are particularly relevant in neurodegenerative disease, where early intervention can improve patient outcomes. High-resolution imaging, for example, as provided by HRCT and MRI, is essential to identifying abnormalities that can preclude successful surgical intervention, such as in findings of cochlear implantation outcomes in children with neurological abnormalities (Aimoni et al., 2015). Moreover, the impact of imaging technology extends beyond treatment and diagnosis into research and has profoundly affected our understanding of neurodegenerative disorders. Higher-level neuroimaging has in recent years been used to uncover the distinctive structural and functional abnormalities that are associated with various forms of dementia, including those due to Alzheimer's disease and alcohol. MRIs ability to detect atrophy within specific areas of the brain has helped to determine the clinical presentation of different dementias and allows researchers to separate their causes based on neuroimaging findings. This has not only improved classification by diagnosis but has also improved prognostic indicators, allowing intervention strategies to be tailored more effectively to individuals (Eberling et al., 1995). With advancing imaging technology, its use in clinical practice and research will definitely increase, leaving doors open for new methods in managing central nervous system disorders.

1.6.2. Integration of AI in Neuroimaging

The use of artificial intelligence (AI) in neuroimaging significantly enhances the potential for early diagnosis and investigation of a wide range of neurological diseases. Routine imaging methods such as computed tomography (CT) and magnetic resonance imaging (MRI) provide vital information about the anatomy of the central nervous system, but may be time-consuming and interpreter-dependent. AI technology, particularly machine learning- and deep learning-based, has been promising for image interpretation, thereby simplifying radiologists' work and improving diagnostic accuracy. These automated systems can learn from vast amounts of data, refining their predictive functions continuously, which is particularly beneficial for identifying underlying abnormalities that may not show up in run-of-the-mill screenings (Figure 1.17).

As neuroimaging advances, AI integration will be crucial to changing how practitioners formulate diagnoses and develop treatment plans in neurology. Moreover, the application of AI in neuroimaging not only includes image interpretation but also has an important role in unraveling neurophysiological factors involved in occupational stress and burnout. Recent studies have identified growing evidence that uses neuroimaging techniques, such as functional MRI (fMRI) and electroencephalography (EEG), to examine the neurobiological processes underlying stress-related illnesses. By using computational models founded on AI, scientists can code complex patterns of information and reveal neurophysiological biomarkers that differentiate burnout from depression.

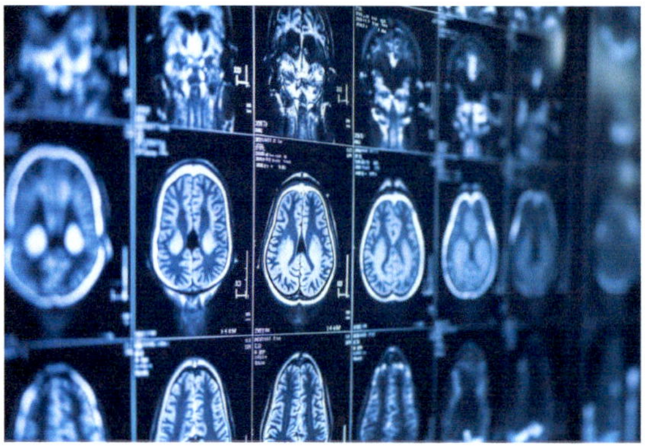

Figure 1.17. Concept image of AI detecting abnormalities in brain scans.

Source: https://neurosciencenews.com/files/2024/10/ai-mri-neurology-neuroscience.jpg.

The ability to correlate these findings with clinical presentation enhances diagnostic specificity and offers new therapeutic avenues better adapted to the individual neurobiological profile. As scientists continue to delve deeper into such integrative approaches, the convergence of AI and neuroimaging can redefine our understanding of mental health disorders and their impact on the central nervous system (Mailles et al., 2010; Masiak et al., 2023). Lastly, AI's ability to integrate data from various neuroimaging modalities is a significant step forward. Integrative analysis involving data from CT, MRI, and PET scans enables whole-brain health and disease monitoring. By employing AI to build multimodal classifiers, clinicians can create more nuanced methods for diagnosis and treatment. For instance, AI can interpret the relationship between structural and functional imaging data to better predict disease patterns and treatment outcomes. With ongoing research, the marriage of AI with neuroimaging technology will not only enhance the diagnostic process but also enable approaches to prevention and early intervention, changing the field of neurological care and opening the doors to personalized treatment pathways (Masiak et al., 2023).

1.6.3. Potential of Personalized Medicine in CNS Disorders

The introduction of personalized medicine into CNS disease is a paradigm shift in models of psychiatric and neurological treatment. Universal one-size-fits-all approaches are often ineffective at delivering effective interventions because they cannot address the diverse neurobiological profiles of individual patients. Neuroimaging techniques such as CT and MRI play an important function in describing these differences between individuals by charting the structural and functional characteristics of the brain. Their ability to identify individual CNS biomarkers makes it possible for clinicians to tailor interventions closely to the neurological and psychological needs of patients. Along with developing research, conjoining behavioral assessments with neuroimaging may increasingly tailor therapy, thereby optimizing total treatment in conditions like depression and anxiety, which tend to co-exist with most neurological diseases, thereby offering some routes for specific therapies (Abelson et al., 2020). The investigation of neuroimaging's role as a personalized medicine tool goes beyond its mere utility for diagnosis; it provides information on how treatment works and if treatment is effective (Figure 1.18).

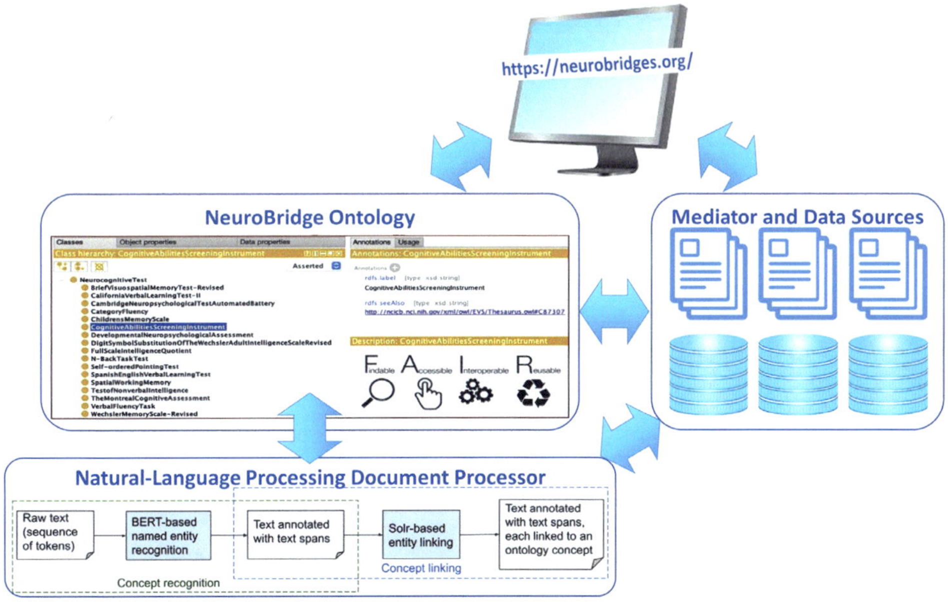

Figure 1.18. Personalized neuroimaging dashboard interface prototype.

Source: https://www.frontiersin.org/files/Articles/1215261/fninf-17-1215261-HTML/image_m/fninf-17-1215261-g001.jpg.

For instance, studies combining structural and functional neuroimaging have begun to elucidate the neurological underpinnings of cognitive changes described in patients with CNS disorders. These kinds of imaging modalities allow for the detection of structural and functional changes to the brain that could be linked to the cognitive impairments often described in relation to specific therapies. A focus on neurobehavioral aspects, such as approach-avoidance behaviors derived from brain functioning, could enhance the efficacy of treatment personalization by determining which patients can benefit most from specific treatment interventions. Placing these findings within clinical practice, neuroimaging does not just progress the understanding of the patient's condition but also improves the precision of interventions, aligning with the objectives of personalized medicine (de Ruiter et al., 2013). In addition, integrating machine learning algorithms with neuroimaging data is a promising approach to developing personalized treatment protocols for CNS diseases. Through the utilization of large datasets from various populations, researchers can establish intricate patterns and precision of treatment outcome. This is particularly beneficial in the context of generalized anxiety disorder, where particular markers of neurobehavior might inform clinicians about the likely efficacy of varied therapeutic approaches. The synergy between neuroimaging and machine learning has the potential to result in a unifying paradigm that reconciles genetic, environmental, and neurobiological determinants of patient outcomes. These advances not only facilitate the development of more refined understanding of CNS disorders but also set the stage for innovative, tailored treatment regimens that leverage neuroimaging technologies to the fullest extent, bringing the field closer to the promise of personalized medicine in psychiatry and neurology (Abelson et al., 2020).

SUMMARY

In conclusion, advances in neuroimaging technology, namely computed tomography (CT) and magnetic resonance imaging (MRI), have transformed our understanding of the central nervous system (CNS). Both modalities enable visualization of both structural and functional brain components, thereby significantly contributing to the comprehension of a variety of neurological disorders. As has been demonstrated in current studies, the integration of neuroimaging along with other clinical data has been effective in identifying certain brain signatures behind conditions such as irritable bowel syndrome (IBS). The finding helps to show the non-linear communication between the brain and gut and points toward the need to further study such complex relationships in CNS pathology (Aziz et al., 2019). Besides that, neuroimaging is crucial in optimizing outcomes for patients undergoing such interventions as cochlear implantation. The identification of anatomical defects in the inner ear and brain using high-resolution CT and MRI exemplifies the critical importance of accurate diagnosis in determining the outcome of such interventions. The results suggest that the knowledge of any underlying brain abnormalities can inform clinical decisions, particularly in assessing candidates for cochlear implants (Aimoni et al., 2015). Thus, neuroimaging is not just crucial to the comprehension of brain anatomy but also to the best choice of treatment strategies for individuals with hearing impairment. In conclusion, the use of CT and MRI together in clinical neuroimaging is a milestone towards a more holistic neurological well-being. The combination of imaging data with genetic and clinical assessment is the kind of multidisciplinary activity to enhance patient care and prognostic capability. To advance research, the creation of standardized protocols for data collection and analysis is required to enable collaborative research at the multi-institutional level. An emphasis on cooperative quest for knowledge by consortia and data repositories will not only drive innovations in neuroimaging but also facilitate a better understanding of the CNS, leading to improved patient outcomes in a range of neurological disorders (Aziz et al., 2019; Aimoni et al., 2015).

CLOSER LOOK

Neuroimaging techniques such as computed tomography (CT) and magnetic resonance imaging (MRI) have revolutionized the diagnostic process and management of central nervous system (CNS) disorders. Imaging technology is of paramount importance in providing accurate estimates of the brain structures, and by using these images, identification of acute and chronic diseases such as strokes, tumors, and neurodegenerative disorders becomes feasible. Advances in imaging acquisition strategies and computational algorithms have dramatically enhanced our ability to analyze complex data sets, enabling researchers and clinicians to identify network features of the brain. This neuroimaging advance is both quantitative and qualitative, as the integration of imaging modalities enables the creation of comprehensive profiles of brain pathology and function, which are essential for optimizing targeted therapeutic interventions. Improved understanding of neuroimaging in recent years is particularly beneficial to the situation of clarifying brain-gut interactions. A combination of structural, functional, and metabolic imaging modalities has enabled clarification of the means by which gut health impacts mental health disorders such as irritable bowel syndrome (IBS). Of special interest has been the capacity of neuroimaging to define neural signatures for IBS that are akin to other chronic pain syndromes with implications for commonalities regarding mechanisms involved. However, despite these advances, there remain challenging issues in defining preclinical vulnerability factors and outcome predictors. Furthermore, the realization of multisite partnerships to harmonize imaging protocols and offer large-scale archives of neuroimaging data will be central to further establishing these intricate interactions that underlie numerous CNS disorders (Aziz et al., 2019). The application of sophisticated imaging in stroke research underscores its value in enhancing both clinical and pre-clinical understanding. The traditional imaging modalities not only exclude non-stroke structural lesions but also allow determination of brain vascular condition, essential for early intervention in ischemic stroke. Further, the use of more advanced imaging modalities, such as angiography and penumbral imaging, offers a translational tool that optimizes trial recruitment and identification of responders to treatment. Despite the fact that there are some limitations, such as increased rates of exclusion and decreased patient enrollment in trials, the benefits of advanced imaging in terms of providing mechanism-based information and permitting real-time assessment of interventions plainly outweigh such limitations (Macrae et al., 2016). As neuroimaging technology continues to advance, the potential to improve treatment strategies will definitely optimize patient outcomes across a broad spectrum of neurological diseases. In neuroimaging, the choice of imaging modality significantly impacts diagnostic accuracy and treatment planning. The decision between magnetic resonance imaging (MRI) and computed tomography (CT) is clinically difficult due to their differences in imaging central nervous system (CNS) structures. CT is largely selected due to availability and speed, particularly in emergency departments for the assessment of acute conditions such as hemorrhagic strokes. However, MRI provides improved soft tissue contrast and thus is required for conditions such as tumors, demyelinating processes, and other CNS pathologies. The selection of the appropriate imaging modality rests finally in the clinical context, patient age, and personal diagnostic need, thereby stressing the need for clinicians to be well aware of the limitations and advantages of each modality. Moreover, the selection of an inappropriate imaging modality can lead to misdiagnosis and inappropriate treatment. Inappropriate imaging can potentially mask significant findings, leading to delay and further jeopardizing outcomes. For instance, in the assessment of stroke, incorrect initial imaging will result in failure to detect ischemic events, an error that can be life-threatening if not corrected in a timely manner. The American Heart Association emphasizes the importance of integrating clinical criteria and modern neuroimaging techniques to facilitate accurate characterization of the cerebrovascular disease spectrum (N/A). Therefore, protection of patient health relies heavily on the correct selection of neuroimaging strategies, selecting the modality according to clinical presentations so that the diagnostic accuracy is enhanced, as well as therapy planning. Besides enhancing diagnostic performance, the right imaging modality will also enable effective patient management and subsequent follow-up. For example, MRI application in CNS disease longitudinal studies explains the pattern of treatment response and disease progression from subtle changes in anatomy. The development in imaging modalities, such as hybrid ones, such as PET-CT, once more highlights the expanding capability for simultaneous functional and structural evaluation, which is ever important in oncology and neurology (Alavi et al., 2009). These methods increase diagnostic accuracy and offer prognostic information useful in formulating individualized treatment plans. The prospect of the future of neuroimaging in medicine is brightening with spectacular growth based on the development of computed tomography (CT) and magnetic resonance imaging (MRI). They promise increased resolution, decreased acquisition time, and improved patient safety, all of which are essential for successful diagnosis and treatment planning of neurological disorders.

With improved neuroimaging, its role in the early diagnosis of conditions such as acute stroke will become more pivotal. For instance, the use of multimodal imaging methods has already revolutionized how practitioners diagnose infarcts and hemorrhages in the central nervous system, highlighting the importance of high-quality imaging in selecting therapeutic options. These advancements can also become the standard checks of silent strokes, which are risky but underrated. Hence, neuroimaging will remain an essential role in deciding early intervention and positive patient outcomes in the years to come (Cheung et al., 2014). Combining artificial intelligence (AI) and machine learning with neuroimaging is another new wave that holds a high potential for the healthcare sector. By analyzing big data generated from neuroimaging studies, AI applications can diagnose diseases more accurately and faster than conventional methods. These technologies have the potential to assist in creating personalized treatment plans by identifying faint patterns in neuroimaging data that would indicate disease progression or drug susceptibility. In addition, as health care systems increasingly recognize the need for equal access to neuro-oncology treatment, integrating advanced neuroimaging with AI may help reduce some of the gaps currently seen in treatment outcomes. Closing these gaps is particularly urgent for countries such as Sub-Saharan Africa, where there are limited health care resources (Banson et al., 2024). The future promise of AI-aided neuroimaging to drive improved diagnostics and treatment delivery could be a paradigm shift in a new health equity for a diverse population. Finally, the future implications of neuroimaging extend beyond diagnostics, with additional studies continuing to demonstrate the significant contribution of imaging approaches to elucidating brain health and disease. The capability to image intricate brain anatomy and functional processes in real time will not only enhance diagnosis but also enable monitoring of disease progression and response to treatment. As the science continues to mature, collaborative ventures between radiologists and neurologists will be required to optimize imaging protocols and review studies. Furthermore, studies investigating the integration of neuroimaging data with clinical data could enable a more holistic strategy to patient care. This cohesive perspective is imperative, especially as we proceed towards a prevention- and precision-medicine-oriented healthcare model. Finally, technological advances in neuroimaging will definitely shape the direction of future healthcare, emphasizing its critical role in improving neurological health outcomes (Cheung et al., 2014; Banson et al., 2024).

REFERENCES

1. Santiago, J., Akeman, E., Kirlic, N., Clausen, A. N., Cosgrove, K. T., McDermott, T. J., Mathis, B., Paulus, M., Craske, M. G., Abelson, J., Martell, C., Wolitzky-Taylor, K., Bodurka, J., Thompson, W. K., & Aupperle, R. L. (2020). Protocol for a randomized controlled trial examining multilevel prediction of response to behavioral activation and exposure-based therapy for generalized anxiety disorder. *Trials*, *21*(1), 17. https://doi.org/10.1186/s13063-019-3802-9Adams, R. J., Albers, G. W., Anthony, A. S., Barber, P. A., Brazzelli, M., Bryan, R. N., et al. (2012). Wide variation and rising utilization of stroke magnetic resonance imaging: Data from 11 states. https://deepblue.lib.umich.edu/bitstream/2027.42/90061/1/22698_ftp.pdf (accessed on 15th July 2025).
2. Afshari, D., Farzizadeh, M., Fatehi, D., Mirfendereski, M., & Fattahi, A. (2015). Traumatic spinal cord injury; theragnostic applications of advanced MRI techniques. https://core.ac.uk/download/143841198.pdf (accessed on 15th July 2025).
3. Aimoni, C., Busi, M., Calzolari, F., Castiglione, A., Ormitti, F., & Tognola, G. (2015). Cochlear implant outcomes and genetic mutations in children with ear and brain anomalies. https://core.ac.uk/download/53523126.pdf (accessed on 15th July 2025).
4. Alavi, A., & Basu, S. (2009). Revolutionary impact of PET and PET-CT on the day-to-day practice of medicine and its great potential for improving future health care. https://core.ac.uk/download/268440994.pdf (accessed on 15th July 2025).
5. Ali, L., Binish, T., Iqrar, A., Karim, M., & Khan, M. (2016). Utility of intraoperative neurophysiological monitoring (IONM) in various surgeries at a tertiary care hospital in Karachi, Pakistan. https://core.ac.uk/download/47264786.pdf (accessed on 15th July 2025).
6. Amirbekian, B., Braunstein, S., Chapman, C., Henry, R. G., Tward, D. J., & McConnell, K. (2019). An open-source tool for anisotropic radiation therapy planning in neuro-oncology using DW-MRI tractography. https://core.ac.uk/download/323063235.pdf (accessed on 15th July 2025).
7. Anand, N., Horner, N., Prater, S., Wei, X., & Nelson, S. J. (2017). Crossed aphasia in a patient with anaplastic astrocytoma of the non-dominant hemisphere. https://core.ac.uk/download/129192526.pdf (accessed on 15th July 2025).
8. Annibali, O., Bernetti, C., Castiello, G., Gangemi, E., Mallio, C. A., Parizel, P. M., Quattrocchi, C. C., et al. (2023). Neuroradiology of acute pathologies in adults with hematologic malignancies: A pictorial review. https://core.ac.uk/download/599505088.pdf (accessed on 15th July 2025).
9. Arunogiri, S., Baldacchino, A., Bates, M. E., Bowden-Jones, H., Lubman, D. I., & Verdejo-García, A. (2019). A roadmap for integrating neuroscience into addiction treatment: A consensus of the Neuroscience Interest Group of the International Society of Addiction Medicine. https://core.ac.uk/download/286356092.pdf (accessed on 15th July 2025).
10. Ashe-McNalley, C., Coveleskie, K., Gupta, A., Kilpatrick, L. A., Mayer, E. A., & Labus, J. S. (2015). Altered functional connectivity within the central reward network in overweight and obese women. https://core.ac.uk/download/323079142.pdf (accessed on 15th July 2025).
11. Aziz, Q., Borsook, D., Elsenbruch, S., Kilpatrick, L. A., Mayer, E. A., & The Rome Foundation Working Group. (2019). Role of brain imaging in disorders of brain-gut interaction: A Rome Working Team Report. https://core.ac.uk/download/323078713.pdf (accessed on 15th July 2025).

12. Bagnato, F., Bakshi, R., Barker, P., Beck, A., & North American Imaging in Multiple Sclerosis Cooperative. (2024). The use of 7T MRI in multiple sclerosis: Review and consensus statement from the North American Imaging in Multiple Sclerosis Cooperative. https://core.ac.uk/download/622529148.pdf (accessed on 15th July 2025).

13. Banson, M., Buckman, V., Darko, K., Totimeh, P., & Osei-Bonsu, E. (2024). Neuro-oncology access in Sub-Saharan Africa: A literature review of challenges and opportunities. https://core.ac.uk/download/613721197.docx (accessed on 15th July 2025).

14. Bargalló Alabart, N., Cervera I Segura, R., & Sarbu, N. (2017). Advanced and conventional magnetic resonance imaging in neuropsychiatric lupus. https://core.ac.uk/download/83829243.pdf (accessed on 15th July 2025).

15. Basu, N., Goni, M., Murray, A. D., Waiter, G. D., & Macfarlane, G. J. (2018). Neural indicators of fatigue in chronic diseases: A systematic review of MRI studies. https://core.ac.uk/download/159067075.pdf (accessed on 15th July 2025).

16. Bernardo-Castro, S., Donato, H., Ferreira, L., Sargento-Freitas, J., & Silva, A. (2020). Permeability of the blood-brain barrier through the phases of ischemic stroke and relation with clinical outcome: Protocol for a systematic review. https://core.ac.uk/download/344687412.pdf (accessed on 15th July 2025).

17. Blanco, E., Carretero González, J., Delgado, J., Fuente, E., & Rodríguez, M. (2003). Morphological and morphometric assessment of the encephalic ventricles using different neuroimaging techniques. https://core.ac.uk/download/610671355.pdf (accessed on 15th July 2025).

18. Bozzao, A., Nicita, F., Paolino, M. C., Parisi, P., & Ursitti, F. (2013). Four-year follow-up study in an NF1 boy with a focal pontine hamartoma. https://core.ac.uk/download/54480786.pdf (accessed on 15th July 2025).

19. Bradford, D. E., Curtin, J. J., Fox, A. S., Hur, J., & Shackman, A. J. (2018). Acute alcohol administration dampens central extended amygdala reactivity. https://core.ac.uk/download/323069596.pdf (accessed on 15th July 2025).

20. Cheung, R. T. F. (2014). A systematic approach to the definition of stroke. https://core.ac.uk/download/38076548.pdf (accessed on 15th July 2025).

21. Ciesielski, M., Janik, A., Markowicz, M., Mikiciuk-Olasik, E., & Mikiciuk, G. (2010). Neuroimaging diagnosis in neurodegenerative diseases. https://core.ac.uk/download/268441030.pdf (accessed on 15th July 2025).

22. D'Arcy, R., Downie, J., Hadskis, M., Kenny, A., & Gagnon, L. (2008). The therapeutic misconception: A threat to valid parental consent for pediatric neuroimaging research. https://core.ac.uk/download/568216503.pdf (accessed on 15th July 2025).

23. de Ruiter, M. B., Deprez, S., McDonald, B. C., Saykin, A. J., & Vandenberghe, J. (2013). Neuroimaging biomarkers and cognitive function in non-CNS cancer and its treatment: Current status and recommendations for future research. https://core.ac.uk/download/46961941.pdf (accessed on 15th July 2025).

24. Doolittle, N. D., Dósa, E., Farrell, B. T., Frenkel, V., & Neuwelt, E. A. (2013). Using iron oxide nanoparticles to diagnose CNS inflammatory diseases and PCNSL. https://core.ac.uk/download/42927168.pdf (accessed on 15th July 2025).

25. Eberling, J., & Jagust, W. J. (1995). Imaging studies of aging, neurodegenerative disease, and alcoholism. https://core.ac.uk/download/323081855.pdf (accessed on 15th July 2025).

26. Farooq, S., Khatri, I. A., & Khatri, M. A. (2016). Preventing stroke at door step–Need for a paradigm shift in delivery of preventive healthcare. https://core.ac.uk/download/47264780.pdf (accessed on 15th July 2025).

27. Happonen, T. (2025). Dizziness and headache in emergency brain MRI: A retrospective analysis of imaging outcomes. https://core.ac.uk/download/645626519.pdf (accessed on 15th July 2025).

28. Hoang, D. M., Pham, P. T., Bach, T. Q., Ngo, A. T., Nguyen, Q. T., Phan, T. T. K., Nguyễn, H. G., et al. (2022). Stem cell-based therapy for human diseases. *Signal Transduction and Targeted Therapy, 7*. https://doi.org/10.1038/s41392-022-01134-4 (accessed on 15th July 2025).

29. Jauch, E. C., Saver, J. L., Adams, H. P., Bruno, A., Connors, J. J., Demaerschalk, B. M., Khatri, P., et al. (2013). Guidelines for the early management of patients with acute ischemic stroke. *Stroke, 44*, 870–947. https://doi.org/10.1161/str.0b013e318284056a (accessed on 15th July 2025).

30. Macrae, I. M., & Muir, K. W. (2016). Neuroimaging as a selection tool and endpoint in preclinical and clinical trials. https://core.ac.uk/download/46164953.pdf (accessed on 15th July 2025).

31. Maffione, A. M., Anagnostou, C., Civitelli, L., Collorone, S., Fantozzi, L., & Zito, G. (2015). Role of brain perfusion SPECT with 99mTc HMPAO in the assessment of response to drug therapy in patients with autoimmune vasculitis: A prospective study. https://core.ac.uk/download/54523723.pdf (accessed on 15th July 2025).

32. Mailles, A., Neves, A. M., Krynska, B., Glaser, C. A., Centers for Disease Control and Prevention, Pohl, D., Kimberlin, D. W., et al. (2010). Advances in pediatric neurovirology. https://core.ac.uk/download/pdf/8391975.pdf (accessed on 15th July 2025).

33. Masiak, J., Mikołajewska, E., & Mikołajewski, D. (2023). Neurophysiological determinants of occupational stress and burnout. https://core.ac.uk/download/587246459.pdf (accessed on 15th July 2025).

34. N/A. (2025). Stroke. https://core.ac.uk/download/619631457.pdf (accessed on 15th July 2025).

35. Omuro, A. (2013). Glioblastoma and other malignant gliomas. *JAMA, 310*, 1842–1842. https://doi.org/10.1001/jama.2013.280319 (accessed on 15th July 2025).

36. Perkins, G. D., Gräsner, J. T., Semeraro, F., Olasveengen, T. M., Soar, J., Lott, C., Van de Voorde, P., et al. (2021). European Resuscitation Council Guidelines 2021: Executive summary. *Resuscitation, 161*, 1–60. https://doi.org/10.1016/j.resuscitation.2021.02.003 (accessed on 15th July 2025).

37. Welch, A., Platt, B., Billings, L., Borchelt, D., Brankack, J., Drzezga, A., Dubois, B., et al. (2012). FDG-PET imaging, EEG and sleep phenotypes as translational biomarkers for research in Alzheimer's disease. https://core.ac.uk/download/370450.pdf (accessed on 15th July 2025).

38. Yu, H. (2016). Deep grey matter volumetry as a function of age using a semi-automatic qMRI algorithm. https://open.bu.edu/bitstream/2144/15336/1/Yu_bu_0017N_10772.pdf (accessed on 15th July 2025).

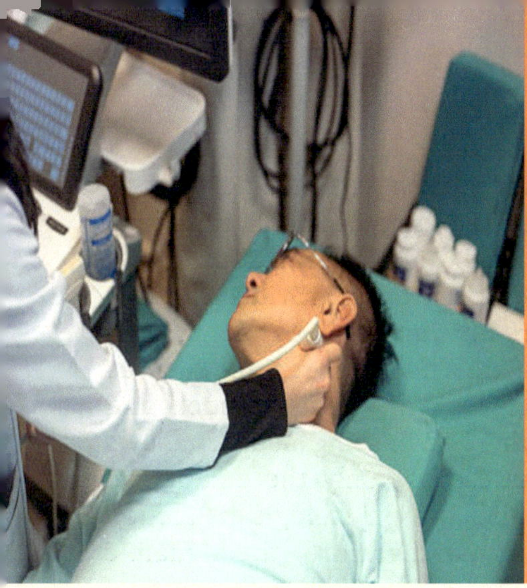

Chapter 2

HEAD AND NECK IMAGING: TECHNIQUES AND APPLICATIONS

Contents

Introduction

Head and neck imaging is a critical component of diagnostic imaging in contemporary medicine, particularly given the intricate anatomical structures and the abundant variation in this region. Such imaging techniques are not merely for visualization but also for longitudinal assessment of various medical diseases, from benign disease to malignant neoplasms. Among the many techniques employed, computed tomography (CT), magnetic resonance imaging (MRI), and positron emission tomography (PET) all have specific strengths and limitations that affect their application in clinical practice. As technology advances, more focus on accuracy, efficacy, and patient safety has led to advancements in imaging techniques. The increasing significance of artificial intelligence (AI) also highlights these developments, resulting in more accurate diagnoses and tailored treatment regimes, which are pivotal in head and neck illness management. In the last few years, AI has emerged to have a revolutionary role in head and neck imaging, particularly enhancing diagnostic capability. Techniques such as machine learning and deep learning have been integrated into imaging procedures, transforming the analysis of CT, MRI, and PET scans. As noted, AI technologies have, in most cases, surpassed the interpretive accuracy of human radiologists, instigating a fundamental shift in diagnostic procedures. In addition, AI's application is not just in image interpretation but also includes automating histopathology and molecular profiling to contribute to efficient tumor characterization and personalized medicine. The development of improved algorithms results in better mutation detection and the identification of biomarkers, ultimately contributing to better patient outcomes. Notwithstanding all that, AIs' use has its drawbacks, which are data standardization and algorithm bias, and these must be addressed to ensure fair healthcare delivery. Furthermore, interdisciplinary collaboration between AI researchers, clinicians, and AI experts is required for the successful integration of these technologies into practice. As indicated, cutting-edge developments in explainable AI, robotics, and real-time monitoring systems are on the horizon. These developments will advance beyond current limitations and expand head and neck imaging capabilities. A multi-pronged approach is called for to create an environment in which AI can thrive, ensuring that new tools not only work well but are also transparent and easy to use. Addressing current challenges will enable healthcare practitioners to unlock the full potential of AI to improve diagnostic methods and deliver personalized therapy. Thus, the future of head and neck imaging is more in cooperative efforts to enhance patient care and outcomes in multiple healthcare environments rather than in developing technology.

2.1. Ultrasound in Head and Neck Imaging

Ultrasound has been found to be a valuable modality in head and neck imaging, with some specific advantages such as real-time imaging and absence of ionizing radiation. Predisposed to a significant extent for the evaluation of soft tissue structures, ultrasound provides valuable information regarding various conditions affecting the head and neck region, such as thyroid disorders, salivary gland infection, and lymphadenopathy. This imaging modality allows operators to assess not only the anatomical structure but also the physiological function of such organs. Furthermore, the dynamic capabilities of ultrasound enable assessment of blood flow in tumors and other lesions, further expanding its utility in the characterization of neoplastic processes. In addition to other imaging modalities, ultrasound offers a useful complementary tool, enhancing overall diagnostic yields and helping clinicians create appropriate treatment plans tailored to the individual patient. The role of ultrasound extends beyond diagnosis, as it is increasingly used to guide interventional procedures such as biopsies and abscess drainage in the head and neck. The ability to perform real-time-guided procedures significantly reduces complications and enhances patient safety. In ultrasound-guided fine-needle aspiration (FNA), for instance, medical professionals can readily target lesions without damaging adjacent vital structures, thus realizing more successful sampling and reducing repeat procedures. Such a feature of ultrasound not only maximizes patient management but also aligns with modern medical practices that emphasize minimally invasive approaches. The integration of ultrasound into routine practice in head and neck imaging reflects its evolving role in optimizing clinical outcomes and overcoming the constraints of conventional imaging techniques. With advancing technology, the role of integrating ultrasound into multidisciplinary teams for the treatment of head and neck cancer has become increasingly essential. Fusion imaging, which combines ultrasound with other imaging technologies such as computed tomography (CT) and magnetic resonance imaging (MRI), also allows for more precise tumor localization and characterization, driving the creation of individualized therapeutic regimens. Through this symbiotic process, the biology and behavior of tumors are more clearly elucidated, mirroring the broader trend towards precision medicine in oncology. Moreover, the multiformity of ultrasounds guarantees that it is instrumental in monitoring treatment outcomes, guiding clinicians to assess treatment effectiveness in real-time. Through its integration of diagnostic and therapeutic aspects, ultrasound plays a pivotal role in comprehensive patient care, further solidifying its place in contemporary head and neck imaging (Feygin et al., 2020; Diva et al., 2023).

2.1.1. Principles of Ultrasound Technology

Ultrasound imaging is at the core of imaging head and neck pathologies due to its accessibility, safety, and ability to provide real-time imaging. It utilizes high-frequency sound waves generated by a transducer in this medical imaging technique, which are directed into the body. When these sound waves interact with different tissues, they bounce back and, upon impacting different interfaces, generate echoes, which are subsequently converted into visual images by the ultrasound equipment. The advantages of using ultrasound for imaging of the neck and head include the absence of exposure to ionizing radiation, making it best suited for certain populations, such as children and pregnant women. Ultrasound is also generally less costly compared to other imaging devices, making it more accessible in the clinic. Its ability to analyze soft tissue structures places it in a special position as a vital tool for the examination of lymph nodes, salivary glands, and thyroid tissues, thereby enhancing diagnostic accuracy in various diseases (N/A, 1987) (Figure 2.1).

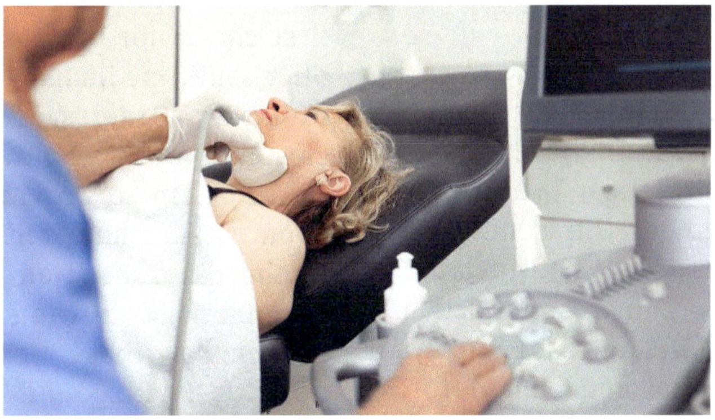

Figure 2.1. Ultrasound machine transducer in contact with the neck surface.

Source: https://assets.medpagetoday.net/media/images/97xxx/97743.jpg.

Another vital aspect of ultrasound technology is its ability to perform dynamic assessments, which is particularly significant in the examination of certain disease conditions. For example, during ultrasound scanning, doctors can see tissue movements and blood flow in real time, enabling them to study abnormalities such as cysts, tumors, or vascular disease. Doppler ultrasound is beneficial here, as it presents details about blood flow patterns that reflect changes in vascular properties that may indicate malignancy or other pathological processes. The dynamic nature of ultrasound enables enhanced diagnostic confidence, particularly in differentiating cystic from solid masses in the head and neck region. For that reason, clinical applications of ultrasound go beyond static imaging and contribute notably to the development of treatment plans tailored to each patient's unique condition (Culp et al., 2019). While it has many strengths, ultrasound technology has limitations that must be considered when imaging the head and neck. Ultrasound is influenced by a range of factors that include the operator's skill, patient anatomy, and the existence of air or bone, which act as barriers to sound waves. As a result, there will be some structures that will be hard to see. For instance, although ultrasound is excellent at soft-tissue imaging, deeper structures may require additional imaging, such as computed tomography or magnetic resonance imaging, to provide sufficient evaluation. Furthermore, interpretation of ultrasound images is not always objective and thus demands specialized training and experience on the part of practitioners to enable proper diagnoses. Therefore, the role of ultrasound in head and neck imaging is best considered as an adjunct to a multimodal imaging strategy, providing critical information complemented by other imaging modalities (N/A, 1987).

2.1.2. Applications in Thyroid and Salivary Gland Assessment

The assessment of thyroid and salivary glands in clinical practice is increasingly reliant on advanced imaging techniques, which are superior to traditional methods. Ultrasound (US) is particularly valuable as it is non-invasive, provides real-time images, and is cost-effective. In the case of thyroid nodules, ultrasound plays an important role in distinguishing benign from malignant lesions, especially when used in conjunction with fine needle aspiration biopsy (FNAB). Such refinements allow more precise staging and treatment planning and therefore better patient outcomes. Furthermore, the integration of ultrasound with other imaging techniques like computed tomography (CT) and magnetic resonance imaging (MRI) allows for a complete assessment of malignancies, overcoming the limitations of individual imaging modalities and overcoming issues of sensitivity and specificity that have been reported using CT and MRI separately (Baatenburg et al., 1990) (Figure 2.2).

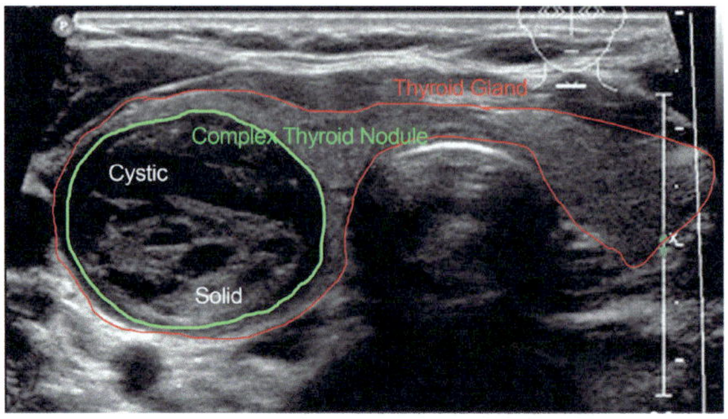

Figure 2.2. Normal versus abnormal thyroid on ultrasound.

Source: https://rfaforlife.com/wp-content/uploads/2022/04/complex-thyroid.png.

Assessment of salivary glands, particularly the parotid gland, also benefits from state-of-the-art imaging technology. This organ of the body is commonly plagued by a variety of disorders that vary from benign to cancerous in nature. Ultrasound, specifically using B-mode and color Doppler techniques, is the imaging method of first choice for evaluation due to its ability to offer real-time imaging with no risk of ionizing radiation. Besides, new techniques such as elastography and contrast-enhanced ultrasound (CEUS) help to provide valuable information about tissue characterization, assisting greatly in the differentiation of neoplastic and non-neoplastic conditions. The exact imaging provided by these techniques benefits clinical decision-making and preoperative planning, emphasizing their major role in modern diagnostic practice (Arduini et al., 2020). The need for accurate imaging of thyroid and salivary gland assessment becomes even more critical when the fallacies of subclinical disease are considered. Routine palpation and clinical examination often lead to misdiagnosis due to the fallacies inherent in physical examinations. Imaging modalities can correct such fallacies by providing a more comprehensive and detailed impression of head and neck anatomy. For example, the use of ultrasound together with cytologic evaluation has shown promise for improving diagnostic accuracy of cervical metastatic disease and effectively eliminating the uncertainties inherent in clinical examinations by themselves. In general, the development of imaging modalities not only improves the detection of pathology but also enables more accurate prognostic evaluation and individualized therapeutic management of head and neck disease (Baatenburg et al., 1990).

2.1.3. Advantages and Disadvantages of Ultrasound

Ultrasound imaging, particularly as used in head and neck imaging, has several advantages that make it a clinician's go-to option. Maybe the greatest advantage is that it is not invasive, allowing real-time visualization of structures without exposure to ionizing radiation. It is extremely useful in pediatric patients and pregnant females, where minimizing exposure to radiation is paramount. Ultrasound also offers high-resolution images of vascular structures and soft tissues, enhancing the assessment of conditions such as thyroid nodules or salivary gland disease. Also, technological advancements, such as CAOS systems with more advanced ultrasound integration, have enhanced its utilization in precise treatment planning and diagnostic applications, and it is now an important component in contemporary imaging strategies in head and neck examinations (Kalová et al., 2019). Despite its many advantages, ultrasound imaging is not without inherent limitations that clinicians must overcome.

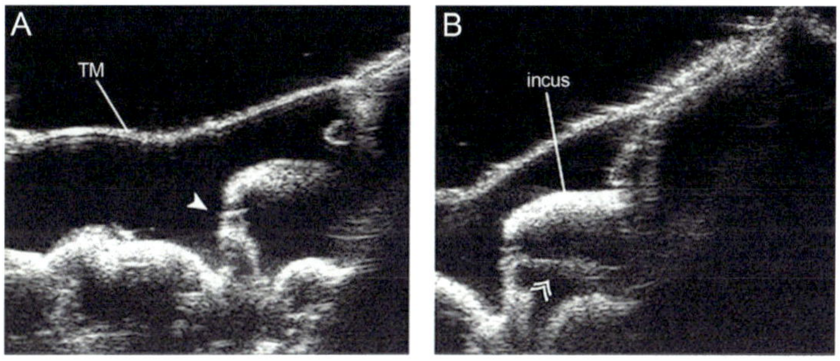

Figure 2.3. Ultrasound imaging of the ear.

Source: https://cdn.dal.ca/content/dam/dalhousie/images/faculty/medicine/departments/department-sites/surgery/earlab/earlab04.jpg.lt_97ab0068e3b874ef8c916f9b3e5c5d81.res/earlab04.jpg.

One of its significant drawbacks is being operator dependent; image quality attained to a large extent depends on how skilled and proficient the technician performing the procedure is. Other factors, such as patient body habitus, can also degrade image quality, making diagnosis more difficult. Furthermore, in comparison with other modalities like computed tomography (CT) or magnetic resonance imaging (MRI), ultrasound is not as effective at assessing bone structures and some anatomically located regions deep within the body. Additionally, although developments such as Fusion Imaging aim to advance diagnosis by combining ultrasonography with CT or MRI, the equipment can require more extensive training and equipment, adding new constraints to daily clinical application (Bellati et al., 2018). The future of ultrasound head and neck imaging is not only in its existing applications but also in its future innovations that can reduce its limitations. Emerging technologies such as 3D ultrasound and advanced imaging techniques are facilitating better visualization of complex head and neck anatomy. Besides, more integration with other imaging modalities, such as in the case of Fusion Imaging, may produce synergistic effects where ultrasound complements the existing strengths of other modalities to enable more comprehensive evaluations. More research can further solidify ultrasound's effectiveness for a broader set of clinical conditions and make it even more reliable and easier to use. Finally, by recognizing both the strengths and the limitations of ultrasound in head and neck imaging, clinicians can make optimal decisions to maximize diagnostic yields and patient safety (Figure 2.3).

2.2. Positron Emission Tomography (PET)

In head and neck imaging, Positron Emission Tomography (PET) has emerged as a pivotal modality, particularly for its ability to provide both structural and functional information about tissues. Such dualism comes in very handy in oncological uses, where an accurate staging of tumors is critical for the successful management of malignancies. The most widely used tracer in PET scans for cancer assessment is 18F-Fluorodeoxyglucose (18F-FDG), which is a radioactive glucose analogue. Research has demonstrated its effectiveness, particularly in delineating tumors in highly vascular head and neck tissue. Surprisingly, 18F-FDG PET is highly sensitive for detecting metastatic nodal involvement, which is critical for selecting appropriate treatment modalities. However, consideration should be taken that despite the impressive sensitivity, specificity may be variable with different research findings, and therefore optimal utilization practices require further work (Culp et al., 2019).

In addition to evaluating primary tumors, PET imaging has demonstrated significant potential for detecting and managing conditions beyond oncology, including inflammation and pain syndromes. For instance, 18F-FDG PET has been validated as beneficial for the detection of periodontitis and infection of dental implants, conditions that are prevalent in the head and neck region. Moreover, the imaging modality supports evaluation of pain and inflammatory disorders via the detection of metabolic activity, indicating tissue reaction to pathology. In addition, the value of 18F-NaF for evaluating tumor bone involvement or metastasis demonstrates PET's wider use beyond its sole role in cancer detection. With ever-evolving technology and PET methods, its applications in head and neck inflammation and pain management are sure to expand further, thereby improving patients' clinical outcomes (Culp et al., 2019). In inherited syndromes such as paraganglioma syndrome type 1, PET is critical in diagnosis since it facilitates the detection and characterization of specific lesions. Application of advanced tracers such as 18F-DOPA PET-CT can yield crucial information on the nature of tumors within genetic syndromes. The technique has been recognized as the gold standard for imaging these neoplasms, facilitating effective clinical management and surveillance. Furthermore, the adoption of 68Ga-peptide PET-CT is gaining momentum due to its greater diagnostic accuracy, particularly in assessing aggressive tumor features. Hence, PET imaging not only supports initial diagnostic assessment but also makes a valuable contribution to real-time monitoring and decision-making in high-risk patient populations. As technology continues to develop, the future of PET as a comprehensive imaging modality in head and neck imaging is bright enough to warrant continued research.

2.2.1. Mechanism of PET Imaging

Positron Emission Tomography (PET) scanning is a sophisticated nuclear medicine technique necessary in the diagnosis and treatment of head and neck cancers. PET achieves its effect by using radiopharmaceuticals, compounds with radioactive isotope markers. These medications emit positrons as they decay after administration into the body. When the electrons are encountered by the tissues, they give rise to pairs of gamma photons that are detected by the PET scanner. The imaging technique is adept at identifying metabolic aberrations characteristic of neoplastic processes because cancer tissue exhibits increased glucose metabolism. By illustrating such metabolic changes, PET provides unprecedented data that helps in the assessment of tumor presence, nature, and response to therapy, and ultimately, enhances patient management for treating head and neck cancers. Furthermore, the integration of PET imaging with other imaging modalities, such as Computed Tomography (CT) and Magnetic Resonance Imaging (MRI), offers strong diagnostic potential. This integration allows for the coupling of metabolic and anatomical information, thereby creating a better image of the tumor. A case in point is PET/CT scans, which synergistically combine the high-resolution anatomical details of CT with the functional imaging capabilities of PET, thereby enabling precise localization of tumors and metastases. Along with that, advances in imaging technologies have seen the development of novel radiotracers to bind to specific receptors or metabolic pathways, further clarifying the biology of tumors (Figure 2.4).

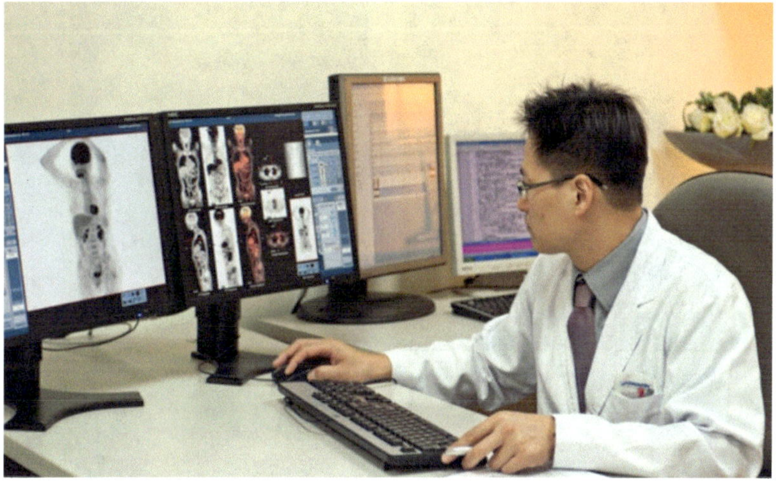

Figure 2.4. PET scanner in use for staging head and neck cancer.

Source: https://kiranpetct.com/wp-content/uploads/2024/05/Understanding-PET-scans-for-stage-head-and-neck-cancer-1-1024x614.png.

In turn, the use of PET imaging in the clinic greatly benefits oncologists, as it enables more refined treatment planning and monitoring of therapeutic response. With continued progress in artificial intelligence (AI), its application in PET imaging has great potential to improve diagnostic performance and treatment tailoring. Machine learning and artificial intelligence algorithms can enable image analysis by segmenting and detecting tumors automatically, minimizing human error and accelerating diagnosis. Further, deep learning algorithms can integrate radio genomic data to provide predictive analytics informing treatment decisions based on individual tumor profiles. While standardization and clinical validation are difficult issues, the potential to complement traditional imaging methods is significant. As noted in recent studies, the combination of AI with PET imaging techniques may identify entry points for more personalized therapies, ultimately leading to improved patient outcomes in the treatment of head and neck cancer (Broggi et al., 2024; Illimoottil et al., 2023).

2.2.2. Role in Oncology for Head and Neck Cancers

The employment of advanced imaging modalities in oncology has dramatically transformed the management of head and neck cancers (HNC). Imaging modalities such as computed tomography (CT), magnetic resonance imaging (MRI), and positron emission tomography (PET) play significant roles in diagnosis, staging, and treatment planning. The precision rendered by these technologies enables clinicians to identify tumor locations, assess metastasis, and establish the extent of local invasion. Accurate imaging not only guides the optimal treatment regimens but also facilitates ongoing tracking of therapeutic effects against cancers. Furthermore, as imaging technology continues to develop, integrating AI is poised to enhance interpretation accuracy and reduce variability among radiologists, enabling timely interventions for patients, as in this highly aggressive form of cancer (Figure 2.5).

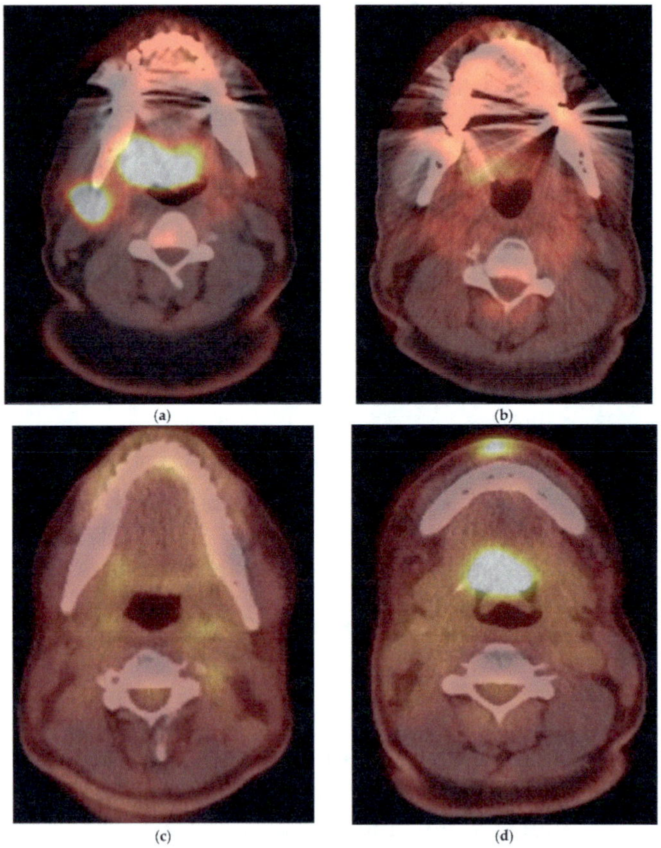

Figure 2.5. Role of PET/CT in oropharyngeal cancers.

Source: https://www.mdpi.com/cancers/cancers-15-02651/article_deploy/html/images/cancers-15-02651-g003a.png.

Artificial intelligence is increasingly being used to augment imaging in head and neck oncology. The use of machine learning algorithms and deep learning techniques has been found to improve the interpretation of complex imaging data significantly. With the application of convolutional neural networks (CNNs), such AI systems can outperform traditional human interpretations in tasks such as tumor segmentation and grading in histopathological images. In addition, AI-based analytics has the ability to enhance workflow efficiency without sacrificing diagnostic quality, opening up more sophisticated treatment personalization depending on patient-specific profiles. The novel applications of AI also find their way into molecular profiling, where computerized systems aid in determining genetic mutations that guide therapeutic selection. With advances in the discipline, these technological innovations promise a new dawn for increased clinical decision-making in HNC care, with the ultimate goal of better patient outcomes. Despite promising advances in AI and head and neck cancer imaging techniques, there are also challenges that must be addressed for them to realize their full potential. That includes data quality and standardization, which are highly challenging to achieve at scale. Algorithmic bias is also of concern because AI systems trained on small or unrepresentative datasets can perpetuate health inequities. An effective strategy, through interdisciplinary collaboration between clinicians, AI researchers, and researchers, is a necessity to overcome these challenges. In addition, the development of explainable AI systems that offer decision-making explanations is necessary to secure trust among healthcare professionals. In the long run, surmounting such hurdles will not only enable AI applications but also make diagnosis and treatment of HNC more evenly developed, ultimately towards better quality care for everyone (Tuan et al., 2024; Broggi et al., 2024).

2.2.3. Integration with CT and MRI for Enhanced Diagnostics

The integration of computed tomography (CT) and magnetic resonance imaging (MRI) technology is a critical innovation in head and neck diagnosis, particularly in addressing the complexity of head and neck pathologies. CT scanning is characterized by its high speed , facilitating precise tumor localization. At the same time, MRI provides clear visualization of soft tissue anatomy and tumor morphology. These complimentary modalities supplement diagnostic accuracy so that clinicians can quantify not only the extent of tumors but also their invasion into adjacent tissues—critical to treatment planning. Furthermore, the integration of CT and MRI aids in evaluating treatment response, as changes in tumor features over time can be fully analyzed with both modalities, ultimately improving patient care in the treatment of head and neck cancers. The application of current imaging technologies, such as dual-energy computed tomography (DECT), is revolutionizing head and neck imaging. DECT utilizes two distinct energy spectra to generate high-resolution datasets in a single scan and has the potential to yield improved material differentiation required in tumor characterization. DECT finds particular utility in head and neck cancers, where accurate discrimination between tumor tissues and neighboring structures can significantly improve diagnostic and prognostic accuracy. Of particular importance, DECT enhances contrast resolution and reduces artifacts that mask valuable anatomical details. More current research highlighted in the literature has underscored DECT's sensitivity for detecting iodine quantification with monochromatic reconstruction, assisting in tumor characterization and response to therapy. Thus, the addition of DECT to routine imaging protocols holds great promise for maximizing the diagnostic potential for head and neck disease (Finizio et al., 2024). More recent molecular imaging technologies that utilize targeted contrast agents further increase the promise of combining CT and MRI in head and neck diagnostics. These new agents amplify the imaging's detection and description of tumors with greater contrast and specificity of imaging, a welcome tool given the region's intricate anatomy as well as the challenges of the blood-brain barrier. By combining the fast imaging ability of CT with the soft tissue information of

MRI, physicians are able to develop a full picture of head and neck tumors that is invaluable for accurate assessment. Targeted contrast agents, for instance, can be formulated to enable dual- or triple-modal imaging and reduce the toxicity and potential bioaccumulation of traditional imaging agents, thereby making diagnostic processes safer for patients. This innovation reflects oncology's shift towards personalized medicine, offering healthcare practitioners advanced tools for customized treatment regimens (Ginat et al., 2024) (Figure 2.6).

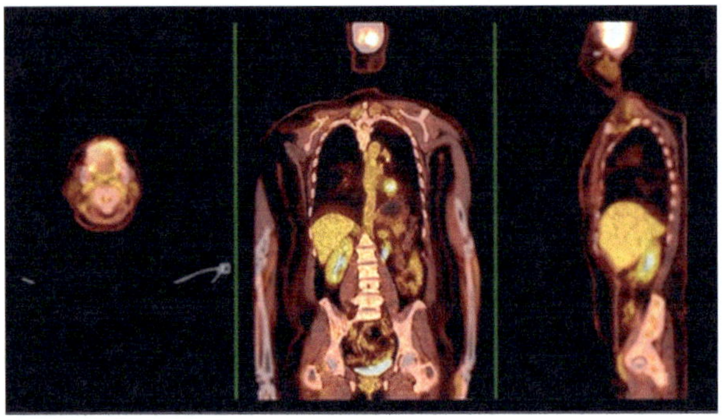

Figure 2.6. Fused PET/CT scan displaying anatomical and metabolic detail.

Source: https://www.shutterstock.com/image-illustration/pet-ct-scan-fusion-image-260nw-2404200427.jpg.

2.3. Contrast Agents in Imaging

In head and neck imaging, the use of contrast agents is key to maximizing the diagnostic performance of many imaging modalities. These agents optimize the visualization of anatomical structures and pathological processes, making the interpretations more precise. Examples include iodine-based contrast for computed tomography (CT) and gadolinium-based agents for magnetic resonance imaging (MRI). Their key function is to increase the contrast between different tissues, particularly where there is a need for differentiation of soft tissue, like in the assessment of tumors or inflammatory illnesses. The choice of contrast agent most often corresponds to the imaging technique used and the clinical situation, emphasizing the need for radiologists to understand the pharmacokinetics and safety profiles of these agents to maximize benefit for patients. Moreover, the safety and tolerability of contrast agents remain the focus of work in clinical settings. High-efficacy iodine-based contrast agents carry risks such as allergic reaction and nephrotoxicity in individuals with pre-existing renal impairment. Pre-screening can prevent adverse reactions, but patients may not always escape them. On the other hand, gadolinium-based contrast media, used predominantly in MRI, have come under scrutiny due to the possibility of causing nephrogenic systemic fibrosis (NSF) in patients with severe kidney damage. Hence, the identification and judicious use of alternative agents, such as those outlined in (N/A, 2005) and (N/A, 1994), have become essential to minimize harm while maintaining high-quality images in the assessment of head and neck disease, such as malignancy and vascular disease. The addition of newer imaging technology has also spurred on the development of novel contrast agents aimed at enhanced diagnostic capability. These agents are engineered to overcome head-and-neck-specific challenges and provide greater sensitivity and specificity in pathogen detection. As an illustration, new compounds are being created to target specific tissues or biomarkers within tumors, enabling enhanced visualization of difficult-to-define lesions with conventional contrast agents. The evolution of these agents underscores the importance of ongoing research and development in radiology practice to improve diagnostic techniques continually. Ultimately, the prudent selection and use of contrast agents for head and neck imaging reflect a broader commitment to optimal clinical outcomes through state-of-the-art technology and customized treatment.

2.3.1. Types of Contrast Agents Used

In head and neck imaging, several contrast agents are employed to optimize diagnostic sensitivity and anatomical information. Most are gadolinium-based in magnetic resonance imaging (MRI) owing to the capacity of paramagnetic agents to elevate the relaxation rates of adjacent protons and, therefore, image contrast. Their utility is perhaps best seen in dynamic contrast-enhanced MRI (DCE-MRI) because they allow tissue vascularity and permeability to be quantified so that tumors may be more accurately characterized and treatment planning directed. Their application is critical in head and neck cancers, as early detection of recurrence significantly affects patient outcomes and therapeutic interventions.

The effectiveness of gadolinium-based agents underscores their vital role in improving diagnostic imaging techniques for this anatomical region (Alzabni et al., 2022). In conjunction with gadolinium-based agents, ultrasound contrast agents, composed of gas or air-filled microbubbles, play a significant role in optimizing the diagnostic value of ultrasound imaging. These agents enhance echogenicity, allowing for enhanced visualization of vascular tissue and lesions associated with a variety of head and neck illnesses. Convenient, particularly for detecting and characterizing thyroid nodules and masses in the neck, ultrasound contrast agents help differentiate between benign and malignant lesions.

These agents are effective because they make sound waves reflect more strongly than within nearby tissues, resulting in more explicit images that help make accurate diagnoses. Consequently, the use of ultrasound contrast agents is increasing in importance, particularly for patients for whom MRI or CT scans are contraindicated or unavailable, thereby enriching the imaging arsenal for physicians (Bec et al., 2019) (Figure 2.7).

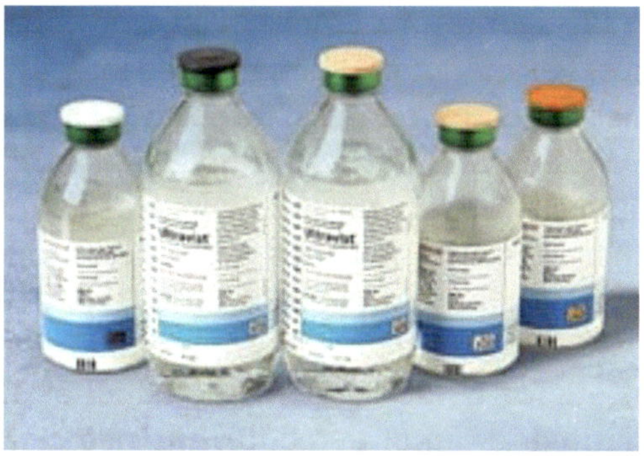

Figure 2.7. Assorted contrast agent vials for CT and MRI procedures.

Source: https://axisimagingnews.com/wp-content/uploads/2006/05/issues_images_MI_2006-05_2006-05_02-1.jpg.

New technologies utilizing new contrast agents are also beginning to reshape head and neck imaging protocols. Time-resolved fluorescence spectroscopy (TRFS) is among those innovations that can make cancerous tissues detectable by their characteristic autofluorescence patterns. It is a technique that is free of exogenous contrast agents, offering real-time assessment of biochemical properties during transoral robotic surgery (TORS) and other surgeries. Integration of TRFS into surgical procedures allows for label-free tissue margin characterization to support better decision-making and possibly enhance surgical success.

As researchers continue to explore the applications of such emerging methods integrated with conventional imaging modalities, the future for improving diagnostic accuracy in head and neck cancer diagnosis and treatment looks more promising. These developments in the creation of contrast agents indicate a dynamic evolution in medical imaging history (Bec et al., 2019).

2.3.2. Importance of Contrast in Enhancing Image Quality

In head and neck imaging, image quality is key to successful diagnosis and treatment planning.

Contrast agents are essential in this improvement by providing better contrast among various tissues. For instance, during tumor imaging, contrast agents are able to highlight malignant lesions against normal vicinal tissue so that clinicians can ascertain neoplasm size and borders, as in the case of head and neck squamous cell carcinoma (HNSCC). This information is important because the majority of patients are diagnosed at advanced stages without readily identifiable pre-malignant lesions, which complicates early detection and treatment. The contrast integration improves the effectiveness of imaging modalities like CT and MRI via visibility enhancement, which is especially important in regard to the complex nature of head and neck pathologies, as suggested in the treatment overview for HNSCC provided (Daniel et al., 2020). In addition, contrast application in imaging is not limited to tumor detection but also includes tracking the course of disease as well as evaluating surgical success. Adequate post-treatment imaging follow-up is crucial for assessing outcomes of multimodal treatment, which may include surgery, chemoradiotherapy, and immunotherapy. Utilizing sophisticated imaging techniques, healthcare providers can better distinguish between differences in tissue characteristics, evaluate possible recurrences, and adjust follow-up treatment based on individual patient needs. This level of precision guides the overall impact of treatment modalities on patients' quality of life, facilitating more informed discussions between clinicians and patients about their pathways of care (David et al., 2020). These evaluations are paramount, particularly following the discovery of new therapeutic targets and biomarkers in HNSCC variant management. Moreover, reliance on contrast-enhanced imaging is aligned with a growing movement towards personalized medicine in head and neck oncology. With advancing imaging technology, radiologists can obtain high-resolution images that not only outline malignancies but also convey information about their biological behavior. This aspect is crucial in differentiating between HPV-positive and HPV-negative HNSCC, given the varied therapeutic approaches required for each subtype. Increased contrast during imaging also enables the capture of intricate interactions between tumors and surrounding structures, thereby benefiting surgical planning and minimizing complications. The intersection of imaging technology and ongoing studies of HNSCC biology underscores the central role of contrast in enabling accurate and effective patient management in the highly technological field of head and neck oncology (Daniel et al., 2020) (Figure 2.8).

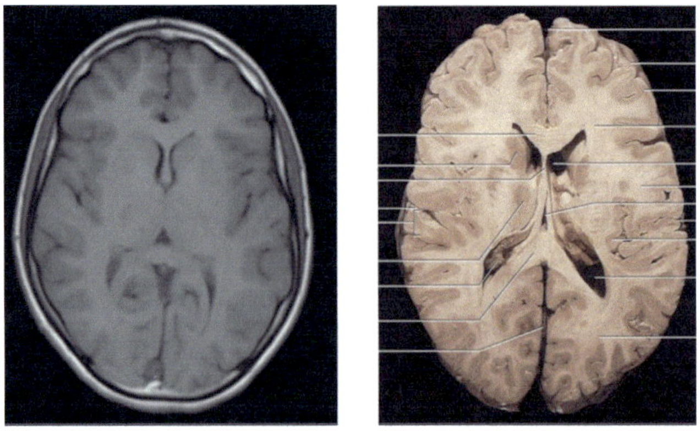

Figure 2.8. Side-by-side brain MRI with and without contrast enhancement.

Source: https://airsmed.com/wp-content/uploads/2023/07/Brain-MRI-and-real-brain-1024x603.png.

2.3.3. Risks and Considerations in Using Contrast Agents

The application of contrast agents in head and neck imaging is a hazardous and risky procedure that has to be properly managed by medical personnel. Contrast agents are typically iodine-based and play a vital role in highlighting blood vessels and tissues in imaging procedures such as CT scans and magnetic resonance imaging (MRI). However, their adverse side effects vary from mild allergic reactions to life-threatening anaphylactic reactions in some individuals. Particularly vulnerable are patients with a history of contrast media allergy or chronic renal insufficiency, with whom they can develop contrast-induced nephropathy. The balancing of the benefits of improved imaging quality against these possible risks becomes the object of clinical decision-making, especially in complex examples like head and neck cancer, when precise imaging is relevant to treatment planning. In addition, one needs to consider the contrast agent application's effect on patient safety and overall care. Due to the growing prevalence of renal dysfunction, particularly among the elderly or comorbid patients, the impact of contrast media on renal function cannot be overestimated. Under certain conditions, the nephrotoxicity of iodinated contrast materials is a concern, especially when serial imaging studies are performed in close proximity. This risk necessitates assessment of renal function prior to contrast use, underscoring the importance of thorough evaluation within the imaging process. Because patients typically present with varying functional status, modifications to approach and protocol that minimize risk while preserving diagnostic effectiveness are essential for delivering optimal patient outcomes in head and neck imaging. Moreover, ongoing innovation in imaging technology, such as the development of synthetic contrast agents highlighted in recent literature, presents both challenges and opportunities. Techniques such as the development of synthetic contrast-enhanced virtual monoenergetic images derived from non-contrast CT scans offer encouraging alternatives that can reduce reliance on traditional contrast media, thereby reducing risks associated with their use. One recent study suggested that deep learning methods may improve imaging quality without the risks associated with iodine contrast agents (Gao et al., 2025). However, the challenges of integrating new imaging technologies into practice remain considerable. This revolution requires rigorous testing under clinical trials to ascertain safety and efficacy in different patient groups and to ensure new techniques are in accordance with the prevailing standards of care of head and neck imaging (Kürten et al., 2024) (Figure 2.9).

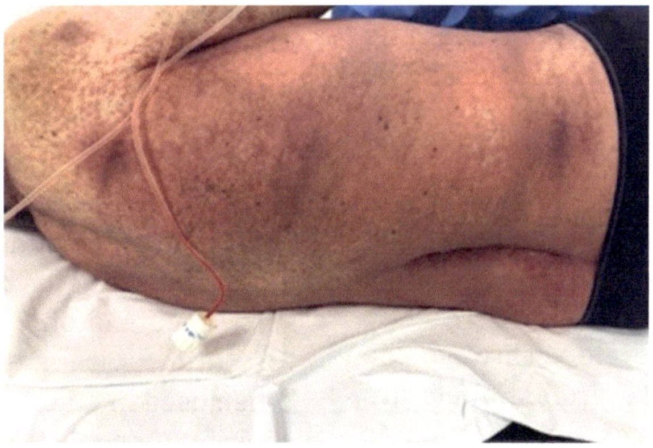

Figure 2.9. Image showing contrast-related allergic reaction risks.

Source: https://jours.isi-science.com/imageXml.php?i=amjcaserep-22-e928930-g001.tif&idArt=928930&w=1000.

2.4. Clinical Applications of Imaging Techniques

The clinical application of imaging techniques in the diagnosis of head and neck disorders plays a vital role in enhancing patient prognosis and therapeutic intervention. Among all imaging modalities, Quantitative Phase Imaging (QPI) has been demonstrated to be an effective non-invasive technique with excellent phase sensitivity, capturing high-fidelity morphological data that is pivotal for assessing cellular responses in cancer. This approach is particularly relevant in the case of head and neck cancer, when information regarding the effect of radiation therapy can be employed to direct treatment. Integration of explainable AI approaches with QPI enables clinicians to better understand deep learning models and associate them with clinical decision-making. These developments have the potential to identify subtle differences in tumor response phenotypes and, hence, to provide actionable biomarkers and enable personalized therapy to evolve with technological progress (Arora et al., 2024).

In addition to QPI, dynamic contrast-enhanced MR lymphangiography (DCE-MRL) has made great strides in visualizing the lymphatic pathway, particularly in the head and neck. This imaging modality provides the detailed insight into lymphatic anatomy and flow that is required for the diagnosis of numerous congenital and acquired lymphatic diseases. The complexity of lymphatic anatomy means that high-tech imaging is needed to effectively visualize and evaluate the pathologies that can develop. Through the use of DCE-MRL, healthcare professionals are able to obtain important insights into lymphatic physiology and also utilize findings in order to maximize treatment protocols. Because it can show both lymphatic morphology and functional flow, DCE-MRL demonstrates how imaging technology can provide detailed diagnostic information, thereby enhancing multidisciplinary management of head and neck illness (Negm et al., 2024). In addition to the diagnostic value, however, is the revolutionizing influence on therapeutic concepts in head and neck medicine. The employment of novel imaging techniques, such as DCE-MRI, facilitates improved understanding of the disease course and increased interventional therapies through providing real-time visualization during the intervention. With increasing access to imaging data, clinicians can make more evidence-based, informed decisions about patient-specific interventions. This development showcases the ability of imaging technologies to not just identify pathology but also to significantly affect clinical workflows and the quality of patient care. Placing emphasis on the continuous evolution of imaging techniques emphasizes the importance of healthcare professionals staying abreast of the updates to ensure that they apply the newest technologies to improve diagnostic accuracy and treatment outcomes in head and neck surgeries (Arora et al., 2024; Negm et al., 2024).

2.4.1. Tumor and Lesion Diagnosis

Diagnostic assessment of head and neck tumors and lesions is closely associated with various imaging modalities, which provide critical information about their nature and behavior. CT and MRI are the most effective modalities employed in the diagnostic evaluation, and they excel in delineating tumor margins, local invasiveness, and potential metastasis to guide clinical management. As a case in point, MRI is particularly effective in the visualization of soft tissue anatomy and offers higher contrast resolution within the head and neck region. When used in tandem, these technologies enable clinicians not only to establish a reliable diagnosis but also to develop treatment protocols based on the unique profile of each patient's tumor presentation (Figure 2.10).

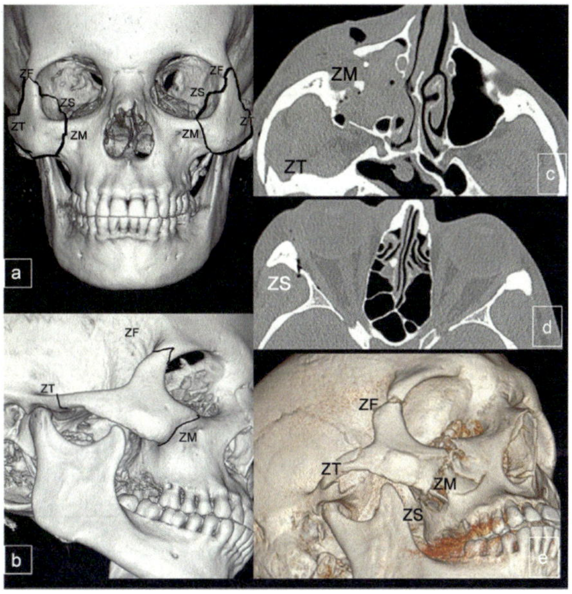

Figure 2.10. CT image illustrating facial bone fracture in trauma evaluation.

Source: https://media.springernature.com/lw1200/springer-static/image/art%3A10.1186%2Fs13244-020-00847-w/MediaObjects/13244_2020_847_Fig11_HTML.png.

New imaging technologies have also contributed to improving the accuracy of tumor diagnosis. Positron emission tomography with specific tracers holds promise in defining metabolic activity in tumors, which can be crucial in distinguishing benign lesions from malignant tumors. In familial paraganglioma syndrome type 1, with problems raised by recent research, diligent imaging strategies, including functional imaging techniques, become imperative. These techniques, such as 18F-3,4-dihydroxyphenylalanine (18F-DOPA) PET-CT, give the highest diagnostic accuracy and are presently the standard of care in evaluating tumor traits and staging. Using multiple imaging modalities also enables thorough evaluation, ensuring that clinicians consider all diagnostic possibilities before reaching a final conclusion regarding the lesions observed (Cantisani et al., 2020).

Specific considerations are to be taken into account when diagnosing rare tumors, such as hypoglossal schwannomas. Lesions will frequently mimic more common pathologies, and the diagnostic evaluation can be difficult, with a high index of suspicion needed in the clinicians' minds. A case worth noting is a hypoglossal schwannoma that was presenting as a carotid body tumor, and it underscores the necessity of newer imaging technologies such as magnetic resonance angiography (MRA) to resolve these diagnoses. The specific features of these imaging tests, such as the use of contrast agents, can significantly influence diagnostic outcomes and surgical planning. These intricacies underscore the need for a multi-disciplinary strategy in managing head and neck tumors, integrating the imaging findings and clinical presentation to formulate an accurate diagnosis and well-informed treatment plan (Abie et al., 2012).

2.4.2. Injuries and Trauma Assessment

There is a need for proper evaluation of trauma and injury in the head and neck region to make an accurate diagnosis and treatment. High-energy blows, such as might be found in motor accidents or sports, can have vast cervical spine and brachial plexus injuries. The complexity of these injuries demands a systematic approach to imaging and evaluation. The initial assessments of these patients typically begin with radiographic imaging techniques, such as computed tomography (CT) and magnetic resonance imaging (MRI), to provide extensive information on both bony and soft-tissue anatomy. Results from radiography may not always accurately reflect the severity of injury, and therefore, the link between imaging findings and clinical evaluations becomes the most important thing. Identification of the association between the mechanism of injury and resulting imaging findings can enhance clinical decision-making and ultimately patient care. Presentation of a 19-year-old male who hurt his shoulder while practicing football highlights the challenge in evaluating head and neck trauma (Figure 2.11).

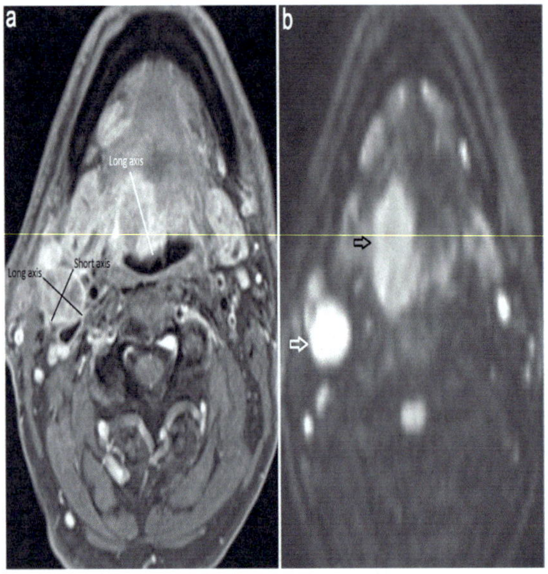

Figure 2.11. MRI in head and neck cancer following chemoradiotherapy.

Source: https://media.springernature.com/lw1200/springer-static/image/art%3A10.1007%2Fs00330-021-07913-x/MediaObjects/330_2021_7913_Fig1_HTML.png.

Despite early MRI findings of a cervical cord contusion, eventual neurological evaluation revealed an upper brachial plexus avulsion injury, which was also confirmed by CT myelogram. This serves to remind us that imaging studies, while useful, can at times be misleading and require a full physical examination to make an adequate diagnosis. In cases of polytrauma patients who may present with traumatic injury of the upper extremity in combination with trauma to the head or cervical spine, exclusive reliance on imaging would lead to second-best management plans. Early surgical intervention and prompt diagnosis are crucial to improving long-term outcomes in this regard (Aversano et al., 2010). Other than the complex mechanisms of cervical spine and brachial plexus injuries, medical professionals must also consider other anatomical structures that are susceptible to trauma, that is, soft tissues. Soft tissue injuries in the surrounding area of the Achilles tendon, for example, pose certain challenges for reconstruction, and hence a multidisciplinary management strategy is required. The free anterolateral thigh (ALT) flap, one of the options in reconstructive surgery, has proved useful for covering soft-tissue loss in traumatic injury. Assessments of various reconstructive modalities underscore the need to understand the advantages and limitations of each. In cases of widespread loss of soft tissue in trauma patients, coordination between systematic imaging strategies and surgical modalities is essential in an effort to optimize functional outcomes and enhance recovery quality for patients. Finally, thorough knowledge about the assessment of trauma in different dimensions is essential in the domain of head and neck trauma (Chou et al., 2013).

2.4.3. Monitoring Treatment Response and Disease Progression

Monitoring head and neck cancer progression and response to therapy has been improved by advances in imaging technology and biomarker evaluation. Invasive conventional methods, such as invasive biopsies and physical examination, are prone to shortcomings due to their inaccuracy and associated distress. These restraints emphasize the worth of other technologies, including liquid biopsies, which enable physicians to gain essential information from non-invasive samples of bodily fluids. The assessment of circulating tumor DNA (ctDNA) and other biomarkers is gaining popularity, as it can more effectively track a patient's cancer status over time without invasive methods. The integration of these cutting-edge monitoring techniques is critical for early identification of progression or recurrence, thereby allowing clinicians to adjust treatment modalities to optimize patients' prognosis (Sami et al., 2024).

Further, the implementation of user-friendly surveillance systems has been of interest regarding cancer progression in head and neck cancer patients. These systems utilize a variety of data inputs—from patient activity levels and clinical histories—to identify early clinical deterioration. An example is the use of wearable technology, which has proven effective in delivering actionable information about a patient's health status. For instance, Fitbit trackers can capture vital signs and activity levels and pave the way for predictive models that signal potential clinical deterioration, such as unplanned emergency presentations or treatment adjustments. Such proactive care is highly compatible with high-stakes oncology care, where timely intervention can significantly reduce the risk of cancer treatment.

Successful use of these technologies indicates the potential to improve the accuracy of treatment response monitoring and to effectively manage the complex treatment protocols for head and neck cancer (Nath et al., 2021). Ongoing advances in imaging modalities and biomarker monitoring, as head and neck oncology evolves, are necessary to maintain successful management of the disease. Combining these modalities with clinical decision-making can offer an enriched, holistic appreciation of disease progression. For example, state-of-the-art imaging modalities such as PET-CT and MRI may offer extensive anatomical and functional data to complement biomarker analysis. These approaches combined enable medical experts to develop their predictive abilities. Therefore, ongoing research into liquid biopsies in conjunction with established imaging techniques holds promise for a better, less invasive system for monitoring treatment response. This adaptive modification is critical, as it not only enhances patient comfort but also contributes to the greater good of enhancing treatment protocols and thus the quality of care in head and neck cancers (Sami et al., 2024).

2.5. Future Trends in Head and Neck Imaging

The evolving landscape of head and neck imaging is strongly influenced by advances in artificial intelligence (AI) and machine learning. These technologies have the potential to enhance diagnostic performance, streamline workflows, and deliver customized treatment plans. Deep learning algorithms, for instance, are being increasingly designed and trained on imaging data to identify tumors and predict patient outcomes with unflinching precision. This integration of AI into imaging protocols not only optimizes early detection but also enables the study of potential biomarkers that can guide treatment decisions. With further development of such systems, high-quality information and multidisciplinary interaction become ever more critical. Addressing problems such as algorithmic bias will ensure that AI applications in head and neck imaging are effective and equitable, therebyensuring an AI-enabled diagnostic future that greatly enhances patient care and treatment outcomes (Tuan et al., 2024).

The future of molecular imaging is also likely to undergo a drastic change, particularly in the intraoperative assessment of head and neck cancers. The development and utilization of targeted near-infrared fluorescence agents have shown promise in this field. Agents such as panitumumab-IRDye800 enable surgeons to visualize cancerous tissue in real time during surgery, thereby achieving negative margins with improved efficiency. The method enhances the accuracy of tumor resections and decreases the risk of recurrence, which is a significant concern in the treatment of head and neck cancer. With increasing research, the uses of these imaging modalities will expand, and rigorous tests of their effectiveness and limitations will be required. In the future, molecular imaging may be more integrated with traditional methods, thereby enabling greater accuracy in surgery and improved patient outcomes in head and neck oncology (Haley et al., 2024). Furthermore, the advent of multi-modal imaging approaches is poised to revolutionize head and neck imaging practice. The combination of different modalities, such as MRI, CT, and ultrasound, enables clinicians to collect extensive information regarding the anatomical and functional characteristics of head and neck organs. The simultaneous observation of both areas is crucial for assessing pathologies, surgical planning, and evaluating treatment outcomes. New technology, such as hybrid imaging, will enable simultaneous acquisition of imaging information, yielding greater sensitivity and specificity for the detection of abnormalities. These technologies will not only enhance diagnostic accuracy but also individualize planning of treatments for each patient's own individual clinical circumstance. With these technologies becoming more advanced, ongoing research and development will be in the forefront of defining the destiny of head and neck imaging, ultimately leading to improved patient outcomes and care within this specialty (Tuan et al., 2024).

2.5.1. Advancements in Imaging Technology

Technological advances in imaging have completely transformed head and neck imaging, enhancing diagnosis and treatment planning for a variety of diseases. The older methods of imaging, such as X-rays and CT scanning, have been rudimentary building blocks; however, newer advances in magnetic resonance imaging (MRI), particularly fat- and water-separation-based methods, have opened new vistas for head and neck pathology. The use of advanced software allows clinicians to differentiate between tissue types with greater precision, providing information that is valuable to both diagnosis and treatment planning. As highlighted in the current literature, the use of such advanced imaging modalities not only enables the detection of occult anatomical changes but also provides a better understanding of the biopsychosocial determinants of symptoms, with the promise of improved patient outcomes through targeted therapy (Crawford et al., 2018) (Figure 2.12).

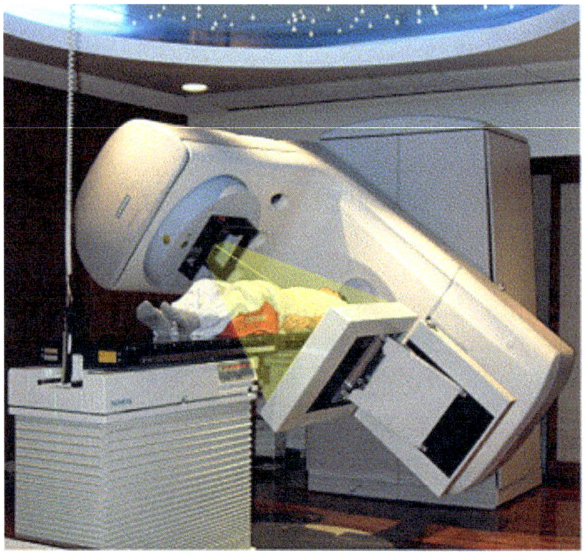

Figure 2.12. Megavoltage cone-beam CT (MVCBCT) system.

Source: https://ars.els-cdn.com/content/image/1-s2.0-S0958394705001962-gr1.jpg.

Additionally, megavoltage cone-beam CT (MVCBCT) is a significant breakthrough in head and neck imaging, yielding high-resolution three-dimensional images that are critical for treatment planning, particularly in oncology. MVCBCT enables real-time imaging during radiation therapy, allowing the treatment plan to be adjusted to maximize dose delivery based on the patient's anatomy at the time of treatment. Despite the advantages, dose calculations are complicated by artifacts in the image data; however, novel correction methods have been developed to improve the quality of images of this type. By mitigating MVCBCT's shortcomings, such as missing data and cupping artifacts, doctors can ensure that imaging accurately represents tumor and organ locations, thereby optimizing treatment efficacy and minimizing collateral injury to nearby healthy tissues. This development holds the promise of new imaging technologies to enhance protocols and enhance standards of care in head and neck treatment paradigms (Aubry et al., 2009). Moreover, interdisciplinary collaboration between radiologists, oncologists, and scientists is important in employing advancements in imaging technology to enhance the care of patients. As new imaging technologies are developed, the integration of clinical data with these technologies creates an environment conducive to revolutionary research and clinical innovation. New technologies have opened the possibility of new diagnostic modalities, enabling more subtle assessment of head and neck disease and the development of innovative treatment approaches. With ongoing investigation and the application of cutting-edge imaging techniques, the potential to untangle complex pathophysiological processes grows, enabling progress toward precision medicine. Therefore, these imaging developments not only grow the diagnostic toolkit but also enable clinicians to implement more individualized treatment regimens that are informed by detailed visual analysis, ultimately improving overall patient quality of life.

2.5.2. Artificial Intelligence's Role in Analysis of Images

The use of artificial intelligence (AI) in imaging analysis has revolutionized head and neck imaging, bringing the diagnostic process to less time-consuming yet more accurate levels. With the implementation of advanced machine learning tools and deep learning systems, AI also enhances the interpretation of complex imaging modalities such as computed tomography (CT), magnetic resonance imaging (MRI), and positron emission tomography (PET).

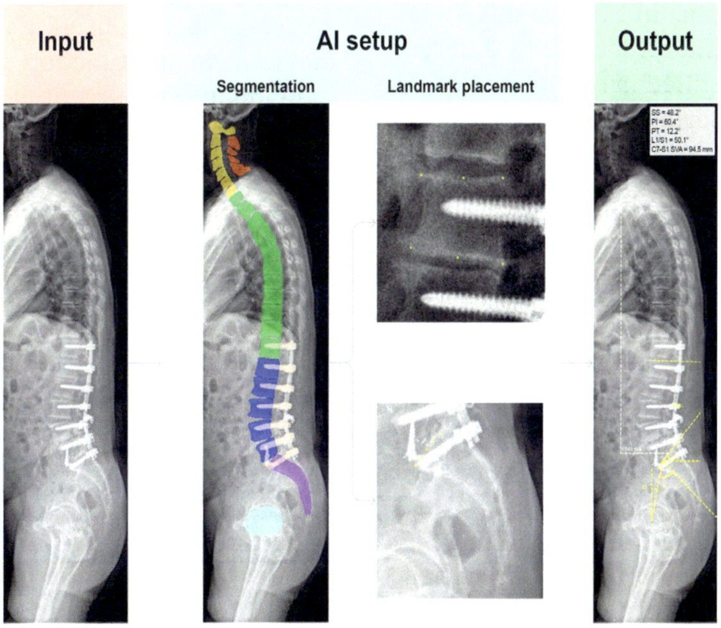

Figure 2.13. Schematic showing AI-based image segmentation in radiology.

Source: https://www.researchgate.net/publication/377463930/figure/fig1/AS:11431281288207690@1730602309803/AI-based-landmark-detection-and-segmentation.png.

Not only do these technologies improve the detection of anomalies, but they also facilitate better information about the anatomical structures that are affected in head and neck pathologies. For instance, AI-enabled solutions can assist radiologists in identifying subtle lesions, leading to earlier intervention and better patient outcomes in head and neck cancer (Broggi et al., 2024). As machine learning continues to develop, its ability to deal with big data sets will shed light that enhances diagnostic precision, confirming the central role that AI plays in our current imaging protocols (Figure 2.13).

Besides, the application of convolutional neural networks (CNNs) in image analysis is an ideal example of innovations in the automation of radiological image interpretation. CNNs have been shown to segment and grade head-and-neck scan tumors efficiently, reducing the subjectivity inherent in traditional evaluation techniques. Not only does this function the time spent on image analysis, but it also allows for higher consistency in interpretations by different radiologists. As highlighted in recent studies, AI algorithms have outperformed human experts on certain diagnostic tasks, demonstrating their potential to be beneficial additions to clinical practice (Tuan et al., 2024). Automation of intensive image assessment work through AI tools positions healthcare professionals to focus on patient care and treatment decision-making rather than being overwhelmed by extensive interpretive tasks. In addition to improving diagnostic capabilities, AI's role in imaging analysis extends to facilitating personalized treatment planning and monitoring patient responses to therapies. By leveraging imaging data alongside molecular profiling and patient health records, AI systems can identify treatment protocols tailored to the unique characteristics of each patient's condition. This unification centers on AI's promise within predictive modeling, developing the capability to forecast treatment results based on successful histories in the past. However, concerns such as data standardization, algorithmic explainability, and interdisciplinarity remain at the core of advancing the use of AI in head and neck imaging. Overcoming these challenges is central to realizing the full potential of AI, enabling groundbreaking advances in how healthcare professionals arrive at diagnoses, treatments, and follow-ups for head and neck cancers (Broggi et al., 2024).

2.5.3. Potential for Personalized Medicine in Imaging

The potential of personalized medicine in the field of head and neck cancer imaging methods is unfolding at a rapid pace, fueled by long-standing advances in diagnostic imaging devices. With patient-specific therapy now emerging as a pillar of modern oncology, the integration of personalized imaging protocols can optimize the precision of therapy. For instance, emerging imaging technologies such as SPECT and PET enable enhanced visualization of tumor metabolism and function, making it possible to individualize treatment plans accordingly. With the use of 3D-printed anthropomorphic phantoms in radiopharmaceutical therapy, researchers can replicate patient-specific anatomy, enabling tailored dosimetry that aligns with the individual biological characteristics of each patient's tumor (Adam et al., 2022). This approach not only enhances the precision of dose delivery but also minimizes damage to the surrounding normal tissues, hence the importance of personalized imaging in optimal treatment of head and neck cancers. Furthermore, personalized imaging and medicine are also used to detect cancer biomarkers and guide treatment (Figure 2.14).

With increasing understanding of the molecular origins of head and neck cancer, personalized therapies are now starting to surface as promising alternatives, particularly for those patients whose cancers harbor specific genetic mutations. With this understanding, it will be feasible to develop imaging agents that can visualize such biomarkers *in vivo*, which will open the doors to more informed and targeted therapeutic interventions. The current interest in the integration of molecular imaging with standard imaging modalities is an adaptation on the potential that personalized medicine has in maximizing patient outcomes in head and neck oncology. Additionally, the use of targeted drug therapies and immunotherapy, coupled with precise imaging techniques, aligns with current advances in cancer treatment regimens (Anand et al., 2022) to provide systematic treatments that extend disease-free survival in patients.

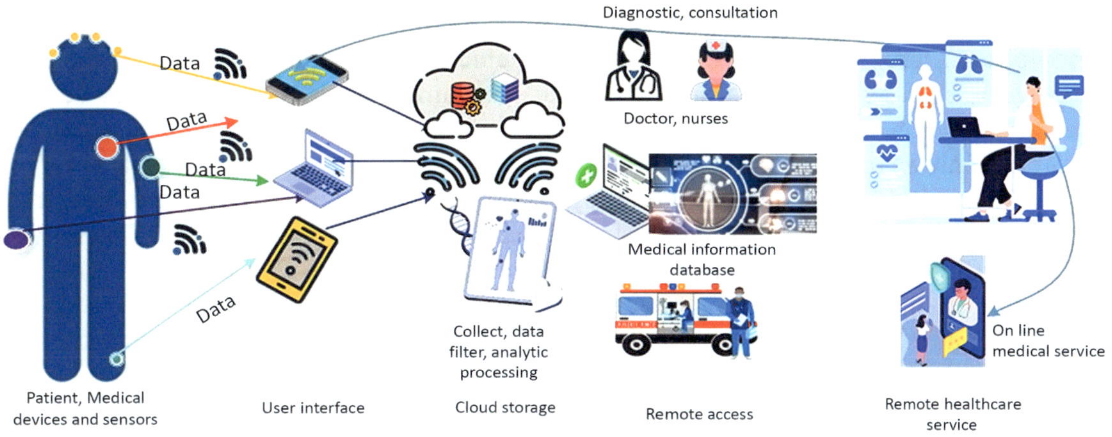

Figure 2.14. Diagram of patient-specific imaging protocols using AI tools.

Source: https://www.mdpi.com/engproc/engproc-70-00054/article_deploy/html/images/engproc-70-00054-g001.png.

The advancement in personalized imaging is also marked by the broad capability to avoid the toxicity of conventional treatment. Chemotherapy is a widely used option for treatment, but it is most likely to have side effects that make patients' quality of life difficult. Personalized diagnostic imaging makes fine-tuning chemotherapy regimens possible by identifying patients who will benefit the most from specific agents and thereby avoid unnecessary exposures. By integrating personalized imaging techniques, such as targeted isotopes in radiopharmaceutical therapy, medical professionals can monitor therapeutic effects in real time and customize treatment strategies based on individual patient data. This dynamic practice not only enhances clinical outcomes but also serves the higher goals of individualized medicine by providing patients with the assurance that they are receiving the best and least harmful therapy possible (Adam et al., 2022). Emphasis on these benefits positions personalized imaging at the forefront of the future treatment of head and neck cancer.

SUMMARY

In conclusion, advances in head and neck imaging modalities have greatly enhanced diagnostic capability, therapeutic planning, and outcomes. A deep understanding of the intricacies of head and neck anatomy and pathology is required to utilize these imaging modalities effectively. Optical imaging, with advances such as optical coherence tomography (OCT), has been a high-resolution, non-invasive technique, enabling real-time visualization of structures. These innovations not only improve disease evaluation but also further our overall knowledge of inherent biological processes, leading to the best clinical outcomes in head and neck disorders like cancers and developmental disorders (Lee et al., 2025). In addition, the marriage of targeted imaging agents, particularly for head and neck cancers (HNC), is an immense improvement. The use of near-infrared fluorescence-guided surgery, such as administering drugs like panitumumab-IRDye800, enables surgeons to enhance the precision of tumor resections and surgical margin analysis (Haley et al., 2024). The equipment not only enables intraoperative detection of malignancies but also helps identify sentinel nodes, a process critical for staging and therapy. As these techniques continue to evolve, they hold great promise for redefining outcomes in surgery and reducing the recurrence of cancer. Finally, ongoing research into head and neck imaging techniques paves the way for future progress and better techniques. Multidisciplinary collaboration between radiologists, oncologists, and surgeons is obviously required to maximize the potential of these imaging techniques. With an emphasis on a holistic patient care strategy, the incorporation of new imaging modalities will ultimately lead to tailored treatment protocols, improve our understanding of disease pathophysiology, and enable early detection mechanisms. Thus, continued exploration of these fronts in head and neck imaging not only has the potential to improve clinical outcomes but also to enhance understanding of complex head and neck pathophysiologies (Lee et al., 2025; Haley et al., 2024).

CLOSER LOOK

HEAD AND NECK IMAGING:

Head and neck imaging is a world of rapidly advancing technology, and the specialty is driven by the need for constant research and development. With imaging technologies as well as diagnostics and outcomes improving, ongoing innovation becomes imperative. The integration of artificial intelligence into image interpretation, for instance, offers real potential to enhance the interpretation of complex cases. Furthermore, advancements in imaging methods, such as MRI and CT scans, require ongoing research to optimize protocols and minimize radiation exposure while maintaining patient safety as paramount. All of these incremental advances are the overall need for a dedication to ongoing refinement in methodology and technology so that practitioners are continually equipped with cutting-edge tools and information within their diagnostic arsenal. Furthermore, the development of new imaging agents and technologies is important in the creation of head and neck imaging technologies. Research and development that enable the production of improved contrast materials capable of improving the detectability of various tissue types play an important role in the diagnostic process. New techniques, such as hybrid imaging modalities combining PET and CT, offer superior information for tumor characterization and treatment planning, allowing for more personalized therapeutic strategies. Similarly, ongoing research to assess the safety and efficacy of these novel agents is important for determining the best way to use imaging to treat head and neck illnesses. All of these advances, individually and collectively, emphasize the need for specialist research and development programs to keep abreast of technological progress and guide evidence-based clinical practice within a constantly evolving healthcare environment. Continued development in healthcare regulations and patient needs underscores the importance of ongoing research and development in head and neck imaging. Technology, such as telemedicine and remote diagnostics, is increasingly taking root, and the demand for efficient imaging strategies has widened beyond traditional clinical settings. The studies must address these evolving situations by considering the accessibility and effectiveness of imaging techniques across various populations, especially the underprivileged. There remains an ongoing need for comprehensive studies that contrast imaging outcomes, safety practices, and patient satisfaction to inform best practices. To this end, researchers have a crucial role in bridging knowledge and practice gaps, so that head and neck imaging continues to be at the vanguard of addressing challenges in modern medicine, thereby leading to improved patient care and outcomes in an ever-changing healthcare environment.

The future of patient outcomes and care for head and neck imaging depends increasingly on technological advancements that enhance diagnostic accuracy and therapeutic strategies. Advances in technologies such as high-resolution CT and MRI enable enhanced visualization of complex anatomical structures relevant to oncology, making improved treatment planning feasible. For instance, the evolution of functional imaging modalities, which are able to quantify biological events at the cellular level, has significantly enhanced cancerous tissue identification. With an evolving understanding of tumor biology, integrating such imaging modalities will enable early intervention techniques, culminating in better patient outcomes and quality of life. Moreover, ongoing research into the molecular and genetic characteristics of head and neck tumors can lead to tailored imaging protocols that are adaptive to individual patient profiles, optimizing both outcomes from therapy and individualized models of care. Additionally, head and neck oncology patient management will be aided by the integration of new imaging modalities and artificial intelligence (AI) and machine learning. These technologies can aid radiologists in identifying patterns and abnormalities that may be challenging to detect with the naked eye. AI algorithms are able to sift through large volumes of imaging data in order to provide predictive information on tumor growth and patient outcomes, which can lead to more informed clinical decisions. For example, as shown by the investigation of head and neck cancer patients at advanced stages and survival trends, surgery has been associated with improved survival compared with non-surgical treatment (Kidwai et al., 2016). Such research underscores the pivotal role of advanced imaging in identifying viable treatment options and the potential to prolong patients' lives through early, effective surgery. In addition to technological innovation, future implications of head and neck imaging for patient care will also emphasize multidisciplinary teamwork and patient-led care. As healthcare systems continue to evolve, the need for collaborative models of care that incorporate input from oncologists, radiologists, surgeons, and allied health professionals becomes increasingly significant. Such a multidisciplinary approach not only enhances the decision-making process regarding treatment options but also respects patient preferences and values. Clinical guidelines for the surgical treatment of stage IVb tumors demonstrate favorable survival and thus justify discussion of aggressive treatment even in situations deemed otherwise unresectable (Kidwai et al., 2016). Furthermore, patient involvement in treatment planning and the use of imaging findings to educate patients regarding their conditions have the potential to empower the patient, facilitating a more holistic model of care that ultimately improves outcomes and satisfaction.

REFERENCES

1. Adam, D. P., Grudzinski, J. J., Bormett, I., Cox, B. L., Marsh, I. R., Bradshaw, T. J., Harari, P. M., & Bednarz, B. P. (2022). Validation of Monte Carlo 131I radiopharmaceutical dosimetry workflow using a 3D-printed anthropomorphic head and neck phantom. *Medical Physics, 49*(8), 5491–5503. https://doi.org/10.1002/mp.15699Alzabni, A. S., Alrashdi, M. M. M., Al Rashidi, S. A., Alzabni, S. H. M., Alqabba, A. H., Alazmi, N. F. G., Alshammari, Y. S. S., et al. (2022). Magnetic resonance imaging (MRI): Emphasis may be placed on new developments in MRI techniques, such as functional magnetic resonance imaging (fMRI) or dynamic contrast-enhancing MRI (DCE-MRI). https://core.ac.uk/download/616775513.pdf (accessed on 15th July 2025).
2. Anand, U., Dey, A., Singh Chandel, A. K., Sanyal, R., Mishra, A., Pandey, D. K., De Falco, V., et al. (2022). Cancer chemotherapy and beyond: Current status, drug candidates, associated risks and progress in targeted therapeutics. *Genes & Diseases, 10*, 1367–1401. https://doi.org/10.1016/j.gendis.2022.02.007 (accessed on 15th July 2025).
3. Arduini, F., Barile, A., Cantisani, V., Cassoni, A., et al. (2020). Narrative review of multiparametric ultrasound in parotid gland evaluation. https://core.ac.uk/download/480109992.pdf (accessed on 15th July 2025).
4. Arora, S., Tandon, A., Ray, S., Rajaram, N., & Barman, I. (2024). A framework for explainable deep learning for aiding clinical applications of quantitative phase imaging. *Proceedings of SPIE, 12852*, 128520H–128520H-4. https://www.semanticscholar.org/paper/b797e5fe3742f4549b3c1c678dc9ccffebfe10f2 (accessed on 15th July 2025).
5. Aubry, J. F., Beaulieu, L., Cheung, J., Gottschalk, A., et al. (2009). Correction of megavoltage cone-beam CT images of the pelvic region based on phantom measurements for dose calculation purposes. https://core.ac.uk/download/323074404.pdf (accessed on 15th July 2025).
6. Aversano, M., Gonzalez-Giraldo, E., Heuer, G. G., Macyszyn, L., et al. (2010). Brachial plexus injury mimicking a spinal-cord injury. https://core.ac.uk/download/323076297.pdf (accessed on 15th July 2025).
7. Baatenburg de Jong, R. J., & Rongen, R. J. (1990). Ultrasound examination of the head and neck. https://core.ac.uk/download/18513420.pdf (accessed on 15th July 2025).
8. Bache, C. E., Harmatz, P. R., Jester, A., Mackenzie, W. G., et al. (2014). Orthopedic management of the extremities in patients with Morquio A syndrome. https://core.ac.uk/download/323062594.pdf (accessed on 15th July 2025).
9. Bec, J., Bewley, A., Dochow, S., Farwell, M., et al. (2019). Autofluorescence lifetime augmented reality as a means for real-time robotic surgery guidance in human patients. https://core.ac.uk/download/323070672.pdf (accessed on 15th July 2025).
10. Bellati, F., Caserta, D., Costanzi, F., De Marco, E., et al. (2018). Real-time virtual sonography in gynecology & obstetrics: Literature's analysis and case series. https://core.ac.uk/download/195777140.pdf (accessed on 15th July 2025).
11. Broggi, G., Maniaci, A., Lentini, M., Palicelli, A., Zanelli, M., Zizzo, M., Koufopoulos, N. I., et al. (2024). Artificial intelligence in head and neck cancer diagnosis: A comprehensive review with emphasis on radiomics, histopathological, and molecular applications. *Cancers, 16*. https://www.semanticscholar.org/paper/47d41fb7b3620b75495be1bbeb8dd88bfc8be899 (accessed on 15th July 2025).

12. Cantisani, V., Colao, A., Di Leo, N., Faggiano, A., et al. (2020). Natural history and management of familial paraganglioma syndrome type 1: Long-term data from a large family. https://core.ac.uk/download/296244529.pdf (accessed on 15th July 2025).

13. Chen, C., Gao, G., Xu, Y., Pu, L., Wang, Q., Wang, L., Wang, W., et al. (2020). SARS-CoV-2–positive sputum and feces after conversion of pharyngeal samples in patients with COVID-19. *Annals of Internal Medicine, 172*, 832–834. https://doi.org/10.7326/m20-0991 (accessed on 15th July 2025).

14. Chou, S., Osman, S., Rosing, J., Sahar, D., et al. (2013). Total posterior leg opens wound management with free anterolateral thigh flap: Case and literature review. https://core.ac.uk/download/323068446.pdf (accessed on 15th July 2025).

15. Crawford, R. J., Elliott, J. M., Hancock, M. J., Smith, A., et al. (2018). Advancing imaging technologies for patients with spinal pain: With a focus on whiplash injury. https://core.ac.uk/download/161704527.pdf (accessed on 15th July 2025).

16. Culp, W. T. N., Spriet, M., & Willcox, J. L. (2019). Role of positron emission tomography in imaging of non-neurologic disorders of the head, neck, and teeth in veterinary medicine. https://core.ac.uk/download/323070037.pdf (accessed on 15th July 2025).

17. Di Finizio, A., Nardi, C., Bicci, E., Treballi, F., Mungai, F., Sica, G., Calamandrei, L., et al. (2024). Head and neck squamous cell carcinoma: Insights from dual-energy computed tomography (DECT). https://core.ac.uk/download/654475049.pdf (accessed on 15th July 2025).

18. Duthoy, W. (2006). Intensity modulated radiation therapy and arc therapy: Validation and evolution as applied to tumors of the head and neck, abdominal and pelvic regions. https://core.ac.uk/download/55748558.pdf (accessed on 15th July 2025).

19. Feygin, T., Khalek, N., & Moldenhauer, J. (2020). Fetal brain, head, and neck tumors: Prenatal imaging and management. *Prenatal Diagnosis, 40*, 1203–1219. https://www.semanticscholar.org/paper/150406043868e0ad23af745469d1133be669ea25 (accessed on 15th July 2025).

20. Gao, Y., Xie, H., Chang, C. W., Qiu, R. L. J., Wang, T., Roper, J., Ghavidel, B., et al. (2025). CT-based synthetic contrast-enhanced virtual monoenergetic images generation using conditional denoising diffusion probabilistic model. *Proceedings of SPIE, 13411*, 134111D–134111D-6. https://www.semanticscholar.org/paper/68595b182fccb71ac41aa75dfb2fc012a983228f (accessed on 15th July 2025).

21. Ginat, D. T., & Neilio, J. M. (2024). Emerging head and neck tumor targeting contrast agents for the purpose of CT, MRI, and multimodal diagnostic imaging: A molecular review. https://core.ac.uk/download/614775487.pdf (accessed on 15th July 2025).

22. Holcman, D., & Hoze, N. (2014). Residence times of receptors in dendritic spines analyzed by simulations in empirical domains. https://core.ac.uk/download/pdf/82192157.pdf (accessed on 15th July 2025).

23. Illimoottil, M., & Ginat, D. (2023). Recent advances in deep learning and medical imaging for head and neck cancer treatment: MRI, CT, and PET scans. *Cancers, 15*. https://www.semanticscholar.org/paper/1d833c1290430ec16880980b2efcff53ea930983 (accessed on 15th July 2025).

24. Johnson, D. E., Burtness, B., Leemans, C. R., Lui, V. W. Y., Bauman, J. E., & Grandis, J. R. (2020). Head and neck squamous cell carcinoma. *Nature Reviews Disease Primers, 6*. https://doi.org/10.1038/s41572-020-00224-3 (accessed on 15th July 2025).

25. Kalová, M., Kubíček, J., Oczka, D., Tomanec, M., et al. (2019). Recent trends, technical concepts and components of computer-assisted orthopedic surgery systems: A comprehensive review. https://core.ac.uk/download/287649034.pdf (accessed on 15th July 2025).

26. Kidwai, N. (2016). Stage T4B head and neck cancer survival outcome comparisons based on treatment modality: Is surgery a viable treatment option? https://open.bu.edu/bitstream/2144/16169/1/Kidwai_bu_0017N_11136.pdf (accessed on 15th July 2025).

27. Kürten, C., & Ferris, R. L. (2024). Neoadjuvante Immuntherapie bei Kopf-Hals-Plattenepithelkarzinomen. *Laryngo-Rhino-Otologie, 103*, S167–S187. https://www.semanticscholar.org/paper/f28345970b22ad940cb58b19686ef52feebcb683 (accessed on 15th July 2025).

28. LeBoff, M. S., Greenspan, S. L., Insogna, K., Lewiecki, E. M., Saag, K. G., Singer, A., & Siris, E. S. (2022). The clinician's guide to prevention and treatment of osteoporosis. *Osteoporosis International, 33*, 2049–2102. https://doi.org/10.1007/s00198-021-05900-y (accessed on 15th July 2025).

29. Lee, E., Chou, L., Chen, Z., & Wong, B. J. F. (2025). Optical imaging of cilia in the head and neck. *Journal of Clinical Medicine, 14*. https://www.semanticscholar.org/paper/4f85a25d35b52e548bb9832b491b0be0e9566f93 (accessed on 15th July 2025).

30. Mendelsohn, A. H., Sidell, D. R., Blackwell, K. E., & Lee, M. K. (2012). Hypoglossal schwannoma masquerading as a carotid body tumor. https://core.ac.uk/download/323079597.pdf (accessed on 15th July 2025).

31. Molga-Magusiak, M., Krawczyk, P., Rzepakowska, A., & Niemczyk, K. (2024). Application of ultrasound shear wave elastography in tumors of head and neck region–A preliminary study and literature review. *Polski Przegląd Otorynolaryngologiczny*. https://www.semanticscholar.org/paper/9d5a1f2f54247a3911117ce79c99b9fa573a2b35 (accessed on 15th July 2025).

32. Nagano, S. Y. M., Chojniak, R., & Porto, G. (2025). Magnetic resonance permeability for the evaluation of head and neck tumors: Parotid and beyond. *Journal of Clinical Imaging Science, 15*. https://www.semanticscholar.org/paper/53859f39d71839e621be6875302548e9f482e9ee (accessed on 15th July 2025).

33. Nassar, S. I., Suk, A., Nguyen, S. A., Adilbay, D., Pang, J., & Nathan, C. A. O. (2024). The role of ctDNA and liquid biopsy in the diagnosis and monitoring of head and neck cancer: Towards precision medicine. *Cancers, 16*. https://www.semanticscholar.org/paper/5837672b53b51d140f149f4773f0a6dd7510ffe1 (accessed on 15th July 2025).

34. Nath, P., Mahadevan, S., Slagle, J., Agarwal, R., Kohutek, Z., Gillaspie, E., Rohde, S., et al. (2021). Using Fitbit data to predict clinical deterioration and unplanned treatment events in cancer outpatients. *Journal of Clinical Oncology, 39*. https://www.semanticscholar.org/paper/adbbc5b0804feff3b9879b5f5f439b508d3e3aa0 (accessed on 15th July 2025).

35. Negm, A., Collins, J. D., Bendel, E. C., Takahashi, E., Knavel Koepsel, E. M., Gehling, K. J., Burke, C. E., et al. (2024). MR lymphangiography in lymphatic disorders: Clinical applications, institutional experience, and practice development. *Radiographic, 44*(2), e230075. https://www.semanticscholar.org/paper/bbebc96758ed6e9aa3d1e583e33bd393f1638120 (accessed on 15th July 2025).

36. Pfister, D. G., Spencer, S., Adelstein, D. J., Adkins, D. R., Anzai, Y., Brizel, D. M., Bruce, J. Y., et al. (2020). Head and neck cancers, version 2.2020, NCCN Clinical Practice Guidelines in

Oncology. *Journal of the National Comprehensive Cancer Network, 18*, 873–898. https://doi.org/10.6004/jnccn.2020.0031 (accessed on 15th July 2025).

37. Pham, T. D., Teh, M., Chatzopoulou, D., Holmes, S., & Coulthard, P. (2024). Artificial intelligence in head and neck cancer: Innovations, applications, and future directions. *Current Oncology, 31*, 5255–5290. https://www.semanticscholar.org/paper/79301386f2ef45ba2dd9501c0b1a9799343a9ada (accessed on 15th July 2025).

38. Shah, D. S., Gehani, A., Mahajan, A., & Chakrabarty, N. (2023). Advanced techniques in head and neck cancer imaging: Guide to precision cancer management. *Critical Reviews in Oncogenesis, 28*(2), 45–62. https://www.semanticscholar.org/paper/defeb13a95f53edee2ab416cfad107c0a366ed9f (accessed on 15th July 2025).

39. Tanaka, F., Umino, M., Maeda, M., Nakayama, R., Inoue, K., Kogue, R., Obara, M., et al. (2022). Pseudo continuous arterial spin labeling: Clinical applications and usefulness in head and neck entities. *Cancers, 14*. https://www.semanticscholar.org/paper/dcfef7b2eed5aaf7898b04ad677d65f36992c84b (accessed on 15th July 2025).

40. White, H. W., Naveed, A., Campbell, B. R., Lee, Y. J., Baik, F. M., Topf, M. C., Rosenthal, E., et al. (2024). Infrared fluorescence-guided surgery for tumor and metastatic lymph node detection in head and neck cancer. *Radiology: Imaging Cancer, 6*(4), e230178. https://www.semanticscholar.org/paper/90c16dcf87662b7dde50cea1719a765052571242 (accessed on 15th July 2025).

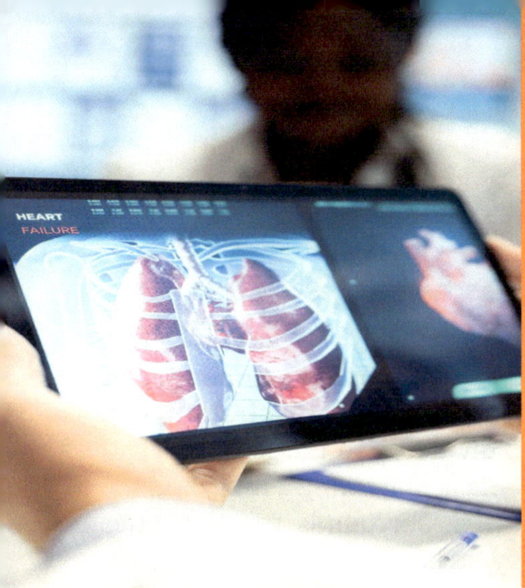

Chapter 3

THORACIC IMAGING: LUNG AND MEDIASTINUM

Contents

Introduction

Thoracic imaging encompasses a range of modalities and techniques used to visualize structures within the thoracic cavity, including the lungs and mediastinum. The specialty is of great significance in diagnosing many conditions, including pneumonia, lung cancer, and cardiovascular diseases. Computed tomography (CT) scans and chest X-rays have been the cornerstone of thoracic imaging because they are widely available and valuable for illustrating structural pathology. But with the development of imaging technology, the scope of thoracic diagnosis has been broadened so that more precise and sophisticated evaluations are possible. With the advent of magnetic resonance imaging (MRI) in thoracic imaging, doctors now have more tools at their disposal that can provide both morphological and functional information about lung diseases. This progression is part of a broader movement toward individualized medicine, in which imaging is central to delivering individually optimized treatment plans. MRIs' inclusion in thoracic imaging is especially notable in certain clinical situations, like cystic fibrosis and pulmonary embolism, where it offers a non-invasive option for young and pregnant women. MRI has been proposed in recent studies to offer unique functional data regarding respiratory mechanics and regional lung perfusion, which could be incredibly valuable for successful diagnoses and therapy planning. In addition, in pediatric illnesses that involve tumoral masses and pneumonia, MRI has been shown to be a viable adjunct or substitute for standard imaging methods, allowing extensive patient assessments.

With progressing supporting evidence, the focus is also to improve the accuracy of thoracic imaging through new applications and advanced protocols. All these advances point towards the future of MRI and how it will revolutionize clinicians' approach to managing thoracic pathologies, bridging the gap between traditional and modern imaging modalities in the clinic (Hebestreit et al., 2011).

The educational content in thoracic imaging continues to expand, providing practitioners with current information on new technological advancements and diagnostic strategies. Publications such as recent open-access volumes provide an elaborate summary of diagnostic as well as interventional imaging applicable to the thoracic cavity, attempting to familiarize radiologists and related professionals with contemporary procedures. These resources encompass a wide variety of modalities, such as conventional radiography, CT, ultrasound, and MRI, and illustrate each modality's role in the diagnostic process. By providing a comprehensive atlas of images for a wide range of chest conditions, they prepare clinicians to use the entire spectrum of imaging modalities they now have available. This anticipatory pedagogy is crucial for attaining a deeper appreciation of disease processes and increased diagnostic sensitivity, which subsequently translate into enhanced patient outcomes in thoracic conditions management (N/A, 2021).

3.1. Anatomy of Thoracic Cavity

The thoracic cavity is a highly complex cavity that has complicated anatomy, which accommodates critical organs that handle respiration and circulation. It is divided into the left and right pleural cavities, each containing a lung, and the mediastinum, which surrounds these cavities and contains key structures such as the heart, major vessels, trachea, and esophagus. The pleura, a double membrane lining the thoracic cavity, enables the lung to expand and contract without restriction during breathing and, at the same time, offers protection against infection. Intrathoracic anatomy plays a crucial role in the comprehension of most medical conditions, particularly those of the cardiovascular and respiratory systems. Imaging of these structures accurately allows clinicians to diagnose pathologies from pneumonia to more critical ones, such as lung cancer or mediastinal mass, and therefore knowledge of thoracic anatomy is vital in the practice of thoracic imaging. The radiologic techniques for imaging the thoracic cavity include X-ray, computed tomography (CT), and magnetic resonance imaging (MRI), each having special virtues and definite circumstances of use. Chest X-rays are often the initial imaging study, providing a quick assessment of the lung fields and cardiac silhouette. They can show pleural effusions and vascular congestion but may fail to provide definitive detail. But CT scanning provides much higher resolution, allowing high-quality images of the lung parenchyma and mediastinal structures to be obtained. The modality permits the detection of very subtle lesions and can help stage malignancies. Moreover, recent research indicates that the use of some fixation devices during chest examinations of children can enhance image quality, particularly in challenging populations where cooperation can be an issue (Apriantoro et al., 2024). Thoracic imaging modalities research exposes not just the structural characteristics but also the functional dynamics of thoracic anatomy. For instance, imaging tests can assess changes in lung volumes, airflow mechanics, and cardiovascular function under stress. Radiographic techniques, when applied proficiently, can outline a changed pulmonary pattern or reveal cardiac abnormalities that would otherwise go undetected. Recent studies, such as those assessing capuchin monkeys, demonstrate the applicability of anatomical assessment using imaging to refine thoracic structural differences and the concomitant implications (Alves et al., 2012). These comprehensive assessments enhance understanding of intricate interactions within the thoracic cavity, underscoring the value of effective imaging for research and practice (Figure 3.1).

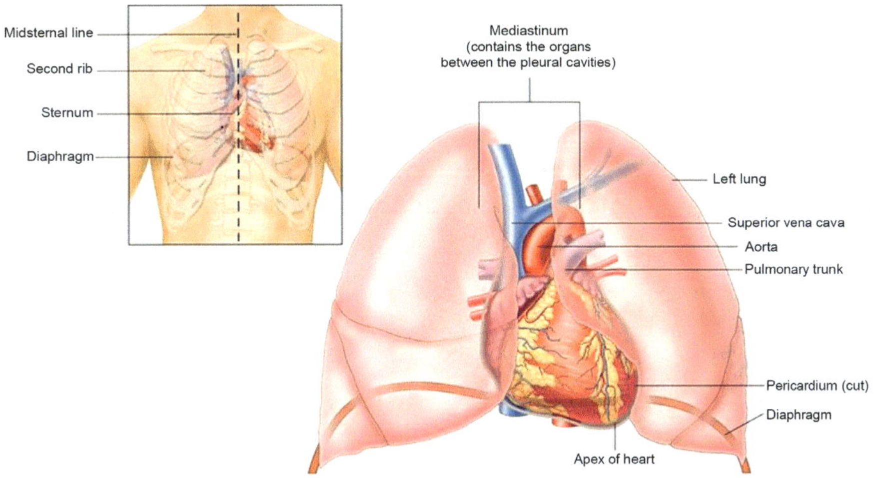

Figure 3.1. Labeled diagram of the thoracic cavity showing lungs, heart, and diaphragm.

Source: https://i.pinimg.com/736x/53/87/de/5387dedb91235cb3664c5540b8819a0d.jpg.

3.1.1. Structure of the Lungs

The lungs, respiratory structures, possess a complex design that allows them to perform their primary functions of ventilation and gas exchange. There are three lobes on the right lung and two on the left, each separated by fissures, which make them more functionally efficient. The bronchial tree, consisting of airways, branches from the trachea to the lungs and ends in alveolar sacs, where gas exchange occurs. This intricate design is necessary to both maximize surface area and reduce the distance that gases have to diffuse, pointing out the lungs' design as evolutionally optimized for respiratory efficiency. Further, the structural integrity of the lungs is provided by pleural membranes that create a pleural cavity, allowing for maximum inflation and deflation with each breath. Understanding this system and the mechanisms of systemic and bronchial circulations, as highlighted by studies using SPECT/micro-CT imaging, may provide information on various pulmonary illnesses and treatment techniques (Clough et al., 2008). Multimodality imaging has significantly increased understanding of lung structure and function, particularly in detecting anomalies and assessing pulmonary diseases. New modalities such as computed tomography (CT), magnetic resonance imaging (MRI), and positron emission tomography (PET) have radically changed thoracic imaging with high-resolution, three-dimensional visualization of lung structure. These technologies can delineate critical information about the size, shape, and integrity of structures in the thoracic compartment, including the mediastinum, central airways, and related blood vessels. For instance, lung tumor staging, which plays a key role in treatment planning, especially for conditions like NSCLC, relies very much on accurate imaging. The use of advanced technology capable of automatically segmenting the lung and mediastinal structures enhances the accuracy of tumor characterization and treatment assessment, highlighting the role of imaging in modern thoracic medicine (Adebahr et al., 2017). Second, the investigation of the lung's vascular architecture has provided significant insights into its physiological role and response to disease. The bronchial circulation, being a lesser but significant constituent of the pulmonary circulation, plays a significant role in supplying the lung tissue, particularly during hypoxia or injury. Recent studies using SPECT/micro-CT methods have demonstrated the adaptive nature of bronchial circulation in response to compromised pulmonary artery function, suggesting intricate interactions between lung health and vascular hemodynamics. For example, adjustment of bronchial blood flow, as observed following pulmonary artery ligation, illustrates the lungs' adaptive mechanism for maintaining homeostasis. These findings have significant implications for thoracic disease pathophysiology and potentially open the door to new therapeutic strategies targeting these vascular responses (Clough et al., 2008). By integrating such information with advanced imaging modalities, clinicians can more effectively guide therapy for thoracic disease (Figure 3.2).

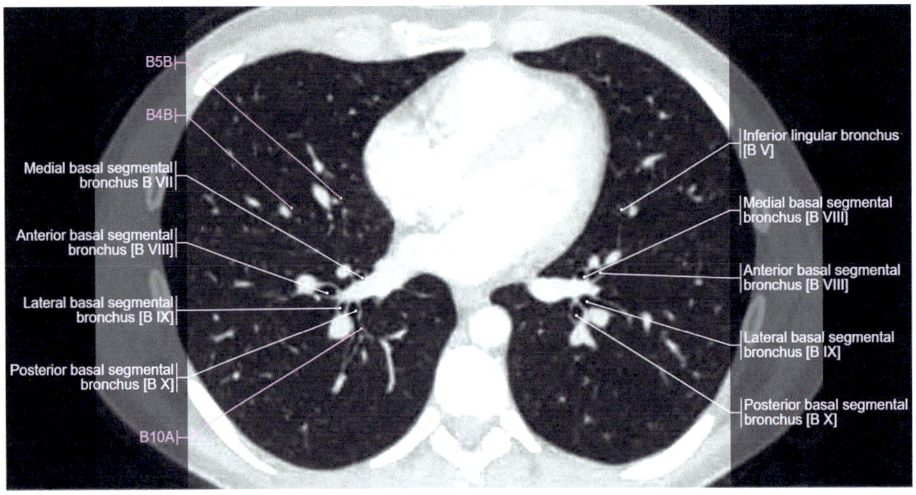

Figure 3.2. Cross-sectional CT image displaying lung lobes and their anatomical orientation.

Source: https://cdn1.imaios.com/i/images/2/2/8/7/477822-10-eng-GB/c6563f5cef30-bronchopulmonary-segments-ct-axial.jpg?caption=1&q=75&w=1280&s=f66f7c7c32fbf3de9b1a9695dbc9add4.

3.1.2. Components of the Mediastinum

The mediastinum between the lungs is a complex anatomical region containing vital structures essential for respiratory and cardiovascular function. The mediastinum is classically divided into upper and lower spaces, each having definitive anatomical components. The superior mediastinum contains significant structures, including the great vessels, trachea, esophagus, and portions of the thymus gland. These organs have critical functions in delivering oxygenated blood and dissolved nutrients to the body and in supplying the airway for respiration. Identification of these structures is important to both clinicians and radiologists since imaging of the thorax provides information about numerous pathologies that affect these organs. Advanced high-resolution imaging modalities can significantly aid the diagnosis and interpretation of entities such as mediastinal tumors and vascular malformations, thereby impacting patient management and treatment strategies. During division of the inferior mediastinum, it is further divided into anterior, middle, and posterior compartments, each having specific anatomical structures. The anterior mediastinum contains only fatty tissue, lymphatic channels, and, at times, thymomas, which are tumors of the thymus. The middle mediastinum is defined principally by where the heart and pericardium, the great bronchi, and large blood vessels that are responsible for communication between the heart and lungs are located. It is imperative to understand the spatial relationships among these organs, particularly in the evaluation of cardiac and pulmonary disease using imaging modalities.

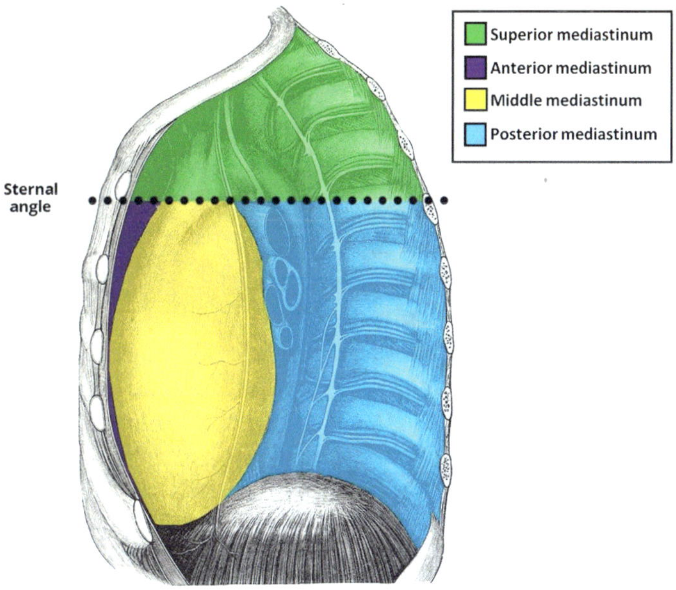

Figure 3.3. Schematic of the superior, middle, and inferior mediastinum, showing boundaries and contents.

Source: https://teachmeanatomy.info/wp-content/uploads/The-Superior-Mediastinum-and-Sternal-Angle-1024x843.jpg.

The posterior mediastinum is filled with the descending aorta, the thoracic duct, and several essential nerve tracts. The discrimination of these spaces on thoracic imaging may enhance diagnostic sensitivity, allowing healthcare practitioners to identify underlying pathology that can compress adjacent structures, potentially leading to severe complications. With ongoing improvements in imaging technologies in thoracic medicine, precise visualization of the mediastinum is increasingly pivotal for diagnosis and treatment. New technology, such as low-dose computed tomography (LDCT), has improved the potential for studying this region with reduced patient radiation. Advances in image processing algorithms, processing capabilities, and computing power, including the artifact-suppressed large-scale nonlocal means method, have also been promising for enhancing image quality by reducing noise and streak artifacts commonly seen on thoracic LDCT scans. These technological developments enhance the visibility of critical mediastinal structures, thereby facilitating accurate interpretation by radiologists, especially in the diagnosis of disorders such as mediastinal masses and lymphadenopathy. Last but not least, the intersection of contemporary imaging modalities and processing techniques not only solidifies insight into the mediastinum's content but also improves patient outcomes through timely and precise interventions (Chen et al., 2012; Bustos et al., 2019) (Figure 3.3).

3.1.3. Relationship Between Thoracic Structures

The intricate interplay of thoracic structures takes center stage in understanding various respiratory and cardiovascular conditions. The thoracic cavity contains essential organs such as the lungs, heart, and major blood vessels, all of which interact closely with one another. This relationship of anatomy is highly prone to pathological processes that can lead to complications, for example, vascular structure compression of the bronchi.

Left mainstem bronchus, for example, can be compromised by vascular anomalies, which compromise airflow and respiratory function. How these interactions are made through advanced imaging techniques, such as CT imaging, enhances diagnostic accuracy and treatment planning for pathologies of these structures. Adequate imaging is critical to diagnose the structural defects that may compromise respiratory function or lead to serious complications in children, whose anatomical variations are more exaggerated in terms of developmental issues. In pediatric medicine, the interaction between thoracic structures becomes more complex, mainly due to anatomical variations as well as the increased presence of congenital anomalies. Vascular rings and other malformations may produce compressive forces on the trachea and bronchi, leading to respiratory symptoms over a range. Imaging techniques such as three-dimensional computed tomography (3D CT) have completely transformed preoperative diagnosis of such conditions by providing clear imaging of the interface among the airway, vascular structures, and adjacent tissues. By accurately defining the anatomy before surgery, clinicians can tailor their surgical approach to alleviate symptoms effectively and minimize invasiveness.

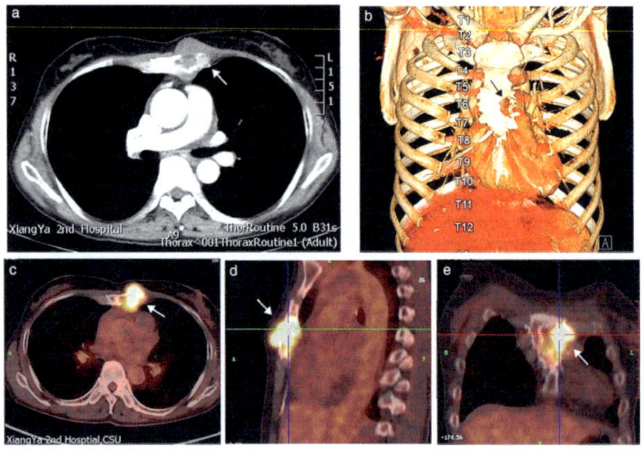

Figure 3.4. 3D reconstruction CT scan delineating spatial relationships of thoracic organs. (a, b) Initial computed tomography (CT) scan of the thorax. White arrow indicates the sternal tumor. (b) 3D reconstruction of the skeleton of the chest. (c–e). Initial positron emission tomography-computed tomography (PET-CT) scan of different sections demonstrated a 4 cm visible increased glucose metabolism sternal mass (max standardized uptake value = 42). White arrow indicates the increased glucose metabolism mass.

Source: https://www.researchgate.net/figure/a-b-Initial-computed-tomography-CT-scan-of-the-thorax-White-arrow-indicates-the_fig1_333138198.

3D imaging has proved to be an incredible resource, not only for diagnosis but also for enhancing surgical success by better appreciating mechanical interactions within the thoracic cavity (Angel et al., 2005). One such intervention in this context is surgical posterior aortopexy to relieve airway compression, which has been effective in children with respiratory issues due to left mainstem bronchus compression. In a study involving 18 children, the surgery alleviated symptoms caused by bronchial compression and demonstrated that consideration of the spatial relationships between the vascular structures and the airways can significantly impact treatment.

The coordination between such thoracic components requires a multidisciplinary approach, often implicating collaborative efforts from pulmonologists, cardiothoracic surgeons, and radiologists. Employing high-technology imaging techniques, doctors are better positioned to navigate the complexities of thoracic pathologies, thereby improving airway management and overall patient outcomes (Arcieri et al., 2016) (Figure 3.4).

3.2. Imaging Techniques for Lung Evaluation

The evaluation of lung pathology necessitates the utilization of a variety of imaging modalities each with a defined use for a unique clinical scenario. Of these imaging modalities, chest radiography is the initial imaging modality, offering a rapid, inexpensive assessment of the thoracic space.

Chest radiography can detect a host of abnormalities, including infections, tumors, and structural disease. However, its deficiency is that it fails to describe lesions effectively and distinguish between pathologies with similar characteristics. Therefore, whenever further evaluation is necessary, more advanced imaging techniques, such as CT, are employed. CT scans offer better anatomical resolution and higher spatial resolution, which are crucial for evaluating complex pulmonary diseases and planning follow-up interventions. In infectious diseases such as tuberculosis, imaging is critical for diagnosis and management. Physicians ought to be expert in recognizing the subtle radiographic features of tuberculosis, especially in regions where the disease is endemic. A modern imaging classification that accommodates variability in presentation between populations, such as between children and adults, is required. Critical imaging features need to be interpreted, particularly in the face of rising drug resistance, as imaging will impact therapeutic planning. There should be communication between radiologists and clinicians to ensure a sophisticated interpretation of imaging results in light of local epidemiological data, including the prevalence of HIV coinfection.

This collaborative approach results in higher diagnostic accuracy and ultimately improves outcomes for patients with tuberculosis (Ahmad et al., 2009). Another advanced imaging technique gaining increasing popularity for thoracic evaluation is magnetic resonance imaging (MRI).

While traditionally relegated to a second-line role in lung disease evaluation by CT, newer technological innovations with improved perfusion and diffusion imaging have broadened its application in certain pulmonary diseases. MRI is particularly valuable for evaluating mediastinal structures, including the thymus gland in MG. It has been found that ectopic thymic tissue can significantly influence clinical outcomes in MG patients following thymectomy. Studies indicate that ectopic thymic tissue is associated with poorer postoperative outcomes, and thus precise imaging to identify this tissue effectively becomes crucial. MRI, hence, can play the role of complementing other imaging methods, providing a comprehensive overview of thoracic anatomy and supporting more informed management strategies (Bauer et al., 2019).

3.2.1. Chest X-Ray: Fundamentals and Interpretation

Knowledge of the principles of chest X-ray imaging is essential for effective interpretation and diagnosis in thoracic disease. A chest X-ray is a valuable first-line imaging modality that allows clinicians to evaluate a variety of lung and mediastinal organ conditions. The picture will typically incorporate both the lungs and heart, as well as bony structures, to allow evaluation of pathologies such as pneumonia, lung tumors, and cardiac enlargement. Proper interpretation relies on a systematic approach, with familiarity of normal and abnormal radiographic anatomy (Figure 3.5).

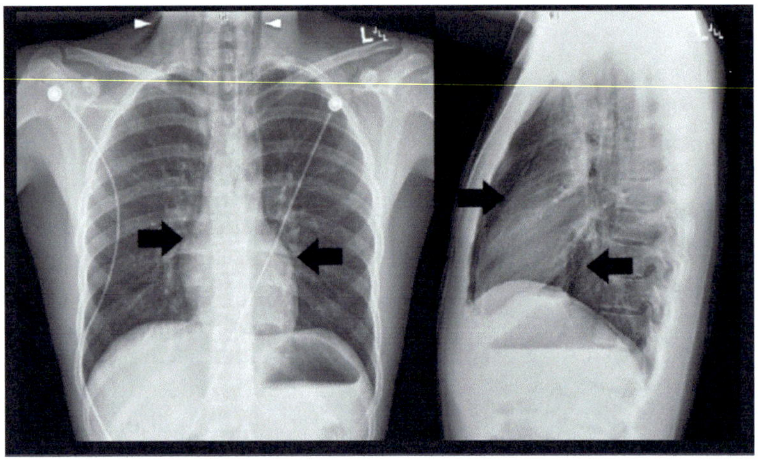

Figure 3.5. Chest x-ray, PA and lateral. PA, posterior-anterior The patient's pneumomediastinum was confirmed on chest x-ray, on the grounds of air dissecting in the mediastinum (arrows) and entering the lower part of the neck bilaterally (arrow heads).

Source: https://www.researchgate.net/figure/Chest-radiograph-PA-and-lateral-views-PA-posterior-anterior-The-patients_fig2_274397046.

Accurate knowledge of typical image characteristics enables clinicians and radiologists to effectively identify abnormalities, thus facilitating early diagnosis and patient care. A good mastery of the basics of chest X-ray interpretation is therefore a must for any clinical expert engaged in thoracic imaging (N/A, 1991). In the context of technological progress, newer imaging equipment, such as the Lodox X-ray system, has made the chest X-ray scene more complex. Originally used for many purposes, the Lodox system has been shown to be an alternative for obtaining high-quality chest radiographs in the trauma setting. Studies have shown that Lodox imaging can acquire higher quality images that delineate structures such as lung parenchyma and mediastinum more effectively than conventional X-ray machines. However, while still inferior in some respects, conventional X-rays are superior in the detection of illnesses such as pulmonary effusion and pneumothorax. This complementary relationship among several imaging modalities underscores the need to use the appropriate system based on clinical indications, thereby re-emphasizing the importance of healthcare professionals staying up to date on advances in imaging technology (N/A, 2022). The success of interpreting chest X-rays also requires knowledge of relevant clinical indications and patient history. Clinicians should correlate radiographic results with clinical symptoms to arrive at a comprehensive diagnosis. For instance, an infiltrate seen on an X-ray compatible with pneumonia will be considered a definite diagnosis only on the basis of clinical correlation with fever or elevated white blood cell counts. The same clinical context is important when utilizing it, particularly for the determination of whether or not ancillary imaging, like CT or ultrasound, is needed. The new imaging rules, especially in trauma settings on machines like Lodox, provide evidence for well-informed decision-making through both radiologic and clinical data. A final grasp of vocational knowledge and technology will optimize the validity of chest X-ray interpretation in thoracic medicine (N/A, 1991).

3.2.2. Computed Tomography (CT) Scans: Strengths and Weaknesses

Computed Tomography (CT) scans are increasingly standard in thoracic imaging, particularly for evaluating the lungs and mediastinum. With the ability to produce high-resolution cross-sectional images, accurate visualization of anatomical details is provided, making it irreplaceable for diagnosing pathologies such as lung cancer and other thoracic diseases. One of the interesting advantages of CT scans is that they are capable of enhancing the definition of tumors and associated structures, a point that is vital in disease staging. As highlighted in more recent studies, advances like the combination of CT with fluorodeoxyglucose-positron emission tomography (PET) have additionally contributed to diagnostic accuracy, yielding valuable information on tumor size as well as metastasis. This alliance enhances planning for therapy interventions and has the potential to normalize treatment for patients undergoing lung cancer assessment (Andía et al., 2006).

Nonetheless, despite numerous advantages, CT scans have limitations as well. One such limitation of them is exposure to ionizing radiation, which also raises questions about long-term risks, particularly in vulnerable populations such as young patients or those requiring multiple imaging tests. Furthermore, CT scans can yield false positives, necessitating further invasive exams, such as biopsies, to confirm diagnoses (Figure 3.6).

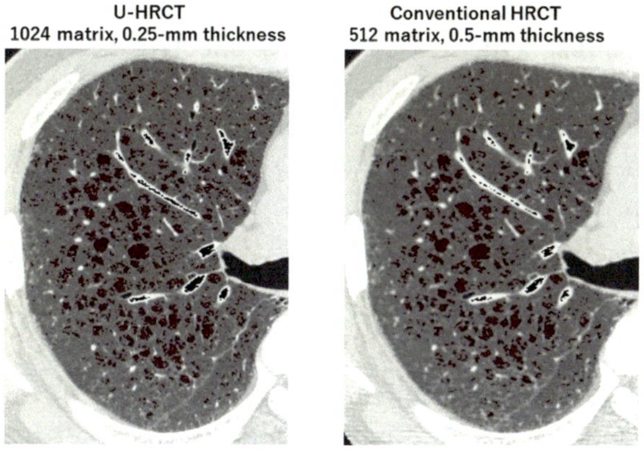

Figure 3.6. Ultra-high-resolution CT (U-HRCT) image compared with a conventional HRCT image for the detection of emphysema. At the threshold setting of <−950 Hounsfield units, emphysematous lesions are identified as dark-red areas on axial images. Some of the very small emphysematous lesions, which is clearly identified on the U-HRCT image (left), cannot be seen on the identical conventional HRCT image (right).

Source: https://www.researchgate.net/figure/Ultra-high-resolution-CT-U-HRCT-image-compared-with-a-conventional-HRCT-image-for-the_fig2_336335963.

This parameter can cause undue stress and potential complications in patients. Additionally, while CT is excellent at detecting larger tumors, it can sometimes miss smaller lesions, making it crucial in the early diagnosis of lung cancer. Thus, while the technical advantage of CT scans in thoracic imaging is notable, physicians must be mindful of these limitations to offer an integrated, patient-centered approach (Bogers et al., 2019). The addition of new technologies, including three-dimensional (3D) reconstruction and virtual reality applications, is already beginning to overcome some of the limitations of traditional CT scans. The latest technologies give a better view of complex thoracic anatomy, which not only assists in diagnosis but also in surgical planning and intervention. For instance, 3D CT application can improve the understanding of the relationships between mediastinal tumors, vasculature, and surrounding tissues, which is central to effective surgical techniques. Beyond that, as technology continues to evolve in thoracic imaging, artificial intelligence will be able to optimize image interpretation, further reducing false-positive outcomes and increasing detection of small lesions. As technology in CT continues to evolve, the balance between its advantages and disadvantages will be critical in shaping future thoracic imaging protocols and, ultimately, enhancing patient care (Bogers et al., 2019).

3.2.3. Magnetic Resonance Imaging (MRI) in Lung Assessment

Magnetic Resonance Imaging (MRI) is now a significant modality for assessing lung disease, particularly the mediastinal structures. MRI is superior to other conventional imaging modalities like chest X-ray and computed tomography (CT) because it offers improved soft tissue contrast, which is particularly useful for the detection of malignant lesion and assessing the extent of disease. MRI's ability to distinguish among tissue types improves visualization of tumors, lymph nodes, and vessels in the thoracic cavity.

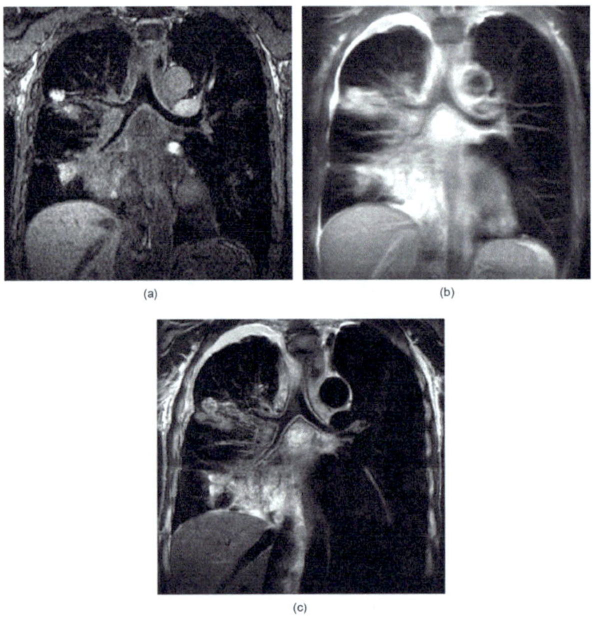

Figure 3.7. T2-weighted magnetic resonance imaging (HASTE [half-Fourier single-shot turbo spin-echo]) at 31 weeks of gestation shows high signal intensity of the enlarged mid and lower lobes of the right lung with compression of the right upper lobe, mediastinal shift to the left side, and flattening diaphragm. Although a mediastinal shift to the left and slight compression of the left lung were observed, the left lung appeared almost normal. Furthermore, the preservation of vascular structure in the right mid and lower lobes (arrowheads) and the retained normal shape of the lobes are depicted.

Therefore, MRI is increasingly used as a non-surgical alternative for precise lung evaluation, particularly in the presence of mediastinal pathology. Nevertheless, its use remains complicated due to inherent difficulties posed by respiratory motion, which can significantly affect image quality and diagnostic reliability. Advancements in cutting-edge techniques continue to address such limitations as well as improve overall diagnostic performance. One such significant advancement in MRI technology for lung assessment is the enhancement of fat suppression techniques. Recent literature has outlined the impact of several vendor-specific protocols, particularly addressing DWI application in freely breathing patients. A comparative analysis of short-tau inversion recovery (STIR) and spectral adiabatic inversion recovery (SPAIR) techniques revealed notable differences in image quality. In specific terms, images created with the STIR fat suppression method were deemed considerably superior in overall quality, with its application for diagnosing mediastinal lymph nodes and providing greater diagnostic confidence in oncological studies. With the application of optimal fat suppression methods, clinicians will be able to visualize malignant and benign lesions more clearly, thus leading to more informed clinical decision-making and earlier intervention (Blackledge et al., 2017).

Source: https://www.researchgate.net/figure/T2-weighted-magnetic-resonance-imaging-HASTE-half-Fourier-single-shot-turbo-spin-echo_fig2_328187200.

Furthermore, the growing body of publications reveals the significant contribution of MRI in a systematic assessment of lung pathology along with other modalities. As the thoracic imaging environment evolves, the coalescence of minimal intervention methods with state-of-the-art imaging modalities is transforming clinical practice. Techniques such as endobronchial ultrasound with transbronchial needle aspiration have transformed the diagnostic pathway for mediastinal patients. While MRI provides superb anatomical detail, multimodal imaging synergizes to enable a thorough assessment of lesions amenable to biopsy for definitive diagnosis. This multimodality approach eventually results in enhanced patient-centered care, with the potential for early diagnosis and tailored treatment regimens, thereby improving patient outcomes. With continued technological advancements, synergy among MRI and other imaging modalities will be vital for maximizing management of thoracic pathologies (Cheng et al., 2024) (Figure 3.7).

3.3. Common Lung Pathologies

In thoracic imaging, one needs to remain aware of common lung diseases to enable effective diagnosis and management planning. Among all lung health diseases, pneumonia stands out due to its prevalence and severity. It is a tissue infection of the lung that leads to inflammation and can be diagnosed on standard radiographic techniques that show definite patterns, such as consolidations and infiltrates. The ability to interpret chest X-rays has the potential to significantly enhance the diagnostic accuracy of pneumonia, alerting healthcare providers to the need for intervention. Based on the large dataset reported by Bustos et al. (2019), images annotated for more than 67,000 patients enable the detection of multiple radiographic signs of pneumonia, enabling management tailored to practice. Another frequent pathology is chronic obstructive pulmonary disease (COPD), and it encompasses emphysema and chronic bronchitis. Characterized by airflow limitation and persistent respiratory symptoms, COPD is typically diagnosed with imaging examinations that identify hyperinflation of the lungs and changes in pulmonary vasculature. Chest X-rays and CT scans are essential in evaluating the severity of lung damage and making treatment decisions. The relevance of accurate imaging is underscored by more recent advances in diagnostic methodology, as outlined in the comprehensive reference manual developed in (N/A, 2021). These advances equip clinicians in any specialty, including pulmonology and radiology, with tools to adequately assess disease progression in COPD patients, thereby maximizing patient outcomes through tailored interventions. Lastly, lung nodules are another obligatory area that must receive focus through thoracic imaging. These tiny, round growths are highly heterogeneous in etiology, varying from benign conditions such as granulomas to neoplasms. Advances in high-resolution imaging modalities have revolutionized the management of lung nodules by enabling improved characterization and, in turn, patient management. The integrative nature of databanks, such as the one presented in (Bustos et al., 2019), helps standardize the classification of these nodules based on imaging characteristics and associate them with patient outcomes. Such unifying approaches are instrumental in determining whether a biopsy or surgical intervention should be undertaken, thereby facilitating early detection and effective treatment of lung cancers, thus significantly impacting patient survival rates.

3.3.1. Pneumonia: Imaging Characteristics

The radiological signs of pneumonia play a critical role in diagnosing and treating this typical lung infection. Chest X-ray remains the imaging study of first choice, and it can reveal classic patterns such as consolidation, an area of homogeneously opacified lung that replaces standard markings. Further, chest X-rays will differentiate between forms of pneumonia, such as lobar pneumonia, which typically appears as segmental or lobar consolidation, and bronchopneumonia, which typically appears as patchy opacities diffusely throughout the lung fields. Although useful initial information is provided by radiography, its limitations necessitate further imaging, particularly in complicated cases. Computed tomography (CT) has also gained sensitivity. It offers useful information about lung parenchyma, enabling detection of secondary complications such as abscess or pleural effusion, which is not apparent on routine X-rays. Radiologists and clinicians need to have a thorough understanding of imaging features in pneumonia, with the multiple presentations depending on the patient population. Understanding imaging features that are unique between adults and children is imperative as children's pneumonia may present different patterns or associated diseases, such as human immunodeficiency virus (HIV) infection, which may make the clinical situation more complicated. Clinicians should be skilled in image interpretation to guide appropriate management strategies and influence appropriate treatment. By encouraging inter-disciplinary collaboration between radiologists and the clinical team, precise diagnostic imaging of pneumonia can be assured, optimizing patient outcomes. Continuing education on evolving imaging techniques, as well as limitations in communication, is key to improving pneumonia management in diverse patient populations.

Current literature emphasizes the importance of integrating advanced imaging technologies to broaden our understanding of pneumonia's complexity. For instance, newer imaging modalities such as positron emission tomography (PET) and magnetic resonance imaging (MRI) have added information, particularly in the evaluation of suspected atypical pneumonia or assessment of lung function. Coupling these newer methods with conventional imaging provides an integrated picture of lung pathology, improving diagnostic accuracy and enabling targeted interventions. Besides, recent research highlights the need for accurate imaging to track response to therapy and detect potential complications throughout the disease course. With continually evolving thoracic imaging technology, it is increasingly critical for practitioners to stay up to speed on advancements to uphold standards of care and address evolving conditions in pneumonia diagnosis and treatment (Figure 3.8).

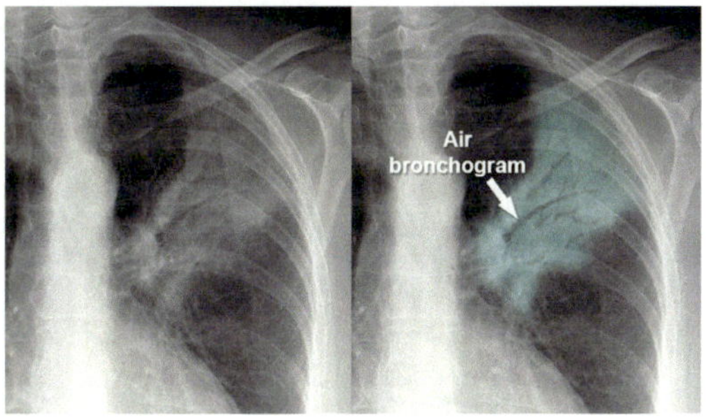

Figure 3.8. Chest X-ray showing air bronchograms indicative of pneumonia.

Source: https://www.radiologymasterclass.co.uk/images/chest-images/gallery-pulmonary/bronchogram_1.jpg?mtime=20210304211317&focal=none.

3.3.2. Lung Cancer: Detection and Staging

The diagnosis of lung cancer remains a high priority for thoracic imaging practice, in large part because the disease is complex and tumors appear so variably. Simple diagnostic imaging techniques such as chest X-rays and CT scans are vital for detecting suspicious pulmonary masses or nodules. It remains a challenge for clinicians to differentiate between malignant and benign lesions. Advances in imaging modalities, including positron emission tomography (PET) and magnetic resonance imaging (MRI), have also improved diagnostic accuracy and staging. These, in combination with traditional methods, enable more medical practitioners to have a global overview of the thoracic environment that determines eventual therapeutic management. It follows that the use of multiple imaging modalities is central to improving diagnostic performance and facilitating timely intervention in lung cancer patients. Once lung cancer is suspected or diagnosed, accurate staging is highly critical to plan an appropriate treatment strategy. Staging refers to determining how far the disease has spread – whether it is localized in the lungs or has extended to nearby lymph nodes or other organs (Figure 3.9).

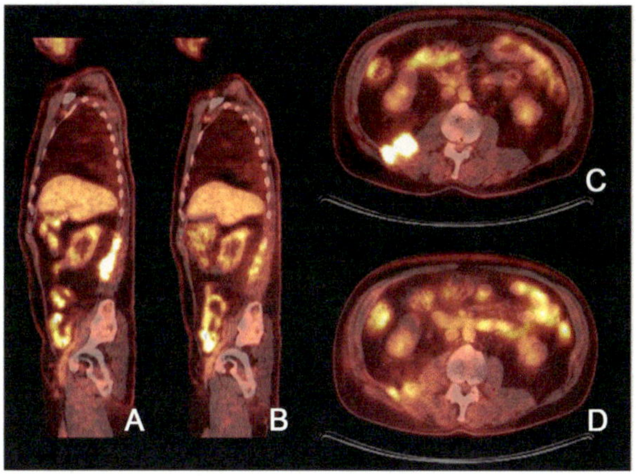

Figure 3.9. PET CT scan images showing changes in metabolic activity at the site of recurrent tumor after starting treatment with concurrent radiotherapy and immunotherapy. (a) and (c) illustrate a high standardized uptake value (SUV) in sagittal and axial sections, respectively. It decreased in the next 12 weeks following therapy as indicated by relatively reduced metabolic activity of the tumor in sagittal (b) and axial sections (d).

Source: https://www.researchgate.net/figure/PET-CT-scan-images-showing-changes-in-metabolic-activity-at-the-site-of-recurrent-tumor_fig2_334781402.

The use of imaging modalities such as CT scans provides accurate evaluation of tumor size, location, and lymphatic involvement. Advances in recent years in minimally invasive staging modalities, such as endobronchial ultrasound-transbronchial needle aspiration (EBUS-TBNA) and endoscopic ultrasound-fine needle aspiration (EUS-FNA), have significantly improved the staging of mediastinal and peripheral lung adenopathy with excellent sensitivity and specificity. These techniques not only enhance diagnostic accuracy but also reduce patient morbidity from more invasive treatments. As such, the role of staging in lung cancer therapy underscores the importance of robust imaging technology to deliver maximum patient care and results. By integrating recent advances in thoracic imaging, clinical practitioners can adjust their approach towards diagnosis and staging of lung cancer to accommodate the evolving landscape of technology and clinical guidelines. Research into new imaging equipment, such as artificial intelligence and deep learning algorithms, promises much for greater understanding of images and diagnostic precision. As outlined in comprehensive reviews of thoracic imaging modalities, including advancements in minimally invasive approaches, these technologies will transform patient flow and simplify care pathways. Additionally, coordinating diagnostic imaging and clinical information allows for an integrated lung cancer management strategy that bridges the gap between radiologic results and clinical presentation. By correlating imaging advancements with current treatment strategies, it is achievable to maximize overall patient outcomes and ultimately redefine lung cancer staging and detection (Cheng et al., 2024; N/A, 2021).

3.3.3. Interstitial Lung Disease: Radiologic Findings

Interstitial lung disease (ILD) is a heterogeneous collection of interstitial inflammation and fibrosis of the interstitium of the lungs and refers to an interstitial pulmonary condition. Radiologic examination plays a crucial role in ILD diagnosis and classification, with critical information on the extent and patterns of the disease. HRCT is the imaging modality of choice because it allows accurate visualization of lung architecture. Common radiological findings in ILD include ground-glass opacities, reticular patterns, and cystic changes, which may mirror the degree of fibrosis or inflammation. The clinician must recognize these patterns and relate them to clinical findings to effectively diagnose. As radiologists become increasingly comfortable with the nuances of these findings, appropriate and timely management strategies can be developed, thereby enhancing patient outcomes in this multifactorial, complex group of diseases (Figure 3.10).

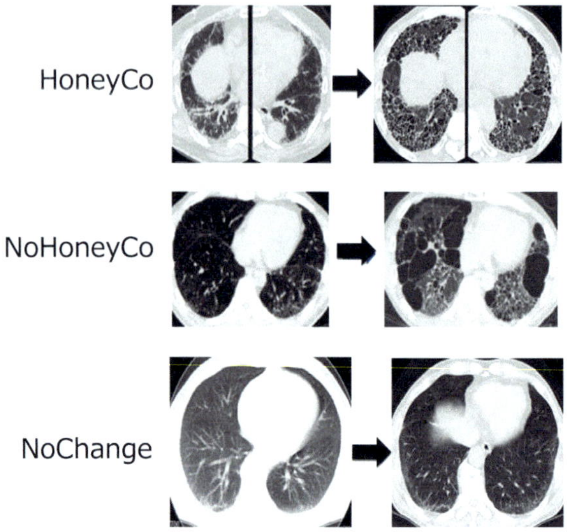

Figure 3.10. Representative HRCT scans from the three patient groups. HoneyCo: Honeycombing became evident on the HRCT scan. NoHoneyCo: Traction bronchiectasis or cysts became evident on HRCT scan. No Change: No significant change in HRCT findings. *Source:* https://www.researchgate.net/figure/Representative-HRCT-scans-from-the-three-patient-groups-HoneyCo-Honeycombing-became_fig4_309876061.

Identification of unique patterns within radiology on various forms of ILD diagnosis remains crucial for accurate diagnosis. For instance, honeycombing would typically be consistent with IPF, while a reticular pattern would tend to indicate diseases such as sarcoidosis and connective tissue disease-associated systemic ILD. This discrimination can be critical in management and prognosis. Advanced imaging modalities and the ongoing increase in large datasets are also responsible for identifying these patterns. As demonstrated by current studies, not only do such data sets enhance information on usual radiologic observations in ILD, but they also enhance the correlation between clinical and imaging data, supporting increased multidisciplinary collaboration among caretakers, particularly in challenging cases in which radiologic interpretation can have a crucial role in impacting management outcomes (Ahmad et al., 2009). Further, the advancements in artificial intelligence and machine learning are set to revolutionize the way radiologic findings of interstitial lung disease are handled. The PadChest dataset is a prime example of this change, with a full dataset of over 160,000 chest X-ray images annotated with a variety of findings that are pertinent to the differential diagnosis of ILD and other thoracic conditions (Bustos et al., 2019). This precious resource is able to facilitate the development of predictive models that assist radiologists in detecting pathologies effectively and accurately. With increasing integration of these tools into diagnostic workflows, the precision of overall ILD diagnoses is likely to improve, and treatment planning is likely to become better, along with patient care. Lastly, the integrated function of radiology and clinical practice will promote an interdisciplinary approach to interstitial lung disease, highlighting the pivotal role of radiological information in the broader context of thoracic imaging.

3.4. Imaging Techniques for Mediastinal Evaluation

Mediastinal assessment is important evaluation of thoracic disease, especially given the intricate anatomical structures within this compartment. Imaging modalities are instrumental in diagnosing and staging processes such as lung cancer and infection. Chest X-ray, as is usually the initial imaging examination, may be insufficient in its capacity to image the organs of the mediastinum. Computed Tomography (CT) scanning, however, has been a more effective tool, offering superior cross-sectional imaging that better delineates the soft tissues, lymph nodes, and vascular mediastinal anatomy. It not only provides precise lesion measurement but also aids in evaluating lymphadenopathy, making it an indispensable first-line tool for mediastinal evaluation that informs subsequent clinical decision-making. In the past couple of years, Endoscopic Bronchial Ultrasound (EBUS) has revolutionized the staging phenomenon in thoracic imaging, particularly in lung cancer staging and assessment of mediastinal masses. By utilizing ultrasound technology during bronchoscopy, EBUS facilitates easier, minimally invasive sampling of mediastinal lymph nodes via transbronchial needle aspiration. The process enhances the accuracy of staging by allowing real-time visualization of the mediastinum and hence fewer invasive procedures. Specificity and sensitivity of EBUS have made it a cornerstone in lung cancer management, particularly its role in diagnosing metastatic lymph node involvement that affects prognosis. The ability to provide cytological specimens at no cost to patient morbidity reinforces the significant role of EBUS in the overall strategy of mediastinal evaluation approaches (Bilocca et al., 2016). Imaging modalities are not limited to CT and EBUS; other imaging modalities, including Magnetic Resonance Imaging (MRI) and Positron Emission Tomography (PET), provide additional information on mediastinal pathologies. MRI is beneficial in cases where soft-tissue recognition is of particular significance, providing high-resolution images of anatomical structures and potential neoplasms. Concurrently, PET imaging, either with CT (PET/CT), provides functional information by identifying regions of metabolic activity associated with malignancies, thereby enabling proper staging and treatment planning. Having insight into the interactions among these imaging methods is essential for clinicians, allowing them to adapt diagnostic strategies to individual patient needs. The addition of new imaging modalities to clinical practice heralds a shift in the mediastinal evaluation paradigm, rendering healthcare providers skilled in managing more complex thoracic diseases (Ahmad et al., 2009).

3.4.1. The CT Contribution in Mediastinal Imaging

Computed tomography (CT) has transformed mediastinal imaging, providing clinicians with accurate anatomical data essential for diagnosing thoracic diseases. The mediastinum is a complex anatomical space that harbors essential structures, including the heart, great vessels, trachea, esophagus, and lymph nodes. With CT imaging, clinicians can reliably identify pathologies, including tumors, infections, and inflammatory diseases. This is an advanced imaging modality that produces high-resolution images and can be tailored with different protocols to maximize visualization of mediastinal components, taking into account factors such as patient size and clinical dilemma (Figure 3.11).

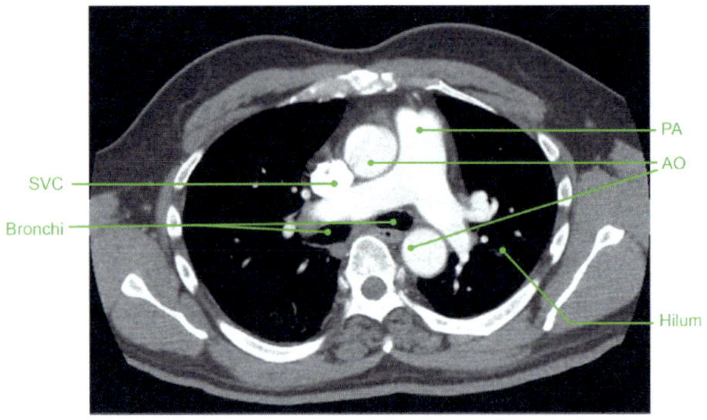

Figure 3.11. Contrast-enhanced axial CT showing anterior mediastinal structures.

Source: https://cdn.lecturio.com/assets/Axial-mediastinal-anatomy-on-CT-post-contrast.jpg.

Optimization of imaging modalities enables clinicians to develop appropriate treatment plans based on accurate localization and characterization of mediastinal lesions, thereby placing CT at the forefront of effective diagnostic pathways for thoracic ailments. Beyond that, CT's role also comes into play as far as staging and evaluating treatment response in mediastinal malignancies is concerned, especially lung cancer. This diagnosis remains a leading cause of death from cancer, and staging helps ensure that it is intervened upon properly. Mediastinal lymph node involvement is a crucial prognostic factor that dictates both therapeutic and patient outcomes. CT aids in determining the presence and extent of lymphadenopathy, which is critical for management planning, particularly in deciding whether to resect or offer systemic treatment to patients. The literature has demonstrated the utility of CT in assessing disease stage and treatment response, thereby solidifying its pivotal role in the multidisciplinary management framework of thoracic oncology and in maximizing survival opportunities for individuals affected (Bilocca et al., 2016). In addition to disease diagnosis and staging, CT imaging facilitates ongoing assessment and triage in various clinical settings, including suspected mediastinal infections such as tuberculosis (TB). It is critical to appreciate these imaging nuances in TB patients, especially the immunocompromised and atypical-presenting ones. The relevance of appropriate imagingonly in the diagnosis of such patients but also in their timely intervention cannot be overstated, as it significantly impacts patient outcomes. Imaging results must be interpreted by radiologists and clinicians collectively accurately to formulate clinical decisions based on both imaging results and overall patient health. The marriage of CT imaging and clinical expertise makes it stronger in mediastinal imaging, ultimately improving patient care and enhancing the detection of complicated thoracic disease (Ahmad et al., 2009).

3.4.2. Use of Ultrasound in Mediastinal Assessment

The integration of ultrasound technologies with mediastinal assessment has revolutionized diagnostic techniques. Traditionally, mediastinal disease diagnosis has centered on imaging techniques such as computed tomography (CT) and magnetic resonance imaging (MRI). Such modalities are inadequate for end-stage tissue diagnosis, leading to invasive procedures such as mediastinoscopy. The advent of techniques such as endobronchial ultrasound (EBUS) and endoscopic ultrasound (EUS) has been a revolutionary step, allowing clinicians to obtain tissue samples with greater invasiveness and lower complication rates. These modalities have significantly improved diagnostic effectiveness, especially in detecting benign and malignant lesions, and have optimized the diagnostic process for patients presenting with mediastinal abnormalities (Cheng et al., 2024). The success of endobronchial ultrasound in mediastinal assessment is attributed by its real-time imaging capability during bronchoscopy. EBUS can effectively localize lymph nodes and other structures, allowing for targeted biopsies that enhance diagnostic yield (Figure 3.12).

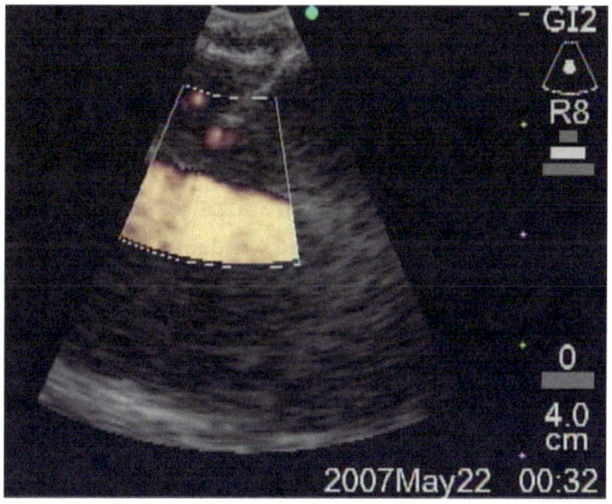

Figure 3.12. Endobronchial ultrasound (EBUS) image of mediastinal lymph node sampling. *Source:* https://www.ctsnet.org/sites/default/files/graphics/experts/Thoracic/d_rice_endobronc_ultrasnd/Figure-6b.jpg.

Researchers have established that EBUS-TBNA (transbronchial needle aspiration) is now vital for staging non-small cell lung cancer, thereby playing a critical role in patient care. The minimally invasive procedure reduces hospitalization and enhances the patient's experience through reduced discomfort and procedure risk. The ultrasound imaging and interventional treatment synergy positions EBUS at the forefront of current lung cancer and mediastinal disease diagnosis practice (Bugalho et al., 2022). Moreover, the evolution of ultrasound technology continues with ongoing innovation, for example, in the development of adjunct imaging modalities such as optical coherence tomography and artificial intelligence. These advancements hold the potential to enhance the accuracy of mediastinal assessment further, potentially adding real-time data analysis and further improving results. As further research continues to validate and improve the use of ultrasound in thoracic imaging, it will likely have a more critical role in mediastinal assessment. With the widening of the diagnostic modalities used, clinicians are better positioned to offer personalized treatment plans that account for the multifactorial nature of mediastinal pathology, leading us toward a future in which non-invasive imaging contributes significantly to patient care (Cheng et al., 2024).

3.4.3. MRI Applications in Mediastinal Pathologies

Magnetic Resonance Imaging (MRI) has now emerged as a valuable tool for evaluating mediastinal pathologies, offering numerous advantages over traditional imaging methods such as computed tomography (CT). The unique advantages of MRI, that is, its improved soft tissue contrast and lack of ionizing radiation, make it particularly suited to the characterization of mediastinal masses. Lymphoma, thymoma, and other tumors in the lung may be reliably diagnosed with MRI, which enables clinicians to identify benign from malignant lesions. The multiparametric nature of MRI also provides detailed tissue characterization, which is important in individualizing management strategies for patients. Technological improvements in MRI equipment, including high-field magnets and advanced sequences, enhance the diagnostic reliability and clinical utility of the technique in the mediastinum (Figure 3.13).

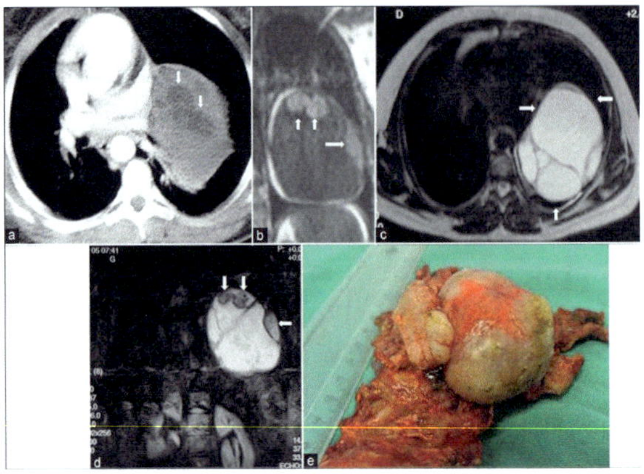

Figure 3.13. Imaging of cystic and cyst-like lesions of the mediastinum with pathologic correlation.

Source: https://clinicalimagingscience.org/content/12/2012/2/1/img/JCIS-2-33-g008.png.

Where the normal imaging modalities fall short, MRI has emerged as a second-line imaging modality of choice in the assessment of congenital heart disease and other thoracic diseases. Its capacity to produce multiparametric and multiplanar images is critical in making diagnoses and displaying associated disease where ultrasound findings are inconclusive. Gating of imaging modalities, that is, ECG gating, has transformed fetal cardiac assessments by synchronizing with heartbeats, thereby improving anatomical and functional evaluation of the thoracic organs. The data acquired through these new MRI techniques not only assists in diagnosing mediastinal disease but also offers a window for investigating resultant complications, thereby moving towards an integrative approach in thoracic imaging (Giancotti et al., 2024). The comprehensive capability of MRI in assessing mediastinal diseases is well established in the literature, for example, in pertinent research where interdisciplinary collaboration between radiologists and clinicians is emphasized. The significant advancement in imaging-guided treatment indicates the pivotal role of MRI in mediastinal disease in enabling precise therapeutic interventions. Imaging fusion of modalities like MRI, CT, and ultrasound provides a clear overview of mediastinal structures in benign and malignant disease. A combined approach boosts diagnostic confidence to stage and plan the treatment accordingly. The usefulness of MRI in this case is highlighted by its role in an overall diagnostic strategy, underscoring its probable benefits not only for radiologists but also for clinicians in oncology, cardiology, and pulmonology (N/A, 2021).

3.5. Common Mediastinal Pathologies

The mediastinum, the middle thoracic cavity compartment, contains a diverse array of structures and is hence susceptible to a diverse array of pathologies. Thymic tumors, lymphadenopathy, and bronchogenic cysts are some of the common mediastinal disorders with typical imaging appearances. Thymic tumors, often in the anterior mediastinum, may appear as well-defined or irregular masses and require proper differentiation from other masses, such as germ cell tumors and lymphomas. Imaging techniques such as computed tomography (CT) play a central part in these differential diagnoses, providing accurate anatomical context to inform clinical decision-making. More imaging modalities, emphasized in recent literature, provide a general view of these pathologies, enabling targeted management strategies in patients with mediastinal illnesses. The integration of high-resolution datasets, such as those reported in studies, enhances diagnostic accuracy by providing a solid basis for the radiologist to examine and validate outcomes (Bustos et al., 2019). Also, mediastinal lymphadenopathy is a critical radiologic finding that can refer to a broad spectrum of underlying pathology, varying from benign infection to malignancy. On imaging, enlarged lymph nodes can present in a highly variable pattern, with some features suggestive of potential etiologies.

For example, CT scan patterns and lymph node morphology can suggest whether the etiology is infectious, such as tuberculosis, or neoplastic, such as lymphoma. Such patterns require a fine understanding of mediastinal anatomy, which is often distorted by the superimposition of features from varying pathologies. Knowledge of these nuances not only aids in the differential diagnosis but also increases the effectiveness of subsequent management options for the patient. Educational resources on imaging interpretation are the principle to it, allowing radiologists and nuclear physicians to enhance their diagnostic abilities in handling prevalent mediastinal abnormalities (Hashmi et al., 2019). In the context of mediastinal imaging, bronchogenic cysts are another extremely prevalent anomaly, typically arising from embryonic development. They may be visualized as well-defined fluid-filled spaces on imaging, most commonly in the mediastinum. Although typically asymptomatic and identified on imaging for other reasons, their potential for complications such as infection or rupture necessitates careful monitoring and management. Radiologists must be able to distinguish these cysts from other mediastinal masses, including neoplastic masses. Advanced imaging techniques, such as MRI and high-resolution CT, supplement the capabilities of the conventional modalities by their ability to provide greater contrast resolution and more accurate delineation of adjacent structures. It is therefore important to recognize the imaging characteristics of bronchogenic cysts to provide an appropriate diagnosis, facilitate appropriate management, and prevent unnecessary invasive procedures (Bustos et al., 2019).

3.5.1. Mediastinal Tumors: Types and Imaging Features

The mediastinum is a complex region of anatomy where a wide variety of tumors exist, from benign to malignant lesions. Thymomas are among the most common mediastinal tumors, are epithelial tumors originating from the thymus gland, and are typically located in the anterior mediastinum. While most often found in this location, thymomas can occur in uncommon sites, as seen in a case where a thymoma arose from the posterior mediastinal pleura (Kalloli et al., 2012). Imaging plays an important role in diagnosing and managing such tumors, and computed tomography (CT) is the preferred modality because it can define tumor characteristics such as size, shape, and relationship to surrounding structures (Figure 3.14).

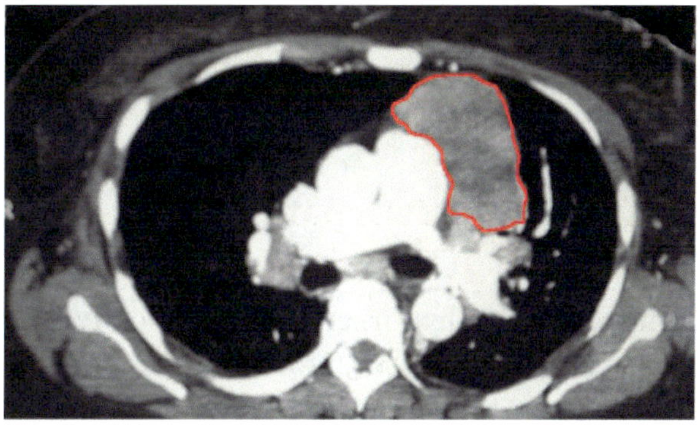

Figure 3.14. CT scan highlighting a large thymoma in the anterior mediastinum.

Source: https://mdsearchlight.com/wp-content/uploads/2024/09/30129-1725897127766-728x420.jpg.

These also include thymomas and other significant mediastinal tumors like germ cell tumors, lymphomas, and sarcomas. Sarcomas are an uncommon group of mesenchymal neoplasms that can occur in any mediastinal structure. Radiological features observed on CT scans are required to differentiate these tumors. For example, sarcomas are traditionally seen to present as large masses with ill-defined margins and heterogeneous enhancement, as highlighted by studies that enumerated the prevalence of such characteristics among intrathoracic masses (Kalloli et al., 2012). Additionally, intratumoral vessels and pleural effusion can also be used by radiologists to distinguish sarcomas from other tumors.

Interpreting imaging findings is a key factor in effective clinical management of mediastinal tumors. Accurate recognition of the characteristic features of a specific tumor guides diagnosis as well as therapy. For instance, sharply delineated, smooth or lobulated borders in a space-occupying mass may suggest a sarcoma, especially when coupled with imaging features such as intratumoral vessels and pleural effusion without significant lymphadenopathy (Heussel et al., 2014). With our growing knowledge of the tumors, integration of advanced imaging modalities with clinical presentation will help progressively enhance the diagnostic potential and therapeutic outcomes for mediastinal tumor patients.

3.5.2. Lymphadenopathy: Causes and Imaging Techniques

Lymphadenopathy, or enlargement of lymph nodes, is a radiologic sign that can be related to a wide range of underlying conditions, ranging from infections to malignancy. Its value in thoracic imaging, including the lung and mediastinum, stems from the roles of the lymphatics in metastasis and protection. Diseases such as lymphoma and tuberculosis tend to present with lymphadenopathy and may be obscured by the thoracic structures on imaging. Detection of mediastinal lymphadenopathy, for instance, may be a key component in diagnosing a tumor or infection and requires adequate knowledge of likely causes. Imaging modalities, therefore, play a crucial role in shedding light on the etiology of lymphadenopathy to help clinicians distinguish malignant from non-malignant illness based on morphology and site of involvement of the lymph nodes (Figure 3.15).

Imaging of lymphadenopathy incorporates conventional and emerging techniques, primarily computed tomography (CT), magnetic resonance imaging (MRI), and positron emission tomography (PET). CT scans are generally used to evaluate lymphadenopathy due to their ability to obtain high-quality cross-sectional images of thoracic anatomy. The ability to assess lymph node size, shape, and enhancement patterns can be used to identify nodes as suspicious or reactive. As highlighted in the literature, communication between clinicians and radiologists is central to effective management, particularly in complex situations such as tuberculosis with human immunodeficiency virus (HIV) coinfection (Ahmad et al., 2009). Categorization of imaging conditions related to lymph nodes must keep improving, with an eye towards maximizing practitioners' diagnostic performance against an ever-changing presentation of disease.

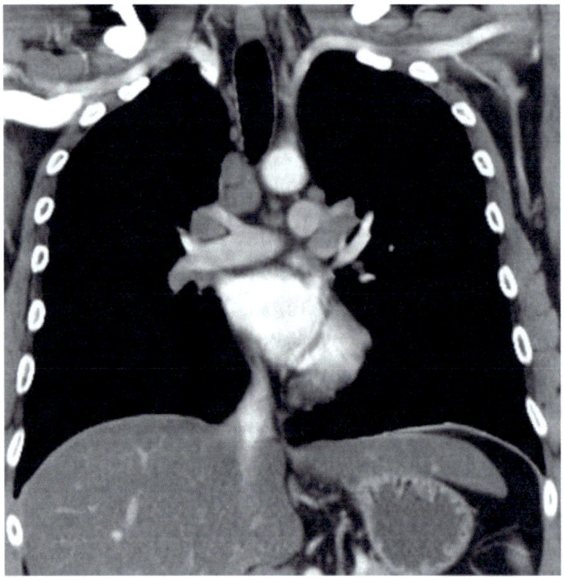

Figure 3.15. Coronal CT scan showing enlarged mediastinal lymph nodes.

Source: https://prod-images-static.radiopaedia.org/images/291140/f4499b68a57cefca837e26b4eac9a0_gallery.jpg.

Minimally invasive techniques such as endobronchial ultrasound (EBUS) and endoscopic ultrasound (EUS) have revolutionized the diagnosis of thoracic lymphadenopathy, particularly mediastinal lymphadenopathy. These techniques allow for accurate lymph node sampling with minimal patient risk, improving diagnostic yields and reducing time to best interventions (Cheng et al., 2024). This evolution in bronchoscopy not only improves the care of patients with suspected malignancies but also facilitates improved care of infections and other diseases with lymphadenopathy. Ongoing advances in imaging technology and methods promise a bright future for the diagnosis and staging of thoracic disease. Ultimately, a multidisciplinary approach that integrates imaging and clinical acumen remains essential to effectively address the complexities of lymphadenopathy.

3.5.3. Aortic Aneurysms: Detection and Implications

The detection of aortic aneurysms is a significant part of thoracic imaging, with significant patient management and outcome consequences. Aortic aneurysms, which can occur in the thoracic and abdominal aorta, are often asymptomatic until they become a specific size or rupture. This silent growth necessitates advanced imaging modalities for early detection and follow-up. Various modalities, such as computed tomography (CT) angiography and magnetic resonance imaging (MRI), enable minute visualization of the aorta's structure and are crucial for detecting aneurysm abnormalities. This role is underlined by their ability to not only identify the size and location of aneurysms but also associated complications, such as dissection, with great impact on treatment planning and patient prognosis. Early detection by quality imaging can greatly improve outcomes for affected patients. Beyond direct patient care, the implications of successful diagnosis of aortic aneurysms extend to public health considerations in general. Early detection of an aneurysm allows clinicians to intervene in a timely manner, which may be through repair by surgery or endovascular techniques, and reduce the risk of lethal rupture. Improvements in imaging technology have also facilitated enhanced risk stratification, allowing clinicians to tailor surveillance intervals based on patient-specific variables and aneurysm features. This individualized approach not only optimizes the use of resources but also ensures patient safety and long-term health as prime priorities. With continually advancing thoracic imaging modalities, science is helping us learn more about aortic pathologies and ultimately standardize diagnostic approaches with enhanced efficacy and clinical practice.

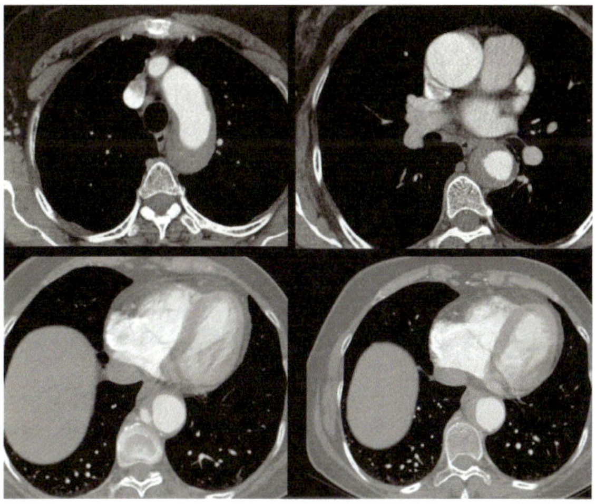

Figure 3.16. Contrast CT showing saccular aneurysm of the thoracic aorta.

Source: https://prod-images-static.radiopaedia.org/multiple_choice_questions/155/aorta_bueno_big_gallery.jpeg.

In addition to imaging technological advances, an interdisciplinary collaboration of radiologists, cardiologists, and vascular surgeons is necessary for effective management of aortic aneurysms. Because of the interdependence of aortic disease, there is a need to integrate findings from thoracic imaging into a planned treatment strategy. Radiologists play a pivotal role through appropriate imaging study interpretation and enabling subsequent clinical treatment. The partnership model is applied to the creation of integrated patient education programs that can support higher levels of awareness of risk factors and the necessity of screening among high-risk groups. In the end, through promoting an integrated process with early detection and team management, healthcare systems are able to improve patient outcomes and equip patients with knowledge regarding their cardiovascular health (N/A, 2021) (Figure 3.16).

3.6. Advances in Thoracic Imaging

Advances in thoracic imaging have significantly enhanced the diagnostic capabilities for most pulmonary diseases, particularly tuberculosis (TB). Recent technological progress made in imaging modalities like computed tomography (CT) and MRI has allowed for the visualization of the satisfactory resolution of lung disease. Current guidelines suggest that a new TB imaging categorization is required that accounts for the now-overlapping presentation across patients of all age groups. Clinicians must learn to recognize imaging features typical of TB to facilitate early diagnosis, especially in settings where radiologists are unavailable. Successful inclusion of imaging in routine clinical practice requires effective communication and coordination between clinicians and radiologists to address local disease patterns, HIV co-infection rates, and practical imaging parameters that affect patient management strategies (Ahmad et al., 2009). This combined approach guarantees that technological advances in imaging are realized in patient benefit and increased clinical confidence. In diagnosing lung cancer, innovations such as endoscopic bronchial ultrasound (EBUS) have transformed traditional practice. EBUS provides minimally invasive methods for obtaining cytology from multiple intrathoracic lymph nodes, enabling accurate staging of lung cancer. This approach has been shown to reduce the demand for more invasive surgical biopsies and to maintain high sensitivity and specificity—a key parameter, given that early and accurate staging is directly correlated with prognosis. In light of lung cancer's contribution to having a heavy burden of advanced-stage diagnoses, advancement in imaging protocols like EBUS is a critical factor to facilitate early intervention. Besides, the excellent safety profile of EBUS renders it a first choice in the clinical setting, consonant with trends towards minimizing surgical risk and maximizing diagnostic yield (Bilocca et al., 2016). Thus, the ongoing development of techniques such as EBUS underscores the importance of integrating new imaging modalities into lung cancer treatment protocols. With continuing advancements in thoracic imaging, it is important to consider the implications of such advancements on public health as well as on clinical practice. Improved imaging modalities not only increase diagnostic precision but may also lead to more effective treatment regimens through early disease detection. Artificial intelligence and machine learning technologies adopted in thoracic imaging have immense potential to enhance diagnostic efficiency by automating image analysis. These technologies could assist radiologists in calling attention to regions of interest for further assessment, thereby reducing diagnostic errors and enhancing patient care overall. Furthermore, the continuous innovation in imaging modalities has the potential to increase access to good-quality diagnostics, particularly in underserved areas. This innovative age of thoracic imaging is not only a technological breakthrough but also a commitment to better patient outcomes in the lung and mediastinum healthcare system.

3.6.1. Innovations in Imaging Technology

Thoracic imaging has made tremendous advances with the advent of newer imaging modalities, setting the stage for improved diagnostic testing for various pulmonary and mediastinal illnesses. Conventional imaging methods, such as computed radiography (CR), have been the workhorse in clinical settings. Newer modalities like low-dose linear-slit digital radiography (LSDR) are revolutionizing the diagnosis of thoracic diseases. One of the major studies found that LSDR received better overall image-quality ratings than CR, at 9.75 compared with CR's 8.16 on a scale of 10 (Szucs-Farkas et al., 2018). This improvement is particularly valuable for delineating anatomical structures within the mediastinum and retrocardiac areas, which are also challenging to evaluate. These developments will lead to enhanced diagnosis and better patient management, ultimately pointing toward a future with innovations that continuously maximize chest imaging quality (Figure 3.17).

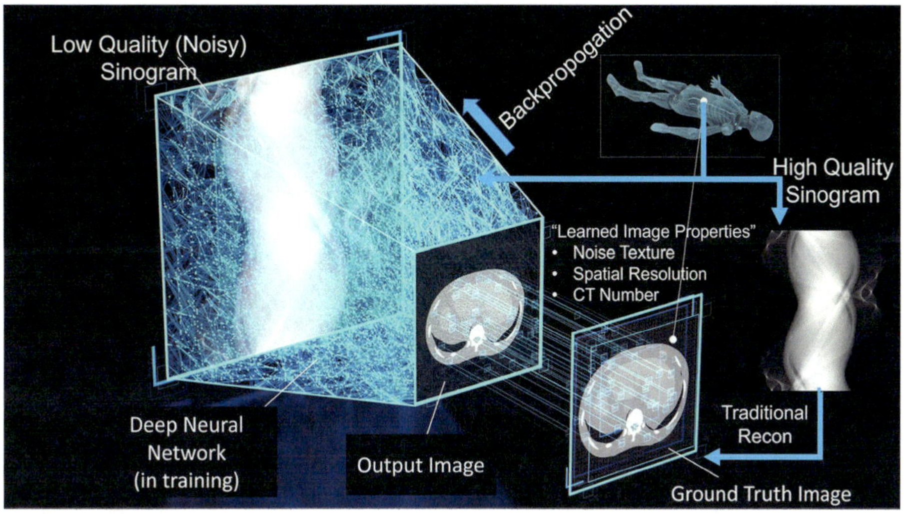

Figure 3.17. An overview of deep learning CT reconstruction.

Source: https://media.springernature.com/lw1200/springer-static/image/art%3A10.1007%2Fs40134-022-00399-5/MediaObjects/40134_2022_399_Fig2_HTML.png.

Human anatomy is inherently complex, particularly in regions such as the thorax, where many important structures are closely packed. Improvements in imaging technology, particularly LSDR, have demonstrated greater proficiency in imaging these complex structures, thus allowing clinicians to base decisions on more informed data. The ability to identify fine anatomical details is essential when evaluating diseases like pulmonary nodules, mediastinal masses, and vascular malformations. The retrospective analysis indicated a statistically significant difference in image quality between CR and LSDR, whereby the latter would be more valuable in detecting meaningful pathological detail, especially where there is high attenuation (Szucs-Farkas et al., 2018). As imaging technologies continue to evolve, it is increasingly important for healthcare practitioners to stay abreast of such developments to get the best outcomes for patients by enhancing diagnostic precision. Besides, the uses of these innovations extend beyond image quality enhancement; they also encompass patient safety and radiation dose exposure. The benefits of low-dose in the LSDR technique are an important step towards minimizing unwanted effects from traditional imaging methods. By combining diagnostic performance with a reduced radiation dose, LSDR is a leap ahead of current health agendas regarding patient safety and ethical practice. This balance is crucial in thoracic imaging, where repeated imaging can be performed for longitudinal assessment. In this manner, these innovations not only promote augmented diagnostic confidence but also promote patient-centered care. The enormous expansion of cutting-edge imaging technologies, like LSDR, positions thoracic imaging at the forefront of medical diagnosis, ushering in opportunities for innovative healthcare provision and patient experience for lung and mediastinum diseases.

3.6.2. Artificial Intelligence in Radiology

The application of artificial intelligence (AI) in radiology has fundamentally changed the practice of thoracic imaging, particularly in the lung and mediastinum. AI algorithms, and more importantly, deep learning models, have helped improve diagnostic accuracy and efficiency in most imaging modalities. For instance, convolutional neural networks (CNNs) are routinely applied to read thoracic radiographs, facilitating the computer-aided detection of diseases such as lung nodules or mediastinal masses. The ability of these models to learn from large datasets makes them more effective at detecting subtle imaging features that human radiologists often overlook. Therefore, the potential of AI to supplement radiological assessment is the promise of earlier and more accurate diagnoses, thereby enhancing patient management in clinical settings (Figure 3.18).

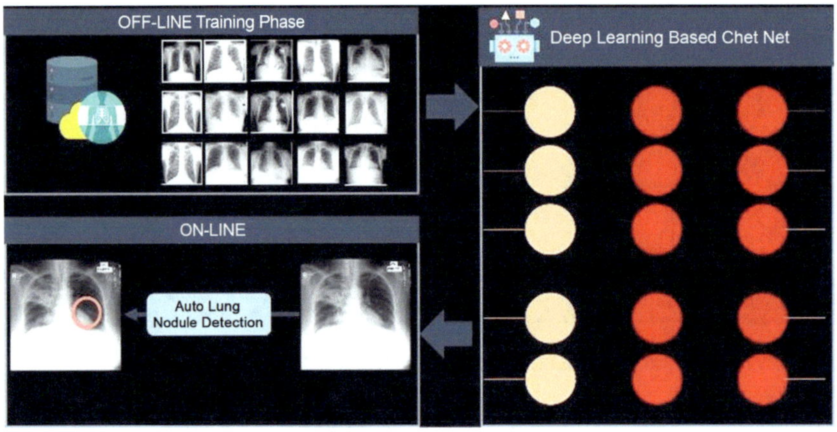

Figure 3.18. Auto lung nodule detection software of samsung electronics.

Source: https://www.researchgate.net/figure/Auto-Lung-Nodule-Detection-Software-of-Samsung-Electronics_fig1_352112867.

In lung imaging, AI has played a significant part in creating systems that assist clinicians in detecting and determining lung conditions more efficiently. Studies based on large datasets of chest X-rays substantiate that AI can identify patterns that are associated with diseases such as pneumonia, chronic obstructive pulmonary disease, and lung cancer. By leveraging AI-driven insights, radiologists can enhance their interpretive accuracy, with AI pointing out atypical findings for closer examination. Furthermore, the analytical power of AI algorithms can facilitate assessment of disease evolution over time, providing key information to guide treatment and improve patient outcomes across a variety of thoracic disorders. Assessment of the mediastinum is difficult due to the variability of disease processes that can occur there. The conventional approaches to diagnosis have included invasive procedures to obtain sufficient diagnoses. Novel technological advances in the form of AI-based imaging modalities of bronchoscopy and other minimally invasive techniques are changing this paradigm. Modality such as endobronchial ultrasound and AI-based imaging have shown high diagnostic yields with minimal complications. Not only are these advancements accelerating the diagnostic process, but they also enhance the overall accuracy of diagnosing mediastinal disease. With the advancement of AI, its integration with traditional diagnostic approaches represents a new era in thoracic imaging that profoundly impacts the diagnosis and treatment of mediastinal diseases in clinical practice (정지원, 2023; Cheng et al., 2024).

3.6.3. Future Trends in Thoracic Imaging

With progressing thoracic imaging, various trends are emerging that are bound to enhance the precision and efficacy of diagnosis and treatment in pulmonary and mediastinal disorders. One such trend is the use of artificial intelligence (AI) in imaging technologies to enable more advanced analysis and interpretation. Computer programs now are more capable of detecting tiny patterns in imaging information that a human reader could overlook, making diagnostic sensitivity for illnesses such as lung nodules and mediastinal lymphadenopathy stronger. As machine learning technology advances, these systems can learn from massive databases, improving their performance over time and allowing radiologists to focus on tougher diagnostics. This trend underscores the need for radiologists to evolve alongside new technologies while continuing to play their critical analytical role in interpreting imaging findings and clinical correlations. The integration of imaging specialists and oncologists is another promising future trend, especially for managing complex thoracic conditions such as lung cancer. Treatment modalities, especially for stage III non-small cell lung carcinoma (NSCLC), must be developed by incorporating a multimodal strategy that harmonizes imaging data and treatment. Emerging imaging modalities, such as better positron emission tomography (PET) and high-resolution computed tomography (HRCT), are transforming staging and monitoring of NSCLC by clinicians. Later advancements have placed greater emphasis on endobronchial ultrasonography in mediastinal staging, which can be pivotal in treatment decision-making (Figure 3.19).

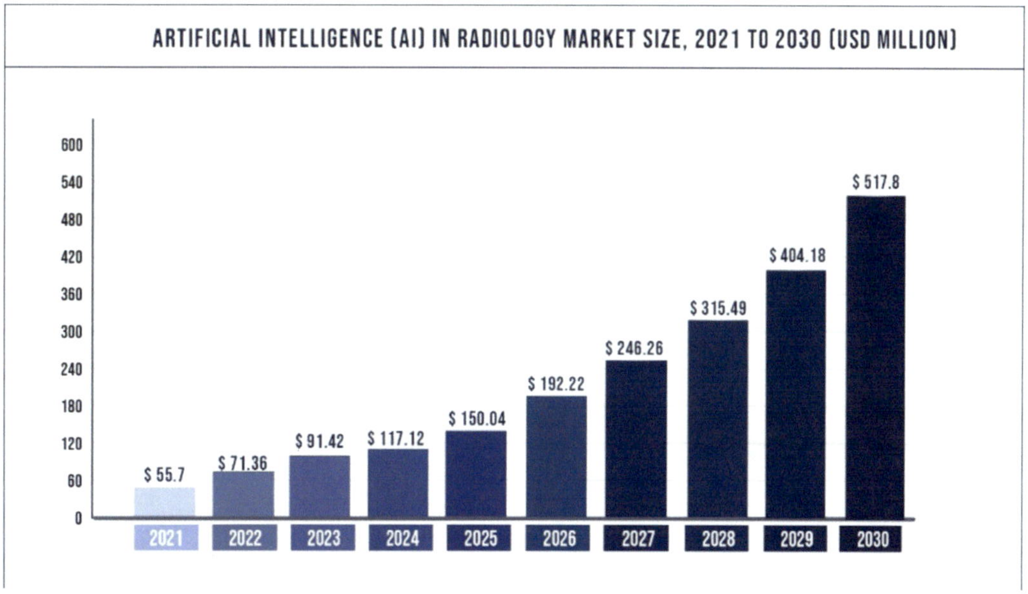

Figure 3.19. Infographic showing artificial intelligence (AI) in radiology up to 2030.

Source: https://www.visionresearchreports.com/reportimg/Artificial-Intelligence-(AI)-in-Radiology-Market-Size-2021-to-2030.jpg.

Such convergence not only enhances patient care but also underscores the necessity of ongoing education in both imaging and oncologic treatment protocols, thus equipping healthcare providers to address the rapidly changing environment of thoracic cancer management. Moreover, the future of thoracic imaging is closely interrelated with the development of personalized medicine, in which treatment plans are tailored to the patient's unique characteristics and tumor biology. New imaging biomarkers constructed from state-of-the-art imaging modalities have the potential to reveal useful molecular and genomic information and provide insights into the behavior of lung cancers and sensitivity to various treatments. This shift towards precision imaging enables more individualized therapeutic modalities in cancers such as NSCLC, including immunotherapy and targeted molecular therapies. This advancement in imaging modalities is necessary to monitor the response to treatment and adjust management plans accordingly. As these trends take shape, there is growing need for radiologists and oncologists working in tandem with one another, so imaging technology as well as treatment protocols both need to evolve in tandem so that patient outcomes for thoracic disease are optimized.

SUMMARY

In conclusion to our review of imaging of the thorax, particularly of the lung and mediastinum, it is worth noting the wide-ranging impact that advances in imaging technologies have had on practice. Mixing high-resolution imaging modalities, for example, chest CT and radiography, has significantly enhanced the detection and diagnosis of a myriad of thoracic conditions, including cancer of the lung and respiratory disease. For instance, the deployment of large databases, such as PadChest, which provide labeled chest X-ray images, enables automated radiographic result exploration and has the potential to improve diagnostic performance and efficiency during patient management (Bustos et al., 2019). This addresses the necessity for continuous innovation in thoracic imaging as a critical component in the face of mounting challenges posed by pulmonary diseases. Furthermore, the application of imaging modalities in the staging and treatment of non-small cell lung cancer demonstrates the pivotal role thoracic imaging plays. Evidence has shown the merits of using chest CT for the precise definition of tumor status, as high sensitivity and specificity values are detailed in the literature (Busroh et al., 2003). Effective preoperative staging ensures optimization of treatment modalities, enabling customized therapeutic modalities, and ultimately optimizing patient outcomes. With the evolving imaging modalities, new methodologies and algorithms should also be refined to decrease the limitations currently faced in terms of specificity and accuracy, primarily concerning different histological subtypes of lung cancer. This evolution will be extremely beneficial to make sure that thoracic imaging still improves standards of care in oncology. While considering the role of thoracic imaging in clinical practice, we can observe that the future also holds fertile ground for novel technologies that leverage developments in artificial intelligence and machine learning. By employing large data sets and developing wise algorithms, the field will be in a position to witness enhanced diagnostic competence that not only complements existing imaging protocols but also surmounts significant challenges, such as the variability of interpretation among radiologists. Last but not least, the ongoing integration of these technologies will redefine the thoracic imaging environment, improving the detection and characterization of thoracic abnormalities and thereby improving the quality of care provided to patients with respiratory diseases. Commitment to research and technological innovation will remain essential in the evolution of thoracic imaging towards meeting the complexity of today's medicine.

CLOSER LOOK

THORACIC IMAGING, LUNG AND MEDIASTINUM

Provide particular diagnostic challenges that require total knowledge of their anatomical complexities. To begin with, lung cancer remains the leading cause of cancer mortality worldwide, and the most frequent subtype is non-small cell lung cancer (NSCLC). Stereotactic body radiation therapy (SBRT) has revolutionized treatment algorithms for stage I NSCLC, particularly in peripheral tumors. The technique offers optimal tumor control with less toxicity but is susceptible to centrally placed lesions due to proximity to crucial structures. To optimize the treatment strategy, a classification that discriminates between central and peripheral lung cancer is essential to ensure that personalized treatment is properly utilized in clinical practice (Adebahr et al., 2017). The posterior mediastinum contains significant structures, including the descending thoracic aorta, esophagus, and variable lymphatic and vascular structures. These anatomic structures are susceptible to a broad range of pathological abnormalities that make the diagnosis challenging. While most abnormalities can be detected by initial diagnostic evaluation on chest radiography, newer imaging modalities, such as computed tomography (CT) and magnetic resonance imaging (MRI), are emerging as useful tools for delineating these mediastinal lesions. Such imaging techniques are beneficial in evaluating the relationship between lesions and adjacent structures, thereby refining differential diagnoses and enhancing the precision of clinical evaluation. This emphasis on modality-specific responses underscores the necessity to adopt some imaging protocols for complete morphological evaluation in the thoracic region (Bankier et al., 2015). In summary, the role of high-tech imaging devices in thoracic imaging, particularly in lung and mediastinal disease assessment, is paramount to improving patient outcomes. The characterization of lung tumors and mediastinal structures must evolve with changes as a function of technological and therapeutic innovation. As with successful clinical applications of SBRT for NSCLC, precise imaging not only aids diagnosis but also plays a crucial role in treatment planning. Lastly, the creation of a multi-disciplinary system that combines these technologies and classification systems will enhance diagnostic accuracy and therapeutic efficacy in the management of complex thoracic diseases (Adebahr et al., 2017; Bankier et al., 2015).

The significance of accurate imaging in the diagnosis of thoracic disorders cannot be overemphasized, as it constitutes the cornerstone of successful medical evaluation and treatment planning. Imaging modalities such as computed tomography (CT) and endoscopic ultrasound are instrumental in detecting and characterizing lung and mediastinal lesions. In lung cancer, for instance, precise imaging allows for assessment of tumor staging, which is invaluable in determining prognosis and therapeutic strategy for the patient. It has been found that failure to precisely discern significant features, such as mediastinal lymph node involvement, can lead to inappropriate treatment regimens, compromising patient outcomes. Therefore, the role of imaging is not merely identification; it dictates the entire clinical pathway, and therefore, there is a need for advanced imaging modalities and specialist interpretation in thoracic medicine. Pursuit of accurate diagnosis involves the integration of various imaging modalities, particularly between neoplastic and inflammatory lesions. Reliance on patient history and physical examination alone is usually inadequate because most thoracic diseases present paradoxically. With the introduction of techniques such as endoscopic bronchial ultrasound (EBUS), lung cancer staging has been revolutionized, with the capability of healthcare practitioners to carry out cytological sampling of intrathoracic lymph nodes in a minimally invasive but highly sensitive manner. This is particularly critical, as early diagnosis and accurate staging are crucial for treatment outcomes. EBUS not only minimizes the need for more invasive surgical biopsies but also enhances overall diagnostic accuracy, often leading to quicker therapeutic intervention and better patient prognoses, thereby emphasizing the interconnectedness of imaging, diagnosis, and effective patient management (Bilocca et al., 2016). Furthermore, the precision of imaging techniques significantly affects decision-making in treatment modalities in thoracic medicine. Computational techniques such as CT-guided fine-needle aspiration (FNAB) and tissue-core biopsy (TCB) are significant determinants in the evaluation of thoracic lesions, as various studies have shown that the imaging modalities combined achieve high diagnostic accuracy. The application of these new methods not only allows for better lesion demarcation but is also useful in the minimization of complications arising from the employment of traditional diagnostic interventions. For instance, results show that while minute risks are associated with FNAB, for instance, pneumothorax or hemorrhage, overall safety profiles are favorable considering the accuracy they present (Felici et al., 2021). In practice, accurate imaging is not just an adjunct to diagnosis; it is a critical component that directly affects clinical outcomes and the success of therapeutic interventions in thoracic management. With the increasing evolution of thoracic imaging, one of the brightest prospects is integrating artificial intelligence (AI) and machine learning into diagnostic protocols. These are likely to improve imaging analysis, making it more precise and effective, particularly for the detection of conditions such as lung cancer and interstitial lung disease. By leveraging vast datasets and sophisticated algorithms, scientists are creating AI models that not only detect abnormalities but also predict patient outcomes based on imaging features. The approach has the promise to reduce diagnosis error and timely interventions, ultimately improving prognostic capability in thoracic medicine. Further, extensive validation studies must be conducted to ensure that such AI software may be seamlessly incorporated into daily clinical practice and enhance the decision-making for pulmonologists and radiologists (N/A, 2000). Advances in imaging modalities, such as 3D printing and virtual reality, also hold promise for future directions in thoracic imaging research. With the potential to revolutionize preoperative planning and interventional treatment, these modalities have the potential to provide precise, patient-specific anatomical models. By creating three-dimensional reconstructions of the lung and mediastinum from imaging data, surgeons can better understand complex anatomical variation and improve the accuracy of procedures such as biopsies or resections. Further, the inclusion of virtual reality as part of surgical training optimizes the learning process for medical personnel in that they can practice techniques on a realistic simulation. These technologies are on the verge of enhancing surgical precision and safety for patients, a paradigm shift for the treatment of thoracic pathology in clinical practice (N/A, 2006). Finally, thoracic imaging is moving towards a personalized medicine paradigm, in which imaging modalities are tailored to patients' specific requirements. The increased understanding of genetic and molecular etiologies of thoracic diseases spurs such an evolution. Researchers are now investigating how imaging biomarkers can be correlated with genetic signatures to enable more targeted therapies and interventions. By combining genomic data with imaging findings, clinicians can better stratify risk and optimize treatment for patients with diseases such as lung cancer. This intersection of thoracic imaging and molecular biology not only holds the promise of further enhancing treatment outcomes but also emphasizes the importance of interdisciplinarity in future thoracic imaging research.

REFERENCES

1. Fechter, T., Dolz, J., Chirindel, A., Schlachter, M., Carles, M., Adebahr, S., Mix, M., & Nestle, U. (2017). Fully Automatic Danger Zone Determination for SBRT in NSCLC. *Journal of Radiation Oncology Informatics*, *7*(1), 1–27. https://doi.org/10.5166/jroi-7-1-26Ahmad, A. N., Andronikou, S., Andronikou, S., Andronikou, S., Andronikou, S., Andronikou, S., et al. (2009). Advances in imaging chest tuberculosis: Blurring of differences between children and adults. https://core.ac.uk/download/pdf/9417669.pdf (accessed on 15th July 2025).
2. Alves, F. R., Ambrosio, C. E., Araujo, A. V. C., Costa, R. C., et al. (2012). Aparência anatômica e radiográfica da cavidade torácica do macaco-prego (*Cebus apella*). https://core.ac.uk/download/pdf/37509683.pdf (accessed on 15th July 2025).
3. Andía, E., Arnáiz, M. D., Cardenal, F., Fernández, R., et al. (2006). PET/CT fusion scan in lung cancer: Current recommendations and innovations. https://core.ac.uk/download/pdf/82071853.pdf (accessed on 15th July 2025).
4. Angel, C., Belli, E., Bruniaux, J., Lambert, V., et al. (2005). Preoperative and postoperative evaluation of airways compression in pediatric patients with 3-dimensional multislice computed tomographic scanning: Effect on surgical management. https://core.ac.uk/download/pdf/82809468.pdf (accessed on 15th July 2025).
5. Apriantoro, N. H., Prasetio, H., Sinaga, C. E., Supriyono, A., et al. (2024). Analysis of pediatric fixation equipment with audio-video for chest radiography examinations. https://core.ac.uk/download/604580482.pdf (accessed on 15th July 2025).
6. Arcieri, L., Assanta, N., Baggi, R., Di Maurizio, G., et al. (2016). The role of posterior aortopexy in the treatment of left mainstem bronchus compression. https://core.ac.uk/download/74319435.pdf (accessed on 15th July 2025).
7. Asmara, O. D., Bouterfas, A., Boerma, C., Hardavella, G., et al. (2024). Stage III NSCLC treatment options: Too many choices. https://core.ac.uk/download/653278752.pdf (accessed on 15th July 2025).
8. Bankier, A. A., Eisenberg, R. L., Franquet, E., Heidinger, B. H., et al. (2015). Imaging the posterior mediastinum: A multimodality approach. https://core.ac.uk/download/326840215.pdf (accessed on 15th July 2025).
9. Bauer, G., Elsner, A., Englisch, J., Ismail, M., et al. (2019). Unraveling the role of ectopic thymic tissue in patients undergoing thymectomy for myasthenia gravis. https://core.ac.uk/download/286567837.pdf (accessed on 15th July 2025).
10. Bilocca, D., Montefort, S., & Vella, C. (2016). Endoscopic bronchial ultrasound in mediastinal staging of lung cancer. https://core.ac.uk/download/46604248.pdf (accessed on 15th July 2025).
11. Blackledge, M., Collins, D., Ap Dafydd, D., DeSouza, N. M., et al. (2017). The influence of fat suppression technique on diffusion-weighted (DW) MRI in lung cancer. https://core.ac.uk/download/322471824.pdf (accessed on 15th July 2025).
12. Bogers, A., Maat, A., Mahtab, E., Sadeghi, B., et al. (2019). The realm of oncological lung surgery: From past to present and future perspectives. https://core.ac.uk/download/322445833.pdf (accessed on 15th July 2025).

13. Bugalho, A., Ribeiro, J. C., Clementsen, P. F., Eberhardt, R., et al. (2022). A comprehensive review. https://core.ac.uk/download/555761972.pdf (accessed on 15th July 2025).

14. Busroh, I., Icksan, A., Syachruddin, E., Yusuf, H., et al. (2003). The diagnostic accuracy of chest CT in the detection of tumor and nodal status in non-small cell lung carcinoma. https://media.neliti.com/media/publications/147363-EN-the-diagnostic-accuracy-of-chest-ct-in-t.pdf (accessed on 15th July 2025).

15. Bustos, A., de la Iglesia-Vayá, M., Pertusa, A., Salinas, J., et al. (2019). PadChest: A large chest x-ray image dataset with multi-label annotated reports. https://core.ac.uk/download/328881801.pdf (accessed on 15th July 2025).

16. Chen, W., Chen, Y., Hu, Y., Li, X., et al. (2012). Thoracic low-dose CT image processing using an artifact-suppressed large-scale nonlocal means. *[No DOI or access link provided]*

17. Cheng, G., Dollin, Y., Fortich, M., Hasteh, F., et al. (2024). Diagnostic modalities in the mediastinum and the role of bronchoscopy in mediastinal assessment: A narrative review. https://core.ac.uk/download/640802665.pdf (accessed on 15th July 2025).

18. Clough, A. V., Gordon, J. B., Haworth, S. T., Molthen, R. C., et al. (2008). Bronchial circulation angiogenesis in the rat quantified with SPECT and micro-CT. https://core.ac.uk/download/213086433.pdf (accessed on 15th July 2025).

19. Felici, A., Ghiraldelli, A., Dettori, A., Miglio, A., Del Signore, F., Simeoni, F., Falerno, I., et al. (2021). Clinical value of CT-guided fine needle aspiration and tissue-core biopsy of thoracic masses in the dog and cat. https://core.ac.uk/download/534179724.pdf (accessed on 15th July 2025).

20. Giancotti, A., Catalano, C., Di Mascio, D., Curti, F., Ventriglia, F., Cundari, G., Rizzo, G., et al. (2024). The new frontiers of fetal imaging: MRI insights into cardiovascular and thoracic structures. https://core.ac.uk/download/621403281.pdf (accessed on 15th July 2025).

21. Hashmi, R. (2019). Sectional anatomy quiz III. https://core.ac.uk/download/604064146.pdf (accessed on 15th July 2025).

22. Hebestreit, A., Kluge, A., Kluge, A., Kluge, A., Bankier, A. A., Henderson, A. C., Brody, A. S., et al. (2011). MRI of the lung (3/3)–Current applications and future perspectives. https://core.ac.uk/download/28969132.pdf (accessed on 15th July 2025).

23. Heussel, C. P., Sommer, G., Kauczor, H. U., Koenigkam-Santos, M., Puderbach, M., Schnabel, P. A., & Safi, S. (2014). Primary intrathoracic malignant mesenchymal tumors: Computed tomography features of a rare group of chest neoplasms. https://core.ac.uk/download/pdf/81585923.pdf (accessed on 15th July 2025).

24. Kalloli, M., Ramachandra, C., Srinivas, C., Vijayakumar, R., et al. (2012). A rare giant pleural thymoma in posterior mediastinum. https://core.ac.uk/download/pdf/13598784.pdf (accessed on 15th July 2025).

25. Szucs-Farkas, Z., & Vock, P. (2018). Image quality of supine chest radiographs: Intra-individual comparison of computed radiography and low-dose linear-slit digital radiography. https://core.ac.uk/download/159152332.pdf (accessed on 15th July 2025).

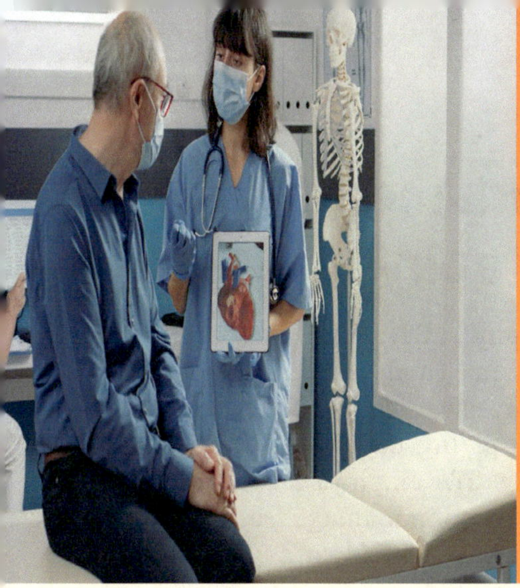

Chapter 4

CARDIOVASCULAR IMAGING: CT ANGIOGRAPHY AND MRI

Contents

Introduction

The field of cardiovascular imaging has advanced significantly in recent years, largely due to the introduction of sophisticated technologies such as CT angiography and MRI. These imaging methods take pivotal roles in diagnosing, evaluating, and treating most cardiovascular diseases and provide clinicians with important information regarding the structure and function of the heart and vascular system. CT angiography, known for its high-quality images and short acquisition times, enables visualization of the coronary arteries and, consequently, the early diagnosis of potentially fatal conditions such as coronary artery disease. MRI, on the other hand, has distinct benefits, especially in evaluating myocardial tissue properties and identifying conditions such as cardiomyopathy or myocarditis, thereby improving diagnostic sensitivity. Establishment of these imaging modalities is a paradigm change in the field of clinical cardiology that necessitates an insider's understanding of their applications, effectiveness, and integration into routine practice. Furthermore, understanding of the limitations and fallacies in currently used imaging modalities is crucial to enhance cardiovascular therapy. Although CT angiography provides adequate anatomical information, it does involve ionizing radiation exposure and does not necessarily well define certain cardiac pathologies. Similarly, although MRI is a highly successful tool for soft tissue evaluation, availability and cost might discourage widespread usage. Both methods also require interpretation by skilled individuals, and therefore, there is a need for ongoing education and training in the field. Advances in deep learning technologies over the recent past should present helpful avenues for the management of some of these problems. By facilitating the processing of large volumes of data generated by imaging studies, deep learning can enhance diagnostic capabilities and streamline workflow for cardiologists while overcoming certain limitations intrinsic to traditional imaging interpretation (Bizopoulos et al., 2021). As the landscape of cardiovascular imaging continues to evolve, it becomes increasingly important to explore future directions to further optimize the use of CT angiography and MRI. The integration of machine learning and artificial intelligence with imaging workflows has the promise to bring significant advances in efficiency and accuracy. These may be the secrets to building predictive models and personalized treatment pathways from patient-specific data, ultimately translating into better cardiovascular disease outcomes. Furthermore, ongoing research into hybrid imaging technologies that combine functional and anatomical information might revolutionize the diagnosis and treatment of cardiovascular diseases. Embracing these advances in technology will most likely redefine the practice of cardiology, providing improved patient care and healthier outcomes in a preventive model. Increased research into cardiovascular imaging will ensure that in-depth knowledge of current practice and emerging technologies is essential for experts in the field in the future.

4.1. Fundamentals of CT Angiography

CT angiography (CTA) is a significant advancement in cardiovascular imaging, enabling non-invasive imaging of blood vessels and organs. Applying computed tomography (CT) technology, CTA employs X-rays to create complex cross-sectional images of the body, revealing both anatomical and pathological structures in the cardiovascular system. The technique begins with intravenous injection of a contrast agent that enhances the visibility of vascular structures. As it travels through the arteries, the contrast agent is used to provide clear demarcation from surrounding tissues, allowing detailed observation of vascular anomalies, occlusions, or obstructions. This capability is particularly important in diagnosing conditions such as coronary artery disease, where rapid and accurate imaging can significantly affect patient management and outcomes. CT angiography can be further optimized by virtue of enhanced image processing and analysis algorithms. Recent developments in deep learning and neural networks have shown promise to improve the precision and efficiency of CTA interpretation. Such technologies offer sophisticated algorithms for segmentation of medical images, enabling better delineation of anatomical structures such as arteries and veins. As has been highlighted in more recent publications, the integration of neural networks in the workflow of CTA offers support in overcoming some common challenges faced in radiology, including the short supply of labeled data to use in model training and generalizability in heterogeneous patient populations. Such advances emphasize the active evolution of cardiovascular imaging, where traditional methods are increasingly complemented by cutting-edge computational techniques that enhance diagnostic accuracy and improve workflow processes (Bai et al., 2025). Most significantly, while CT angiography is today an effective tool in cardiovascular imaging, its advantages need to be weighed against disadvantages, including radiation. The utilization of X-rays to make CTA is problematic, particularly in specific populations where serial imaging could become obligatory. However, the advantages of rapid diagnosis and visualization of complex vascular beds usually trump. Relentless innovations in technology aim to reduce radiation doses while maintaining excellent image quality, thereby enhancing patient safety. As researchers explore new techniques to limit exposure, the future of CTA will be redirected through the integration of the most up-to-date techniques and methodologies that align with today's standards of cardiovascular diagnosis and intervention (Jiang et al., 2010).

4.1.1. Principles of Computed Tomography

The principle behind computed tomography (CT) is the use of X-ray technology to produce high-quality cross-sectional views of the body. A CT scan produces these views by scanning an X-ray source in a circle around the patient, and detectors located opposite the source collect the radiation that has traveled through the body.

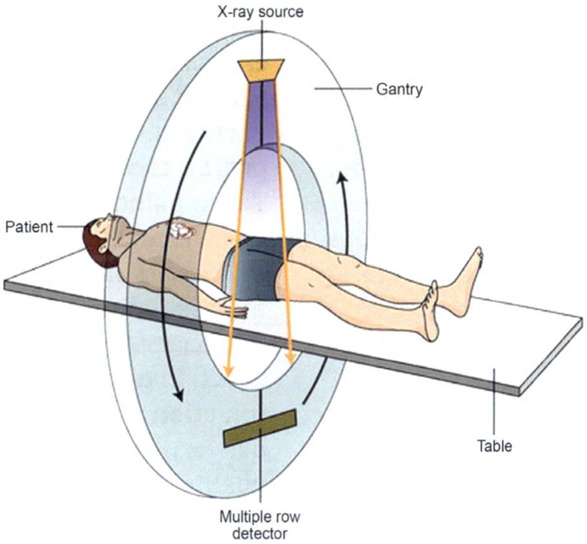

Figure 4.1. A diagram illustrating the rotational gantry mechanism in computed tomography with X-ray source and detectors positioned in a circular path around the patient.

Source: https://www.researchgate.net/profile/Richard-Garnett-4/publication/343519170/figure/fig1/AS:941550649483264@1601494576068/Figure-demonstrating-the-main-components-of-a-CT-machine-including-gantry-x-ray-tube.jpg.

This rotational technique allows data collection from different directions, which are then reconstructed into images by complex algorithms. CT has important advantages across various areas of cardiovascular imaging, especially for assessing coronary artery disease. With the thorough visualization of cardiac structures and blood vessels, CT angiography facilitates the diagnosis of disorders such as blockages and abnormalities, and is a valuable tool in contemporary cardiology. Another significant aspect of CT imaging is the ability to enhance diagnostic accuracy through the use of contrast agents. In CT angiography for cardiac tests, intravenous contrast medium is administered to improve visibility of blood vessels. This agent differentially absorbs X-rays to allow better differentiation of blood vessels and adjacent tissues. This function is critical for assessing conditions such as aortic aneurysms, pulmonary embolism, and other vascular malformations, as it improves overall image quality. The rapid acquisition times of newer CT scanners also eliminate motion artifacts, which can reduce image quality, thereby solidifying the role of CT angiography as the gold standard in non-invasive vascular imaging (N/A, 2003). The complementarity of sophisticated reconstruction algorithms and post-processing software has also improved the speed of CT imaging in cardiovascular operations. Multi-detector row computed tomography (MDCT), for example, facilitates the production of high-quality images with reduced radiation doses, addressing long-standing concerns about patient safety. Advances in technology enable cardiologists to use tools such as three-dimensional (3D) reconstructions to enhance visualization of complex vascular anatomy. This not only facilitates pre-operative planning but also improves the accuracy of diagnostic evaluation. For that reason, CT angiography remains a significant modality in cardiac imaging, particularly when combined with magnetic resonance imaging (MRI), an attacking-together approach to evaluate cardiovascular health and disease (N/A, 1996) (Figure 4.1).

4.1.2. Contrast Agents Used in CT Angiography

Contrast agent utilization in CT angiography is crucial for the improvement of visibility of blood vessels to enable more accurate diagnosis and assessment of cardiovascular illnesses. The agents consist predominantly of iodine-based compounds containing high atomic numbers with the ability to attenuate X-ray beams effectively, thereby providing improved contrast between tissues and blood vessels. When intravenously administered, contrast media rapidly move through the bloodstream, delineating areas of interest on imaging. The efficacy of these agents relies on their ability to provide maximum vascular opacification with the least risk for unwanted effects. Creating more sophisticated formulations to ensure improved quality in imaging and maximum safety to the patient will continue to advance with technological progress (N/A, 2008). In addition, the choice of contrast media in CT angiography has direct implications on diagnostic outcomes and patient experiences. Recent years have seen the increasing popularity of low-osmolar and iso-osmolar iodinated contrast media due to their improved safety profiles, resulting in fewer cases of contrast-induced nephropathy, especially among high-risk patient populations, such as those with existing kidney dysfunction. Furthermore, the use of nonionic agents is proven to reduce the risk of allergic reactions. These points emphasize the need to know the pharmacokinetics and pharmacodynamics of the agents in order to facilitate the choice of the best one for individual patient selection by physicians. Besides, the enhancement of contrast injection technique, such as by use of automated injection systems, has improved contrast delivery accuracy, which ultimately makes the quality of CT angiographic examination better (N/A, 1999). Future developments of contrast agents for CT angiography will also be directed towards considering patient-specific variables such as age, renal status, and chronic conditions in order to tailor personalized imaging protocols. New substitutes, including gadolinium-based contrast, more commonly employed in MRI, are being engineered to provide complementary vascular imaging with reduced nephrotoxicity risk. Moreover, there is growing interest in the application of biomarker-specific contrast agents that are capable of tracking real-time pathological alterations within the vascular circuit. These advances are centered on improving image quality and CT angiography's diagnostic capabilities to facilitate more precise treatment planning in cardiovascular disease. With continuous improvement, an equitable solution with efficacy, safety, and patient-centered treatment is still essential in optimizing the use of contrast agents in cardiovascular imaging (N/A, 2008) (Figure 4.2).

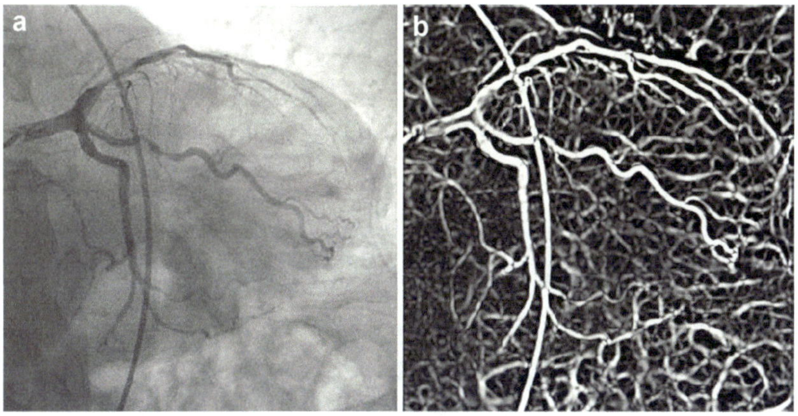

Figure 4.2. Image of iodine-based contrast medium being injected intravenously for vascular enhancement during a CT angiogram.

Source: https://www.researchgate.net/profile/Daniel-Ruijters/publication/40769016/figure/fig1/AS:341462953807877@1458422520691/a-X-ray-image-of-the-coronary-arteries-Iodine-contrast-medium-is-injected-in-the.png.

4.1.3. Indications for CT Angiography in Cardiovascular Assessment

The use of CT angiography (CTA) in cardiovascular assessment has been increasingly focal, particularly in diagnosing and assessing various cardiac conditions. Being non-invasive and offering enhanced resolution, this technique allows clinicians to visualize the coronary arteries completely, which is essential for accurate diagnosis. One of the major uses of CTA is the evaluation of suspected coronary artery disease (CAD) patients, where standard stress testing is non-diagnostic. CTA is a good choice, delivering high-resolution anatomical information that could aid in further management. Also, in Kawasaki disease, CTA plays a vital role in the identification of coronary artery aneurysms. The late cardiac sequelae, such as myocardial ischemia in Kawasaki disease patients, need close follow-up and prompt diagnosis, highlighting the use of CTA in children and adults, as pointed out in recently published guidelines for treatment of the condition (Brogan et al., 2020) (Figure 4.3).

Another important indication of CT angiography is the assessment of renal artery stenosis (RAS). Such patients with resistant hypertension or occult renal dysfunction are typically the optimal candidates for CTA, which optimizes renal artery anatomy and potential stenosis visualization. Though RAS can be a result of pathologies such as fibromuscular dysplasia and atherosclerosis, the use of CTA plays an essential role in determining the optimal management protocol. In particular, atheromatous RAS is associated with a high cardiovascular complication and death risk, which underlines the need for proper assessment. Current controversy in clinical practice concerns the selection of patients who may be candidates for intervention, indicating that CTA could be a valuable tool for identifying patients at high risk and in need of further therapeutic interventions, as demonstrated by recent evidence (Losito et al., 2014). Additionally, the CTAs' value extends to pre-operative assessment and follow-up post-procedure in various cardiovascular procedures. Pre-operative CTA will provide invaluable insights into coronary anatomy for patients undergoing coronary artery bypass grafting or valve replacement. Post-procedure, CTA is well-suited to check graft patency, establish newly formed coronary connections, and identify complications such as stenosis or occlusion. As cardiovascular diseases are multifactorial in origin, incorporation of CTA as a part of routine clinical assessment is highly advantageous. With advancement in cardiovascular pathology and with continuous technological changes in CTA technology, improved imaging capability is ensured, further reinforcing its application in cardiovascular assessment and management in diverse patient groups.

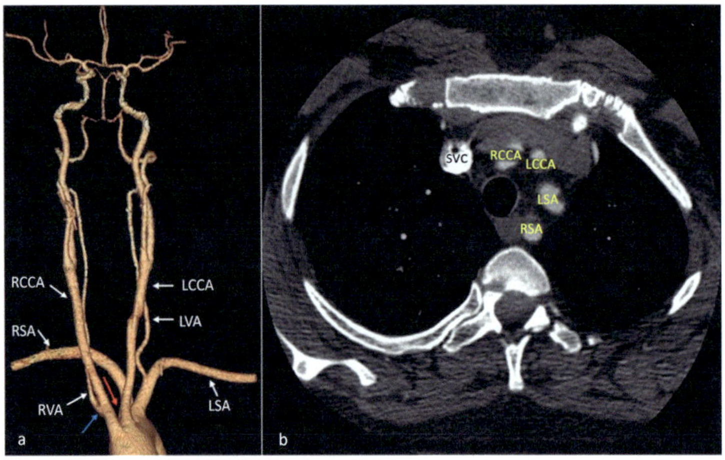

Figure 4.3. CT Angiography for aortic arch anomalies.

4.2. MRI Fundamentals in Cardiovascular Imaging

Magnetic resonance imaging (MRI) is a central modality in cardiovascular imaging, with unique strengths that are critical for diagnosing and monitoring heart disease. Unlike traditional imaging techniques, MRI employs powerful magnetic fields and radio waves to generate images, which provide rich information on the heart's function and structure. This technique is particularly beneficial for examining soft tissues, allowing clinicians to assess cardiac morphology, detect myocardial ischemia, and evaluate the integrity of cardiac chamber walls. Moreover, MRI's ability to capture real-time functional information makes it an essential tool for the comprehensive evaluation of cardiac dynamics, such as ventricular volumes and ejection fraction, thus informing treatment decisions and patient management strategies. Apart from its ability to image structure, MRI can be further enhanced by using contrast agents, which make the coronary arteries and myocardial perfusion more visible. Imaging techniques such as myocardial perfusion imaging allow assessment of blood supply to the heart muscle, enabling determination of crucial information related to ischemia and myocardial health. The combination of advanced imaging technologies, including stress MRI and late gadolinium enhancement, makes diagnosing cardiac conditions more accurate by separating viable myocardium from scar tissue. Furthermore, MRIs' non-invasive nature can be a significant advantage compared to other imaging equipment, particularly for populations that require repeated testing, such as patients with heart disease or those undergoing therapeutic monitoring. With advances in cardiovascular imaging, MRI technologies are enhancing cardiovascular evaluation specificity and accuracy. Recent advances have led to the development of techniques to improve image resolution and contrast. Application of newer MRI sequences and post-processing methods has allowed for detailed visualization of atherosclerotic plaques and, by extension, enhanced plaque characterization. As accentuated in recent research, continued investigation into MRI applications in cardiovascular diseases has the potential to deliver important information regarding atherosclerosis and related complications. With advancements, there is potential for the fusion of MRI and computational modeling to enhance diagnostic accuracy and personalized treatment planning, marking an innovation in the successful management of cardiovascular disease (Berti et al., 2024; Buckler et al., 2022).

4.2.1. Principles of Magnetic Resonance Imaging

The idea behind magnetic resonance imaging (MRI) is based on the fundamentals of nuclear magnetic resonance (NMR). Essentially, MRI uses powerful magnetic fields, radiofrequency pulses, and gradient coils to manipulate the magnetic properties of hydrogen nuclei, which are predominantly found in water and fat throughout the body. When left in a magnetic field, the nuclei would orient themselves in the direction of the field. By using radiofrequency pulses, the nuclei are temporarily displaced from their position, and then relax back to their equilibrium location. It is this relaxation process that produces signals which are detected by the MRI system and converted into images. These images can be manipulated by adjusting parameters such as repetition time (TR) and echo time (TE) to enable detailed visualization of cardiac structures (N/A, 1996).

Moreover, MRI's inherent property of distinguishing between different types of tissues is especially useful in cardiovascular imaging. In contrast to the x-ray transmission-based CT angiography, MRI contrast phenomena involve T1 and T2 relaxation times, susceptibility effects, and diffusion imaging. This allows for the detailed depiction of the anatomy, function, and any disease processes present within the heart, for example, myocardial infarction or cardiomyopathy.

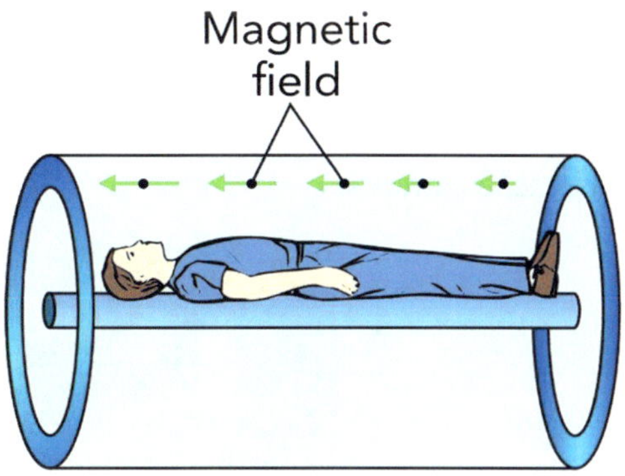

Figure 4.4. Illustration of hydrogen proton alignment and realignment in a magnetic field, depicting the principle of MRI signal generation.

Source: https://people.iitism.ac.in/~sarun/notes/pho303/figs/pic28/c13.jpeg.

Moreover, newer MRI techniques, including contrast-enhanced imaging and functional MRI (fMRI), provide insight into myocardial perfusion and viability, enabling clinicians to assess coronary perfusion to the heart muscle in greater detail. Accordingly, MRI is as good a tool for visualizing the structure of the heart as it is for determining its functional ability and diagnosing illness early on in its development (N/A, 2003). The use of MRI for cardiovascular imaging is validated by its lack of ionizing radiation, an actual advantage over CT angiography. This feature enables imaging to be performed more safely, especially in sensitive populations such as pregnant women and children. MRI also offers wide functionality in assessing dynamic aspects of cardiac function, including wall motion and ejection fraction, without exposing the patient to harmful radiation. The improving techniques in MRI, such as stress testing and dual-energy imaging, also contribute to its application in the treatment and diagnosis of cardiovascular conditions. The inclusion of MRI in everyday clinical practice has transformed cardiovascular imaging by providing discrete, accurate information that is invaluable for making informed clinical decisions and patient care (N/A, 1996) (Figure 4.4).

4.2.2. Types of MRI Sequences Relevant to Cardiovascular Imaging

Among cardiovascular imaging methods, magnetic resonance imaging (MRI) employs several sequences to enhance the visualization of cardiac anatomy and blood flow kinetics. Among the most used is the steady-state free precession (SSFP) sequence, due to its ability to produce high-resolution images of the heart and the vessels surrounding it. SSFP sequences excel at blood-pool imaging, with bright signal in regions of flowing blood and good tissue contrast. This sequence is especially useful for assessing cardiac chamber size and function, enabling clinicians to make accurate assessments.

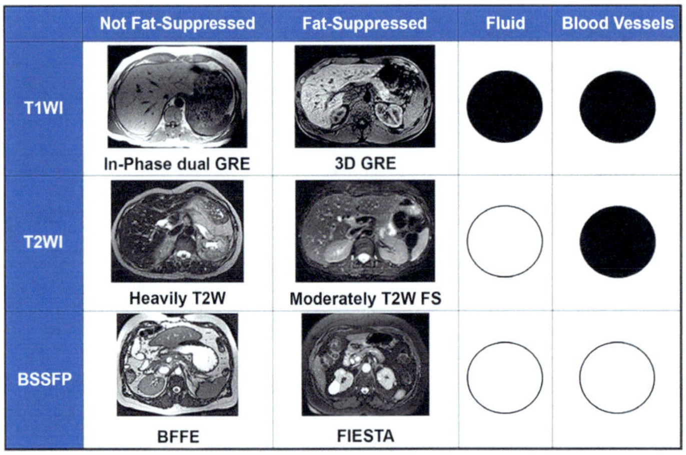

Figure 4.5. Side-by-side comparison of MRI pulse sequences, including T1-weighted, T2-weighted, and gradient-echo sequences.

Source: https://www.researchgate.net/publication/305521773/figure/fig28/AS:391682592919562@1470395815496/Diagram-illustrating-how-to-differentiate-T1-weighted-T2-weighted-and-balanced.png.

Through the application of SSFP, cardiologists can now visualize both anatomical structures and functional indices, with the latter demonstrating its utility in comprehensive cardiovascular disease assessment. The late gadolinium enhancement (LGE) method is another important MRI sequence for detecting myocardial ischemia and fibrosis. Following the injection of gadolinium, areas of scar tissue exhibit typical enhancement relative to normal myocardium, thereby identifying regions at risk for ischemic events. The sequence relies upon differential behavior of gadolinium in T1-weighted imaging for differentiation between viable and non-viable myocardium. Research illustrates the importance of LGE in the risk stratification of patients with established coronary artery disease, as it informs myocardial viability and has been linked to poor outcomes. Thus, LGE is a crucial modality in informing therapeutic choices and personalizing patient care in cardiovascular practice. Further MRI sequence diversification for cardiac imaging is time-of-flight (TOF) and phase-contrast (PC) imaging, which are very helpful for cerebral and peripheral vascular disease evaluation. TOF imaging uses flow-encoding techniques to generate images of blood vessels with minimal background noise, enabling good visualization of vessel patency and morphology without contrast agents. Conversely, PC imaging is used to quantitatively assess blood flow direction and velocity, which are crucial for evaluating conditions such as aortic stenosis or valvular inadequacy. When these two methods are utilized together, doctors can obtain a whole scenario of vascular health and function. The use of such sophisticated MRI sequences in the clinical arena significantly enhances diagnostic accuracy, providing greater insight into cardiovascular pathology, which is crucial for effective management and treatment (Bizopoulos et al., 2021; Balu et al., 2018) (Figure 4.5).

4.2.3. Indications for MRI in Cardiovascular Assessment

In cardiovascular imaging, magnetic resonance imaging (MRI) has emerged as an essential tool across various clinical scenarios. One significant indication for MRI in cardiovascular assessment is the need for non-invasive evaluation of vascular conditions, particularly in patients with underlying renal issues. The use of traditional imaging techniques, such as contrast-enhanced CT, poses inherent risks for those with advanced kidney disease due to potential nephrotoxicity. MRI offers a feasible alternative, particularly with the use of innovative contrast agents such as ferumoxytol. This superparamagnetic iron oxide preparation, administered intravenously, has demonstrated effective diagnostic capabilities without the adverse effects typically associated with conventional contrast materials. With its ability to produce high-quality vascular images, MRI is a valuable option for assessing vascular integrity and suitability for procedures such as kidney transplants, ultimately enhancing patient safety and diagnostic accuracy (Hennessy et al., 2017). Another prominent indication for employing MRI in cardiovascular assessments lies in the evaluation and characterization of coronary artery disease. Compared to CT angiography, which is often the preferred method for ruling out significant stenosis, MRI can provide a complementary approach for non-invasive visualization of coronary plaques. Its ability to assess plaque integrity, combined with the absence of ionizing radiation, positions MRI as a crucial second-line imaging modality, especially in specific patient cohorts where radiation exposure should be minimized. Recent consensus recommendations endorse MRI's role as a supplementary option to CT angiography, particularly in experienced centers, thereby broadening access to advanced imaging techniques for coronary artery evaluations (Alkadhi et al., 2023). This positioning exemplifies the growing recognition of MRI's capabilities in enhancing the diagnostic workup of coronary artery disease while promoting patient-centered care. Moreover, MRI extends beyond typical assessments by enabling comprehensive evaluation of myocardial conditions. In particular, MRI excels at visualizing myocardial ischemia, infarction, and structural abnormalities, enabling detailed analysis of cardiac tissue. Its high spatial resolution and functional imaging capabilities would allow clinicians to assess not only the structural integrity but also the physiological function of the heart. This dual functionality is critical for patients presenting with atypical symptoms or those with complex clinical histories, where conventional imaging may fall short. Additionally, MRI provides valuable insights into myocardial tissue characteristics, such as edema and fibrosis, enhancing the understanding of pathological processes. Consequently, MRI's ability to deliver intricate details about both the vascular and myocardial conditions collectively underscores its integral role in comprehensive cardiovascular assessments, paving the way for informed clinical decision-making and tailored patient management strategies (Figure 4.6).

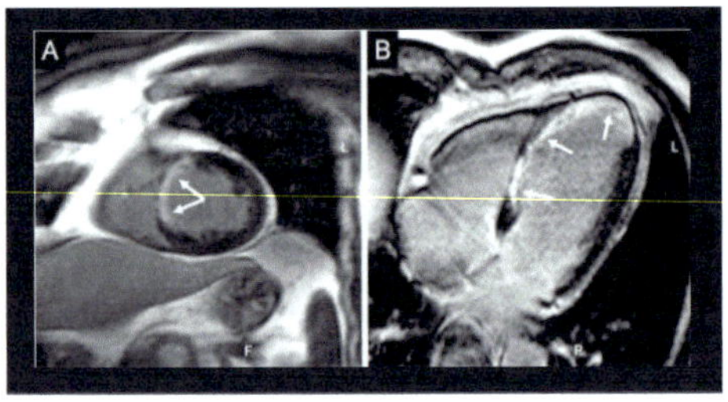

Figure 4.6. Late gadolinium enhancement images of a patient with chronic myocardial infarction of the septal ventricular wall, including the apex (white arrows). Images in basal short-axis view (A) and 4-chamber view (B) at 3 T acquired 15 minutes after injection of 0.15 mmol gadolinium/kg body weight.

Source: https://www.researchgate.net/profile/Sebastian-Kelle-2/publication/45441135/figure/fig3/AS:203197080707080@1425457367331/Late-gadolinium-enhancement-images-of-a-patient-with-chronic-myocardial-infarction-of-the.png.

4.3. Advantages of CT Angiography

The advantages of computed tomography (CT) angiography are numerous, particularly if one considers its use in the diagnosis and evaluation of cardiovascular conditions. Among the most significant advantages is its speed and efficiency; CT angiography can rapidly produce good-quality images of blood vessels, an application that is crucial when dealing with emergencies. This rapid imaging capability allows doctors to make important decisions quickly, especially in the case of acute cardiac conditions, thus potentially salvaging lives. Additionally, the non-invasive nature of CT angiography minimizes the risks associated with more invasive procedures, making it a safer option for patients requiring vascular evaluation. This harmony of speed, efficiency, and safety underscores the utility of CT angiography as the first-choice imaging modality for cardiovascular imaging. In addition to its speed and minimally invasive technique, CT angiography also offers the advantage of producing high-resolution images that allow visualization of vascular structures in detail. With this advantage, clinicians are able to diagnose a wide range of pathologies like aneurysms, stenoses, and vascular malformations precisely. Unlike traditional angiography, which typically involves catheterization of blood vessels, CT angiography provides a complete view of the vascular system in one sitting. Also, in clinical scenarios where conventional imaging techniques are to be compromised, such as in those with advanced kidney disease, when conventional procedures would be extremely risky and hazardous, CT angiography is an acceptable substitute that does not distort diagnostic reliability. With the integration of state-of-the-art imaging equipment, CT angiography expands the possibilities for vascular assessment, offering improved, broad-based insights to inform future therapies. Another significant advantage is in CT angiography's ability to evaluate the arterial and venous systems in a single sitting, which is a significant advancement over some other imaging modalities. This aspect is particularly useful for comprehensive evaluation and treatment planning in conditions like peripheral artery disease or coronary artery disease. In addition, the technique can be used to guide interventional procedures because it provides real-time imaging that facilitates accurate instrument positioning in minimally invasive procedures. In line with advances in cardiovascular imaging, CT angiography aids not only in addressing immediate diagnostic needs but also supports long-term treatment plans through its extensive, comprehensive imaging. The synergy between these abilities positions CT angiography as a critical element in the global picture of cardiovascular imaging, complementing other modalities such as MRI and enhancing patient treatment and diagnostic precision.

4.3.1. Speed and Efficiency of the Procedure

In contemporary cardiovascular imaging, the speed and efficacy of diagnostics such as CT angiography and MRI are prime considerations in clinical decision-making. The modalities have evolved significantly to yield rapid results that provide crucial information about cardiovascular health. CT angiography stands out for its ability to produce high-resolution images in a matter of minutes, reducing the time required for diagnosis compared to traditional angiography methods.

This quick imaging feature allows clinicians to make timely decisions regarding patient care and thus enhance overall treatment. Quick image acquisition enables faster response times in emergency medical scenarios, where prompt action can be the difference between life and death for a patient. The effectiveness of procedures of these imaging techniques is further enhanced by the technological developments, particularly those concerning deep learning algorithms. By using computer-aided image analysis, physicians can lower the interpretation time of complex data sets generated through imaging by a significant degree. Deep learning assists in revealing intricate patterns with the large volumes of data generated during CT and MRI scans, transforming the diagnostics process. This technological shift not only accelerates diagnosis but also improves the overall accuracy of measurements, enabling the development of more uniform treatment plans at high speed. Such integration points towards a direction of more effective cardiology procedures that end up benefiting patients through timely intervention (Bizopoulos et al., 2021). Moreover, the cooperative function of CT angiography and MRI in cardiology facilitates thorough examination of cardiovascular disease, which enhances procedural efficacy. By providing supplementary information on blood flow, vessel shape, and tissue composition, these imaging modalities help streamline diagnostic protocols. As an illustration, the combined approach can facilitate one patient visit that offers a complete image of cardiovascular well-being, thus diminishing the need for scanning duplication. This integrated practice not only saves time for patients and clinicians alike but also optimizes the use of resources within healthcare systems. The growing trend towards integrative imaging practices indicates a broader appreciation for efficiency in modern medicine and for rapid, accurate diagnosis in fast-paced clinical environments of today (N/A, 2007) (Figure 4.7).

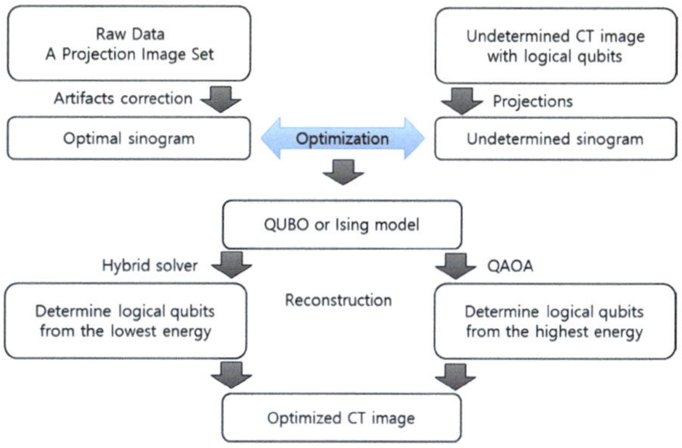

Figure 4.7. Flowchart of the process of obtaining a CT image. To reconstruct a CBCT image, the entire 3D sinogram is needed. To reconstruct a parallel-beam CT image, a sinogram at a single axial level is required. In this case, optimization must be applied to all axial levels to obtain 3D CT images.

Source: https://www.researchgate.net/figure/Flowchart-of-the-process-of-obtaining-a-CT-image-To-reconstruct-a-CBCT-image-the-entire_fig3_373600301.

4.3.2. High-Resolution Images and Detail

High-resolution imaging is of utmost significance in cardiovascular diagnostics, particularly with the assistance of advanced modalities such as CT angiography and MRI. These imaging modalities will record the subtle, fine details of the cardiovascular structures, allowing accurate judgments of anatomical abnormalities and pathological states. High-resolution images allow clinicians to observe minute details, such as the very minute changes in vessel anatomy or plaque composition, which will directly affect therapeutic interventions. This level of detail is critical in the prompt diagnosis of coronary artery disease and other cardiovascular pathologies because it would permit early intervention and tailored treatment regimens. As imaging technology continues to advance, the emphasis on high-resolution imaging ensures that the diagnostic capabilities of these modalities not only persist but are enhanced, ultimately improving patient outcomes in cardiovascular medicine (Figure 4.8).

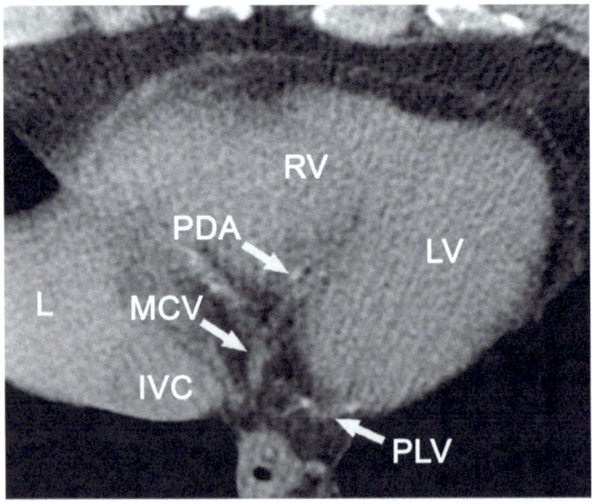

Figure 4.8. Electron beam CT of the coronary arteries cross-sectional anatomy for calcium scoring.

Source: https://ajronline.org/cms/10.2214/ajr.177.6.1771437/asset/images/12_ab0572_10b.jpeg.

The infusion of advanced methods within the cardiovascular imaging environment paves the way for more effective diagnostic modalities. High-resolution images obtained through CT angiography and MRI enable thorough examination of intracardiac flow dynamics and myocardial structure. The strongly accelerating demand for precise visualization has prompted the integration of computational fluid dynamics (CFD) simulations that require high-fidelity 4D meshes for biomechanical analysis with reliability. These meshes, extracted from high-resolution datasets, provide valuable information on ventricular function and energetics by accurately mimicking blood-flow dynamics. The fact that this can be obtained with the help of semiautomatic morphing tools that enable the creation of these structured meshes is an indication of the technological advancements in imaging modalities. It transforms complex medical images into quantifiable data that increases insight into cardiac function and therefore significantly enhances patient-specific diagnostic practice. Finally, the applications of high-resolution imaging extend to the research community and foster innovation in the treatment of cardiovascular disease. The synergistic combination of imaging modalities and CFD not only enables diagnosis but also enhances understanding of the physiological basis for cardiovascular health. Quantification of aneurysms, stenosis, and other vascular malformations is highly facilitated by the resolution of images produced by CT angiograms and MRIs. Highly resolved images enable scientists and clinicians to quantify physiological quantities and apply them in various clinical contexts, thereby enhancing patient care. Recent studies keep moving the automation of meshing algorithms and utilization of high-resolution imaging in diverse datasets, as revealed in 4D data analysis in different ultrasound, MRI, and CT modalities. Such breakthroughs underscore the importance of high-resolution images in the improvement of our knowledge of cardiovascular dynamics and improving clinical outcomes among individuals at cardiovascular risk (N/A, 1996; Bertrand et al., 2018).

4.3.3. Non-Invasive Character and Patient Comfort

The non-invasive nature of new cardiovascular imaging devices such as CT angiography and MRI dramatically altered the diagnosis situation for patients with suspected coronary artery disease. Unlike traditional invasive procedures, these imaging devices allow high-resolution imaging of coronary arteries without catheterization (Figure 4.9).

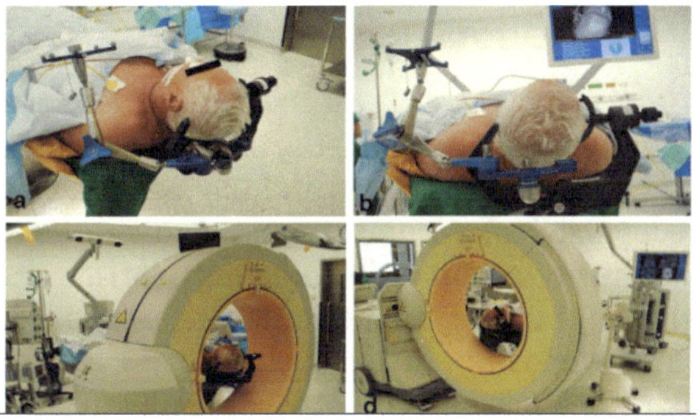

Figure 4.9. a, b Patient positioning in a supine position. Head fixation in a radiolucent Mayfield clamp. c, d The 3-D fluoroscope (O-Arm, Medtronic GmbH, Meerbusch, Germany) position during the hair shaving and surgical disinfection.

Source: https://www.researchgate.net/figure/a-b-Patient-positioning-in-a-supine-position-Head-fixation-in-a-radiolucent-Mayfield_fig1_352106019.

This non-invasive technique significantly reduces the risks of complications such as bleeding and infection with invasive angiography. In the avoidance of such risks, patient safety is considerably enhanced, and CT angiography and MRI offer preferable alternatives, in line with the increasing demand for safer diagnostic devices in clinical practice. Additionally, the reduction in physical invasiveness facilitates simpler monitoring and more rapid assessment of patients without hospitalization, thereby ultimately improving patient outcomes and streamlining care pathways. Patient comfort is a crucial consideration in the acceptance of any medical imaging modality. Research demonstrates a high preference for CT angiography over MRI by patients, largely due to its speed of performance and lower distress. The study revealed that, while both CT and MRI provide a non-invasive alternative to traditional angiography, patients with CT imaging reported fewer problems and an overall better experience (Leber et al., 2007). The non-invasive character of CT angiography allows patients to be assessed in a less stressful fashion because it does not involve protracted immobilization or potential anxiety due to claustrophobia generally associated with MRI imaging.

Therefore, patient comfort levels can be a significant factor in deciding on the imaging modality, thereby advocating for CT angiography as the initial-line diagnostic tool. In examining overall patient acceptance, the comparative study of CT angiography and MRI delineates important observations on pain sensing and satisfaction. Significantly, most participants in the studied population expressed eagerness to repeat CT angiography, attesting to its perceived painlessness and effectiveness (Leber et al., 2007). By comparison, invasive coronary angiography was marked by significant discomfort, reducing the rates of patient satisfaction. The most compelling advantages attributed to CT angiography are its fast-throughput rate, non-invasive nature, and greater degrees of comfort, serving the dual function of yielding diagnostic dependability while prioritizing patient experience. As a result, growing demand for non-invasive imaging technologies like CT angiography is reshaping standards of care for cardiovascular diagnosis, moving beyond functional imperatives to incorporate patient-centric priorities that are at the heart of contemporary healthcare.

4.4. Advantages of MRI in Cardiovascular Imaging

Magnetic resonance imaging (MRI) has a wide variety of advantages in cardiovascular imaging that significantly enhance diagnostic precision. The most important one could be the capability to produce superior volumetric detail and exceptional tissue characterization. It does not use ionizing radiation, unlike other traditional imaging modalities, so it is safer for patients, particularly those who require repeated imaging. Furthermore, MRI is more effective for imaging both structural and functional elements of the heart and, as such, can be used to assess myocardial viability, perfusion, and anatomical defects. The comprehensive approach helps clinicians make informed decisions about treatment and disease management, ultimately leading to better patient outcomes. An additional important advantage of MRI in cardiovascular imaging is the capability to assess vascular states without the inherent risks associated with contrast media typically used in computed tomography (CT). In patients with pre-existing kidney disease, for example, use of conventional contrast media poses a significant risk due to the risk of nephrotoxicity. Recent studies have explored other contrast agents like ferumoxytol, demonstrating that MRI can safely and effectively augment vascular imaging without such harm. Specifically, ferumoxytol-enhanced magnetic resonance angiography (FeMRA) has shown promising results for aorto-iliac vessel evaluation in renal transplant patients since it performs arteriography and venography in a single, harmless test (Hennessy et al., 2017). Such advancements demonstrate the potential of MRIs to improve diagnostic performance, with top priority given to patient safety. Moreover, integrating newer technologies such as deep learning into MRI procedures makes it more useful in cardiovascular imaging. Deep learning models can handle the vast amounts of data from MRI scans to make diagnoses more accurately and predictively. Such uses not only make interpretation easier but also reveal complex patterns in imaging data that are hard to detect with traditional methods (Bizopoulos et al., 2021). The synergy created through MRI's high-resolution images and the ability of deep learning to analyze has tremendous promise for cardiovascular diagnostics in the future. As the technology advances, it has the potential to introduce more specific treatment protocols and better patient outcomes for those suffering from cardiac disease.

4.4.1. No Ionizing Radiation Exposure

The significance of applying imaging modalities that do not use ionizing radiation is increasingly recognized in cardiovascular medicine. Both magnetic resonance imaging (MRI) and ultrasound are significant alternatives for cardiovascular disease diagnosis without exposing patients to the harmful effects of ionizing radiation. It is particularly significant in susceptible groups of patients, including pregnant women and children, who are most sensitive to the harmful effects of radiation exposure. In addition, MRI creates high-resolution images of cardiac anatomy and dynamics of blood flow, allowing clinicians to precisely evaluate a wide range of cardiovascular conditions. Prioritizing imaging methods that do not use ionizing radiation helps healthcare professionals ensure patients' safety while maintaining effective diagnostic capability that is congruent with ethical medical practice and improves patient care. Despite the advantages of non-ionizing radiation imaging techniques, clinicians are still confronted with the intricacies of image interpretation that is obtained. MRI, for instance, although it offers greater contrast resolution, could be a challenge to radiologists' interpretation due to differences in the quality of the image and the heterogeneity of cardiovascular diseases. Such complexity of the imaging process brings to the foreground the need for frequent updates and training for those performing cardiovascular imaging. Furthermore, as the subspecialty evolves, so too does the demand for newer techniques, such as contrast-enhanced MRI, which, though nonionizing, introduces its own concerns regarding contrast media and safety profiles. This evolution in cardiovascular imaging calls for a balanced approach that maximizes diagnostic efficiency without enhancing patient risk, once more emphasizing the utility in employing modalities free from ionizing radiation. The debate regarding the ethical implications of radiation exposure also supports the move towards non-ionizing imaging techniques. The literature in the area indicates that patient autonomy and informed consent not only constitute a straightforward debate about potential risks associated with various imaging modalities, but also about the long-term risk of cancer related to ionizing radiation exposure (Finestone et al., 2007). Where patients, on occasion, are not well-informed about such risks, inclusion of the non-ionizing imaging modality promotes an ethical practice that prioritizes their safety and well-being. With laws that promote justified and optimized use of ionizing radiation, there is a comprehensive practice that promotes the non-ionizing techniques in cardiovascular imaging (Bhuiyan et al., 2023). Thus, an imperative to employ imaging methods that do not utilize ionizing radiation not only contributes to enhanced patient outcomes but also aligns with contemporary-day ethical aspects in medicine, ultimately developing a patient safety and informed consent culture.

4.4.2. Improved Contrast of Soft Tissues

The significance of high soft tissue contrast in cardiovascular imaging cannot be overstated, as it is very crucial in the field of enhanced diagnostic accuracy and therapeutic planning. Traditionally, imaging modalities such as ultrasonography provided poor resolution in distinguishing between soft tissue structures.

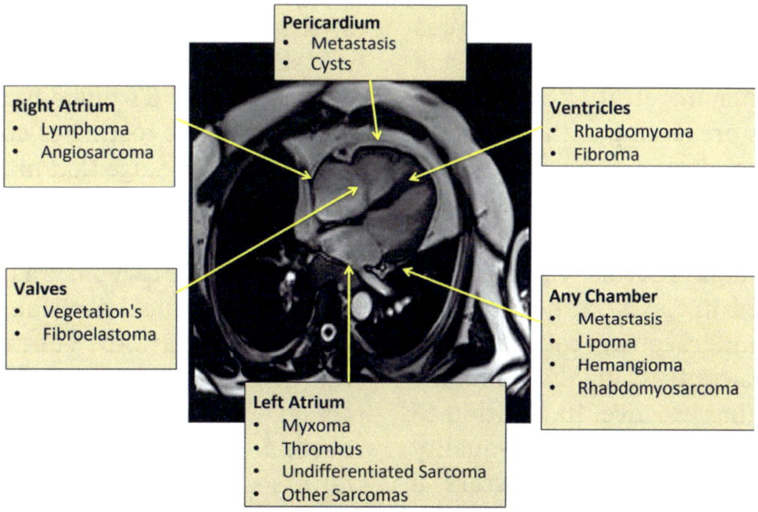

Figure 4.10. MRI scan showing detailed cardiac muscle tissue and adjacent vascular structures with superior soft tissue contrast.

Source: https://www.frontiersin.org/files/Articles/1009411/fcvm-10-1009411-HTML/image_m/fcvm-10-1009411-g001.jpg.

Advanced technologies, such as magnetic resonance imaging (MRI), on the other hand, perform better using a combination of powerful magnetic fields and radio waves to provide high-resolution images. This soft tissue discrimination ability enables the detection of minute anatomical differences, for example, between normal and abnormal vascular tissues. Significantly, soft tissue contrast is particularly valuable in assessing disorders such as atrial fibrillation, where high-resolution imaging is likely to influence ablation therapy planning and delivery. As noted in current research, advancements in imaging tools have improved the characterization of cardiac anatomy and, consequently, treatment outcomes (D'Silva et al., 2011). Furthermore, the integration of advanced imaging modalities, such as CT angiography, has emphasized the benefits of enhanced soft-tissue contrast for evaluating carotid artery health (Figure 4.10). CT angiography, compared to conventional ultrasound, has substantial excellence in identifying features associated with plaque vulnerability, like intraplaque hemorrhage and lipid-rich necrotic cores. The imaging results that agree with the histological features of carotid plaques provide vital information to ASCVD risk assessment (Fleischmann et al., 2020). More specifically, patients presenting with particular plaque characteristics require more aggressive management strategies to prevent dangerous cardiovascular events. The application of advanced imaging thus goes beyond visualization; it is actively involved in risk stratification and tailored therapy, underscoring the need for enhanced soft-tissue contrast in contemporary cardiovascular imaging practice. In addition to enhancing diagnostic proficiency, high-quality contrast of the soft tissues also fosters a culture of ongoing research and innovation in cardiovascular imaging. In the quest for better patient outcomes, technologies for imaging like MRI and CT angiography are being refined to gain increasingly precise information regarding the structural and functional integrity of the cardiovascular system. Such ever-changing adaptability is most important in the diagnosis of complex pathologies, such as those that accompany atrial fibrillation or carotid artery atherosclerosis, where accurate anatomical information is central to successful treatment. By bridging the gap between clinical need and the technical capability of imaging equipment and software, enhanced soft tissue contrast not only assists diagnosis but also makes larger research projects possible with the aim of developing new therapeutic interventions. Ultimately, continued advances in imaging technology will reshape the future of cardiovascular care, allowing for more strategic decision-making and improved patient outcomes (D'Silva et al., 2011; Fleischmann et al., 2020).

4.4.3. Ability to Assess Cardiac Function and Viability

The ability to assess cardiac viability and performance is at the heart of cardiovascular imaging, particularly with newer technologies such as CT angiography and MRI. These imaging technologies provide unrivaled detail of the heart's anatomy and physiology, which is essential for diagnosing coronary artery disease (CAD). CT angiography, for one, excels at non-invasive testing of coronary arteries for stenosis or blockage that may result in ischemic states. Its diagnostic applicability extends to the detection of significant coronary artery lesions warranting interventions like angioplasty, supporting clinical decision-making in patients with suspected CAD. Contrast-enhanced CTCA can also provide vital information about the vessel wall, enabling comprehensive evaluation beyond plain obstruction, which is essential for assessing myocardial viability and function (Cochet et al., 2010). At the same time, cardiac MRI provides a powerful alternative to assess heart viability, performing effectively to quantify myocardial perfusion and function following ischemic damage. It is particularly well-equipped to visualize cardiac anatomy and quantify tissue properties, allowing for the detection of myocardial scarring and loss of viability. The non-invasive nature of MRI, along with its ability to achieve good-quality images, makes it a great choice for assessing patients with advanced CAD. With the resolution of myocardial viability, MRI aids physicians in determining the most suitable therapeutic strategies to achieve optimum cardiac outcome. The complementary pairing of CT and MRI deepens the clinical toolkit for cardiovascular disease treatment, that measurements of cardiac function are accurate and detailed (Cochet et al., 2010). Additionally, recent evidence has suggested a future role for positron emission tomography (PET) in the imaging toolkit for myocardial viability. Compared to traditional modalities such as single-photon emission computed tomography (SPECT), PET is of higher diagnostic value, especially in detecting perfusion abnormalities in CAD. In comparison, the research reflects that PET can provide superior information about myocardial metabolism, enabling a more delicate understanding of cardiac viability in patients with severe coronary disease. With less invasive imaging, integrating various techniques like CT, MRI, and PET offers cardiologists a useful method for assessing cardiac viability and function and ultimately improving patient management and outcomes in cardiovascular practice (Figure 4.11).

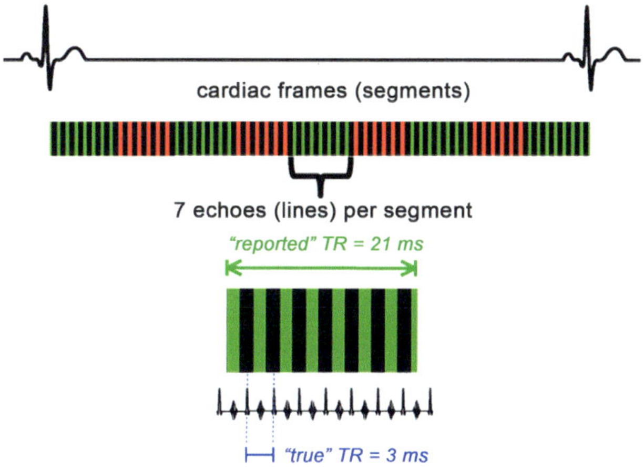

Figure 4.11. MRI cine sequence demonstrating dynamic cardiac function and chamber movement across the cardiac cycle.

Source: https://mriquestions.com/uploads/3/4/5/7/34572113/257644_orig.gif.

4.5. Shortcomings of CT Angiography

Despite CT angiography (CTA) having revolutionized vascular imaging by providing rapid, non-invasive assessment of the blood vessels, it is not without its drawbacks. One major drawback is that it relies on iodinated contrast media, which are harmful to patients with renal insufficiency. Contrast-induced nephropathy is a source of concern in patients with pre-existing renal disease. As has been demonstrated in patient imaging with severe renal disease, other imaging modalities such as ferumoxytol-enhanced MRI avoid these risks altogether by preventing the use of nephrotoxic agents altogether (Hennessy et al., 2017). While CTA is an institution in cardiovascular imaging, its application may be contraindicated in those at higher risk of renal compromise, necessitating careful weighing of benefit against risk when selecting imaging modalities. Also, the diagnostic competence of CTA can be compromised by several image quality and patient-related factors. Artifacts from motion, usually due to heartbeats or patient motion, can obscure the vascular structures and lead to misinterpretation. While technological development has improved temporal resolution, a high or irregular heart rate is still a cause for suboptimal imaging findings. In addition, the presence of calcifications in the vessel walls can complicate accurate examinations, particularly in patients with atheromatous disease. Research has indicated that calcification can hinder accurate visualization of the arterial lumen, thereby affecting the overall reliability of the diagnosis (Losito et al., 2014). These elements need careful preparation and consideration of patient-specific features to improve the efficacy of CTA. Furthermore, the impact of CTA can be restricted when analyzing some vascular diseases comprehensively. For instance, CTA has been found to be less sensitive for identifying renal artery stenosis (RAS) than other imaging modalities, particularly in fibromuscular dysplasia, when greater sensitivity is required for accurate diagnosis. The clinical relevance of RAS is extremely high, given its link with resistant hypertension and declining renal function. While CTA is useful for screening, findings often require follow-up to determine the clinical relevance of stenotic lesions (Losito et al., 2014). Thus, use of CTA alone can lead to less than comprehensive assessment and attendant delay in proper intervention. At the same time, cardiovascular imaging advances, the incorporation of multimodality will provide the optimal diagnostic capability in a patient-specific format.

4.5.1. Radiation Exposure Concerns

In cardiovascular imaging, the use of computed tomography (CT) angiography and magnetic resonance imaging (MRI) offers significant benefits but comes at the cost of radiation exposure. CT angiography itself uses ionizing radiation to generate high-quality images of the vascular system, raising concerns about radiation exposure over time. The long-term effects of radiation exposure are an elevated cancer risk and thus demand a careful evaluation of the indication for imaging and the clinical necessity of such practices (Figure 4.12).

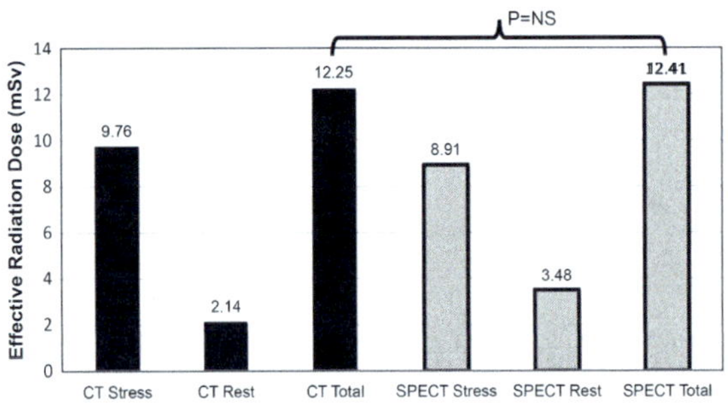

Figure 4.12. Radiation exposure of CT perfusion versus SPECT-MPI. Estimated effective radiation dose in millisievert (mSv) is displayed for CTP (solid bars) and SPECT (striped bars). The total effective radiation dose was not statistically different between the two modalities.

Source: https://www.researchgate.net/figure/Radiation-exposure-of-CT-perfusion-versus-SPECT-MPI-Estimated-effective-radiation-dose_fig3_40030127.

With advances in technology, practitioners are increasingly focusing on the principle of as low as reasonably achievable (ALARA) in radiation dose regulation, so that patients receive diagnostic CT benefits with minimal harmful exposure. Moreover, the innovation of alternative imaging techniques, such as ferumoxytol-enhanced magnetic resonance angiography (FeMRA), offers promising insights for mitigating radiation exposure. FeMRA is a potentially useful alternative, especially for patients with contraindications to standard imaging modalities, such as those with end-stage kidney disease (Hennessy et al., 2017).

This new technique utilizes a non-nephrotoxic contrast agent to visualize vascular anatomy with diagnostic accuracy, without exposing patients to the risks of ionizing radiation. In addition, the application of FeMRA has been successful in enhancing the visualization of arterial and venous compartments, without the restrictions typically encountered in CT angiography, confirming its place as a safe alternative in selected patient populations. Finally, the increasing recognition of long-term sequelae in certain medical disorders, including Kawasaki disease (KD), further underlines the utility of cautious imaging protocols.

The rising incidence of KD and its potential to cause coronary vascular complications warrant timely and effective imaging to guide treatment, particularly in the transfer of patients to the adult care system (Brogan et al., 2020). However, caution in these imaging protocols is also necessary because of the risk of increased lifetime radiation exposure to worsen health outcomes for vulnerable populations. Thus, ongoing education and research into the best imaging techniques will be necessary in improving outcomes while balancing radiation exposure concerns, thereby facilitating a balance between diagnostic efficacy and patient safety in cardiovascular imaging.

4.5.2. Shortcomings of Soft Tissue Characterization

Characterizing soft tissues is a key challenge in cardiovascular imaging, particularly with modalities such as CT angiography and MRI. One of the major limitations is the inherent contrast resolution of these imaging modalities. CT angiography, as excellent as it is at demonstrating vascular anatomy, performs poorly in differentiating between various soft tissues because it relies upon differences in attenuation, and in certain conditions, these are limited. This is most pronounced in the presence of atherosclerotic plaques, which themselves may vary subtly in composition, making their stability or likelihood of rupture unclear without unambiguous demarcation from surrounding tissues. The capacity to make accurate assessments of soft tissue pathology remains constrained by the shortcomings of contemporary imaging technologies, potentially compromising suboptimal clinical decision-making in the management of cardiovascular disease (Figure 4.13).Further, the use of multimodal imaging methods has been meant to surmount some of these obstacles, but is itself fraught with issues. Although breakthroughs in imaging tools such as MRI, which excels at outlining soft tissue, can lead to poorer data quality due to issues related to image acquisition time and patient movement. Notably, MRI's susceptibility to artifacts, particularly in the case of metallic implants, renders soft tissue properties progressively more problematic to interpret. In addition, the sophistication of the biological and pathological processes implicated in diseases such as peripheral artery disease necessitates concurrent use of molecular markers for an integrated analysis. As highlighted in recent criticism, while techniques such as CT and MRI have advanced, they still pose challenges that hinder a thorough description of soft-tissue dynamics within the cardiovascular environment (Chan et al., 2023). The level of cardiovascular imaging is marked by an acute need to develop more advanced methods to overcome these challenges in soft-tissue description. The union of molecular imaging with traditional imaging modalities is an exciting area for further research. New evidence indicates that incorporating molecular markers of inflammatory processes or plaque vulnerability may potentially enhance the predictive performance of imaging for cardiovascular risk prediction (Erta et al., 2020). Validating such molecular markers and standardizing them for clinical implementation pose a significant challenge. Pointing towards the necessity of interdisciplinary convergence, future research must not just concentrate on technological innovations in imaging modalities but also on the coordination of imaging findings with molecular biomarkers to achieve a holistic understanding of cardiovascular health. These gaps must be bridged in order to enhance the outcome of patients and maximize the treatment protocols for cardiovascular conditions.

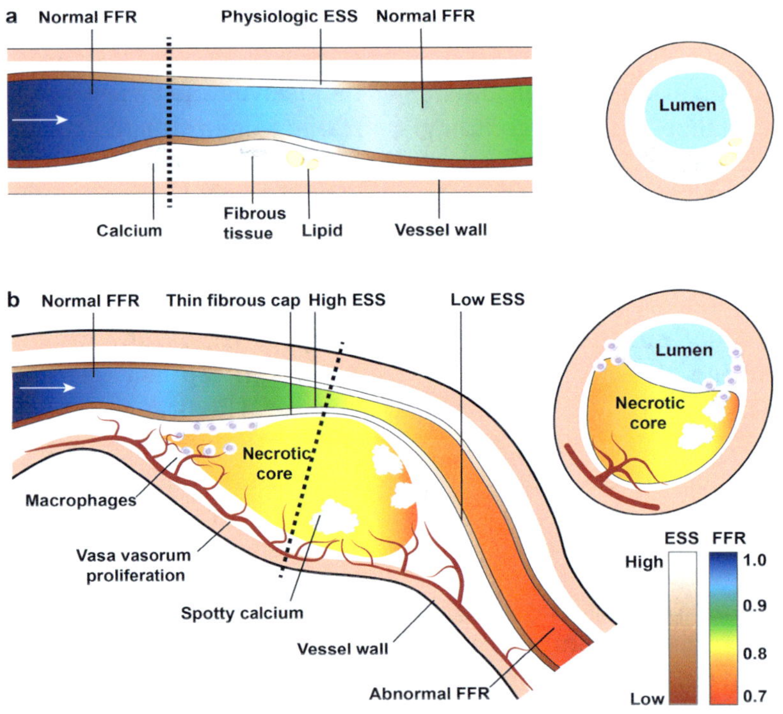

Figure 4.13. Comprehensive plaque assessment by coronary CT angiography.

Source: https://media.springernature.com/m685/springer-static/image/art%3A10.1038%2Fnrcardio.2014.60/MediaObjects/41569_2014_Article_BFnrcardio201460_Fig1_HTML.jpg.

4.5.3. Risk of Contrast-Induced Nephropathy

Contrast-induced nephropathy (CIN) remains a serious concern in cardiovascular imaging, particularly with computed tomography (CT) angiography and magnetic resonance imaging (MRI). CIN, defined as an acute increase in renal function following the administration of contrast agents, can complicate the patient's care, most notably those with pre-existing renal impairment. While the incidence of CIN appears low, especially in patients with preserved renal function, it carries serious consequences for those at high risk, such as the elderly or patients with established kidney disease. Clinicians must weigh the benefit of diagnostic imaging against potential damage to renal function. So robust pre-screening practice must establish those at risk of this complication and provide appropriate interventions. Recent literature indicates a nuanced understanding of contrast-induced acute kidney injury (AKI), with skepticism towards its occurrence and development (Figure 4.14).

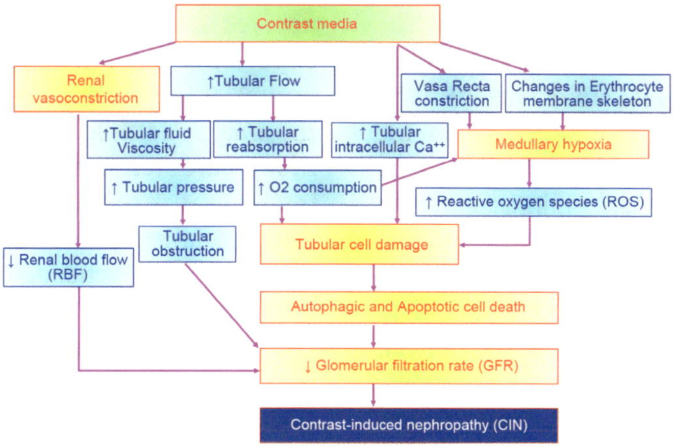

Figure 4.14. Infographic illustrating the contrast-induced nephropathy mechanism from iodinated contrast agents used in CT scans.

Source: https://www.researchgate.net/publication/323400344/figure/fig4/AS:598334771302400@1519665534740/The-detailed-molecular-mechanisms-of-contrast-induced-nephropathy.png.

The historical perspective attributed a higher prevalence of CIN to confounding factors, countering earlier assumptions of a direct causal role for the contrast agent. Animal studies have re-underscored the problems of nephrotoxicity associated with contrast exposure, with implications for potential deficits in clinical protocol for hydration and other prophylactic considerations. Pre-procedure hydration has provided variable outcomes, and the necessity for standardized protocols centered on individual patient risk is most crucial. As research continues to advance, ongoing examination of effective preventive strategies remains necessary to minimize the adverse consequences of contrast utilization during cardiovascular imaging procedures (Hoste et al., 2019). The nature of renal artery stenosis (RAS) renders the discussion concerning CIN even more difficult when cardiovascular imaging is at stake. RAS, especially that caused by atheromatous disease, is an emerging pathology associated with augmented cardiovascular mortality and thereby directing attention to the potential renal impact of imaging agents. Physicians face the challenge of maximizing the use of effective imaging, at the risk of compromising renal function in patients with RAS or other such conditions. There is evidence that selected patient involvement in interventions is critical, particularly among high-risk patients with the indication of accelerated deterioration of renal function or treatment-resistant, severe hypertension. Hence, imaging utilization in this context must be the outcome of a cautious weighing of the benefits against the inherent risks of contrast-induced complications in at-risk patient populations (Losito et al., 2014).

4.6. Limitations of MRI in Cardiovascular Imaging

Magnetic resonance imaging (MRI) is also increasingly recognized as a vehicle for cardiovascular imaging but has certain limitations that influence its clinical usefulness. One of the main limitations is the need for patients to remain immobile during imaging sequences, which may be challenging, especially in populations of patients with conditions such as heart failure or respiratory distress. The longer acquisition time of MRI can also lead to challenges in the creation of high-resolution images of dynamic organs, such as the heart, which can be compromised by respiratory motion.

The inherent complexity of MRI technology also contributes to inconsistent image quality, requiring expert-level technicians and radiologists to achieve optimal outcomes. This limitation poses a constraint in clinical settings where timely decision-making is necessary, potentially slowing the diagnostic process relative to faster imaging modalities such as CT angiography. Moreover, MRI contrast media, even though generally safer than iodinated agents used in CT scans, present unique challenges and risks. Such patients as those with impaired renal function, for instance, are threatened by contrast media containing gadolinium, like nephrogenic systemic fibrosis, an illness that affects susceptible populations. This is particularly the case in patients with end-stage kidney disease, when they may require vascular imaging for vascular assessment, where traditional methods are not feasible. Recent advances, such as the use of ferumoxytol as an MRI contrast agent, can circumvent these constraints, enabling effective imaging without nephrotoxicity, as demonstrated by clinical trials in aorto-iliac vascular imaging in the high-risk population (Hennessy et al., 2017). However, the availability and use of alternative contrast media remain limited in clinical settings. Lastly, the efficacy of MRI can be compromised by artifacts, which may obscure significant anatomical details required for successful diagnosis and treatment planning. For instance, patients with implanted devices, such as pacemakers and defibrillators, experience complications during MRI due to potential interactions between the devices and the magnetic fields generated during imaging. Also, calcifications may interfere with the imaging of vascular structures, leading to poor image quality. While MRI has the potential to provide high soft tissue contrast and potentially be of critical value in the assessment of specific cardiovascular diseases, it is usually utilized in combination with other imaging machines, such as CT, to provide more comprehensive information. Multimodality is especially essential with complex conditions such as atrial fibrillation, where imaging using multiple technologies may result in improved procedural success (D'Silva et al., 2011). Finally, although MRI is highly valuable in cardiovascular imaging, understanding its limitations is essential for maximizing patient care and outcomes.

4.6.1. Longer Acquisition Times

In cardiovascular imaging, prolonged acquisition time poses challenges as well as opportunities for diagnostic precision and patient comfort. Both MRI and CT angiography are important imaging modalities for imaging vascular structures, but their respective imaging protocols require different patient acquisition times. Increased patient acquisition times, particularly for MRI, could lead to patient discomfort due to the static nature of the process as well as prolonged breath-holding times. Also, in patients with difficult anatomical presentation or comorbidities, this discomfort can lead to rescans or degraded image quality due to motion artifacts (Figure 4.15).

These factors, combined, underscore the importance of careful assessment of acquisition parameters to achieve the optimal trade-off between image quality and patient experience. However, it must be pointed out that longer acquisition time is generally associated with higher imaging quality and better ability to obtain more complicated vascular information. For instance, in patients with end-stage kidney disease, the use of ferumoxytol as an MRI contrast agent has been shown to improve both arterial and venous imaging without the nephrotoxicity of traditional agents, albeit at longer acquisition times for optimal benefits (Hennessy et al., 2017).

The added time provides for enhanced evaluation of arterial and venous spaces, resulting in more accurate diagnoses and patient management. Such developments indicate the central role of time in achieving integrated vascular assessments and allude to how longer acquisition times can improve diagnostic potential in focused patient populations. CT versus MRI modality comparison also indicates how longer acquisition times might be impacting overall diagnostic pipelines.

Although CT angiography provides quick image acquisition, its increased processing time for complex reconstructions can slow interpretation relative to MRI methods, which provide more complete data within one exam (Achenbach et al., 2015). With advancing imaging technology, integrating measures to reduce acquisition times without sacrificing quality will be crucial in balancing clinical efficiency and patient throughput. Research into optimal acquisition protocols, such as exploring anesthetic and sedation doses, and technological developments, such as faster imaging sequences, will be essential to minimizing the constraints imposed by increased acquisition time while further enhancing the benefits they offer to cardiovascular diagnostic imaging.

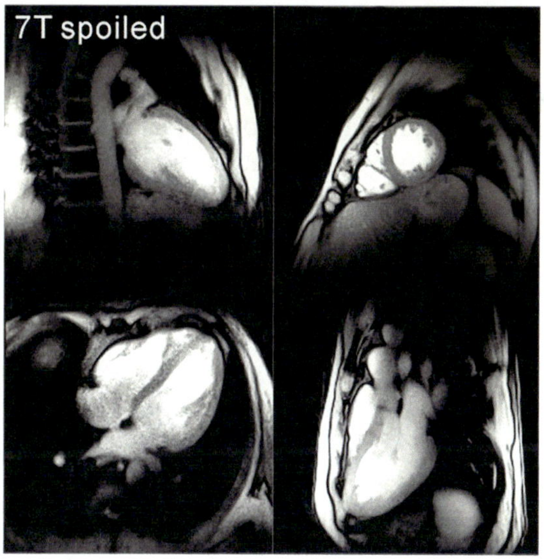

Figure 4.15. Visual representation of longer scan durations in cardiac MRI vs CT angiography in a clinical time chart.

Source: https://www.researchgate.net/profile/Jens-Frahm/publication/267506746/figure/fig3/AS:392072763854851@1470488839232/Real-time-cardiac-MRI-with-T1-contrast-at-7-T-33-ms-End-diastolic-images-of-a-healthy.png.

4.6.2. Patient Incompatibility Problems (e.g., Claustrophobia, Metallic Implants)

Advances in cardiovascular imaging modalities, particularly CT angiography and MRI, have greatly improved diagnostic accuracy; however, patient compatibility remains a significant drawback. Claustrophobia, an emotional disorder, is the most important issue that has been recognized. Claustrophobia prevents patients from undergoing MRI scans. The closed environment of MRI units exacerbates anxiety and feelings of panic, and these can produce motion artifacts, hence compromising image quality. Thus, health care providers should take this issue seriously and offer alternatives, such as open MRI systems, that can minimize patient discomfort while still providing adequate diagnostic information. Pre-interventional treatments, such as sedation or relaxation, may also be employed to enhance patient compliance and satisfaction during imaging, making it a safer and more effective cardiovascular assessment. Another such pressing issue regarding compatibility arises when patients have metallic implants, which are detrimental to the safety and efficiency of MRI imaging. Certain metallic materials, particularly ferromagnetic implants, pose risks during the scan and can create image distortions or even harm the patient (Figure 4.16).

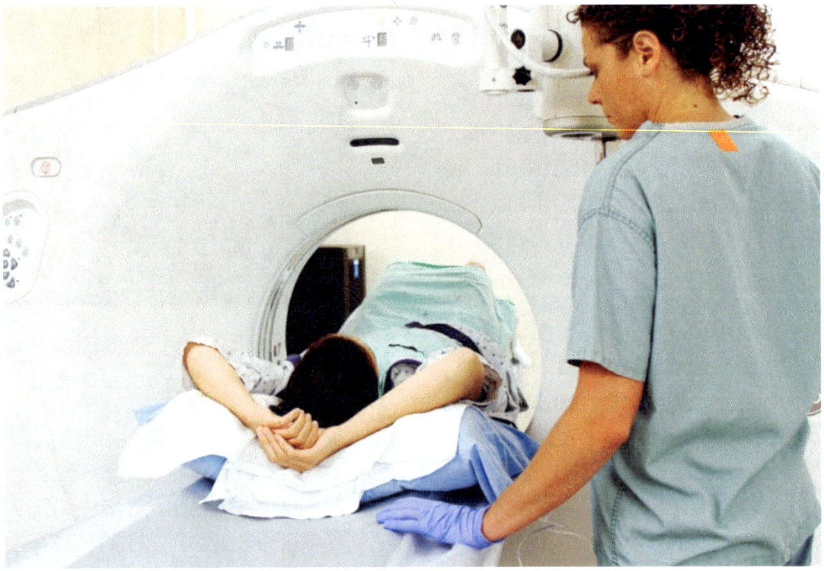

Figure 4.16. Patient in an MRI bore expressing discomfort, with annotations indicating space constraints and warnings about metallic implants.

Source: https://www.healthimages.com/content/uploads/sites/2/2019/07/mri-scan.jpg.

The metal-on-metal (MoM) hip implant regulatory recalls highlight the complexity of these devices, which have been associated with adverse effects, including cardiotoxicity due to elevated circulating cobalt levels, which has been investigated in relevant studies. Though recent developments have shown that non-invasive MRI techniques can detect tissue metal deposition without significant cardiotoxicity at lower blood levels of cobalt, doctors need to remain cautious in the case of patients with such types of implants to present them with appropriate imaging modalities that are safe for the patient (Berber et al., 2019). Hence, awareness of the effect of metal implants is required to optimize cardiovascular imaging procedures. Furthermore, these patient compatibility issues are not confined to personal distress or safety but carry far-reaching implications for the accuracy and reliability of cardiovascular imaging findings. The use of artificial intelligence (AI) in imaging interpretation processes has been proposed as a vehicle to enhance diagnostic accuracy but has its own bag of problems with possible automation bias in decision-making. As such, the development of checklists to accompany AI-aided interpretations has been a prominent alternative solution. The checklists can minimize cognitive bias, based on evidence demonstrating their advantage to accuracy and confidence in diagnosis (Bond et al., 2023). By establishing an environment in which established imaging workflows and new AI assistance converge symbiotically, the field of cardiovascular imaging can deliver more accurate, patient-specific diagnostic solutions, ultimately improving clinical outcomes for patients with heterogeneous compatibility issues.

4.6.3. Limited Availability and Higher Costs

The effectiveness of cardiovascular imaging, such as CT angiography and MRI, is often limited by access and cost. While these advanced imaging modalities are paramount to accurate diagnosis and treatment of cardiovascular diseases, they are not available uniformly across all medical centers. For instance, sub-center clinics and rural hospitals might lack the facility or personnel to conduct such high-level imaging techniques. Hence, such patients who require the same diagnostics are sent to urban regions, which not only increases the diagnostic time but also broadens the scope of healthcare expenditure through the use of transportation expenses and even treatment delay. Thus, the lack of access ultimately leads to unequal health outcomes, particularly for those who reside in underprivileged populations with high percentages of cardiovascular disease. Beyond issues of availability, the expense of MRI and CT angiography poses a significant barrier to widespread application. It is expensive to operate and keep high-tech imaging hardware up to date. In addition, the fees for the procedures themselves are not necessarily covered by insurance and are therefore the patient's out-of-pocket expense. (Buxton et al., 2014) highlights the need to assess the cost-utility of different imaging approaches, finding that while non-invasive cardiac imaging can be cost-effective relative to standard angiography, initial capital and ongoing operating costs may be prohibitive for most healthcare centers.

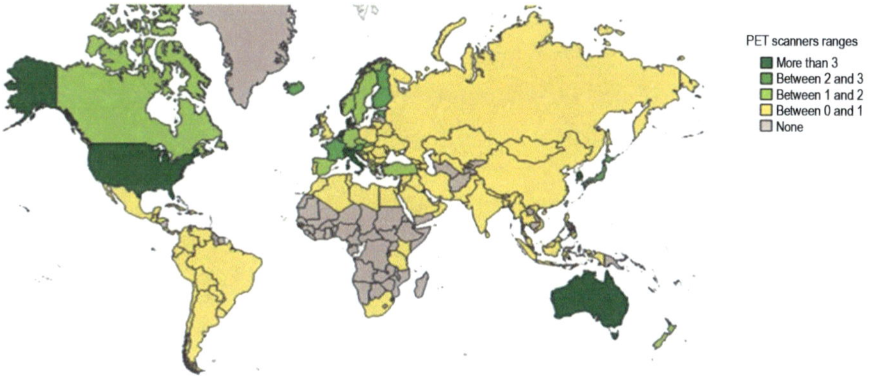

Income group	Population	Total number of PET or PET/CT scanners	Avg. PET scanners (per 1 mil)
High Income	1211232813	4062	1.664
Upper-middle income	2653710742	846	0.287
Lower-middle income	3018336082	352	0.100

Figure 4.17. Global map showing disparities in MRI machine availability per capita across countries.

Source: https://media.licdn.com/dms/image/v2/D5612AQHaKeSHDUhZAA/article-cover_image-shrink_720_1280/B56ZXFnDygHEAM-/0/1742777106241?e=2147483647&v=beta&t=hLGxGEumEYyX1ri_D66A2kGQeY9MqSzJyN3IJSB9MaM.

Therefore, for hospitals and clinics, the decision to implement such imaging techniques depends not only on the promise but also on a careful weighing of economic considerations. Furthermore, the dynamic nature of cardiovascular diagnostics necessitates the re-evaluation of current practices to enhance cost-effectiveness and accessibility. The integration of novel cardiac biomarkers and risk stratification tools may optimize patient care with less reliance on expensive imaging tools. (Berry et al., 2015) underscores that initiatives to rationalize emergency treatment of undifferentiated chest pain, such as the potential use of high-sensitivity troponin assays, can alleviate some economic burdens while retaining diagnostic accuracy. Ultimately, addressing these challenges with limited availability and added cost is crucial to achieving benefits in cardiovascular imaging that extend to all patient groups, promoting health equity in addition to overall diagnostic performance (Figures 4.17; 4.18).

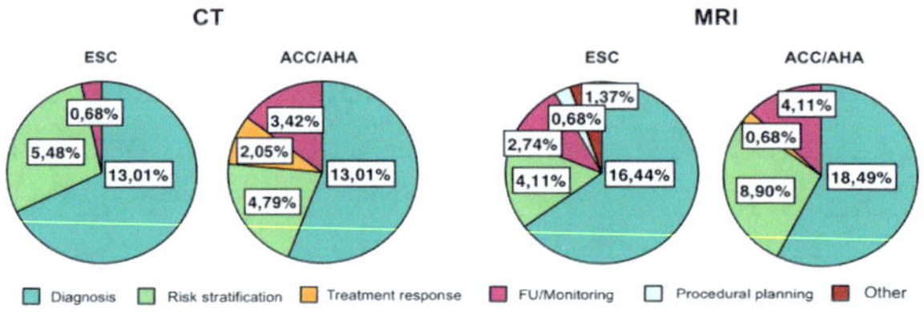

Figure 4.18. Pie chart comparing costs between CT angiography and cardiac MRI, factoring in procedure, staff, and post-processing.

Source: https://www.researchgate.net/publication/344369665/figure/fig1/AS:983361149489154@1611462976828/Rates-of-recommendations-for-CT-and-MRI-by-indication-purpose-in-ESC-and-ACC-AHA.png.

SUMMARY

In summary, the evolution of cardiovascular imaging technology has significantly improved our ability to assess vascular health, especially with CT angiography and MRI. Both imaging modalities have their own advantages, enabling clinicians to achieve precise visualizations of the cardiovascular system with stunning accuracy. CT angiography is superior for speed and is particularly useful in emergency cases, where rapid diagnosis can guide vital interventions. Conversely, MRI offers a non-invasive alternative without nephrotoxicity and can be employed, thus emerging as the first option in patients with contraindications to traditional contrast media. As the recent studies on ferumoxytol in end-stage kidney disease patients requiring vascular imaging indicate, the strength of new contrast agents revolutionizes the boundaries of MRI utilization in the clinical setting (Hennessy et al., 2017). Furthermore, imaging aortic morphology and wall-motion dynamics with these modalities provides important information on cardiovascular risk factors. For instance, studies comparing aortic shape deformation to the cardiac cycle indicate that hypertension and diabetes considerably impact aortic distensibility (Croccia et al., 2012). Such a morpho-functional assessment not only enhances diagnostic precision but can also serve as a preventative measure by identifying vascular changes that happen prior to morphological changes. Secondly, integrating risk assessment with planning imaging protocols helps optimize patient surveillance, making interventions timely and tailored. Lastly, the integration of CT angiography and MRI within cardiovascular diagnosis represents a shift in paradigm toward patient-centeredness. By combining the best of the two modalities, clinicians can develop multimodal imaging strategies that not only offer precise diagnosis of cardiovascular diseases but also trace the course of disease over time. As more research unmasks the complexities of vascular health, the role of advanced imaging modalities will certainly expand, bringing us closer to improved prevention, diagnosis, and treatment of cardiovascular diseases. Lastly, these advancements call for ongoing education and modification of clinical practices to realize optimal patient outcomes.

CLOSER LOOK

CARDIOVASCULAR IMAGING: CT ANGIOGRAPHY AND MRI

CT angiography and MRI are primary imaging modalities used in cardiovascular imaging that enable improved assessment of a wide variety of cardiovascular disorders. Dual imaging modalities enable the clinician to obtain reliable morphological and hemodynamic information about the blood vessels. CT angiography, which is recognized for rapid acquisition and high-quality images, is particularly good at visualizing arterial disease, including coronary artery disease and peripheral artery disease. Meanwhile, MRI offers unparalleled soft-tissue contrast and is thus particularly valuable for evaluating cardiac structure and function. Collectively, these modalities provide the comprehensive evaluation of cardiovascular health, enabling timely and accurate diagnosis, which is paramount for effective intervention and management of cardiovascular disease. The significance of identifying conditions such as renal artery stenosis (RAS) and peripheral artery disease (PAD) in cardiovascular imaging cannot be overstated. RAS remains a dynamic clinical problem with varying approaches to diagnosis and management. Fibromuscular dysplasia, a common underlying cause, demands cautious diagnostic attention, particularly in young hypertensive patients. Conversely, atheromatous RAS is linked with increased cardiovascular risk and therefore a shift in practice away from routine intervention to aggressive medical treatment. This nuanced recognition of RAS reflects evolving practices in cardiovascular therapy and emphasizes the benefit in applying imaging technologies to gather information better for directing interventions. Similarly, advances in the application of multi-modality imaging for PAD identify the central interaction between new technology and improved patient benefits in the management of this crippling disease, as noted in recent research publications.

Furthermore, the future integration of molecular markers with traditional imaging methods offers an exciting direction for cardiovascular imaging. The pathogenesis of conditions such as peripheral artery disease is increasingly understood to be driven by molecular mechanisms, including inflammation and oxidative stress. With the ongoing development of CT and MRI, the incorporation of such molecular markers will offer the potential to gain insight into disease development and mechanisms, thereby enhancing diagnostic specificity. There are still several challenges, though, such as the need to identify new markers and the limitations of existing imaging modalities. Resolution of these challenges will be key to advancing cardiovascular imaging and ultimately improving risk stratification and management. These integrative strategies will not only maintain but also improve the level of cardiovascular care in the future.

REFERENCES

1. Drees, R., Johnson, R. A., Stepien, R. L., Del Rio, A. M., Saunders, J. H., & François, C. J. (2015b). QUANTITATIVE PLANAR AND VOLUMETRIC CARDIAC MEASUREMENTS USING 64 MDCT AND 3T MRI VS. STANDARD 2D AND M-MODE ECHOCARDIOGRAPHY: DOES ANESTHETIC PROTOCOL MATTER? *Veterinary Radiology & Ultrasound*, *56*(6), 638–657. https://doi.org/10.1111/vru.12269Al Moudi, M. Z. (2014). Diagnostic value of nuclear cardiology in coronary artery disease. https://core.ac.uk/download/195631955.pdf (accessed on 15th July 2025).
2. Alkadhi, H., Biavati, F., Botnar, R. M., Channon, K., et al. (2023). Clinical quantitative coronary artery stenosis and coronary atherosclerosis imaging: A consensus statement from the Quantitative Cardiovascular Imaging Study Group. https://core.ac.uk/download/567722990.pdf (accessed on 15th July 2025).
3. Argiro, R., Bezzi, M., Corona, M., De Rubeis, R., et al. (2018). Arms down cone beam CT hepatic angiography: Are we focusing on the wrong target? https://core.ac.uk/download/231748226.pdf (accessed on 15th July 2025).
4. Bai, W., Chen, C., Duan, J., Qin, C., et al. (2025). Deep learning for cardiac image segmentation: A review. https://core.ac.uk/download/266989979.pdf (accessed on 15th July 2025).
5. Balu, N., DeMarco, J. K., Fan, Z., Hatsukami, T., et al. (2018). Carotid artery wall imaging: Perspective and guidelines from the ASNR Vessel Wall Imaging Study Group and expert consensus recommendations of the American Society of Neuroradiology. https://core.ac.uk/download/158170701.pdf (accessed on 15th July 2025).
6. Berber, R. (2019). Clinical and imaging assessment of metal-on-metal hip patients. https://core.ac.uk/download/323198132.pdf (accessed on 15th July 2025).
7. Berry, C., Corcoran, D., & Grant, P. (2015). Risk stratification in non-ST elevation acute coronary syndromes: Risk scores, biomarkers and clinical judgment. https://core.ac.uk/download/42364231.pdf (accessed on 15th July 2025).
8. Berti, S., Bossone, E., Cademartiri, F., Cau, R., et al. (2024). Spectral photon-counting computed tomography: Technical principles and applications in the assessment of cardiovascular diseases. https://core.ac.uk/download/614061489.pdf (accessed on 15th July 2025).
9. Bertrand, P. B., Canè, F., De Beule, M., De Santis, G., et al. (2018). From 4D medical images (CT, MRI, and ultrasound) to 4D structured mesh models of the left ventricular endocardium for patient-specific simulations. https://core.ac.uk/download/147044809.pdf (accessed on 15th July 2025).
10. Bhuiyan, M. M. H., Gupta, K. D., Hossain, I., Islam, M. S., et al. (2023). Introduction of medical imaging modalities. https://arxiv.org/abs/2306.01022 (accessed on 15th July 2025).
11. Bizopoulos, P., & Koutsouris, D. (2021). Deep learning in cardiology. https://arxiv.org/abs/1902.11122 (accessed on 15th July 2025).
12. Bond, R. R., Hughes, C., McConnell, J., McFadden, S., et al. (2023). An evaluation of a checklist in musculoskeletal (MSK) radiographic image interpretation when using artificial intelligence (AI). https://core.ac.uk/download/613687946.pdf (accessed on 15th July 2025).
13. Brogan, P., Burns, J. C., Cornish, J., Diwakar, V., et al. (2020). Lifetime cardiovascular management of patients with previous Kawasaki disease. https://core.ac.uk/download/323066717.pdf (accessed on 15th July 2025).

14. Buckler, A. J. (2022). Linking quantitative radiology to molecular mechanism for improved vascular disease therapy selection and follow-up. https://core.ac.uk/download/541039881.pdf (accessed on 15th July 2025).
15. Buxton, M., CECaT Study Group, Crean, A. M., Dyer, M., et al. (2014). Cost-effectiveness of initial stress cardiovascular MR, stress SPECT or stress echocardiography as a gate-keeper test, compared with upfront invasive coronary angiography in the investigation and management of patients with stable chest pain: Mid-term outcomes from the CECaT randomized controlled trial. https://core.ac.uk/download/29139485.pdf (accessed on 15th July 2025).
16. Cabrelle, G., Crimi, F., Gambato, S., Lupi, A., Pepe, A., Perazzolo, A., Quaia, E., et al. (2023). Medical radiology: Current progress. https://core.ac.uk/download/614221390.pdf (accessed on 15th July 2025).
17. Chan, D. Y. S., Chong, T. T., Gan, J., Hausenloy, D. J., et al. (2023). Multi-modality imaging of atheromatous plaques in peripheral arterial disease: Integrating molecular and imaging markers. https://core.ac.uk/download/573841607.pdf (accessed on 15th July 2025).
18. Cochet, A., Huber, A., Schmermund, A., Mahnken, A. H., et al. (2010). MRI and CT in the diagnosis of coronary artery disease: Indications and applications. https://core.ac.uk/download/pdf/8670855.pdf (accessed on 15th July 2025).
19. Croccia, M. (2012). Influence of cardiovascular risk factors on aortic wall motion after repair of type A aortic dissection: An ECG-gated CT study. https://core.ac.uk/download/14705456.pdf (accessed on 15th July 2025).
20. D'Silva, A., & Wright, M. (2011). Advances in imaging for atrial fibrillation ablation. https://core.ac.uk/download/29469518.pdf (accessed on 15th July 2025).
21. Erta, M., Gupta, A., Murgia, A., Saba, L., et al. (2020). CT imaging features of carotid artery plaque vulnerability. https://core.ac.uk/download/541242797.pdf (accessed on 15th July 2025).
22. Finestone, A., ABIM Foundation, American Board of Internal Medicine, Einstein, A. J., Lee, C. I., Committee to Assess Health Risks from Exposure to Low Levels of Ionizing Radiation, Loré, C., Picano, E., et al. (2007). Radiological informed consent in cardiovascular imaging: Towards the medico-legal perfect storm? https://core.ac.uk/download/pdf/7797032.pdf (accessed on 15th July 2025).
23. Fleischmann, D., Hom, J., Jiang, B., Li, Y., Porcu, M., Rodriguez, F., Saba, L., et al. (2020). Carotid plaque imaging and the risk of atherosclerotic cardiovascular disease. https://core.ac.uk/download/541242956.pdf (accessed on 15th July 2025).
24. Hennessy, M., Kasthuri, R., Kingsmore, D. B., Mark, P. B., et al. (2017). Ferumoxytol-enhanced magnetic resonance angiography for the assessment of potential kidney transplant recipients. https://core.ac.uk/download/83960454.pdf (accessed on 15th July 2025).
25. Hoste, E., & Vandenberghe, W. (2019). Contrast-associated acute kidney injury: Does it really exist, and if so, what to do about it? https://core.ac.uk/download/225020701.pdf (accessed on 15th July 2025).
26. Jiang, J., Ren, J., & Trundle, P. (2010). Medical imaging analysis with artificial neural networks. https://core.ac.uk/download/9031176.pdf (accessed on 15th July 2025).

27. Leber, A. W., Hamm, B., Kondo, C., Herborn, C. U., Ropers, D., Schnapauff, D., et al. (2007). Patient acceptance of noninvasive and invasive coronary angiography. https://core.ac.uk/download/pdf/7541708.pdf (accessed on 15th July 2025).

28. Losito, A., Persu, A., Cragg, A. H., Severn, A., Antiplatelet Trialists' Collaboration, Chade, A. R., Hirsch, A. T., et al. (2014). Renal artery stenosis—When to screen, what to stent? https://core.ac.uk/download/30661796.pdf (accessed on 15th July 2025).

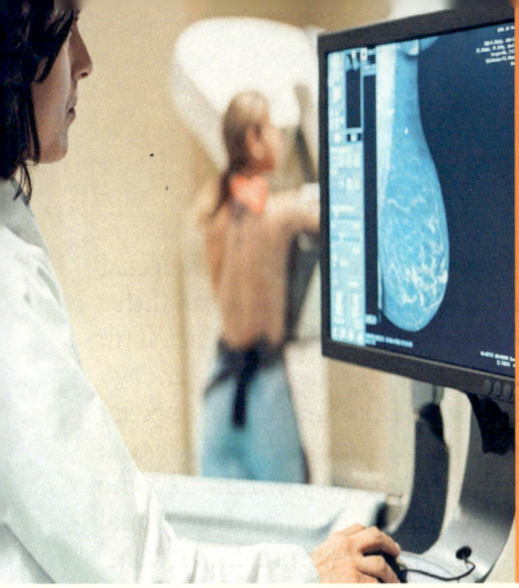

Chapter 5

BREAST IMAGING: MAMMOGRAPHY TO MRI

Contents

Introduction

In breast cancer diagnostics, imaging technologies have advanced dramatically, enabling earlier diagnosis and improved therapy. Mammography has long been the preferred modality for breast cancer screening, due to widespread availability in numerous clinics and demonstrated effectiveness. Its utility has been constrained by poorer sensitivity for dense breasts, hence the development of other imaging modalities. Emerging technologies such as photoacoustic (PA) imaging hold great promise as alternatives that could enhance or even replace mammography for certain diagnostic purposes. Leveraging the combined effect of light and sound, PA imaging allows for low-cost, non-invasive detection with minimal risk while keeping patients comfortable. This emerging technology highlights efforts to improve diagnostic accuracy in breast cancer, as many studies have shown its potential effectiveness at both initial and advanced stages, including its use in combination with traditional imaging methods like MRI (Hilgerink et al., 2011).

Although mammography remains imperative in breast cancer screening, it is imperative that it be complemented by techniques like magnetic resonance imaging (MRI) to improve the capability to diagnose. MRI is the most sensitive modality for the detection of breast cancer, particularly in high-risk individuals and complex cases where mammography is suboptimal.

Breast MRI sensitivity and specificity are improved by the use of newer contrast media, permits greater visualization of tumor characteristics. This agent, due to high r1 relaxivity, enhances diagnostic precision in breast MRI, thereby optimizing assessment and treatment planning (Kirchin et al., 2015). The integration of these advanced imaging technologies enables health practitioners to deliver tailored approaches to managing breast cancer that align with the global objective of maximizing patient outcomes through tailored diagnostic modalities.

With further advancements in breast imaging technologies, it is important to understand the individual strengths and weaknesses of each to enable effective clinical implementation. Mammography to MRI shows the trend towards diversified diagnostic approaches driven by the need for more accurate diagnosis and patient-centric treatment.

While looking at recent literature on newer technologies like PA imaging and MRI methodological advances, one can see clearly that there is no end to innovation here. With doctors and healthcare professionals now using such new imaging methods more and more, research and ongoing education play a very important role in equipping professionals with the appropriate knowledge to apply the best practices. Hence, the future for breast cancer detection is bright, as these developments pave the way for increased detection rates and, eventually, better survival rates for the patients.

5.1. Mammography

Mammography remains a cornerstone in breast cancer screening as it can detect abnormalities in their earliest stage, allowing successful treatment. Mammography uses low-energy X-rays to produce clear images of breast tissue, allowing radiologists to detect potential tumors much earlier than they would become palpable. While extremely popular, traditional X-ray mammography has inherent limitations, including false positives and negatives, which complicate diagnosis. Further, more compact breast tissue can obscure lesions, resulting in false negatives or unnecessary biopsies. Because breast cancer incidence is still relatively high, particularly among women, continuous innovation and refinement of mammographic approaches are necessary to assist with accuracy and outcome enhancement for patients. Advances in imaging technology have created interest in complementary and alternative techniques to standard mammography. For instance, photoacoustic imaging is a promising modality that offers a possible alternative or complement to ultrasound and X-ray mammography for early diagnosis. It is a technology that relies on the release of ultrasound waves following light absorption by tissues and permits high-resolution imaging without ionizing radiation. Research shows that the addition of photoacoustic imaging to the diagnostic protocol is more acceptable to patients and reduces risks associated with it while maintaining competitively diagnostic efficiency relative to other options available (Hilgerink et al., 2011). Further research and clinical validation of photoacoustic imaging have the potential to transform practice significantly for breast cancer screening, particularly in women with dense breasts. Other research on novel imaging techniques includes microwave imaging, which exploits the inherent electromagnetic properties of breast tissue to distinguish between malignant and benign cells. The technique, assisted by a synthetic reference beam, offers advantages such as low cost and ease, making it an appealing alternative to standard mammography (Elsdon et al., 2010). Even though early findings in breast phantoms are promising, the transition to the clinical setting needs cautious validation and optimization. The integration of these innovative imaging technologies with standard mammography might eventually provide a complete diagnostic arsenal against breast cancer, allowing individualized benefits based on patient-specific characteristics and choices.

5.1.1. Types of Mammography (Screening Versus Diagnostic)

The imaging of the breast encompasses a variety of techniques, and among them, mammography remains a standard for both screening and diagnostic imaging. Screening mammography, for the most part, is reserved for asymptomatic women and is performed annually or biennially, depending on age and risk factors. Its primary goal is early detection of breast cancer, hopefully before clinical presentation. This approach not only reduces mortality from breast cancer but also allows for less extreme interventions should the malignancy be detected early. The guidelines that have been established for screening mammography have worked, with conclusive evidence existing for its capacity to lower breast cancer mortality through the earlier detection of malignancy. Therefore, as one of the methods of breast imaging, screening mammography is the initial defense against breast cancer and has a significant impact on women's health outcomes. Diagnostic mammography, on the other hand, is for a specific reason and to evaluate associated particular symptoms such as lumps or changes detected during a screening routine. This category is characterized by its dedicated imaging technique, often using additional views or enhanced imaging techniques to better visualize into suspect areas. Diagnostic mammography is essential for further assessing abnormalities identified by a screening test. Its application is particularly important for women with a family history of breast cancer or those with evidence of potential malignancy. With advances in ancillary imaging techniques, diagnostic mammography complements screening by providing a more accurate assessment of breast tissue. It therefore plays a significant role in handling cases and management following preliminary screening with pathological findings.

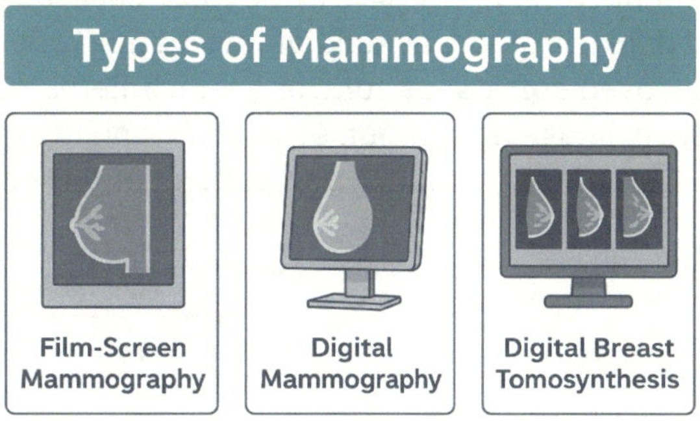

Figure 5.1. Types of mammography.

Source: https://cdn.prod.website-files.com/655dcbf19753fff0028b249d/68183c87e86f67f9a4bccc1b_20336150-b3f9-4237-8969-2fb321ffd42b.png.

In the continuous process of breast imaging, emerging technologies like photoacoustic imaging (PA) are being explored as potential alternatives for established methods like X-ray mammography. While PA imaging is still in the research stage, its non-invasive nature and lower risks compared to conventional methods make it an attractive option for early detection. Studies have shown that PA imaging can be a helpful adjunct tool to improve diagnostic performance in addition to x-ray mammography and ultrasound. Conversely, magnetic resonance imaging (MRI) is still the most sensitive imaging modality for breast cancer detection, particularly when using advanced agents like gadobenate dimeglumine, which has demonstrated improved diagnostic performance in research. The multidimensional use of such imaging techniques places a demand for a tailored approach to the diagnosis of breast cancer, ultimately leading healthcare providers to optimal clinical decisions regarding patient management (Hilgerink et al., 2011; Kirchin et al., 2015) (Figure 5.1).

5.1.2. Procedure and Technology Used

Breast imaging technologies' evolution has significantly transformed early detection and breast cancer diagnosis. Mammography using X-rays has long been the classic breast imaging mainstay, which enables clinicians to visualize the inner details of breast tissue. Nevertheless, the valuable technique, as it is, has its limitations in terms of sensitivity, particularly for dense breasts. In response to these restraints, advancement has seen alternatives such as ultrasound and magnetic resonance imaging (MRI) adopted. Each of these has its advantages; for instance, ultrasound is particularly good at further evaluating abnormal findings on mammograms, and MRI provides improved soft tissue contrast, which helps better visualize malignancies in challenging situations. Hence, image integration of various imaging modalities is crucial for optimal breast cancer detection and treatment planning for individual patients (Figure 5.2).

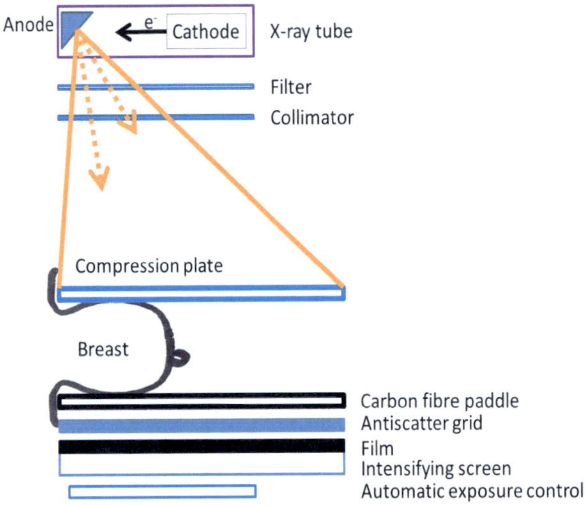

Figure 5.2. Diagram of the mammography procedure, including breast compression plates and X-ray detector.

Source: https://screening.iarc.fr/BreastPici/technique001.jpg

In the quest for diagnostic advancement, photoacoustic (PA) imaging has emerged as a burgeoning technology that offers a non-invasive means of breast cancer detection. A recent review has identified PA imaging's benefits over conventional X-ray mammography and ultrasonography in early diagnosis, and for its application together with MRI in late diagnosis. A multi-criteria analysis of costs, diagnostic efficiency, patient comfort, and risks leans towards the conclusion that PA imaging has highly desirable features, particularly its affordability and the absence of risks in procedure deployment. Although the expected differences in diagnostic capability were not significant, PA imaging's advantages position it as a modality that could complement traditional imaging methods, especially with further advances in its design technology (Hilgerink et al., 2011). The efficiency of any imaging modality greatly depends on the technology and procedural design that form the core of it. For PA imaging, recent research has focused on reducing the quality of the reconstruction algorithm, detector sensitivity, and wavelength diversity to improve diagnostic utility. These advancements might lead to greater clinical acceptance and entry into routine breast cancer diagnostics. As the medical profession grapples with the numerous imaging options, understanding the specific roles and technological underpinnings of each becomes obligatory. The transition from traditional imaging techniques to newer ones signals a new paradigm in which patient-specific treatment is prioritized. In the future, continued technological progress and innovation in imaging will undoubtedly play a part in shaping diagnostic pathways for breast cancer management (N/A, 2007).

5.1.3. Benefits and Drawbacks of Mammography

Mammography is a mainstay of breast cancer screening, primarily because it can detect tumors early, even before symptoms have emerged. This renders it highly likely to treat and improves general survival rates. Technology in the form of low-dose X-rays enables clinicians to detect abnormalities, such as microcalcifications, which may indicate malignancy. Furthermore, the extensive utilization and established effectiveness of mammography make it a readily available choice for population screening programs. Despite these benefits, certain limitations must be considered. Conditions such as breast density can influence the sensitivity of the methods and cause women with denser breasts to be more likely to experience false negatives (Elsdon et al., 2010). Additionally, the tension between screening outcomes and the risk of overdiagnosis raises ethical issues in the application of regular mammography screening. Despite advances in mammography technology, certain constraints still hinder its effectiveness (Figure 5.3).

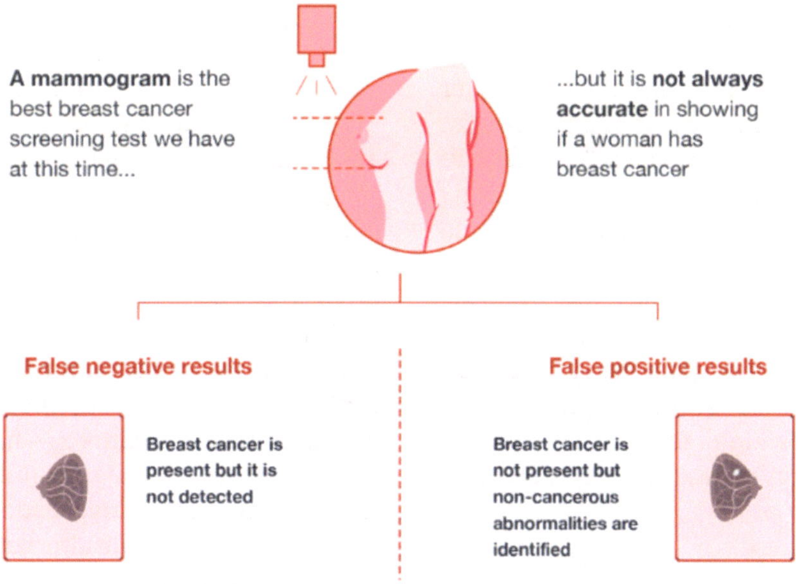

Figure 5.3. Infographic outlining the advantages and limitations of mammography, including detection rate and false positives.

Source: https://assets.hse.ie/media/images/Mammogram-pic.width-1534_PWBew3G.png

While mammograms are usually accurate, they are not perfect; false positives lead to excessive concern, additional testing, and expense for patients. The psychological impact of a false-positive result is gigantic, most often leading to distress and emotional turmoil for patients who must wait for follow-up testing. Additionally, mammography is not perfect at detecting all types of breast cancer, particularly those that are not able to produce calcium deposits, also making it even more challenging to diagnose (Matijaš et al., 2023). These limitations call for the need for other imaging modalities or techniques that are capable of providing comprehensive evaluations of the breast tissue, especially in women who are at high risk or who have dense breasts. To address the limitations of traditional mammography, other imaging techniques, such as contrast-enhanced mammography (CEM) and magnetic resonance imaging (MRI), have been found to be valuable adjuncts. CEM, for example, uses a contrast agent to increase the visibility of abnormalities, thereby improving the detection rates of multifocal lesions and microcalcifications. MRI, by contrast, yields high-resolution images that create detailed information about breast tissue architecture and lesions. But even these options have their drawbacks: MRI and CEM involve higher radiation doses, potential reactions to contrast media, and higher operating costs. These factors imply a delicate balance between employing these advanced technologies and traditional methods of mammography, ensuring that patients are provided with the most accurate and least intrusive diagnostic options available in today's breast imaging (Matijaš et al., 2023). The ongoing process of developing breast imaging techniques highlights the urgency for an overall approach towards early detection of cancer.

5.2. Breast Ultrasound

Breast ultrasound is a critical modality in the breast imaging arsenal, employed alongside conventional mammography, to a significant degree, under specific clinical conditions. Unlike mammography, which is based on the application of ionizing radiation, ultrasound uses sound waves to produce images of breast tissue. It thus is safer to employ in younger women and women with dense breasts in whom mammograms would be less effective. Its non-invasiveness and ability to image lesions in real time in the breast add to its value during diagnosis. It is also highly beneficial for biopsy guidance, allowing precise targeting of the area of concern. It is beneficial but does not replace mammography but rather is an adjunct imaging modality that facilitates a more comprehensive evaluation of breast abnormality, providing an accurate diagnosis when correlated with other imaging modalities. The implementation of breast ultrasound in practice not only enhances the diagnostic accuracy but also lowers the risk of inappropriate interventions. According to studies, breast lesions that are diagnosed as benign on ultrasound can often be managed conservatively, saving patients from unnecessary anxiety and risks of overtreatment. Ultrasound also detects lesions that mammography would likely miss, particularly in the dense breast tissue seen in young patients. By differentiating cystic and solid masses, ultrasound plays an essential role in triaging patients for further diagnostic evaluation. As more personalized breast cancer treatment is sought after, the role of ultrasound in diagnosis becomes more prominent, with clinicians being able to tailor the management plan based on each individual's distinct features and risk factors. New technologies such as photoacoustic imaging and microwave technology have potential for enhancing breast imaging ability. For instance, the evaluation of photoacoustic imaging suggests that it offers a possible alternative to traditional imaging technologies by offering a low-risk, low-cost, non-invasive method that is as good for diagnostics. Similarly, holographic-based microwave imaging can provide additional options for breast cancer detection, especially in cases where mammography and ultrasound yield inconclusive results. As these emerging techniques are further developed, their integration into existing imaging platforms has the potential to increase rates of early detection and patient benefit profoundly. Thus, the constantly evolving profile of breast imaging modalities and the particular role of breast ultrasound are key to enhancing the diagnosis and management of breast cancer and thus enhancing patient outcomes among various population groups.

5.2.1. Role of Ultrasound in Breast Imaging

Ultrasound is now a crucial modality in breast imaging due to its ability to augment mammography and address its limitations. While mammography is the device of choice for the screening of breast cancer, it is not very good at sensitivity, particularly in cases of dense breast tissue, in which its effectiveness drops to a level as low as 7–26% in identifying pathologic nipple discharge (PND) conditions (Panzironi et al., 2019).

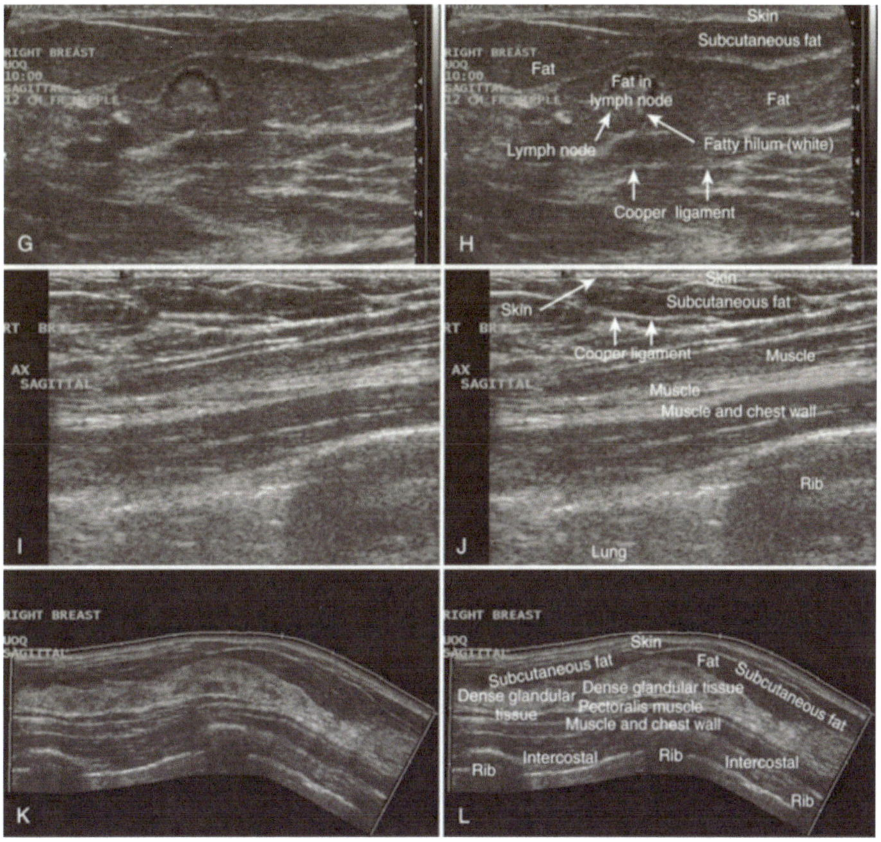

Figure 5.4. Ultrasound image of a breast cyst compared to surrounding tissue with labeled annotations.

Source: https://radiologykey.com/wp-content/uploads/2015/12/B9780323051989000056_f1gl.jpg

On the other hand, ultrasound has been shown to achieve significantly higher sensitivity, ranging from 63% to 100%, and is thus a valuable tool in the evaluation of breast abnormalities. The higher sensitivity not only means more accurate diagnoses but also contributes to risk stratification, guiding further management and potentially eliminating the need for invasive investigations such as biopsies. The value of ultrasound in breast imaging is further highlighted by its use in assessing clinical indications, such as PND. The subtlety of PND is evident, given that even though the initial procedure remains mammography for women above 39 years, the limitations in sensitivity often necessitate the incorporation of ultrasound (Panzironi et al., 2019). This modality enables better visualization of intraductal structures, helping detect lesions not visible on mammography. Additionally, ultrasound is beneficial in real-time evaluations, allowing for guided biopsies to be conducted on suspicious lesions directly. Therefore, the introduction of ultrasound into diagnostic practice not only enhances the quality of results but also facilitates a more penetrating approach to breast pathology management. Advances in ultrasound technology, including the introduction of contrast-enhanced ultrasound, have also expanded its applications in breast imaging. Recent studies indicate that such innovations are as sensitive as MRI, particularly in PND, with sensitivity levels up to 96% (Panzironi et al., 2019). This kind of advancement places ultrasound as a possible substitute for more intrusive procedures like galactography, which are normally accompanied by pain and limited diagnostic capability. Furthermore, the accessibility and non-ionizing nature of ultrasound serve as an attractive tool for patients and further solidify its place in breast imaging models. As advancements in breast imaging technology continue, the role of ultrasound will most certainly be a determining factor in improving diagnosis and patient care (Figure 5.4).

5.2.2. Indications for Breast Ultrasound

Breast ultrasound's role in the diagnostic workup of breast lesions is twofold, primarily as a mammography ancillary. The imaging modality is beneficial for characterization of palpable masses that are less visible on mammography. In dense breast patients, in whom mammography can yield false-negative examinations, breast ultrasound is crucial to enhance detection rates (and, thereby, management decisions). In addition, ultrasound has a role in guidance of fine needle aspiration biopsies, thereby enabling adequate histopathologic examination of breast lesions in a suspicious case. The complementarity of ultrasound to mammography lends itself to its growing application in whole-breast imaging schemes, as per recent recommendations suggesting the use of ultrasound in addition to mammography for certain high-risk groups (Figure 5.5).

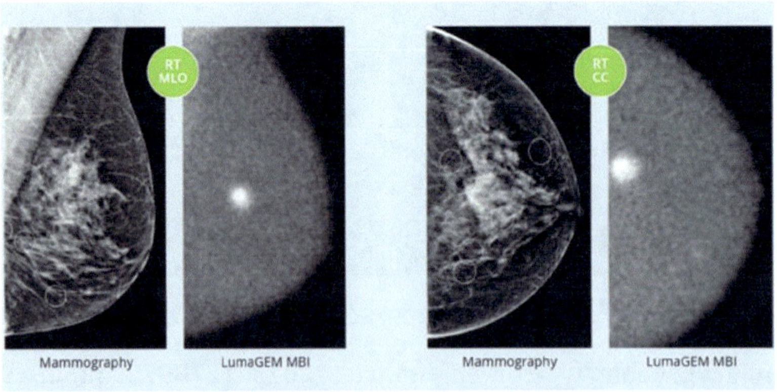

Figure 5.5. A side-by-side comparison of mammography vs. molecular breast imaging.

Source: https://www.itnonline.com/sites/default/files/field/image/Mammo-and-MBI-copy.jpg

In addition to its role in diagnosis, breast ultrasound is also important in the follow-up and assessment of treatment responses, such as neoadjuvant chemotherapy. Breast ultrasound thus can contribute to a multidisciplinary management of breast cancer patients in providing real-time and non-invasive information on tumor dynamics over time. New imaging modalities, such as contrast-enhanced ultrasound, are further improving the role of traditional ultrasound by providing functional and perfusion information on the modality that can rival MRI. This advance not only differentiates benign from malignant lesions but also aids in evaluating treatment response. Studies on comparative effectiveness across imaging modalities continue to support the use of ultrasound in clinical settings, especially in scenarios where patient tolerance and availability are critical considerations. It must be remembered that while there are many benefits to breast ultrasound, its drawbacks must also be highlighted. The operator dependency and complexity of breast tissue architecture also influence ultrasound sensitivity. Thus, although it provides valuable added information, it is not intended to replace mammography but as a complement to it. Comparative studies of ultrasound accuracy relative to other modalities, such as MRI, have found that, though a potent detector of breast lesions, independent ultrasound may be lacking in complete diagnostic capability. For example, very high MRI sensitivity but low specificity, as recorded in some tumor-size estimation studies, suggests that ultrasound be used as part of a broad imaging strategy that may incorporate MRI where appropriate, particularly in pre-surgical evaluation and follow-up (Anidjar et al., 2017; Evans et al., 2021).

5.2.3. Advantages and Disadvantages Compared to Mammography

Mammography is a mainstay of breast cancer screening, particularly in women over 40 years, providing critical early detection. Its main advantage is that it can detect abnormalities such as microcalcifications or tiny tumors that are typically not visible on physical examination. Heightened sensitivity has been singled out as an advantage; however, while popularity has been unmatched, so too have been some of its limitations. Sensitivity ranges from 7% to 26% in some scenarios, like pathologic nipple discharge (PND), which equates to a high likelihood of false negatives. Under such situations, other imaging tools like ultrasound and breast MRI have begun supplementing mammography, offering better sensitivity in most cases, particularly for highly vulnerable groups. The limitations of mammography underscore the importance of continuous improvement and research into alternative approaches to increase diagnostic accuracy and patient benefit. The evolution of breast MRI has become a significant alternative to traditional mammography, particularly in high-risk groups and symptomatic patients such as those with nipple discharge. Its higher soft-tissue contrast and sensitivity are the strengths of MRI, with detection rates up to 96% noted in some conditions, such as PND, especially when compared with mammography and galactography. This is made possible by more accurate visualization of breast tissue, which can help differentiate malignant from benign lesions. However, despite these advantages, MRI has limitations. Its deterrents are cost, accessibility, and the need for advanced technical skill. As such, MRI's incorporation into practice must balance its high diagnostic yield against the logistical realities of the majority of healthcare settings. In addition, increased enthusiasm for alternative imaging technology continues to fuel disputes over the physiological and economic costs of breast screening methods. Microwave imaging, for instance, holds promising advantages as an adjunct or complement to mammography, with simplicity and lower cost. Evidence indicates that the technology might supplant traditional methods seamlessly, particularly considering its success in experiments using breast phantoms, as already shown. However, adoption of such new methods will be contingent on rigorous validation and clinical acceptance. With advances in breast imaging technology, there is a need to weigh the potential advantages of newer technologies against established practices such as mammography so that patients can receive the most effective and comprehensive care at minimal economic cost (Figure 5.6).

Factor	Mammogram	Sono Mammogram (Ultrasound)
Technology Used	Low-dose X-rays	High-frequency sound waves (ultrasound)
Breast Compression	Yes	No – painless, no compression
Radiation Involved	Yes (minimal)	Women under 40, dense breasts, pregnancy
Best For	Microcalcifications, solid tumors	Cysts, fluid-filled lumps, fibrous tissue
Limitations	Less clear for dense tissue	May miss small calcifications

Figure 5.6. Comparative table showing the pros and cons of ultrasound versus mammography in breast cancer detection.

Source: https://uniscansstrapi.mocerohealth.com/uploads/8f8fa7f1_3471_49db_93a0_656cbcb8f2be_b99664faba.png

5.3. Magnetic Resonance Imaging (MRI)

The evolution of breast imaging has fundamentally changed how doctors today approach diagnosis and treatment planning. Among the range of modalities, Magnetic Resonance Imaging (MRI) has emerged as an unavoidable option, particularly in the imaging of breast pathology. MRI is renowned for its high sensitivity score, as much as 96%, and is most beneficial wherever conventional methods such as mammography yield indefinite results. For instance, patients presenting with pathologic nipple discharge, typically representing intraductal lesions, have been assisted by this new imaging technique. With sensitivity as low as 7–26% for mammography, MRI can provide better definition of breast tissue abnormalities, enabling earlier and more targeted interventions for lesions ranging from benign intraductal papillomas to malignancies (Panzironi et al., 2019).

One of the interesting uses of MRI is in the treatment of pathologic nipple discharge (PND), which was a problem of diagnostic quandary in the past. Contrast-enhanced breast MRI has proven to be helpful not only in increasing the rate of diagnosis but also in assisting surgical planning. Traditional forms of diagnosis, including ductoscopy and galactography, while beneficial, are limited by pain and suboptimal performance. Not only does MRI surpass these methods in sensitivity, but it also facilitates detailed pre-surgical planning through an accurate visualization of intraductal anatomy. With the augmented use of MRI in clinical practice, it underscores our need to revise diagnostic paradigms to incorporate these latest technologies (Panzironi et al., 2019). While MRI boasts a number of benefits over routine imaging, it is also important to consider its limitations within the broad context of breast imaging modalities. Integration of new techniques, such as photoacoustic imaging, indicates promising progress in this field aimed at enhancing patient outcomes. Relative to this, photoacoustic imaging was recognized for its cost advantage and non-invasive feature, which made it a potential alternative to MRI in certain diagnostic uses. Yet MRI still is a cornerstone of advanced breast imaging due to its better diagnostic performance, particularly in challenging cases. As researchers and clinicians collaborate to optimize imaging strategies better, use of multimodal techniques will provide clinicians with a flexible set of tools with which to provide personalized treatment paths tailored to individual patient needs.

5.3.1. Indications for Breast MRI

The application of breast MRI has increasingly become integral in breast imaging, particularly due to its great sensitivity for the identification of breast lesions. Mammography traditionally has served as the imaging method of choice for the screening of breast cancer. However, at times, mammography can result in false-negative findings, hence the need for further evaluation by MRI. This is most important in high-risk patients, for example, those with a family history of breast cancer or genetic risk factors, such as BRCA mutations. Anatomical resolution and functional information provided by MRI allow improved characterization of breast masses and may aid in determining disease spread, thereby influencing therapy planning. Recognition of these factors is vital to clinicians in determining the correct use of MRI in the diagnostic sequence because this is directly tied to patient outcomes and customized therapy. Breast MRI is also extremely useful for evaluating treatment response and identifying recurrences. After surgery or after chemotherapy, MRI becomes an unobtrusive method to determine residual disease. This capability is particularly valuable for mastectomy patients since standard imaging devices may not be able to give effective information in the absence of breast tissue. Regular MRI tests can determine if additional procedures or changes in treatment plans are necessary based on the imaging findings. This adds greater significance to breast MRI beyond its initial diagnostic application, turning it into an agent employed for the long-term care of breast cancer survivors. Through its skilled ability to differentiate between malignant and benign processes, MRI is a cornerstone for personalized patient care in the oncology setting. MRI also plays an important role in diagnostic workups, particularly in indeterminate cases when mammography and ultrasound findings are not conclusive. In cases involving suspicion of microcalcification or architectural distortion seen in mammograms, MRI can further clarify to differentiate between benign and malignant breast disease. It is particularly beneficial in women who have dense breasts, in which case mammography may be concealing tumors behind. With progressing knowledge of breast imaging, MRI use has been expanded to preoperative planning to make surgical procedures as efficient and less invasive as possible. Inclusion in the diagnostic process underscores the importance of MRI in current breast imaging, enabling earlier detection and treatment across different patient groups (N/A, 1994; N/A, 2003) (Figure 5.7).

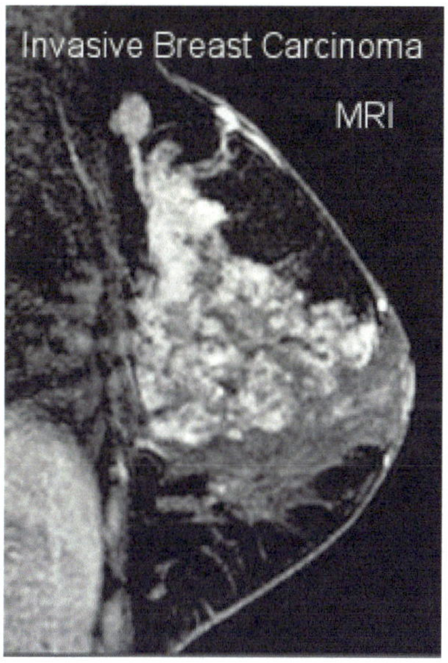

Figure 5.7. MRI image of the breast with contrast enhancement revealing a lesion.

Source: https://breast-cancer.ca/images/breast-carcinoma-mri-image1.jpg

5.3.2. Procedure and Technology Used

The evolution of breast imaging technologies has significantly transformed the procedure of detecting and diagnosing breast cancer. Traditionally, mammography has been the gold standard, employing low-energy X-rays to create detailed images of the breast tissue. The technical step involves compressing the breast to minimize motion and achieve maximal image clarity and exposing the tissue to radiation for a portion of a second. This straightforward process allows the identification of tumors and calcifications, which could indicate malignancy. However, while mammography is successful, especially in the instance of early breast cancer, there are drawbacks, including false negatives in dense tissue and the potential for the patient to feel pain through compression. With the evolving technology, understanding the advantages and disadvantages of mammography is necessary to pave the way for more sophisticated imaging modalities, such as MRI and photoacoustic imaging (Figure 5.8).

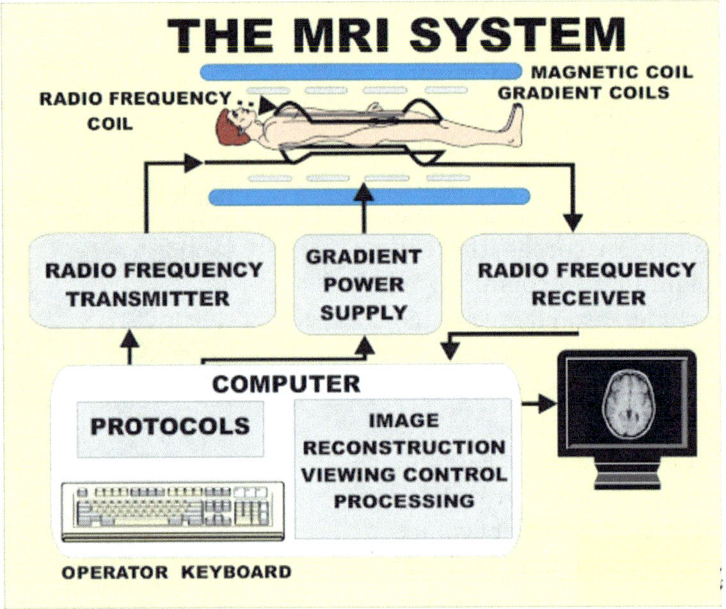

Figure 5.8. Schema of MRI procedure equipment setup including magnet bore, breast coil, and contrast injection line.

Source: https://lh3.googleusercontent.com/proxy/fYUdfkHCaBYRk0iAc6Tdz_RBCgTj3QPTud_6mjD8u8LlojzFERNSrR-sSM8i0VCpwdMplsAg-_wDBjQjZ_vbgxaVdFY

MRI (Magnetic Resonance Imaging) has become an important breast cancer imaging procedure, especially in women with high-risk or dense breast tissue, where mammography is inadequate. Unlike mammography, which is based on ionizing radiation, MRI uses magnetic fields and radio waves to create extremely detailed images of the breast. This technique is better than measuring disease extent and response to treatment, since it provides excellent soft-tissue contrast. MRI is also very valuable in the identification of tumors not palpable on mammography and, therefore, is very valuable in staging and preoperative planning. The patient usually has to remain in a confined space, which may cause anxiety, but the examination is basically safe and nontraumatic. The introduction of MRI to routine breast cancer screening procedures is a significant breakthrough in the pursuit of enhanced diagnostic precision without compromising patient well-being and comfort. Advances in recent technology that enable breast imaging, such as photoacoustic imaging (PA), point toward a promising future for diagnostic techniques. PA integrates optical and ultrasound imaging to provide real-time, high-resolution reconstructions of breast tissue based on the special properties of light absorption by biological tissues. PA has been found to have potential for early cancer detection, providing a non-invasive alternative to standard methods such as X-ray, mammography, and ultrasound. PA imaging is cost-effective, convenient for the patient, and low-risk compared to other imaging modalities, yet offers equal diagnostic ability (Hilgerink et al., 2011). Maximizing the design and use of such technology as medical imaging evolves will become essential to increasing diagnostic capacity and patient care in breast cancer treatment. The application of technologies such as PA imaging may eventually lead to improved early detection and treatment strategies, ultimately proving breast imaging technology successful.

5.3.3. Benefits and Limitations of MRI in Breast Imaging

Breast imaging with magnetic resonance imaging (MRI) has several major advantages, especially for high-risk groups and in situations where standard imaging methods, including mammography, tend to be inadequate. Perhaps the greatest strength of MRI is its powerful capability for generating high-contrast images of soft tissues, enabling clear visualization of tumors and adjacent structures. This is especially helpful in detecting invasive breast cancer that may not be visible on mammogram or ultrasound. MRI plays a crucial role in determining disease extent, particularly in multifocal or bilateral disease, enabling clinicians to make sound therapeutic decisions. The increased sensitivity of MRI has been invaluable in complex cases, adding to the diagnostic process and allowing the identification of breast abnormalities in the early stages that may otherwise be overlooked (Figure 5.9).

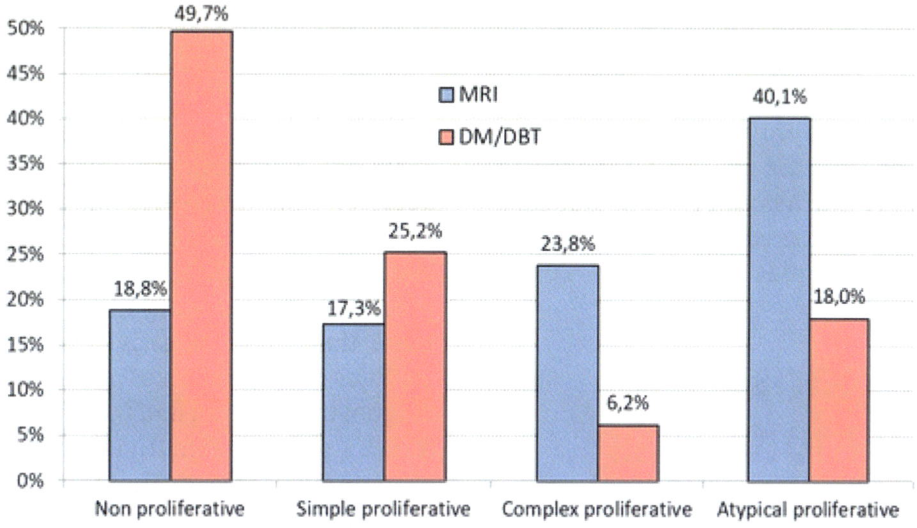

Figure 5.9. Graph comparing detection rates and false positives between mammography, ultrasound, and MRI.

Source: https://media.springernature.com/lw685/springer-static/image/art%3A10.1186%2Fs13058-018-0937-7/MediaObjects/13058_2018_937_Fig3_HTML.gif

Despite its advantages, MRI in breast imaging is not without drawbacks. One significant drawback is its availability and cost, as MRI equipment is typically more expensive and less readily available than other imaging modalities, such as mammography. Moreover, MRI examinations are typically longer than other imaging examinations, which can be an issue in high-volume clinical practice. Furthermore, the presence of contraindications, for instance, the presence of certain metal implants or patient claustrophobia, may restrict MRI use in some instances. Additionally, even though MRI is highly sensitive, specificity remains an issue since benign lesions may be confused with malignant ones, thereby precipitating unwarranted biopsies or patient anxiety prior to them actually happening (Elsdon et al., 2010). The addition of MRI to the breast imaging paradigm holds the potential for a potential opportunity for more complete diagnostic pathways while highlighting the need for careful examination of when and how to use this technology. The use of MRI advantages, particularly in the high-risk group or for evaluating difficult cases, can significantly complement conventional methods such as mammography. But it is essential that the healthcare professionals keep these benefits in mind against the limitations of MRI use. With a multimodal approach that integrates mammography, MRI, and emerging modalities such as contrast-enhanced mammography (CEM), patient outcomes in breast cancer detection and surveillance can be improved. The dual use not only optimizes diagnostic performance but also capitalizes on the intrinsic shortcoming of each modality to optimize the collective performance of breast imaging methods (Elsdon et al., 2010).

5.4. Comparison of Imaging Modalities

The landscape of breast imaging has evolved considerably over time from traditional techniques such as mammography to advanced modalities such as magnetic resonance imaging (MRI). Mammography is the standard for screening for breast cancer, but its sensitivity can be decreased considerably in women with dense breasts. It is reported that mammography's sensitivity ranges from 7% to 26% for pathologic nipple discharge, which is a concern given its potential for earlier detection (Panzironi et al., 2019). On the other hand, ultrasound is more sensitive, ranging from 63% to 100%. This innovation heralds a critical gap in the conventional paradigm of breast imaging, prompting clinicians and patients alike to seek other modalities that can provide more information regarding breast health, and thus forcing a close scrutiny of imaging protocols within clinical practice. The continuous evaluation of imaging modalities leads to the pursuit of newer techniques, such as photoacoustic imaging (PA) and MRI, that hold promising prospects for the diagnosis and treatment of breast cancer. PA imaging offers a non-invasive alternative that achieves high diagnostic performance while also reducing patient discomfort and risk compared to conventional X-ray mammography and ultrasonography. Based on a multi-criteria analysis, PA imaging has been deemed by experts the best course of action for early diagnosis, on the basis of cost-effectiveness, among other factors, and general patient comfort (Hilgerink et al., 2011). With the optimization of system configurations—for example, enhancing algorithm quality and detector sensitivity—PA imaging can radically change the standard of clinical diagnosis, with a good case for its integration into breast imaging protocols. The imaging modality to be used is more than mere sensitivity and specificity; it includes consideration of patient experience and diagnostic clarity. Though MRI is now favored due to greater sensitivity and visualization of complex breast anatomy, complications like access to technology and cost restrict widespread use. Meanwhile, newer evidence indicates that the inclusion of ductoscopy and breast MRI is the way forward in the best approach to dealing with complaints such as pathologic nipple discharge. Combined, these have been shown to surpass more traditional methods, with sensitivity rates as low as 96% (Panzironi et al., 2019). With further research still seeking combinations of modality, the focus remains on the delivery of accurate, timely diagnosis, together with sensitivity to patient-centered medicine that both honors efficacy and comfort. This continuous innovation in breast imaging represents a promising direction towards greater health outcomes.

5.4.1. Sensitivity and Specificity of Each Modality

The evaluation of sensitivity and specificity in breast imaging techniques is paramount for effective cancer detection and treatment. Digital mammography, as the standard modality, has a sensitivity of approximately 72.4% in breast lesion case detection. While still a standard modality, this modality's diagnostic specificity is limited, at only 46.4%. These findings indicate that while mammography can identify a large proportion of breast cancer, it is also associated with a high rate of false positives. This limitation necessitates the study and use of more sophisticated imaging technology to increase early detection rates and prevent unnecessary operations on patients, thus once again highlighting the necessity for a critical appraisal of novel modalities. Breast magnetic resonance imaging (MRI) has greater sensitivity at 93.1%, indicating a strong ability to identify lesions compared to digital mammography. With this greater sensitivity, MRI can prove to be an effective tool, especially in those at high risk or with dense breasts, where regular mammography is not as effective. MRI's specificity is less at 60.7%, which again shows a trade-off between sensitivity and specificity with imaging technologies (Figure 5.10).

Imaging modality	Sensitivity	Specificity
Mammography	~72%	~47%
MRI	~93%	~61%
Ultrasound	~61%	~87%
PET	~77-100%	~69-80%
CT	~71%	~83%
Thermography	~39%	~82%
3D (Tomosynthesis)	~100%	~75%

Figure 5.10. Comparative sensitivity and specificity matrix of mammography, ultrasound, and MRI modalities.

Source: https://encrypted-tbn0.gstatic.com/images?q=tbn:ANd9GcRHBCEb0_P9jTadUEX1VNUdy_ZqLce3TS7dsQ&s

The data suggest that while in some instances breast MRI may be an excellent adjunct, the incidence of false-positive results may trigger unnecessary anxiety and unneeded follow-up tests for patients. Therefore, knowledge of the specific indications and limitations of MRI in breast imaging is important for radiologists and oncologists. The advent of breast tomosynthesis has revolutionized the landscape of breast imaging by imparting valuable gains in sensitivity and specificity. Recent studies have revealed that breast tomosynthesis can achieve a 100% sensitivity as well as a 75% specificity. This innovation has the potential to reduce false-positive rates associated with digital mammography, and thus it is becoming an increasingly sought-after modality for screening and diagnostic evaluation. The receiver operating characteristics (ROC) curve analysis emphasizes the diagnostic advantage of breast tomosynthesis over MRI and traditional mammography, and points to it as a more reliable option. The significant performance measure differences highlight tomosynthesis's potential to enhance early detection, ultimately generating better patient outcomes in the treatment of breast cancer, as seen in earlier findings (Pavic et al., 2015).

5.4.2. Cost-Effectiveness and Accessibility

In the current healthcare setting, cost-effectiveness of modalities used in breast imaging is a key determinant of their global use and access. Mammography, as a lead diagnostic modality for detecting breast cancer, benefits from the praises of comparative affordability and broad accessibility, contributing mostly to early detection rates. However, inequities in access to mammography persist, often driven by socioeconomic factors, local factors, and patient awareness. This provides an uneven ground for the diagnosis and treatment of breast cancer, calling for interventions that ensure equal access. Further, the use of new technologies, such as artificial intelligence for mammographic screening, has the scope to enhance diagnostic efficiency and accuracy and, ultimately, be an affordable option by reducing rates of false positives and unnecessary follow-up visits, thereby reducing both patient and healthcare system costs, as in the innovation in (Hilgerink et al., 2011). The invention of novel imaging techniques, such as photoacoustic (PA) imaging, reflects continuous progress in diagnosing breast cancer, and cost-effectiveness is a critical consideration. PA imaging is non-invasive in nature and has fewer related risks than traditional mammography and ultrasonography, and, therefore, is a sensible choice for the detection of early stages (Figure 5.11).

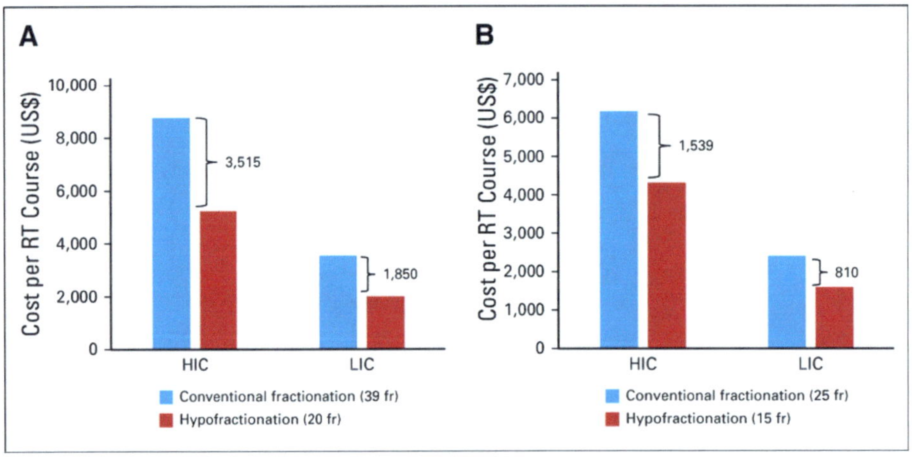

Figure 5.11. Bar graph showing average costs of each imaging modality in various systems of healthcare.

Source: https://www.researchgate.net/profile/Ahmed-Elzawawy-2/publication/340992888/figure/fig2/AS:885482829398016@1588126966763/Bar-graphs-of-A-a-comparison-of-the-cost-reduction-per-radiation-therapy-RT-course.png

Yet, their adoption must be balanced with the need for stringent clinical testing of their diagnostic precision. As seen in Hilgerink et al. (2011), while PA imaging holds promise, its cost-effectiveness remains contingent on improving the sensitivity of its detectors and reconstruction algorithms. Therefore, careful evaluations that incorporate elements such as patient comfort, risks, and relative diagnostic performance are essential to determine the true value of PA imaging as an alternative or supplement to existing practices, while maximizing the utilization of healthcare resources. Mitigating the disparities in breast imaging access requires specialized measures that integrate technology with cost-effectiveness. Recent advances, including 3D tomosynthesis, have proved to be more sensitive in dense breasts among women, making diagnostic exams more thorough and precise (Kukuła et al., 2024). The newer imaging modalities, however, cost more, which might further limit access for the underserved. Health policy efforts to educate about the importance of routine screenings must be undertaken in areas with low participation rates. In addition, intersessions between policymakers, healthcare professionals, and community organizations can make integration of state-of-the-art technologies in current frameworks feasible in a way that all patients, regardless of their socioeconomic status, can have access to advanced breast imaging techniques. The complementarity of cost-effectiveness and accessibility in breast imaging is critical to reducing mortality rates and improving overall patient outcomes.

5.4.3. Patient Experience and Comfort Levels

The comfort of patients and their experience with breast imaging examinations have a profound influence on the efficiency of overall diagnosis and the psychological well-being of the patients. Mammography, as the long-standing pillar of breast cancer screening, tends to be uncomfortably compression-induced. This unpleasantness can discourage women from undergoing routine examinations, which emphasizes comfortable patient management. The integration of imaging technology innovations, such as photoacoustic imaging, offers promising avenues to reduce distress without sacrificing diagnostic precision. The features of new technologies, such as reduced risk and non-invasiveness, point to their potential to enhance the patient experience appreciably and support screening adherence recommendations (Hilgerink et al., 2011). Comfort includes not just physical aspects, but psychological problems such as fear and anxiety regarding diagnoses too. Excessive worry is bound to impact the patient's cooperation with compulsory imaging. In this context, clinicians play an important role in guaranteeing a good experience (Figure 5.12).

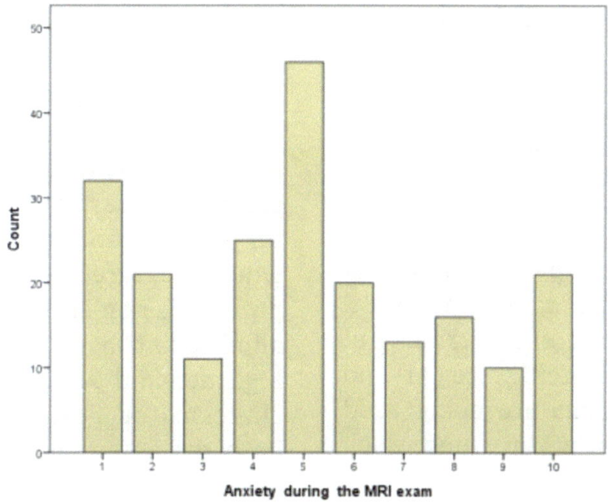

Figure 5.12. Survey results displaying patient preferences on imaging comfort, duration, and anxiety levels.

Source: https://ars.els-cdn.com/content/image/1-s2.0-S1687850723002674-gr2.jpg

Open communication, reassurance, and the provision of educational material about the imaging process can alleviate fear and enhance comfort. Second, bringing the imaging facility as a reassuring and comforting place is significant. As patients are well-informed about advances in breast imaging technologies, they may be more empowered to actively participate in their health care decisions, thereby enhancing their experience. Provision of patient comfort and experience also includes the consideration of different imaging modalities based on their respective advantages and limitations. New technologies, as outlined above, offer extra options for patients, combining effective screening with less discomfort. Emphasizing the core of patient-centered care, the healthcare system should appreciate innovations allowing comfort and accurate diagnosis. A multi-criteria approach used for photoacoustic imaging considers key parameters such as cost, diagnostic quality, and, most importantly, patient comfort (Hilgerink et al., 2011). Applying these findings to practices in breast imaging has the potential to revolutionize patient experiences by fostering a culture that respects their needs and values their preferences, ultimately leading to better health outcomes and higher rates of participation in screening programs.

5.5. Future Directions in Breast Imaging

The breast imaging landscape is evolving at a fast rate, primarily due to technological advancements and increased understanding of breast pathology. Artificial intelligence (AI) and machine learning algorithms are being used to evaluate imaging data, a key trend. Such technology has the potential to make diagnosis more precise by identifying subtle patterns on mammograms and MRIs that may go unnoticed to human perception. AI's ability to process enormous amounts of data can drive more tailored imaging protocols, which fundamentally transform the way clinicians will deal with breast cancer screening and diagnosis. Moreover, AI integration can simplify workflows, enabling radiologists to focus on challenging cases that require human expertise. As health care systems continue to embrace these technologies, the future of breast imaging will move away from conventional techniques toward more technologically advanced methods, promoting better patient outcomes and earlier malignancy detection (Kolari et al., 2011). Another pattern that is redefining the future of breast imaging is the emergence of hybrid imaging modalities. The combination of modalities such as positron emission tomography (PET) with magnetic resonance imaging (MRI) or ultrasound enhances the diagnostic potential of breast imaging. The combination offers an improved assessment of breast lesions, enabling doctors to examine anatomical as well as metabolic characteristics. Hybrid imaging could greatly improve the detection rate of very small tumors, which is critical for successful early treatment. Besides, the technique can distinguish benign from malignant lesions, reducing unnecessary biopsies. As these techniques become more accepted in clinical practice, they are likely to lead to less invasive, more effective management strategies for individuals with high-risk breast cancer (Hospital et al., 2023). In combination with technological developments, other imaging modalities, such as thermography, are gaining interest due to their potential utility for breast cancer detection. Thermography, which measures heat changes in breast tissue, provides a non-surgical alternative for use as an adjunct to conventional imaging methods. The high demand for thermographic signs among clinicians suggests that such methodologies have the potential to increase early detection rates, particularly in women with tightly packed breast tissue, where mammography may be less efficient. Research has established a correlation between thermographic signs and tumor characteristics, particularly in its potential for diagnosis (Kolari et al., 2011). As research continues to verify the reliability of thermography, it could become a standard part of breast cancer screening programs. The use of such new technology is part of the broader trend toward personalized medicine, which aims to tailor breast imaging to the patient's individual needs (Hospital AKU et al., 2023).

5.5.1. Advances in Imaging Technology

Technological improvements in imaging have dramatically changed the treatment of breast cancer, increasing early detection rates and enabling more tailored treatment.

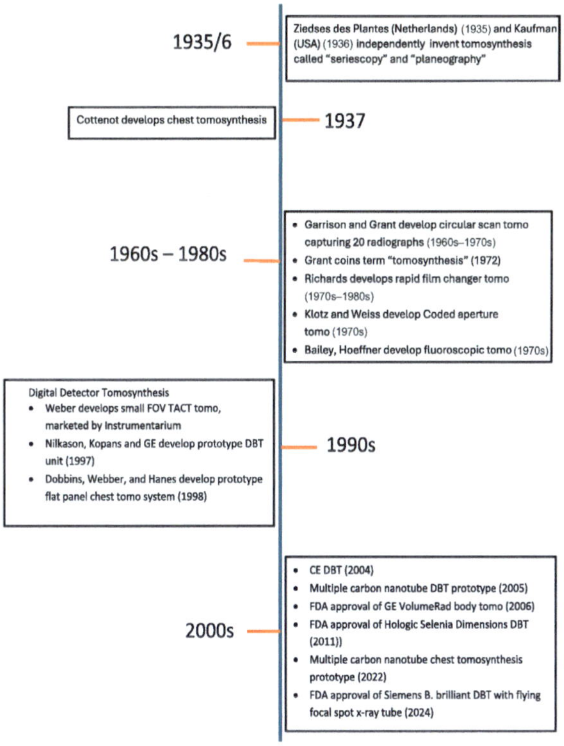

Figure 5.13. Timeline showing the evolution of breast imaging technologies from analog to digital and tomosynthesis.

Source: https://www.spiedigitallibrary.org/ContentImages/Journals/JMIOBU/12/S1/S13012/FigureImages/JMI_12_S1_S13012_f004.png

Among numerous modalities, mammography has long been the gold standard. Nevertheless, the limitations of this modality, particularly for malignancy in women with dense breasts, have promoted ongoing research into additive imaging strategies. This paradigm shift is essential since breast cancer remains the most frequent cancer among women and, in the UK alone, over 45,000 new cases are diagnosed annually. Continuous advances aim to find new technologies that can replace or complement routine mammography for the effective detection of masses in breasts, bypassing the drawback of dense tissues and hard interpretations of results. Magnetic resonance imaging (MRI) is now a valuable adjunct to mammography, especially in the high-risk population and for pre-treatment assessment of the magnitude of clinical findings (Figure 5.13).

MRI's ability to provide superior soft tissue contrast facilitates the detection of early-stage breast cancers that may elude standard mammography. Furthermore, it is increasingly being recommended for routine screening in specific high-risk groups due to its sensitivity and specificity in tumor detection. However, the technique has drawbacks, including high costs and the need for intravenous contrast media, which limits its accessibility in some healthcare settings. Despite such challenges, the pursuit of new non-invasive imaging technologies remains a priority as health care systems strive to enhance early detection capabilities while minimizing the limitations presented by existing techniques (N/A, 2007). New developments in imaging technology have seen promising advancements such as improved digital infrared thermal imaging (DITI), which leverages advanced infrared radiation detection capacity and advanced computational software. Initial research in rodent models indicates the potential to detect elevated vascularization associated with tumor development before detection with conventional imaging techniques. With ongoing research in breast cancer, integration of DITI into practice has the potential to provide a non-invasive means of early detection. This evolving situation emphasizes the necessity of continued investment in research and technology for developing reliable substitutes to support or complement traditional imaging modalities to facilitate more effective screening and diagnosis for more people at risk of breast cancer (N/A, 2007).

5.5.2. Artificial Intelligence Integration in Imaging

Breast imaging with the advancements in artificial intelligence (AI) is a significant step forward in technology that is bound to improve diagnostic efficiency and streamline clinical processes. Early diagnosis is the key to controlling breast cancer, and mammography has been an essential component of its management for years. New advancements, particularly since the introduction of AI, are transforming conventional imaging paradigms. Computer-aided detection (CAD) software programs are now able to identify lesions and abnormalities at very high speeds and accuracy, which aids radiologists in tumor identification in the early stages. According to Naser et al. (2024), the ongoing development of such AI technologies not only improves cancer detection rates but also aids radiologists in interpreting complex imaging findings, with the potential to improve patient management and tailored treatment protocols (Figure 5.14).

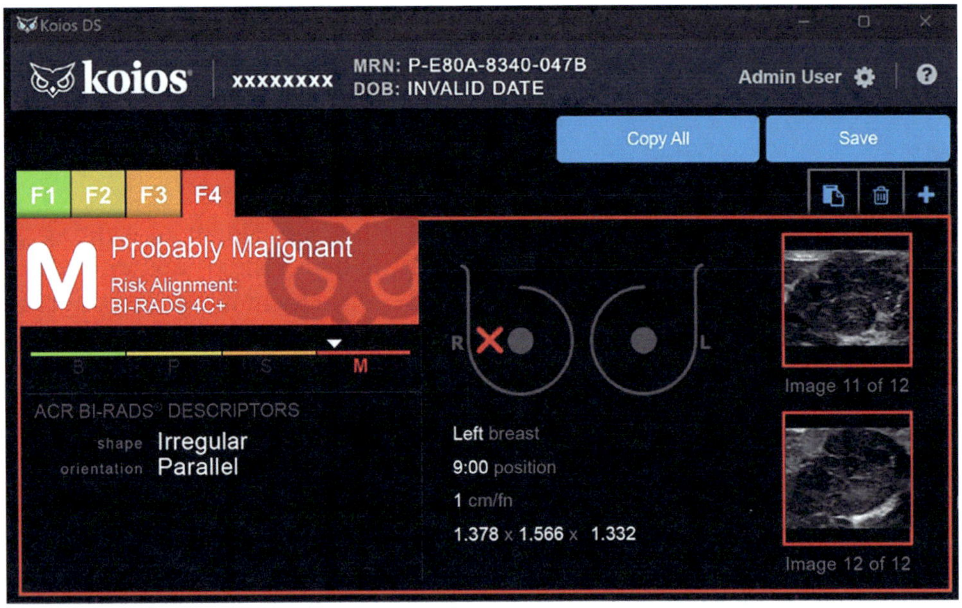

Figure 5.14. Example interface of an AI-assisted breast imaging software with lesions detected.

Source: https://cdn.agilitycms.com/applied-radiology/publishhub/AR-54-2-0075/AR-54-2-0075-F001.jpeg

The application of AI in the clinic extends far beyond mammography to even advanced imaging technologies such as magnetic resonance imaging (MRI). AI platforms can evaluate multiparametric MRI scan data to provide detailed information on tumor characteristics, aiding the clinician in making informed decisions about the best treatment options. In particular, AI can assist in distinguishing between benign and malignant findings, essential in reducing unnecessary biopsies and ensuing patient distress. As Kukuła et al. (2024) theorized, such advancements hold promise for AI-enhanced mammographic sensitivity and improved outcomes, particularly among women with dense breasts. By removing mundane tasks, AI allows radiologists to focus on more complex analyses, ultimately benefiting healthcare professionals and patients alike. Despite its potential, effective deployment of AI in breast imaging also demands tight management of integration with existing clinical systems and the development of robust legal frameworks. AI systems need to be developed that augment, rather than replace, human radiological skill. Future research should also aim to continuously optimize algorithms to support complex patient populations and scenarios in clinical practice. Education campaigns directed at the public also help explain to patients the benefits of AI-based imaging approaches. As Kukuła et al. (2024) have proposed, enhancing participation rates for screening programs could also help achieve higher early detection, along with streamlining disparities in access to quality care. Internationally, the use of AI in breast imaging is a revolutionary shift, which will usher in more precise diagnoses and improved patient care over the next few years (Figure 5.15).

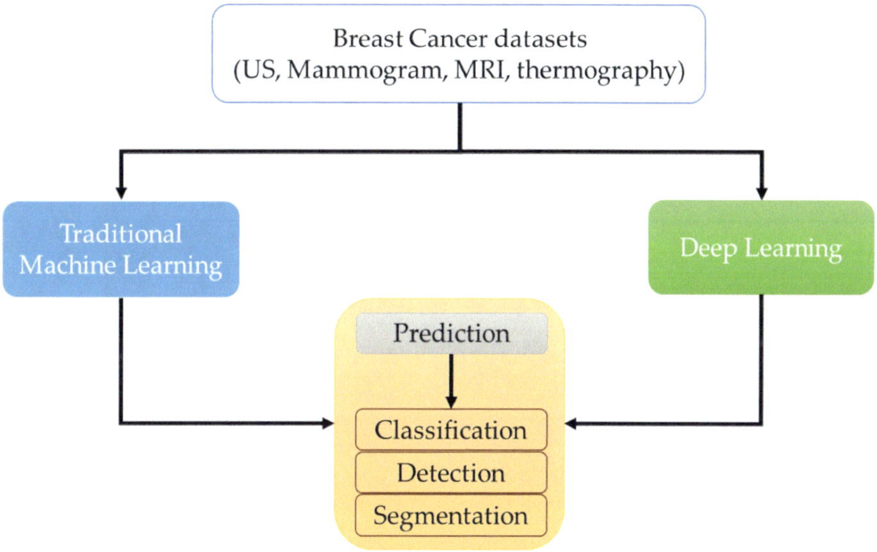

Figure 5.15. AI decision support system in breast imaging illustrating algorithm probability scores and risk stratification.

Source: https://www.mdpi.com/tomography/tomography-10-00055/article_deploy/html/images/tomography-10-00055-g001.png

5.5.3. Potential for Personalized Breast Cancer Screening

Individualized breast cancer screening is at the forefront with the role of developing technology and a better understanding of genetic risk factors redefining traditional approaches to diagnosis. By referencing knowledge about patient-specific risk factors, clinicians can tailor screening modalities to each patient's unique profile. Such individualization may involve the addition of genetic test findings, family history, and lifestyle determinants to imaging modalities such as mammography and MRI. This specific screening might enable the earlier detection of breast cancer, particularly in individuals at elevated risk, and thereby optimize the efficacy of treatment while considerably reducing mortality. The promise of uniquely identifying the patient likely to benefit from heightened surveillance is significant, as highlighted by current efforts to develop customized screening regimens that would replace the omnipresent one-size-fits-all norm that currently dominates the clinical environment. New technologies, including artificial intelligence (AI) and imaging modalities, are central to realizing the potential of personalized breast cancer screening. Imaging methods such as contrast-enhanced mammography (CEM) and radiomics enable more subtle evaluation of breast tissue, thereby permitting sophisticated analyses that are better placed to inform screening decisions. Machine learning algorithms can also process large datasets to identify patterns that would be undetectable to clinicians, leading to improved risk stratification (Figure 5.16).

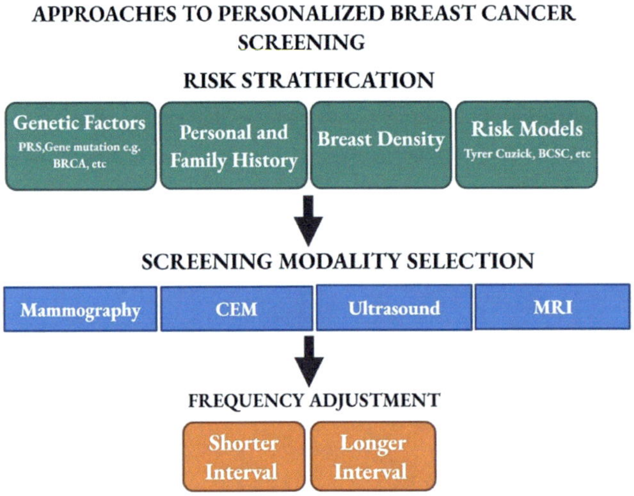

Figure 5.16. Conceptual diagram of personalized breast cancer screening by imaging history and genetic risk.

Source: https://media.springernature.com/lw1200/springer-static/image/art%3A10.1186%2Fs43055-025-01654-3/MediaObjects/43055_2025_1654_Fig3_HTML.png

These developments in breast imaging technologies can improve the effectiveness of screening, especially in women with dense breasts, where standard mammography is not as effective. Therefore, the combination of advanced imaging technologies with individualized risk predictions could transform breast cancer screening, paving the way for personalized and efficient detection methods that have the potential to save lives in the future. The shift in breast cancer screening from standard to personalized practice does not rely solely on technological advancement but also on a revolution in clinical practice and public health policy. Health care providers and patients must be informed about the advantages and restrictions of tailored screening technologies. Moreover, implementation of such individualized approaches demands a robust infrastructure that supports data transfer along with interdisciplinary coordination involving oncology, radiology, and genetic experts. These multidisciplinary partnerships will be indispensable in developing thorough guidelines that integrate personal risk and technology potential. Lastly, the journey towards personalized breast cancer screening will make healthcare a system where preventive and anticipatory care are embraced, hence translating imaging advances into tangible benefits for patients as well as limiting the societal impact of breast cancer, as highlighted by the historic overview of screening efficacy discussed in contemporary literature (Bhushan et al., 2021; Abbate et al., 2023).

SUMMARY

Lastly, the shift of breast imaging technologies from traditional mammography to advanced modalities such as MRI attests to the importance of accuracy in diagnosis and patient care in breast cancer. The conventional application of X-ray mammography, although the most prevalent method of early detection, reflects inherent sensitivity and specificity limitations, particularly in dense breasts. As outlined in various research, the introduction of photoacoustic imaging technologies promises to bridge these gaps, providing a more comprehensive diagnostic setting. Innovations like photoacoustic imaging, combining the virtues of conventional imaging without much risk, are a step forward toward a more personalized approach that prioritizes patient comfort and cost-effectiveness alongside diagnostic efficacy (Hilgerink et al., 2011). In addition, the critical assessment of emerging technologies, like microwave imaging, highlights significant improvements in detection techniques that may shortly be equivalent to conventional means. The advantages inherent in microwave imaging, namely its cost-effectiveness and simplicity, may bring crucial benefits to clinical settings, especially to low-resource centers. Experimental demonstrations are positive with breast phantoms, suggesting that further research can confirm its value as a practical substitute for conventional imaging equipment (Elsdon et al., 2010). With ongoing progress in these areas, their incorporation into standard practice is probable, potentially leading to better outcomes for patients in the detection and treatment of breast cancer. In the end, the future of breast imaging lies in combining various methodologies to create a robust, interdisciplinary approach to cancer diagnosis. As the healthcare industry evolves, there is a need to continue testing and integrating new technologies responsive to the multifaceted needs of patients. The incorporation of approaches like photoacoustic and microwave imaging can serve as a model for other diagnostic equipment that is efficient yet affordable. With the incorporation of such advances, the clinical practice can render the detection of breast cancer more precise, ultimately affecting treatment and survival rates in various populations of women. This kind of ongoing emphasis on development promises much for the future of breast cancer eradication, hence rendering the exploration of new imaging modalities a core part of continuing research and clinical practice.

CLOSER LOOK

BREAST IMAGING: MAMMOGRAPHY TO MRI

The development from mammography to MRI for breast imaging represents significant improvements in the detection and management of breast cancer. Mammography has long been a routine method of breast cancer screening, providing crucial data by detecting microcalcifications and tumors. Despite its widespread application, its limitations in sensitivity, particularly in women with dense breasts, have elicited continued research in other imaging modalities. MRI, with its improved soft-tissue discrimination and the ability to detect lesions not easily imaged by mammography, has emerged as an important adjunctive modality. This development underscores the requirement for the use of multiple imaging modalities to allow maximum diagnostic precision and enhance early detection rates, in turn impacting therapeutic strategies and patient outcomes in the treatment of breast cancer. At the center of breast imaging efficacy lies accurate measurement of breast volume, which is of utmost importance during surgery. Studies have found significant inconsistencies in the accuracy of different volume measurement techniques. Systematic reviews have demonstrated that MRI performs well relative to other techniques, with error measurements below 10% across different breast sizes (Choppin et al., 2016). This precision is particularly vital during preoperative planning, when understanding of breast volume can guide surgical technique and reconstruction options. Even in an increased-cost, out-of-routine environment, the precision of MRI in breast volume assessment might make its application acceptable in selected clinical contexts, further solidifying the role of MRI as an adjunct to more traditional imaging methods such as mammography. Compounding the complexity of breast imaging is the built-in challenge of interpreting imaging in that high sensitivity does not always translate into high specificity. While MRI gives advanced visualization for tumor detection enhancement, it is also associated with risks of undue tumor size overestimation (Anidjar et al., 2017). These include clinical T-stage and histologic subtype and can significantly affect the correlation between MRI-derived measures and actual tumor size, leading to potential mismanagement in treatment planning. This calls for ongoing research to develop better imaging technologies and their application in the clinical setting. By deducing the impact of various parameters on MRI output, medical practitioners are better equipped to handle the subtleties of breast cancer diagnosis and to improve the accuracy of tumor size estimates.

REFERENCES

1. Nicosia, L., Gnocchi, G., Gorini, I., Venturini, M., Fontana, F., Pesapane, F., Abiuso, I., Bozzini, A. C., Pizzamiglio, M., Latronico, A., Abbate, F., Meneghetti, L., Battaglia, O., Pellegrino, G., & Cassano, E. (2023). History of Mammography: Analysis of Breast Imaging Diagnostic Achievements over the Last Century. *Healthcare, 11*(11), 1596. https://doi.org/10.3390/healthcare11111596Aga Khan University Hospital, Karachi. (2023). *LABRAD, 48*(1), July 2023. https://core.ac.uk/download/578442137.pdf (accessed on 15th July 2025).
2. Ambrosio, M., Bocchi, G., Bramesfeld, A., Deandrea, S., Dimitrova, N., Lerda, D., Neamtiu, L., et al. (2017). Report on the call for feedback about the scope of the European guidelines for breast cancer screening and diagnosis: European Commission Initiative on Breast Cancer. https://core.ac.uk/download/84886790.pdf (accessed on 15th July 2025).
3. Bhushan, A., Gonsalves, A., & Menon, J. (2021). Current state of breast cancer diagnosis, treatment, and theragnostic. https://core.ac.uk/download/427549643.pdf (accessed on 15th July 2025).
4. Brenner Anidjar, R. D. (2017). Correlation between ultrasonography and magnetic resonance imaging with pathology-measured tumor size in women with recently diagnosed breast cancer: Optimizing tumor-size estimation with imaging techniques for higher precision. https://core.ac.uk/download/132092463.pdf (accessed on 15th July 2025).
5. Choppin, S., Gee, M., Goyal, A., Wheat, J., et al. (2016). The accuracy of breast volume measurement methods: A systematic review. https://core.ac.uk/download/42542002.pdf (accessed on 15th July 2025).
6. Elsdon, M., Fdo, M. J., Leach, M., Smith, G., et al. (2010). Breast cancer detection using microwave holography. https://core.ac.uk/download/4148312.pdf (accessed on 15th July 2025).
7. Evans, A., Purdie, C., Savaridas, S., Vinnicombe, S., et al. (2021). Contrast enhanced digital breast tomosynthesis for the monitoring of response to neoadjuvant chemotherapy: Preliminary results. https://core.ac.uk/download/619595990.pdf (accessed on 15th July 2025).
8. Hilgerink, M. P., Hummel, J. M., IJzerman, M. J., & Manohar, S., et al. (2011). Assessment of the added value of the Twente Photoacoustic Mammoscope in breast cancer diagnosis. https://core.ac.uk/download/pdf/11481011.pdf (accessed on 15th July 2025).
9. Kirchin, M., Luciani, M. L., Pediconi, F., Telesca, M., et al. (2015). Clinical utility of gadobenate dimeglumine in contrast-enhanced MRI of the breast: A review. https://core.ac.uk/download/141692117.pdf (accessed on 15th July 2025).
10. Kolarić, D., Karlović, K., Banić, M., Borojević, N., Antonini, S., Kuliš, T., Ferenčić, Ž., et al. (2011). Simplified description and interpretation of pathological thermography signs in malignant breast lesions. https://core.ac.uk/download/14444478.pdf (accessed on 15th July 2025).
11. Kukuła, P., Marschollek, J., Pachana, M., Piersiak, T., et al. (2024). Mammography in breast cancer screening–Current knowledge, challenges, the impact of artificial intelligence, and effectiveness with a focus on Poland. https://core.ac.uk/download/636385484.pdf (accessed on 15th July 2025).
12. Matijaš, T., & Teklić, J. (2023). Usporedba između magnetne rezonancije dojki i kontrastne mamografije. https://core.ac.uk/download/598041749.pdf (accessed on 15th July 2025).

13. Naser, M., Nasr, M. M., & Shehata, L. H. (2024). Advances of AI in breast cancer: Review. https://core.ac.uk/download/636457352.pdf (accessed on 15th July 2025).

14. Panzironi, G., Pediconi, F., & Sardanelli, F. (2019). Nipple discharge: The state of the art. https://core.ac.uk/download/188829787.pdf (accessed on 15th July 2025).

15. Pavic, D., Stojanov, D., Djilas, D., Roganovic, D., & Vujnovic, S. (2015). Breast MRI, digital mammography and breast tomosynthesis: Comparison of three methods for early detection of breast cancer. https://core.ac.uk/download/88559715.pdf (accessed on 15th July 2025).

16. Refahi, S., Behrouzkia, Z., & Hadadi, G. (1931). What are differences between medical imaging modalities for assessment of the breast. https://core.ac.uk/download/11686067.pdf (accessed on 15th July 2025).

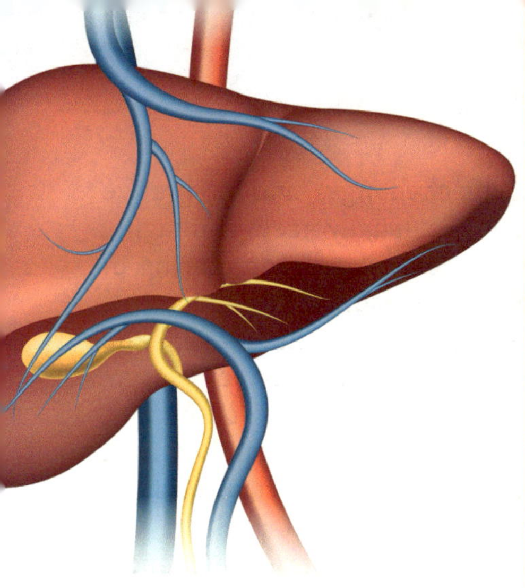

Chapter 6

ABDOMINAL IMAGING: LIVER, BILIARY, AND PANCREAS

Contents

Introduction

The field of abdominal imaging has made tremendous advancements, particularly in the liver, biliary, and pancreatic sectors. Abdominal imaging plays a significant role in the diagnosis and treatment of diseases of these organs, which are essential to gut function. With imaging techniques such as ultrasound, computed tomography (CT), and magnetic resonance imaging (MRI), clinicians can accurately detect abnormalities in patients, thereby instigating timely intervention. As pathological states are increasingly understood, imaging procedures have evolved to offer increased resolution and specificity. This evolution is not only required to detect tumors or obstructions but also to characterize inflammatory disease and evaluate chronic conditions that can threaten organ function. An integrated approach that combines imaging data with clinical context is required to maximize patient care, as fostered by interprofessional collaboration between clinics and radiologists. Furthermore, integrating imaging findings with clinical markers is particularly pertinent for complex conditions such as IgG4-

related gastrointestinal disease. The condition often presents diagnostic challenges, and integrative clinical evaluation, serologic testing, and multimodal imaging workups are usually needed. Imaging serves not only a detection purpose but is also used in ongoing management and monitoring of treatment efficacy. In symptomatic subjects, especially those with obstructive jaundice or abdominal pain, timely and accurate imaging is crucial for treatment decision-making. The guidelines for the management of IgG4-related diseases emphasize the necessity of a multi-disciplinary approach, with the reiteration that any imaging abnormalities should prompt serious consideration of therapy. These guidelines emphasize the role of imaging not only in diagnosis but also as a cornerstone in therapeutic decision-making, reflecting its pivotal role in patient outcomes. Furthermore, appreciation of the complexity of imaging modalities and their application to the diagnosis of liver, biliary, and pancreatic disease can contribute significantly to clinical practice. The emphasis on evidence-based guidelines, as in current literature, offers a systems-based perspective that aids clinicians in understanding the complexity of infectious and non-infectious processes of these life-sustaining organs. As a point of illustration, the microbiology of intra-abdominal infections demands careful selection of imaging studies to guide diagnostic methods, illustrating how imaging is a component of the broader diagnostic process. With a systematic approach in streamlining the diagnostic process, medical professionals can access the full potential of abdominal imaging. This facilitates them to make quicker and improved medical decisions, ultimately leading to improved health outcomes and improved patient care through an informed understanding of abdominal pathology.

6.1. Anatomy of the Liver

The liver is a vital organ in the human body that plays a substantial role in a wide array of metabolic processes, detoxification, and the secretion of bile. Its intricate anatomy is crucial for understanding how it functions and the impact of disease on it. The liver is divided into anatomical lobes, with the right being significantly larger than the left. The surface of the liver is covered by a fibrous layer referred to as Glisson's capsule, which protects the underlying tissues and surrounds the organ, separating it into lobules that represent functional units. The hepatocytes and lobules are the primary cells for most biochemical reactions (Figure 6.1).

The hepatic supply is unique; it is oxygenated by the hepatic artery and nutrient-supplied by the portal vein, highlighting its dual role in metabolism and digestion. In an abdominal imaging scenario, understanding liver anatomy is crucial for accurate diagnosis of hepatic pathologies. Imaging modalities such as ultrasound, computed tomography (CT), and magnetic resonance imaging (MRI) are highly useful for assessing liver structure and function. Every imaging technique has its advantages; for example, ultrasound is a non-invasive method for examining liver structure without radiation, while MRI offers superior contrast resolution, helpful in differentiating various hepatic lesions. The use of these imaging modalities enables a complete assessment, especially in complex cases where evaluation with a single modality may be insufficient. Radiologists must be able to recognize normal liver anatomical landmarks to diagnose pathology and have extensive knowledge of its intricate anatomy (Baccari et al., 2016). Novel imaging technologies, such as CEUS, are revolutionizing the evaluation of liver lesions. Although traditionally applied to adults, subsequent studies have demonstrated the use of CEUS in pediatric populations, especially for the assessment of focal liver lesions. The potential of CEUS is its ability to image vascular flow without exposing patients to ionizing radiation or nephrotoxic contrast agents. This is particularly beneficial to children because it makes the diagnostic environment safer. Clinical guidelines by organizations like the European Federation of Societies in Ultrasound and Medicine (EFSUMB) promote the use of CEUS not just in pediatric imaging but also for further research for expanded use in liver evaluations (Cantisani et al., 2016). By making such imaging techniques more accurate, healthcare professionals can enhance diagnostic outcomes and achieve optimal patient outcomes, particularly when treating liver-related disease.

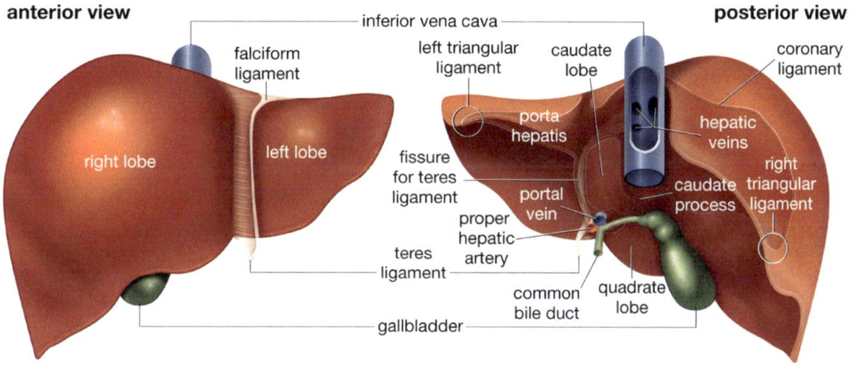

Figure 6.1. An annotated diagram showing the anterior and posterior surfaces of the liver with lobar divisions.

Source: https://www.researchgate.net/profile/Mehmet-Ayyildiz/publication/276386700/figure/fig11/AS:667885735256074@1536247776627/Liver-a-anterior-and-b-posterior-views-14.jpg.

6.1.1. Liver Structure and Function

The liver, being the organ of maximal significance in the human body, is maximally organized to perform an enormous number of vital functions. The most significant feature of the liver is its bi-circulatory character, where oxygenated blood is supplied by the hepatic artery and nutrient-rich blood by the portal vein. This unique circulatory structure enables the liver's primary function in metabolism and detoxification, enabling it to control blood sugar levels, metabolize lipids, and filter toxins from the blood. The liver also consists of functional units called lobules, which contain hepatocytes, bile ducts, and blood vessels. This structural organization enables efficient biochemical processes and contributes to the liver's ability to regenerate after injury. It is critical to understand the liver's purpose-built structure to appreciate its functional capacity, particularly in the context of disease that may be present within the organ. Image modalities play a critical role in assessing liver structure and function, particularly in the diagnosis and management of hepatic disease. Advanced imaging technologies such as ultrasound, computer tomography (CT), and magnetic resonance imaging (MRI) have a key role in revealing the anatomy of the liver, facilitating the detection of abnormalities such as tumors, cirrhosis, and fatty liver. For instance, imaging can show changes in the size, texture, and circulation of the liver, which are essential for early diagnosis and treatment planning. Current guidelines emphasize the applicability of elaborate imaging protocols in preoperative staging of liver tumors, underlining interdisciplinary care to avoid complications and enhance patient outcomes. The greater the integration of imaging information into clinical treatment, the more in line with the evolving hepatology landscape in which measurements of different imaging modalities play an integral role is the scenario (Cannavale et al., 2016). To this, an appreciation of how liver anatomy corresponds to its related functions has led to conditions such as hepatic steatosis and biliary diseases being researched. Non-invasive imaging techniques, including measurement of the hepatic surface area, have been enormously important in therapeutic planning for conditions such as hiatal hernias and related disorders (Boru et al., 2017). These methods provide helpful information about the pathological changes in the liver without the necessity of invasive procedures. The ability to evaluate and monitor liver function through imaging not only aids in diagnosing current conditions but also enables active management plans that can enhance patients' quality of life. As science advances, the role of imaging in liver disease is expected to grow, making personalized treatments possible and improving overall patient care.

6.1.2. Blood Supply and Drainage of the Liver

The liver receives blood supply from two main sources: the portal vein and the hepatic artery. The hepatic artery supplies the liver with approximately 25% of the hepatic blood supply, delivering oxygenated blood from the abdominal aorta. In contrast, the portal vein delivers the other 75% of the liver's blood supply, delivering blood rich in food from the gastrointestinal system and spleen. This dual supply system is critical to the liver's intricate functions, including metabolism, detoxification, and protein synthesis. The intricate vascular architecture of the liver permits efficient filtration and processing of blood, with hepatocytes functioning at the core of several biochemical conversions. Abdominal imaging modalities such as contrast-enhanced ultrasound (CEUS) and magnetic resonance imaging (MRI) are of great utility for imaging this vascular system and thus enhance knowledge of liver pathology and surgical planning (Figure 6.2).

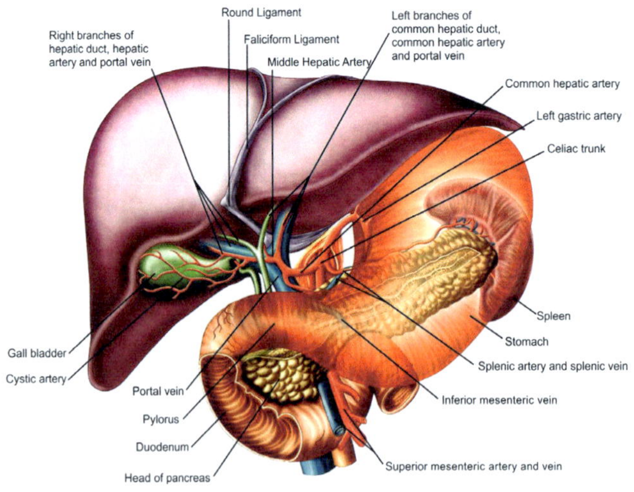

Figure 6.2. Vascular map of hepatic artery.

Source: https://www.verywellhealth.com/thmb/j0wmLfw7Qyr8qQCdRXYB6HyxmCA=/1500x0/filters:no_upscale():max_bytes(150000):strip_icc()/GettyImages-188057933-623b26f9e4c74d5c8dc30c7af642a7d0.jpg.

The hepatic veins are the primary drainage of blood from the liver that culminates in the inferior vena cava. The system is vital for maintaining hepatic venous pressure and preventing complications such as portal hypertension. The liver's ability to regulate its blood supply by constricting or dilating these vessels is instrumental in its response to physiological changes. Complications of disordered drainage are serious health risks, including ascites and variceal hemorrhage, which must be immediately addressed with medical care. Abdominal imaging techniques play a crucial role in assessing hepatic vein patency and function. Non-invasive techniques are utilized to detect pathology within the hepatic venous system, which guide clinical and operative management of liver disease or malignancy. Surgical therapies like liver resection are increasingly being used to cure hepatocellular carcinoma and metastases of other cancers. Successful liver surgery relies not only on skilled technique but also on absolute preoperative imaging that defines patterns of liver blood supply and drainage. Developments like Kelly clamps enhance surgical precision, allowing meticulous control of hemostasis and biliostasis intraoperatively. While liver resections have been proven to significantly improve long-term survival in patients with specific liver disease, they carry the risk of postoperative complications such as liver insufficiency, biliary leakage, and ascites. Understanding the vascular anatomy of the liver using advanced imaging is therefore essential for surgical teams to mitigate such complications and improve patient outcomes for the management of liver disease (Grazi et al., 2007).

6.1.3. General Anatomical Variations

Anatomical variation is the norm and part of the complexity seen in abdominal imaging, such as of the liver, biliary system, and pancreas. Vascular anatomical variations, such as celiac trunk configurations, are common and significantly impact surgical and interventional procedures. For instance, according to a descriptive retrospective study with multidetector computed tomography angiography (MDCTA), abnormalities such as the hepatogastrosplenic trunk were seen in 93% of the studied patients, along with less frequently occurring formations, including the coeliac mesenteric trunk, that were found in only 1.1% of the cases (Balthazar et al., 2009) (Figure 6.3). Understanding these anatomical variations is relevant because they are significant in preoperative planning and may contribute to surgical or interventional success. Anatomical variations, on the part of the pancreas, are of particular value when diagnosing illnesses such as pancreatitis or pancreatic pseudocysts. Such variations complicate the interpretation of imaging studies, leading to difficulty in discrimination between benign and malignant processes. A case study was presented, which showed the difficulty in differentiating between an eroded pancreatic pseudocyst into the splenoportal venous confluence and an arterial aneurysm, highlighting the need for accurate imaging techniques in such cases (Balthazar et al., 2009). Proper imaging modalities like ultrasound, computed tomography, and magnetic resonance imaging should be practiced with complete knowledge of anatomical variation so that there is no misinterpretation and the patient receives the most preferred results. Furthermore, intersubject variation in biliary anatomy also underscores the need for careful imaging evaluation. The occurrence of accessory bile ducts, variations in bile duct drainage, and gallbladder morphologies may affect the success of some surgical procedures, such as cholecystectomy. Understanding these variations allows clinicians to anticipate potential complications, thus enhancing procedure safety. Radiological assessments, according to research, enable visualization of such intricately related anatomy and enable individualized intervention to each patient's anatomy (Czyżowski et al., 2021). As anatomy variations continue to be discovered with imaging studies, they highlight the importance for healthcare practitioners to pay attention to these complexities when diagnosing and treating liver, biliary, and pancreatic illnesses.

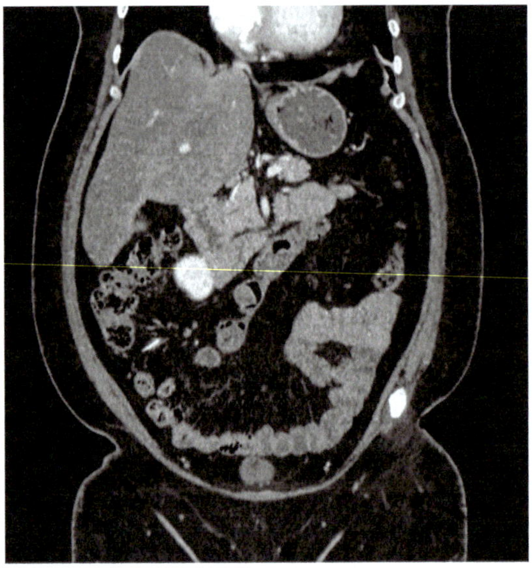

Figure 6.3. CT image showing a common anatomical variation: Riedel's lobe of the liver. *Source:* https://prod-images-static.radiopaedia.org/images/34702811/d95b18d45414156161f28dc146d74591481ccf0595284d69f70172a5c9d14c09_big_gallery.jpeg.

6.2. Imaging Modalities for the Liver

Liver disease diagnosis, in principle, relies on imaging modalities to achieve the organs' pathology, structure, and function. Of the primary modalities, ultrasound (US), computed tomography (CT), and magnetic resonance imaging (MRI) all possess distinctive strengths. The US is commonly the first imaging choice due to its availability, absence of invasive techniques, and ability to detect abnormalities such as masses and bile duct obstruction. CT, by contrast, provides high-resolution images instrumentals in the detection of liver tumors, including hepatocellular carcinoma and metastatic disease. Furthermore, advanced CT imaging can quantify hepatic vascular anatomy, which aids surgical planning. However, while CT is effective in general assessments, ultrasound is generally better suited for real-time studies, particularly when dealing with acute pathology like biliary obstruction or gallstones, which are necessary for patient care (Boskoski et al., 2025). MRI has become an increasingly important tool in the diagnosis of liver disease due to its improved soft-tissue contrast and lack of ionizing radiation. MRI is best suited to describe focal liver lesions and to distinguish benign from malignant lesions. With specific sequences, diffusion-weighted imaging and liver-specific gadolinium-based contrast media enhance diagnostic accuracy. MRI is also crucial in assessing diseases such as primary sclerosing cholangitis (PSC), where traditional modalities have proved insufficient for defining bile duct involvement (Oikarinen et al., 2001). Further, magnetic resonance cholangiography (MRC) complements MRI in that it gives high-quality images of the biliary tree, thus enabling the detection of obstruction of the biliary and strictures that can complicate liver disease (Oikarinen et al., 2001). Proper integration of these imaging techniques into a consistent diagnostic strategy is paramount to optimum patient care. Synergistic merging of the strengths of US, CT, and MRI by clinicians can allow for better overall evaluation of liver pathology. In addition, advances in imaging technology and the adoption of multidisciplinary strategies, including the use of artificial intelligence, promise to further enhance imaging's capacity for diagnosis. Each imaging modality not only reveals characteristic features of liver disease but also allows for crucial differential diagnoses, guiding treatment planning and interventional techniques. A multidisciplinary strategy that emphasizes the strengths of each imaging technique will improve clinical outcomes in patients with liver disease, yielding timely interventions and reducing delay-related complications (Boskoski et al., 2025).

6.2.1. Ultrasound in Liver Imaging

The role of ultrasound in imaging the liver is pivotal, as it offers a cost-effective and non-invasive approach to the evaluation of hepatic pathologies. The imaging process uses high-frequency sound waves to generate real-time images of the liver for analysis of its structure and function. Some of the significant advantages of ultrasound are that it can detect liver pathology, such as tumors, cysts, and cirrhosis, without exposing the liver to the dangers of invasive techniques, such as biopsies. In addition, as Doppler ultrasound is now an option, hepatic vasculature can be inspected to diagnose conditions such as portal hypertension. Thus, ultrasound is not merely the initial imaging of choice but also a valuable adjunct to decision and management and continuation with further examination of liver disease (Al-Haddad et al., 2014) (Figure 6.4).

In addition, ultrasound success in liver imaging relies significantly on operator skill and patient factors, including bowel gas and body habitus, which can obscure image clarity. Advances in ultrasound technology, such as contrast-enhanced ultrasound (CEUS), enhance the detectability of liver lesions by providing dynamic perfusion patterns to separate malignant from benign tumors. CEUS employs microbubble contrast agents to define vascular structures in the liver, improving diagnostic accuracy. This technique is a breakthrough in hepatology because it allows doctors to make more precise decisions during diagnosis and treatment. Since liver pathology is multifaceted and precise imaging modalities are required, the evolution of ultrasound techniques remains a key issue in improving diagnostic capabilities in abdominal imaging (Illanes et al., 2017).

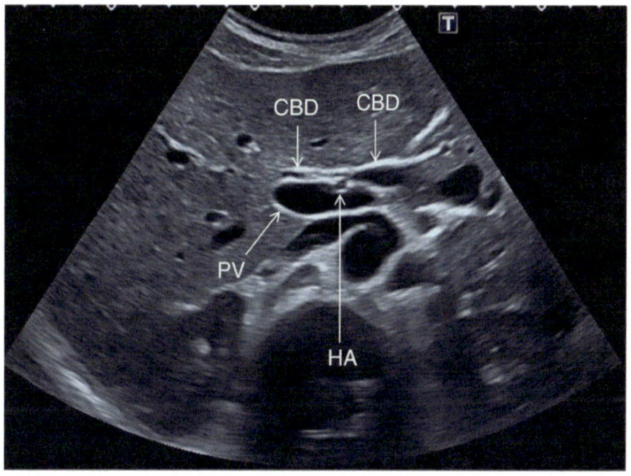

Figure 6.4. Abdominal ultrasound image demonstrating normal liver echotexture and landmarks. *Source:* https://radiologykey.com/wp-content/uploads/2024/02/c03f008.jpg.

Moreover, ultrasound, along with clinical presentation, is a key aspect of optimal management of liver pathology. For instance, in hepatocellular carcinoma surveillance in patients with chronic liver disease, routine ultrasound scans are critical for timely detection. Ultrasound's characteristic of providing immediate feedback regarding the liver's status allows real-time assessment of disease progression and resolution after therapeutic interventions. Furthermore, ultrasound enables therapeutic interventions to be guided, such as draining fluid or performing biopsies, thereby optimizing patient management. Because health professionals are increasingly employing ultrasound in the evaluation of the liver, studies that focus on its applications and advances can help make its diagnostic and management contributions to liver, biliary, and pancreatic diseases a part of the broader canopy of abdominal imaging (Al-Haddad et al., 2014).

6.2.2. CT Scan and MRI for Liver Evaluation

Liver diseases have traditionally been evaluated using a multi-modality imaging approach, with CT scans and MRI widely accepted as pillars. CT scans are rapid and provide accurate cross-sectional images of the liver, allowing identification of hepatic masses, vascular abnormalities, and hepatic morphology. The modality is useful in acute conditions, where rapid diagnosis and treatment plans are made. Contrast-enhanced CT has been shown to have higher sensitivity for detecting malignant lesions and is thus a cornerstone of oncologic evaluation. Furthermore, the capability of CT scans to depict the degree of liver disease, that is, cirrhotic changes and portal hypertension, is crucial in treatment planning and prognosis. Conversely, MRI has evolved as an adjunctive modality for liver assessment, with advantages such as characterization of hepatic lesions (Figure 6.5).

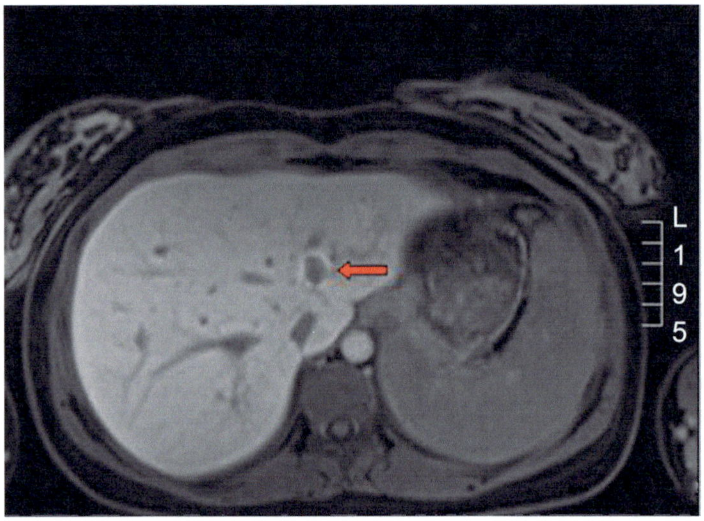

Figure 6.5. T1-weighted MRI of the liver showing high-resolution contrast of hepatic parenchyma. *Source:* https://www.researchgate.net/profile/Kor-Woi-Tiang/publication/260834691/figure/fig2/AS:496422836944896@1495367835089/T1-weighted-MRI-axial-view-Liver-lesion-consistent-with-focal-nodular-hyperplasia.png.

The use of various MRI sequences can enhance the distinction between malignant and benign tumors, providing even better soft-tissue contrast than CT. In addition, MRI is very useful in evaluating conditions like fatty liver disease and iron overload, where specific sequences can provide information on the liver's biochemical environment. The non-invasive nature of MRI and the fact that it is not based on ionizing radiation make it an option, especially in patients undergoing multiple imaging studies, such as those with chronic liver disease. Multimodality imaging enables complete evaluation, with improved diagnostic performance and patient care. A combination of both CT and MRI is crucial in the overall treatment of liver disease. Each modality has unique strengths; CT is often the first imaging modality of choice due to its rapid acquisition and assessment of complex cases. MRI increasingly has been employed as a problem-solving tool, especially when

CT findings are non-diagnostic or additional characterization of liver masses is required. This combination of imaging modalities enhances the diagnostic process, enabling differentiation and staging of various liver pathologies and guiding optimal treatment interventions. Finally, the combination of CT and MRI not only enhances diagnostic accuracy but also supports a patient-centered approach to the management of hepatic diseases, highlighting the importance of tailored imaging strategies in practice.

6.2.3. Role of Elastography in Liver Disease Evaluation

Elastography has emerged as a prominent non-invasive imaging method with a significant role in the evaluation of liver disease. Elastography provides beneficial information regarding the degree of fibrosis and cirrhosis using liver stiffness measurement, which are central determinants of liver disease prognosis and treatment. This imaging modality has several advantages over traditional methods, including the ability to perform the test at the bedside and in real time, enabling efficient clinical decision-making. With the increasing prevalence of chronic liver disease, the use of elastography in routine clinical practice enhances the accuracy of fibrosis staging, thereby aiding the tailoring of therapeutic strategies (Figure 6.6).

Therefore, elastography has become universally accepted as a standard part of the diagnostic evaluation for liver disease, particularly in evaluating patients with hepatitis and non-alcoholic fatty liver disease, where prompt treatment can significantly alter disease course (Nydegger et al., 2010). The reliability and validity of elastography are also boosted with advances in technology. Techniques such as Acoustic Radiation Force Impulse (ARFI) and Transient Elastography have enabled clinicians to accurately assess liver stiffness non-invasively. For instance, ARFI has been central to differentiating the various stages of liver fibrosis and to ensuring proper monitoring and treatment of patients at risk of developing liver complications (Majaz et al., 2012). Studies indicate that elastography can also distinguish between the causes of liver disease, a distinction that clinicians would prefer to base treatment decisions on. Furthermore, its application is broadening into the field of monitoring response to treatment because changes in liver stiffness can portend therapeutic response, thereby providing a dynamic assessment of patients' liver status over time.

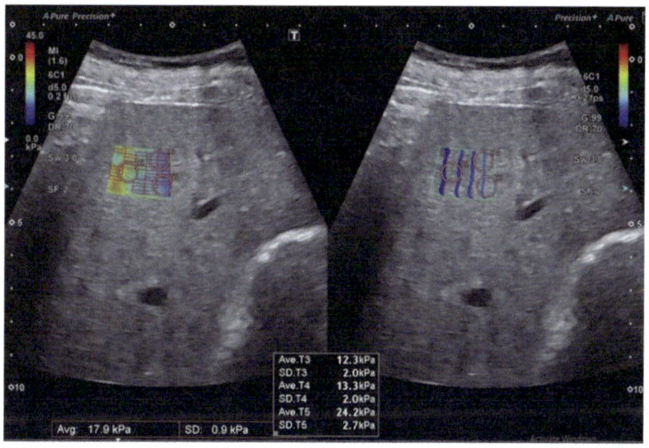

Figure 6.6. SWE image showing liver fibrosis stage F4 with average median value of liver stiffness of about 17.9 kpa.

Source: https://www.researchgate.net/profile/Mahjabeen-Liaqat/publication/354237888/figure/fig2/AS:1062785442119680@1630399203773/SWE-image-showing-liver-fibrosis-stage-F4-with-average-median-value-of-liver-stiffness-of.jpg.

In addition to its use in fibrosis measurement, elastography also assists clinicians in obtaining information regarding the overall status of the liver and its functioning capacity. The technique has been beneficial for characterizing conditions such as portal hypertension and hepatocellular carcinoma, which are critical for guiding patient management. Because multifaceted presentations accompany liver disease most of the time, elastography supports a more comprehensive assessment that can help identify conditions such as steatosis, which may be accompanied by fibrosis. Adding elastography to protocols for abdominal imaging, thus, represents an innovation in the treatment of liver disease because it supports a superior holistic care strategy for patients. As growing evidence supports its effectiveness, elastography can be poised to further revolutionize the diagnosis and management of liver diseases within the broader paradigm of modern medicine (Nydegger et al., 2010).

6.3. Common Liver Diseases

Liver diseases are a public health concern due to their commonness and overall effect on health. Some of the most prevalent liver diseases include hepatitis, cirrhosis, and fatty liver disease, which often arise from a multitude of risk factors like alcohol consumption, viral hepatitis, and metabolic disease. Hepatitis, particularly chronic hepatitis B and C, causes inflammation, which progresses to cirrhosis when left unattended. Cirrhosis has traditionally been defined as fibrosis and is often the ultimate stage of chronic liver disease, significantly increasing the risk for liver failure as well as hepatocellular carcinoma. Thus, regular imaging, such as ultrasound or CT scans, becomes a valuable diagnostic procedure, enabling early detection and treatment of these diseases. With enhanced imaging modalities, clinicians can more precisely assess liver morphology and guide treatment, thus improving the treatment results of patients with liver disease. Cirrhosis, being an adaptive response to chronic liver damage, is a critical turning point in the progression of liver disease. Cirrhosis can be caused by a broad spectrum of etiologies, including viral hepatitis, autoimmune diseases, and alcoholism. Imaging has a role in cirrhosis evaluation, measuring the amount of liver scarring or complications such as portal hypertension and variceal hemorrhage. MRI and CT are two of the abdominal imaging techniques that can identify characteristic findings, such as a nodular liver border or splenomegaly, which are indicative of advanced fibrosis. These imaging techniques provide not only information about cirrhosis severity but also help in surveillance for the development of hepatocellular carcinoma, as patients with cirrhosis are at much greater risk of this cancer. The addition of abdominal imaging to the cirrhosis treatment plan is thus important for both diagnosis and follow-up surveillance, enabling early intervention. Non-alcoholic fatty liver disease (NAFLD) is the most prevalent liver disease associated with obesity and metabolic syndrome. NAFLD is characterized by the accumulation of triglycerides in hepatocytes, and it can progress to non-alcoholic steatohepatitis (NASH), leading to fibrosis, cirrhosis, and hepatocellular carcinoma if not controlled. Diagnostic imaging is essential for assessing liver steatosis and its complications. Ultrasound is generally the first imaging modality due to its accessibility and sensitivity in showing liver fat accumulation. More sensitive data on liver stiffness and inflammation levels, which are necessary for differentiation from other liver diseases, are provided by advanced imaging techniques such as elastography and MRI. The rising burden of NAFLD necessitates reassessing imaging strategies to avoid missing opportunities for early detection and prevention of long-term complications of liver disease (Boru et al., 2017; Abberbock et al., 2017).

6.3.1. Hepatitis and Its Imaging Characteristics

Knowledge of hepatitis and radiological characteristics is crucial in order to diagnose and treat liver disease correctly. Hepatitis, an inflammatory disease of the liver, can be caused by viral hepatitis, autoimmune conditions, alcoholism, and other causes. Imaging modalities such as ultrasound (US), computed tomography (CT), and magnetic resonance imaging (MRI) play an important role in assessing liver anatomy and detecting hepatitis-related complications (Figure 6.7).

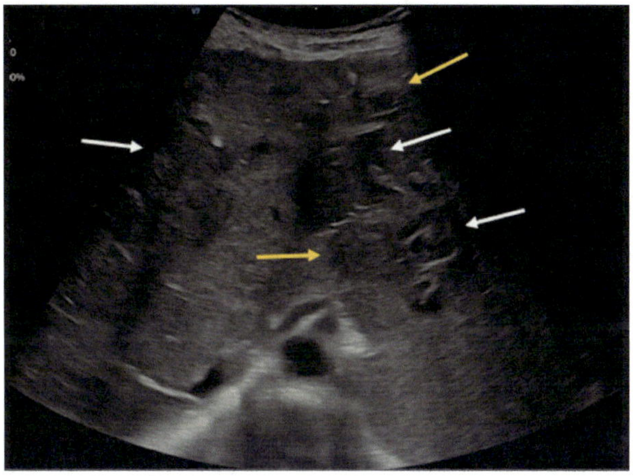

Figure 6.7. Multiple hypoechoic lesions are scattered throughout the liver parenchyma (white arrows). Some lesions show a target ring appearance that is a central hypoechoic area surrounded by hyperechoic rims (yellow arrows).

Source: https://www.researchgate.net/publication/376082616/figure/fig1/AS:11431281214996066@1703897277146/On-ultrasound-multiple-hypoechoic-lesions-are-noted-scattered-throughout-the-liver.ppm.

These imaging techniques not only allow visualization of liver enlargement and textural abnormalities but also allow lesion detection that can point towards complications such as cirrhosis or hepatocellular carcinoma. In particular, non-ionizing modalities such as US and MRI are used to avoid radiation exposure while obtaining detailed information on hepatic status, underscoring the importance of imaging in assessing the complex nature of hepatitis (Nydegger et al., 2010). Apart from identifying hepatic structural changes, imaging also plays a vital role in classifying hepatitis. For instance, acute hepatitis is often disclosed by some imaging characteristics such as hypoechoic patterns on ultrasound, while chronic hepatitis is disclosed by more heterogeneous echotexture and increased liver echogenicity. The more advanced imaging techniques, such as MRI using liver-sensitive contrast agents, give a clearer view of liver lesions and fibrosis. This becomes particularly relevant because liver disease severity can guide therapy decisions and prognostic evaluation. Thus, understanding these imaging characteristics aids physicians not only in the diagnosis of hepatitis but also in determining the extent of liver damage and possibly in altering appropriate therapeutic regimens, making radiological assessment part and parcel of the treatment of hepatitis (Nydegger et al., 2010). Secondly, integrating imaging characteristics into practice reinforces the need for structured training within HPB fellowship programs. Given the variability in training curricula in surgical oncology, transplant surgery, and HPB fellowships, a shared consensus on hepatitis imaging would significantly enhance outcomes. With the implementation of current imaging guidelines and protocols, future HPB surgeons will be able to treat hepatitis with a vast body of knowledge that will remain equally applicable to general surgery residency and subspecialties. The addition of a consensus-based curriculum not only prepares residents and fellows for the complexity of the management of liver disease but also emphasizes the critical importance of imaging in hepatitis diagnosis and treatment as well as the management of complications.

6.3.2. Liver Cirrhosis and Complications

Cirrhosis of the liver is a progressive and multifactorial disorder entailing irreversible fibrosis of liver tissue, typically due to chronic secondary liver disease attributable to alcohol consumption, viral hepatitis, or non-alcoholic fatty liver disease. Cirrhosis of the liver may lead to severe long-term complications, one of which is portal hypertension that occurs due to increased resistance to blood flow through the liver. This increased blood pressure can initiate a chain reaction, which creates esophageal varices, or dilated veins that make individuals susceptible to potentially fatal bleeding. Effective management of these complications demands accurate and timely imaging techniques, such as ultrasound, computed tomography (CT), and magnetic resonance imaging (MRI), that play a crucial role in the diagnosis of the late manifestations of liver cirrhosis, ensuring proper interventions are done to patients before complications worsen to worse outcomes (Nydegger et al., 2010). Liver cirrhosis patients are also at risk for other complications like hepatic encephalopathy and ascites. Hepatic encephalopathy is a neuropsychiatric disease caused by the accumulation of toxins in the bloodstream, usually secondary to liver disease (Figure 6.8).

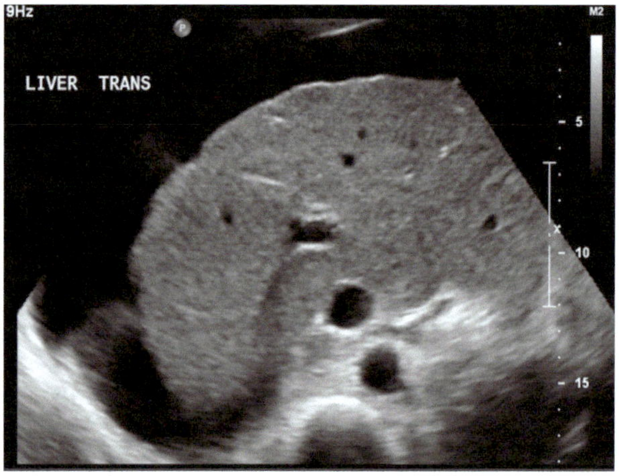

Figure 6.8. CT scan illustrating nodular contour and ascites typical of advanced liver cirrhosis.

Source: https://prod-images-static.radiopaedia.org/images/52960248/62a1c8acbdc687e44700270b71f18f_big_gallery.jpeg.

It is characterized by a range from mild confusion to being completely unconscious, which is detrimental to the quality of life in a patient. Ascites refers to the abnormal accumulation of fluid in the abdominal cavity and is due to portal hypertension and decreased oncotic pressure resulting from low serum albumin. These complications add to the clinical picture of cirrhosis and require periodic imaging studies to track their course, guiding therapeutic maneuvers such as paracentesis for drainage of ascites or interventions for control of encephalopathy through dietetic management or pharmacologic interventions (Gordon et al., 1988). Liver cirrhosis also significantly increases the risk for hepatocellular carcinoma (HCC), a significant liver malignancy. Cirrhotic individuals with cirrhosis have a substantially higher rate of HCC incidence and thus need regular surveillance imaging to detect tumors in the earlier, more treatable stages. Abdominal ultrasound every six months, as guideline-suggested surveillance, is a suggested form of surveillance for at-risk populations, emphasizing imaging's vital role in earlier, proactive detection of cancer. Where imaging does reveal suspecting lesions, more advanced techniques such as MRI and CT might be employed to characterize tumors and measure the extent of their seriousness, ultimately influencing the management alternatives such as liver transplantation or resection. The use of abdominal imaging is thus an intrinsic component of overall patient management for cirrhosis, both for the initial detection of complications and for surveillance of disease severity (Gordon et al., 1988).

6.3.3. Liver Tumors: Benign and Malignant

The liver is a vital organ that can be infested with numerous tumor types, which can be classified as benign or malignant. Benign tumors such as hemangiomas, focal nodular hyperplasia (FNH), and adenomas tend to be less aggressive and are often asymptomatic in nature. Their diagnosis also frequently relies on imaging modalities such as ultrasound, computed tomography (CT), and magnetic resonance imaging (MRI), which enable high-resolution visualization and characterization of such lesions. Benign tumors in most cases may not require surgical excision unless symptomatic or complicated. However, these benign lesions should be differentiated from malignant neoplasms, which, like hepatocellular carcinoma (HCC) and metastatic liver disease, are of significant health risk and require different management. Strong imaging techniques are a vital component of this diagnostic process and have implications for treatment planning and patient outcomes. Malignant liver tumors are more likely to represent a more complex issue for diagnosis and treatment since they are associated with worse outcomes and more intense treatment requirements (Figure 6.9).

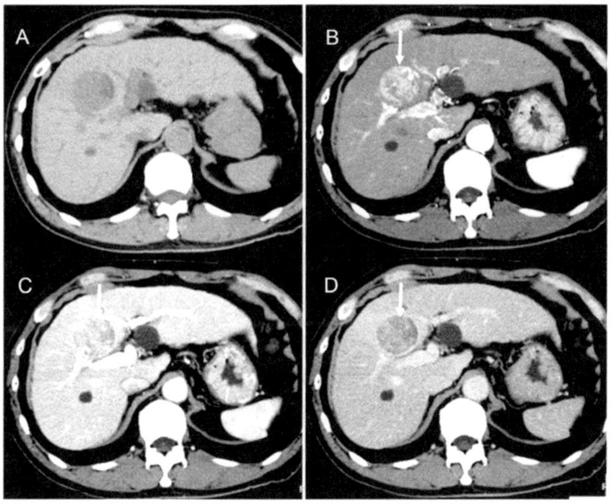

Figure 6.9. Hepatocellular carcinoma. Liver dynamic CT: (A) CT, unenhanced phase, (B) CT, arterial phase, (C) CT, portal venous phase, (D) CT, equilibrium phase. The intrahepatic tumor in liver segment 4/8, which shows low attenuation at the unenhanced phase, shows early stain in the arterial phase (arrow) and washout in the portal to the equilibrium phase (arrows). The tumor is surrounded by a capsule showing delayed enhancement with low attenuation in the arterial phase and high attenuation in the equilibrium phase.

Source: https://www.mdpi.com/gastroent/gastroent-15-00068/article_deploy/html/images/gastroent-15-00068-g001-550.jpg.

Hepatocellular carcinoma (HCC) remains the second most common primary liver cancer, particularly in individuals with underlying liver disease such as cirrhosis or hepatitis. Detection of HCC largely relies on advanced imaging techniques, such as dynamic CT or contrast-enhanced MRI, which can reveal characteristic findings, including arterial enhancement and venous washout. The role of artificial intelligence in helping with such cases is also increasingly relevant to the scenario. Multimodal AI model performance, like that of GPT-4V, is being evaluated for its capacity to aid diagnostic processes and enhance accuracy during benign versus malignant liver lesion differentiation. This technology interface could transform patient care by maximizing diagnostic accuracy and optimizing treatment, thus offering new hope in the battle against liver cancers. Liver tumor treatment, whether benign or malignant, is a multidisciplinary approach of ongoing observation, surgery, and potentially pharmacologic therapy. Benign lesions can be observed without intervention, especially asymptomatic lesions in which there is no indication for treatment. Malignant tumors, however, typically require a more aggressive approach, with options being surgical resection, liver transplant, or targeted therapy. Continuing innovations in imaging modalities are needed to maximize monitoring and treatment decision-making. The future of liver tumor treatment will probably rely heavily on the intersection of sophisticated imaging and artificial intelligence-guided approaches to enable earlier detection and improved treatment planning, as there is an increasingly general trend toward personalized medicine. The potential for innovations in this area can reshape the paradigms of diagnosis and therapy of liver tumors, and hence, there is a requirement for ongoing research and development in abdominal imaging modalities (N/A, 2021; Lei et al., 2023).

6.4. Biliary Anatomy

The biliary apparatus, which consists of the gallbladder, bile ducts, and associated anatomic structures, plays a crucial role in digestion and the regulation of bile. Bile, produced by the liver, passes through a network of ducts referred to as the intrahepatic bile ducts before being collected in the common hepatic duct. The apparatus then empties into the common bile duct, which transports bile to the duodenum, where fats are emulsified. Understanding of this anatomy is crucial in the interpretation of imaging modalities, particularly abdominal imaging. A precise assessment of the anatomy of the biliary tree will reveal cholecystitis or cholangitis, which could manifest as biliary tree obstruction or inflammation.

As imaging technology advances, so too does the precision with which clinicians can diagnose and treat biliary disease, underlining the necessity of careful anatomical knowledge in daily practice. Imaging modalities play a leading role in evaluating the biliary system, with methods such as ultrasound (US), computed tomography (CT), and magnetic resonance cholangiopancreatography (MRCP) being well-known for their diagnostic value. Ultrasound, a highly accessible and non-invasive modality, offers real-time imaging of the bile ducts and gallbladder. Its limited application in morphologic evaluation, however, necessitates complementary imaging in most cases. CT scans provide greater cross-sectional imaging, improved visualization of complex biliary anatomy, and aid in the detection of malignancies, such as gallbladder carcinoma, as observed in studies highlighting CT's sensitivity in identifying biliary disease (Oikarinen et al., 2001). Although MRCP has proved to be a useful aid in biliary imaging, allowing for visualization of bile duct structures without the use of contrast media, it thus detects potential obstructions or anatomical variations with high sensitivity and specificity. The intricate biliary anatomy also presents particular challenges to treatment and diagnosis. Conditions such as primary sclerosing cholangitis (PSC) and biliary fistulas need precise imaging techniques to help enable correct clinical decision-making. For instance, PSC patients occasionally undergo a series of imaging examinations, including ultrasound and MRCP, to assess for changes in the bile ducts and complications. A study emphasized that MRCP is highly effective in demonstrating the anatomical changes associated with PSC, though it may potentially miss some mild dilatations (Alseidi et al., 2021). Thus, a multimodal imaging approach is typically necessary to provide comprehensive evaluation. Lastly, biliary anatomy is a subject of ongoing research and clinical attention, as its understanding is critical to the development of therapeutic techniques and improved patient outcomes in the treatment of biliary disease.

6.4.1. Structure of the Biliary Tree

The biliary tree plays a crucial role in the human digestive system, facilitating the transport of bile produced by the liver to the duodenum. This intricate network comprises several components, including the hepatic ducts, cystic duct, and common bile duct. The structure begins with the right and left hepatic ducts, which emerge from the respective liver lobes and converge to form the common hepatic duct. Alongside this, the cystic duct branches off to connect the gallbladder, a storage organ for bile. The fusion of the common hepatic duct and the cystic duct results in the formation of the common bile duct, which further extends to enter the duodenum at the ampulla of Vater. Understanding this anatomical structure is vital for imaging professionals, as it allows for the detection and evaluation of biliary pathologies, including obstructions and inflammation. Imaging modalities such as ultrasound, CT, and MRI serve as fundamental tools for assessing the biliary tree's integrity. Ultrasound, being non-invasive, is often the first-line investigation due to its ability to visualize gallstones and evaluate bile duct dimensions. CT imaging provides a more comprehensive view of the biliary anatomy and surrounding structures, helping detect tumors and vascular abnormalities (Figure 6.10).

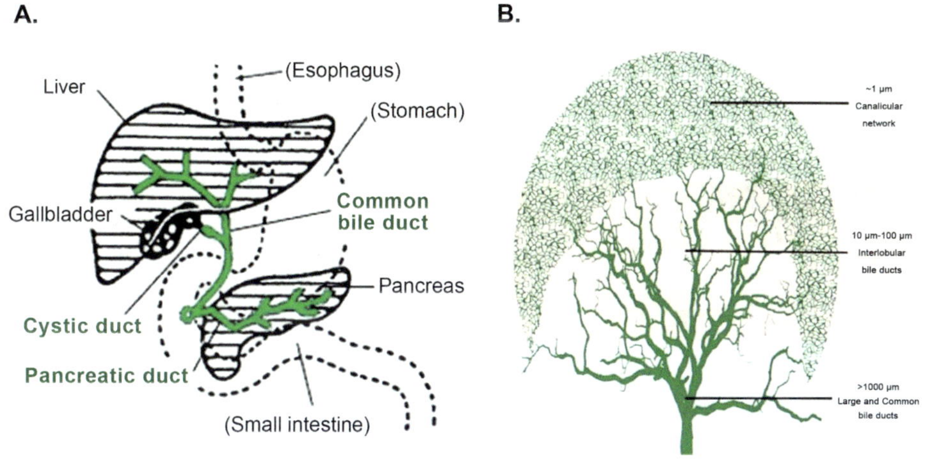

Figure 6.10. Diagram showing the intrahepatic and extrahepatic components of the biliary tree. *Source:* https://www.researchgate.net/profile/Aya-Ali-10/publication/340279249/figure/fig6/AS:874772925800460@1585573526672/Structure-of-the-biliary-tree-A-Intrahepatic-and-extrahepatic-parts-of-the-biliary.jpg.

MRI, particularly with cholangiopancreatography (MRCP), is increasingly used for its greater ability to visualize the biliary ducts noninvasively. Each imaging modality has its own unique strengths that aid clinicians in detecting biliary obstruction, dilatation, or other pathology of the biliary tree. A complete evaluation requires a combination of these imaging modalities, used together, to enable accurate diagnosis and treatment planning. Apart from this, knowledge of pathologies that affect the biliary tree is important in abdominal imaging. Biliary stricture, cholangitis, and malignancy are some of the pathologies that would lead to morbidity if not diagnosed early. Anatomical variation of the biliary tree can complicate the clinical picture and should be kept in mind during imaging. For instance, the presence of variant biliary anatomy may affect the planning of procedures such as ERCP or surgery. Image technology could also increase the ability to separate benign from malignant biliary tree disease, ultimately with a positive outcome for the patient. Knowledge of normal anatomy and potential pathology is crucial for healthcare providers navigating the complex realm of abdominal imaging focused on the liver, biliary, and pancreatic systems.

6.4.2. Gallbladder and Bile Duct Function

The gallbladder is also significant in fat digestion and absorption because it serves as a reservoir for bile, a product of the liver. When it enters the small intestine, especially fats, the gallbladder contracts and releases bile to the duodenum through the bile ducts. The fats are emulsified so they become easier for pancreatic enzymes to digest. Normal gallbladder and associated bile duct functioning is critical; if the bile does not empty on time or in an adequate amount, then it produces digestive issues such as malabsorption and gastrointestinal issues. Moreover, any gallbladder dysfunction may require further imaging studies to confirm suspected conditions such as gallstones, inflammation, or other biliary disease, emphasizing the importance of understanding the anatomy and physiology of this system when imaging the abdomen. Bile ducts, both intrahepatic and extrahepatic, facilitate bile transport from the liver to the gallbladder and eventually to the small intestine (Figure 6.11).

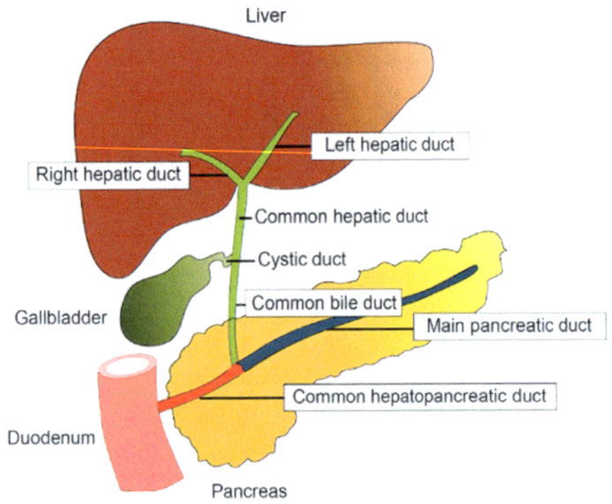

Figure 6.11. Functional schematic of bile storage and secretion involving the gallbladder and ducts.

Source: https://lh3.googleusercontent.com/proxy/q vXgnu9hk9brK0XM j9ty6EpgcZGunMITdO bVD FUnvmWuk0o7APv7Pse BnRHuXK 6GuXf0V4M tL00sB2ZnE QE_GJiv4tUn9YZNLXm dTe9d2gxFk6gX.

The intricate system of bile ducts facilitates bile to be efficiently transmitted, and any obstruction can be identified by imaging techniques like ultrasound, CT scans, or MRIs. Obstruction of the bile ducts can lead to serious issues like cholestasis, where bile in the liver gets accumulated and results in liver failure. Imaging tools play a critical role in assessing bile duct patency and identifying abnormalities such as strictures or malignancies. The compatibility of advanced imaging modalities has maximized diagnostic accuracy for various biliary tract disorders, enabling timely interventions that are vital to patient outcomes, especially for biliary cancer, which may be challenging to diagnose in its early stages (Bartoș et al., 2017). Furthermore, the association of the gallbladder with the bile ducts has extensive implications in neoplastic conditions. Biliary malignancies, though rare, will have cataclysmic consequences if they are not diagnosed early. The anatomical location of the gallbladders with respect to the bile ducts means that any condition in either will significantly impact the other. A case in point is when gallbladder cancer advances to the extent of obstructing bile flow, leading to jaundice and complicating patient management strategies. Accurate imaging is central to staging and treatment planning in abdominal cancers, highlighting the role of radiologic knowledge in distinguishing benign from malignant processes within the biliary tract (N/A, 2020). Accordingly, identification of gallbladder and bile duct roles and interdependence notifies clinicians of strategies for daily digestion while also highlighting the value of careful imaging follow-up when abnormalities are found.

6.4.3. Liver and Biliary System Relationship

The liver and the biliary system are closely related, and they act as a single unit that is significant in metabolism and digestion. The liver produces bile, which plays a vital role in emulsifying fat in the digestive system so nutrients can be absorbed. Bile is channeled through a network of bile ducts to the gallbladder for storage. When fats are ingested, the gallbladder secretes bile into the duodenum, which explains the importance of this connection in normal digestion. Diseases in this system, such as liver disease or biliary obstruction, have significant clinical implications. The interrelationship between the two organs necessitates the use of imaging modalities, such as ultrasound and MRI, to assess abnormalities in bile flow and liver function. Accurate imaging is very important in the evaluation of hepatic and biliary disease, permitting effective intervention and improved patient outcomes in abdominal imaging (Figure 6.12).

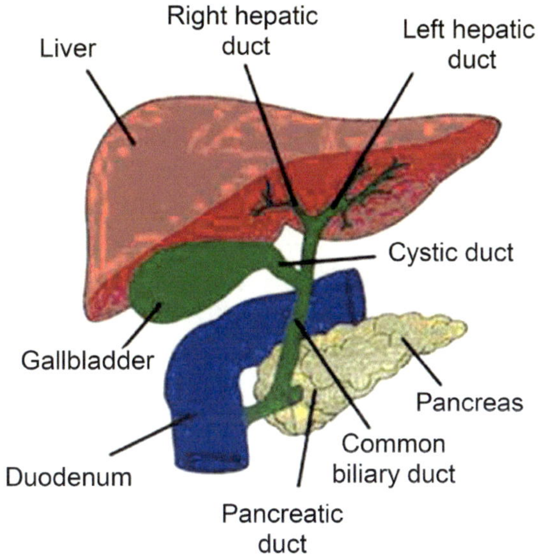

Figure 6.12. An anatomical drawing illustrating the convergence of hepatic ducts with liver lobes.

Source: https://www.researchgate.net/profile/Alex-Kuchumov/publication/260477319/figure/fig3/AS:669969373220884@1536744554541/Color-online-Anatomy-of-the-biliary-system.png.

Imaging lies at the core of understanding the relationship between the biliary tree and the liver, particularly with the advent of newer modalities such as magnetic resonance imaging (MRI) and multidetector computed tomography (MDCT). Both modalities provide superb visualization of anatomical detail and the dynamic function of the liver and biliary tree. For instance, they are able to identify complications such as biliary strictures, stones, or tumors that affect bile duct patency and, consequently, liver function. Imaging of interventional procedures such as hepatobiliary surgery or percutaneous biliary drainage also largely relies on such imaging modalities. Advances in imaging modalities enhance the ability to detect pathological changes and are hence essential for preoperative planning and postoperative follow-up. With advances in techniques, they can offer an enhanced understanding of the dynamics of liver-biliary interaction, which would be crucial for abdominal imaging practitioners. The interaction between the biliary system and the liver is also underscored by some clinical conditions, such as the application of the Associating Liver Partition and Portal vein ligation for Staged Hepatectomy (ALPPS). This new surgical procedure, designed to enhance future liver remnant (FLR) in the context of severe liver disease, underscores the critical interdependence of these systems. Proper staging with MDCT or MRI, for instance, is paramount in determining the liver viability following biliary modification procedures. These imaging modalities can accurately assess liver hypertrophy and detect possible complications arising from deranged bile drainage or liver metabolism. The blending of surgical practice and imaging technology focuses on highlighting the importance of understanding the hepatobiliary relationship in advancing surgical development. The implication of research in this field with advancement is that the relationship between the liver and the biliary system gains more influence over clinical practice and the practice of surgery, showcasing the dynamism of medical knowledge in abdominal imaging, supported by the evidence of Girometti et al. (2017) and Alseidi et al. (2021).

6.5. Imaging Techniques for the Biliary System

The biliary tract, which encompasses the gallbladder and bile ducts, is of prime importance in the process of fat digestion and absorption. Biliary abnormalities are assessed using a variety of imaging studies, each with its own strengths and weaknesses. Ultrasound (US) is generally the first imaging option due to its availability, non-invasiveness, and absence of ionizing radiation. It rapidly identifies gallstones, biliary dilatation, and other abnormalities and helps achieve an accurate first diagnosis. Its performance is occasionally suboptimal due to patient-related factors such as obesity and gas interference. In more complex situations or when initial ultrasound results are inconclusive, secondary imaging modalities may be necessary to achieve a complete evaluation of the biliary apparatus.

Following ultrasound, computed tomography (CT) and magnetic resonance imaging (MRI) are valuable in the investigation of biliary disease. CT is of particular value in the diagnosis of biliary obstruction and pancreatitis complications, providing good cross-sectional images of the abdomen. It does, however, expose patients to ionizing radiation, which is a valuable consideration in patient management. By contrast, MRI, specifically magnetic resonance cholangiopancreatography (MRCP), is a powerful imaging modality for imaging the biliary tree without radiation exposure. With its enhanced soft-tissue contrast, MRI distinguishes among various biliary lesions and complications, thereby enhancing diagnostic sensitivity. Further, MRCP is exceptionally useful in delineating stricture or stones within the bile ducts and is thus essential in preoperative staging and follow-up imaging. One of the new and increasingly encountered imaging modalities for the biliary system is contrast-enhanced ultrasound (CEUS). CEUS provides real-time visualization of the biliary tree and its components, with dynamic assessment of function. CEUS is becoming increasingly popular due to its reduced use of ionizing radiation and iodinated contrast media, though it is as sensitive as other modalities, especially among pediatric populations, in whom normal imaging may be more dangerous. In the evaluation of biliary neoplasia or biliary obstruction, CEUS can provide critical data on lesion characterization and perfusion patterns. CEUS is promoted by the European Federation of Societies for Ultrasound in Medicine and Biology (EFSUMB) for a variety of applications in the biliary tree, suggesting its implementation into practice can enhance the safety and effectiveness of biliary imaging procedures to result in improved patient outcomes (Cantisani et al., 2016; Baccari et al., 2016).

6.5.1. Cholangiography: Indications and Methods

Cholangiography is a pivotal imaging modality for evaluating the biliary tree, providing detailed visualization of both intrahepatic and extrahepatic ducts. Indications for cholangiography are numerous, including biliary obstruction, choledocholithiasis, and cholangitis. In clinical practice, this imaging technique is crucial for providing diagnostic clarity in the presence of jaundice or unexplained abdominal pain. The procedures facilitate the identification of strictures or lesions and guide therapeutic interventions. Additionally, cholangiography can reveal the presence of malignant biliary tumors, which require careful staging and management considerations before surgical resection. Therefore, the method's ability to significantly influence treatment pathways underscores its vital role in abdominal imaging focused on the liver, biliary system, and pancreas (Figure 6.13). Several methods are used for cholangiography, and each has specific advantages and clinical applications. The traditional approaches are percutaneous and endoscopic retrograde cholangiopancreatography (ERCP). Both these approaches have direct visualization of the bile ducts. ERCP is not only performed for diagnostic purposes but also has therapeutic options in terms of stone extraction and stenting. Percutaneous cholangiography is reserved for cases in which endoscopic methods become tedious or insufficient. In the last few years, imaging technology has led to the development of magnetic resonance cholangiopancreatography (MRCP).

This non-invasive modality provides high-quality images without contrast. It has been universally accepted among pediatric and adult patients due to its safety profile and its ability to delineate biliary anatomy, making it a useful tool in cholangiography. The clinical utility of cholangiography is also enhanced in the management of malignancy, particularly malignant biliary tumors (MBTs). Proper preoperative staging and follow-up are crucial to maximize the benefits of therapy, necessitating extensive knowledge of the role of cholangiography in this scenario. New guidelines published by international societies within recent times have maximized imaging protocols, and it is thus important that practitioners remain current with the evolving techniques.

This parallels an increasing interest in imaging-guided multidisciplinary treatment of MBTs, with imaging both guiding surgery and targeted therapy. Sophisticated cholangiography modalities like CEUS are emerging as useful adjuncts, offering novel insights while keeping the risks associated with traditional imaging modalities to a minimum. The potential for increased diagnostic accuracy justifies the ongoing development and research of cholangiographic methods, particularly in abdominal imaging (Cantisani et al., 2016; Cannavale et al., 2016).

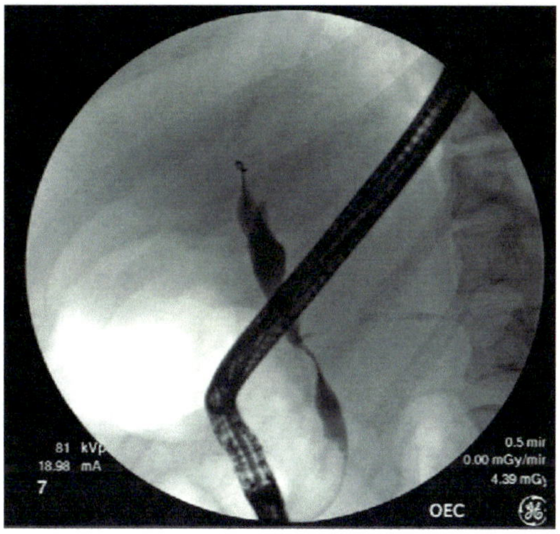

Figure 6.13. Cholangiography showing a biliary stricture involving the hilar region and the middle of the common bile duct.

Source: https://www.researchgate.net/publication/326269057/figure/fig1/AS:714023255425025@1547247818879/Cholangiography-showing-biliary-stricture-involving-in-the-hilar-region-and-middle-of.png.

6.5.2. Ultrasound Role in Biliary Imaging

Ultrasound scanning has significantly improved the diagnosis of biliary disease, providing a readily accessible, non-invasive imaging technique for evaluating biliary anatomy. It is optimally suited to diagnose conditions such as choledocholithiasis, cholangitis, and biliary obstruction. With real-time scanning, ultrasound is able to well delineate gallstones in the gallbladder and common bile duct, an important diagnostic imperative in jaundiced or symptomatic patients. The technique's potential for dynamic imaging makes it extremely useful, as it can detect changes in biliary dilatation and regional lymphadenopathy, which may be suggestive of underlying illness. The technique can evaluate immunologic or infectious illnesses affecting the biliary tree, making it a first-line imaging study in most clinical contexts (Figure 6.14).

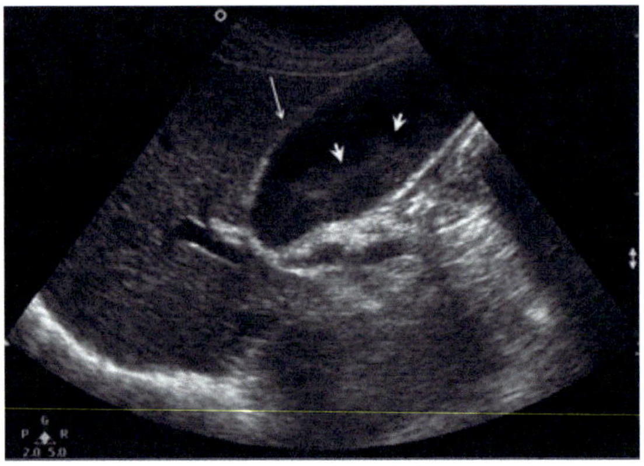

Figure 6.14. Abdominal ultrasound reveals a distended gallbladder (9 × 3.8 cm) with echogenic material (short arrows) in the dependent portion of the gallbladder. The wall thickness of the gallbladder was about 22 mm (thin arrow).

Source: https://www.researchgate.net/profile/Der-Cherng-Tarng/publication/26819909/figure/fig1/AS:394220503355394@1471000900765/Abdominal-ultrasound-reveals-a-distended-gallbladder-9-38-cm-with-echogenic-material.png.

New ultrasound technologies, including contrast-enhanced ultrasound (CEUS), have further enhanced diagnostic capabilities in biliary imaging. CEUS uses microbubble contrast agents to improve visualization of vascular structures and lesions that are poorly visualized with conventional ultrasound. This technique is especially beneficial for evaluating focal liver lesions and biliary disease and is an effective tool for diagnosing and treating complicated cases. While in the past, CEUS was underused in children, increased evidence is available to attest to the safety and efficacy of CEUS in children due to reduced radiation exposure and a more patient-friendly imaging study. Notably, the European Federation of Societies in Ultrasound and Medicine (EFSUMB) recognizes the need for greater use of CEUS, promoting its application in clinical settings as essential in minimizing reliance on ionizing radiation. This expanded ability illustrates the potential of ultrasound technology to expand to meet extensive patient care needs while maintaining clinical utility (Cantisani et al., 2016). Ultrasound plays a critical role in pancreatic disease, not only in initial diagnosis but also in guiding therapeutic intervention, including biliary drainage. Because management of pancreatic cancer is multidisciplinary, accurate imaging to direct decisions for surgery, chemotherapy, and other palliative therapy is needed. Ultrasound allows for real-time guidance during procedures, which makes them safer and more effective. The role of ultrasound extends beyond diagnosis to helping in minimally invasive interventions that decompress biliary obstruction and alleviate symptoms. Moreover, by facilitating timely interventions, ultrasound can improve global patient outcomes and support research efforts to understand the epidemiology and clinical management of diseases involving the biliary system. Through its many uses, ultrasound is a key tool for the integrated imaging method in abdominal and biliary diseases, meeting the complex needs of patient care in this area (Agarwal et al., 2017).

6.5.3. CT and MRI Cholangiography

The roles of computed tomography (CT) and magnetic resonance cholangiography (MRC) in assessing biliary pathology are significant, given the complex nature of biliary anatomy and the pathology that involves it. CT, particularly multidetector CT (MDCT), can provide useful information on the localization and dissemination of biliary carcinomas, which is useful for surgical planning. It is crucial in diagnosing obstructive jaundice conditions, the presence of tumors in the bile ducts, and gallbladder cancer. However, as has been indicated, conventional imaging fails to be effective in the early diagnosis of gallbladder cancer because most are already advanced due to the absence of special early symptoms, so additional reliance on enhanced imaging techniques to outline tumor characteristics distinctly becomes inevitable (Oikarinen et al., 2001). MRI, especially when in the form of MRC, is beneficial in the demonstration of biliary obstruction and other pathologies with improved soft tissue contrast compared with CT. It gives a more accurate visualization of the bile duct and associated structures and is particularly suited to primary sclerosing cholangitis and complicated bile duct strictures (Figure 6.15).

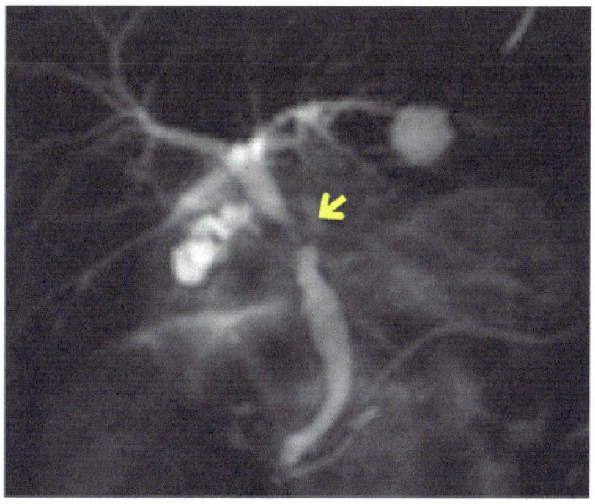

Figure 6.15. MRCP image clearly depicting common bile duct and pancreatic duct in 3D reconstruction.

Source: https://www.researchgate.net/publication/313632435/figure/fig2/AS:460986181263361@1486919078439/A-MRCP-image-shows-sever-stenosis-in-the-middle-common-bile-duct-arrow-Gallbladder-was.png.

MRC can display the intricate biliary tree, highlighting abnormalities that may be overlooked by CT. However, despite its benefits, MRC has the potential to underdemonstrate certain dilatations or provide meticulous measurements that need adjunctive investigations, thus highlighting that diagnosis must be from a multi-dimensional evaluation (Oikarinen et al., 2001). The use of these imaging modalities together, therefore, enhances sensitivity in evaluating biliary disease. Relative efficacy of MRC and CT highlights the importance of matching the imaging method with the optimal clinical setting. Therefore, while CT is the first test due to its rapid acquisition time and ability to reveal related abdominal pathology, MRC is chosen when detailed visualization of the biliary tree is required. Thus, the application of both modalities can provide comprehensive information on biliary tract pathology, allowing greater diagnostic accuracy and outcomes in patients. Also, ongoing advancements in imaging technology further contribute to these methods, making them beneficial for diagnosing and managing complex biliary disease states, ultimately contributing to improved therapeutic interventions for biliary carcinomas and obstruction (Chaube et al., 2025).

6.6. Common Biliary Disorders

Biliary disease is a group of disorders of the bile ducts, gallbladder, and surrounding structures that play a significant role in liver and pancreas function. One of the more common conditions is cholangitis, inflammation of the bile ducts, most frequently caused by obstruction by gallstones or tumors. Imaging plays a critical role in the diagnosis of cholangitis; ultrasound and magnetic resonance cholangiopancreatography (MRCP) are both effective for imaging the biliary tree and detecting obstructive lesions. Immediacy of treatment for cholangitis cannot be overstressed, given its potential to develop into sepsis, a potentially life-threatening infection, if not treated. The patient's symptoms and preliminary imaging findings guide the planning of appropriate treatment modalities, underscoring the absolute necessity of thorough evaluation in the context of suspected biliary obstruction. Cholecystitis, gallbladder inflammation, is another common biliary disease that is usually caused by gallstone obstruction. The clinical presentation is usually dominated by pain in the upper abdomen, particularly in the right upper quadrant, and often accompanied by fever and nausea. Ultrasound remains the imaging modality of choice for evaluating suspected cholecystitis, particularly for its sensitivity in demonstrating gallstones and gallbladder wall thickening or pericholecystic fluid collection. Early diagnosis of cholecystitis is imperative, as the condition can advance to perforation and therefore contribute to increased morbidity and necessitate surgery. The coupling of clinical assessment with imaging examinations accentuates the utility of an integrated approach to care of patients with biliary disease and ultimately impacts outcomes and efficacy of therapy. Lastly, primary sclerosing cholangitis (PSC) is an autoimmune disease that results in chronic inflammation and fibrosis of the biliary tree, often associated with inflammatory bowel disease. PSC diagnosis relies primarily on imaging techniques such as MRCP, which is a non-invasive technique for imaging bile duct pathology and strictures characteristic of the disease. Moreover, screening for complications like cholangiocarcinoma becomes necessary in PSC patients due to the augmented risk with long-standing biliary damage. Management for PSC needs a multi-disciplinary approach involving gastroenterologists and radiologists to formulate treatment plans tailored to the patient's disease course. Therefore, effective imaging and early treatment are crucial for alleviating the detrimental effects of this complex biliary illness, underscoring their relevance to the broader issue of abdominal imaging.

6.6.1. Cholelithiasis and Its Imaging Findings

Cholelithiasis, or gallstones, is a frequent condition that consists of the formation of crystalline material within the gallbladder. They can be of different sizes, composition, and quantity, and are generally incidental but can cause debilitating pain and complications like cholecystitis or pancreatitis. Imaging plays a central role in diagnosing cholelithiasis and associated conditions, and ultrasound (US) has emerged as the first-line imaging modality. The US allows for a non-invasive evaluation of gallstones and can reliably detect the stones and any resulting complications. The sensitivity of US for detecting gallstones is usually in excess of 80% and forms an invaluable clinical tool in the assessment of patients with biliary symptoms (Nydegger et al., 2010) (Figure 6.16).

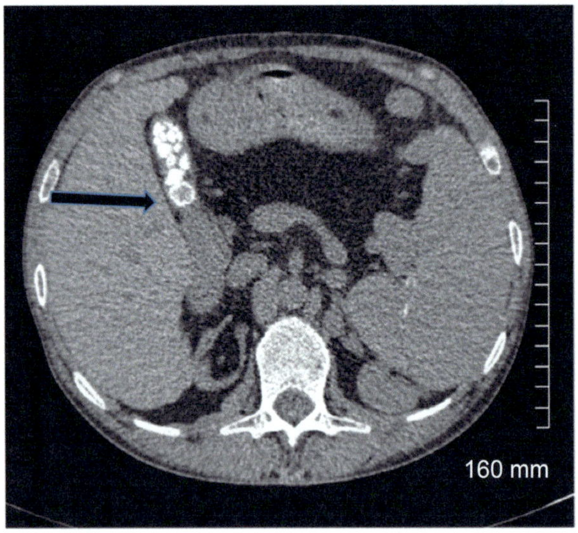

Figure 6.16. Axial CT showing Gallstones top to toe.

Source: https://media.springernature.com/lw685/springer-static/image/art%3A10.1186%2Fs13244-019-0825-4/MediaObjects/13244_2019_825_Fig4_HTML.png.

In addition to ultrasound, computed tomography (CT) and magnetic resonance imaging (MRI) provide complementary data on the biliary system. CT is particularly useful for detecting cholelithiasis complications, such as pancreatitis or biliary obstruction, as it can provide a good view of abdominal structures. While it does utilize ionizing radiation, CT's high resolution of the gallbladder and adjacent organs makes it a diagnostic asset in emergent settings. MRI, specifically magnetic resonance cholangiopancreatography (MRCP), is beneficial for depicting the biliary tree without exposure to radiation. MRCP can distinguish small anatomical details and identify conditions such as choledocholithiasis, in which stones within the common bile duct occur, to further aid management decision-making (Nydegger et al., 2010). The association between cholelithiasis and other biliary diseases highlights the importance of complete imaging evaluation. Patients with cholelithiasis can have a variety of complications, such as choledocholithiasis, biliary strictures, and choledochal cysts, which require proper evaluation using several imaging modalities. Based on recent literature, diseases such as choledochal cysts pose distinct imaging challenges because they can present as cystic dilatations of the biliary tree. The interaction between these pathological conditions highlights the importance of proper imaging so as not to confuse them with other conditions and to administer proper treatment accordingly. In general, it is important to understand the imaging features of cholelithiasis to ensure proper diagnosis and treatment within the broader context of abdominal imaging, especially in cases involving the liver, biliary, and pancreatic systems.

6.6.2. Biliary Obstruction: Causes and Imaging Features

Bile obstruction is a significant clinical syndrome with the impairment of bile passage by one or more intrinsic diseases. Gallstones, malignant illness (e.g., carcinoma of the bile duct or gallbladder), strictures, and infection, such as cholangitis, are some frequent etiologies. In particular, gallstones are a common cause and often present as acute or chronic cholecystitis because they can block the cystic duct or common bile duct. Malignancies also pose special diagnostic challenges because they can cause extrinsic compression of the bile ducts or invade neighboring structures, thereby causing obstruction. Awareness of these causative factors is crucial for early diagnosis and management, as left untreated, biliary obstruction will lead to jaundice, pancreatitis, and potentially life-threatening complications such as cholangitis or hepatic failure. Imaging plays a vital role in the diagnosis of biliary obstruction, with ultrasound (US), computed tomography (CT), and magnetic resonance imaging (MRI) the most frequently used modalities utilized (Figure 6.17).

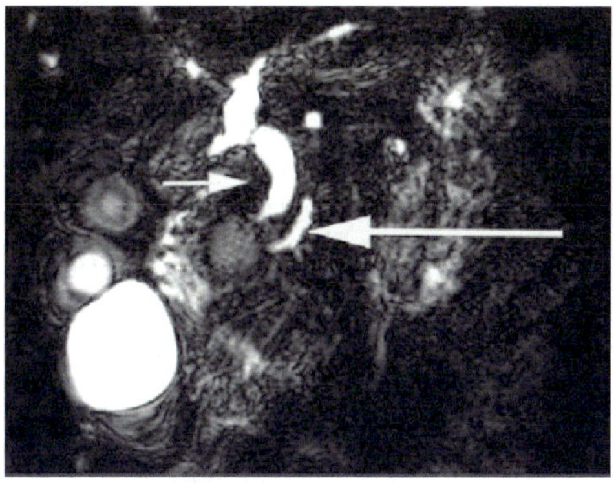

Figure 6.17. MRCP image, demonstrating that the proximal common bile duct was mildly dilated and the distal bile duct was slightly narrow (small arrow). A mildly dilated main pancreatic duct was also present (large arrow). Accessory pancreatic duct was not demonstrated on the MRCP image. MRCP, magnetic resonance cholangiopancreatography.

Source: https://www.researchgate.net/publication/318324080/figure/fig5/AS:631675197353996@1527614511152/MRCP-image-demonstrating-that-the-proximal-common-bile-duct-was-mildly-dilated-and-the.png.

Ultrasound is typically the modality of first choice because it is readily available, low-cost, and non-ionizing. It is excellent at showing gallstones and bile duct dilatation. CT and MRI excel in the demonstration of occult malignancy and complicated relationships of structures. For instance, CT scans may depict the extent of a burdening mass or delineate related vascular structures. At the same time, MRI and magnetic resonance cholangiography (MRC) are better suited to demonstrate bile ducts. The understanding of the imaging modalities is complemented by their comparison of sensitivity and specificity in diagnosing a specific etiology of biliary obstruction, as witnessed by relevant studies that emphasize the inherent strengths and limitations of each method (Nydegger et al., 2010; Oikarinen et al., 2001). Treatment of biliary obstruction typically depends on the underlying etiology, while imaging findings guide the treatment modality. Where malignancy is found, interventions like endoscopic retrograde cholangiopancreatography (ERCP) can be indicated for stent placement or decompression of obstructed bile ducts. Surgical possibilities, on the other hand, could be investigated in symptomatic cholecystolithiasis or benign strictures. The use of metallic stents for malignant biliary obstruction has varied in success, with complications such as stent migration and infection requiring close follow-up and monitoring. By correlating imaging findings with clinical presentations, clinicians can most appropriately design management plans to achieve the best possible outcome for patients with biliary obstruction (Oikarinen et al., 2001). Such a combined approach is paramount to enhancing diagnostic accuracy and therapeutic success in the multifaceted setting of hepatobiliary illness.

6.6.3. Cholangiocarcinoma: Diagnosis and Staging

Diagnosis of cholangiocarcinoma, which is a cancer of the bile duct, is extremely difficult because most of the time it is asymptomatic until very late in the illness. An abdominal ultrasound is typically the first test that will reveal biliary obstruction. Advanced imaging studies are essential for making a definitive diagnosis and for staging. Enhanced computed tomography (CT) and magnetic resonance cholangiopancreatography (MRCP) are particularly important, as they provide invaluable detail for visualizing tumor localization, extent, and metastatic spread. These modalities, though valuable in the diagnosis, tend to fail in early detection (Figure 6.18). The lack of clear markers also makes this process more demanding, requiring a comprehensive diagnostic approach that includes clinical suspicion and advanced imaging techniques (Chaube et al., 2025). Ultimately, early and accurate imaging is paramount in an effort to improve outcomes, given that patients tend to have widespread disease due to delayed diagnosis. Staging cholangiocarcinoma is essential for treatment and prognostic evaluation, as it determines treatment and prognostic evaluation. The correct assessment of the size of the tumors is vital in deciding surgical candidacy, particularly since surgical resection is the only potentially curative treatment. Staging is typically according to the AJCC system, in which the disease is staged based on the depth of invasion, lymph node status, and distant metastasis. Advanced imaging tests, i.e., MDCT and MRCP, are significant in providing accurate details regarding tumor characteristics. They help evaluate lymphatic dissemination and vascular invasion, which are crucial for planning surgery and diagnosing tumor resectability (Chaube et al., 2025). Accurate staging not only influences treatment planning but also has significant implications for the patient's prognosis and survival. The overall prognosis of cholangiocarcinoma remains poor, primarily due to its late presentation along with its virulent nature. The identification of imaging findings related to early disease can have tremendous implications for maximizing patient outcomes. Literature demonstrates that while ultrasound can provide preliminary information, it is less sensitive than CT and MRCP for detecting cholangiocarcinoma, particularly intrahepatic lesions. In addition, the availability of abnormal liver function tests or obstructive jaundice may invoke additional imaging evaluation that allows earlier diagnosis (Chaube et al., 2025). Moreover, imaging technologies have become non-invasive, enabling improved diagnosis and staging models. More recent imaging tools can distinguish between malignant and benign lesions more effectively, potentially allowing intervention at an earlier stage that can improve the survival rates of patients with cholangiocarcinoma.

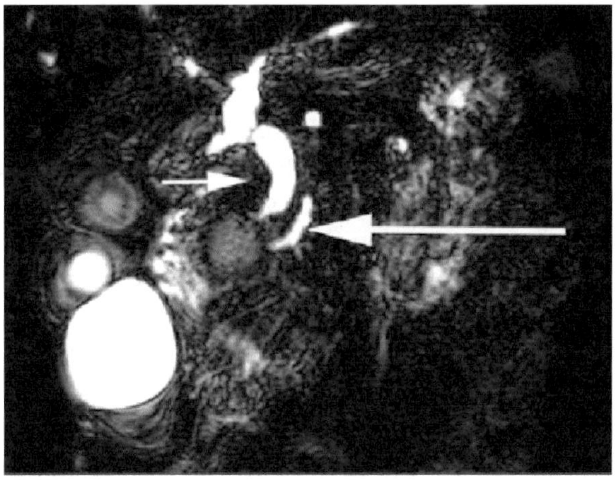

Figure 6.18. T2-weighted MRI showing an irregular mass in the biliary confluence suggestive of cholangiocarcinoma.

Source: https://encrypted-tbn0.gstatic.com/images?q=tbn:ANd9GcTPiVYdj957r3KIkDtfV_ni8SHatFK8P5Jx4Q&s.

SUMMARY

Overall, technological advances in abdominal imaging have improved our understanding and management of liver, biliary, and pancreatic disease. Techniques such as multiphasic computed tomography (CT) and magnetic resonance imaging (MRI) have revolutionized diagnostic and treatment precision. With visualization of anatomical structures and pathological alterations being feasible non-invasively, these imaging methods not only contribute to precise diagnosis but also to effective surgery. With the use of sophisticated imaging modalities, physicians can better delineate malignancies, assess biliary tract dysfunction, and identify chronic inflammatory processes of the pancreas. Such a capability underscores the role of abdominal imaging as a cornerstone in the present-day management of hepatobiliary and pancreatic pathology. The inclusion of sophisticated imaging technologies also extends beyond mere visual examination. As demonstrated by current studies, new methods, such as HSA calculation using multiplanar multislice CT scans, provide essential preoperative information for planning surgical interventions for complex hiatal hernias. This not only supports the imaging function in the management of established disease but also the preventative correction of predicted complications and surgical failures. The ability to correlate imaging results with intraoperative findings yields greater patient benefit and a better understanding of the interplay among symptoms, imaging, and therapeutic response. Consequently, as technology continues to evolve, the potential for abdominal imaging to influence clinical decision-making remains high. Given these advances, future research efforts should seek to optimize imaging protocols and further improve the understanding of imaging findings and clinical outcomes. The application of technologies such as artificial intelligence and sophisticated imaging algorithms can enable even more accurate diagnosis and predictive modeling of hepatobiliary and pancreatic disease. These developments can further optimize patient management strategies, particularly in resource-limited institutions where access to extensive imaging is restricted. In addition, future research needs to validate conventional imaging methods and explore new methods with the potential to transform our knowledge of abdominal pathology. Finally, with the dynamic evolution of medical imaging, these innovations must be corralled into clinical practice to gain optimal advantage for patients with complicated liver, biliary, and pancreatic diseases.

CLOSER LOOK

ABDOMINAL IMAGING: LIVER, BILIARY, AND PANCREAS

In abdominal imaging, evaluation of the liver, pancreas, and biliary tree plays a vital role in diagnosing most pathologies and determining therapeutic interventions. High-resolution imaging methods such as MRI, CT scans, and ultrasound are essential in the revelation of the anatomy as well as the functional integrity of these organs. For instance, imaging can differentiate effectively between benign and malignant liver masses, allowing for earlier interventions in hepatocellular carcinoma or metastatic disease. New imaging technologies also allow visualization of bile duct obstruction or pancreatitis complications, offering essential information that impacts treatment. The imaging findings correlation with clinical data remains significant in the development of effective management plans in patients with complex abdominal disease, highlighting the significance of abdominal imaging in contemporary clinical practice. Management of pancreatitis and biliary illness is typified by peculiar challenges, particularly in determining the nature of injury and the appropriate treatment. Injuries of the biliary system, both traumatic and iatrogenic, should be examined with caution because of their uncommon but impactful occurrence. Iatrogenic damage is much more common than its traumatic counterpart and is usually caused by surgery or diagnostic testing of the liver and pancreas. It is essential to determine the etiology and clinical presentation of these injuries since they are likely to produce serious morbidity and extended health care expenses. Proper imaging is vital in such cases, revealing the extent of injuries and guiding interventions, including biliary reconstruction or other surgical corrections, underscoring that strategic imaging strategies must align with expert clinical insight to ensure optimal patient outcomes (Bazdulj et al., 2018). Technological progress in surgical techniques, particularly those relating to the treatment of pancreatic cancer, has expanded indications for resection in patients with locally advanced disease. Arterial reconstruction in the modified Appleby procedure is a prime example of one such advancement. By preserving collateral blood flow in a delicate manner, these procedures enable margin-negative tumor resections that were previously not considered resectable. As reported, findings from the application of this technique are consistent with beneficial trends in patient recovery, further supporting the evolving field of surgical oncology. These individualized practices serve not only to improve the care of individual patients but, as a cumulative offering, contribute to the growing body of evidence for optimal abdominal imaging and surgical treatment of pancreatic and biliary disease (Lamb et al., 2016).

REFERENCES

1. Machicado, J. D., Amann, S. T., Anderson, M. A., Abberbock, J., Sherman, S., Conwell, D. L., Cote, G. A., Singh, V. K., Lewis, M. D., Alkaade, S., Sandhu, B. S., Guda, N. M., Muniraj, T., Tang, G., Baillie, J., Brand, R. E., Gardner, T. B., Gelrud, A., Forsmark, C. E., . . . Yadav, D. (2017b). Quality of Life in Chronic Pancreatitis is Determined by Constant Pain, Disability/Unemployment, Current Smoking, and Associated Co-Morbidities. *The American Journal of Gastroenterology*, *112*(4), 633–642. https://doi.org/10.1038/ajg.2017.42Adin, C., Allen, A., Alvaro, D., Cardinale, V., Fornoni, A., Lee, C. S., & Ricordi, C. (2022). Patch grafting of organoids of stem/progenitors into solid organs can correct genetic-based disease states. https://core.ac.uk/download/551305305.pdf (accessed on 15th July 2025).
2. Agarwal, D. M., DeWitt, J., Eagleson, M., Easler, J., Gukovskaya, A., & Hines, O. J. (2017). A multidisciplinary approach to pancreas cancer in 2016: A review. *Pancreas*. https://core.ac.uk/download/129149165.pdf (accessed on 15th July 2025).
3. Akinoğlu, A., Akkiz, H., Demiryürek, H., Ergün, O., Gültekin, S., Karasu, Z., & Yüce, G. (1997). Endoscopic retrograde cholangiopancreatography in the diagnosis and management of choledochal cysts. *Turkish Journal of Gastroenterology*. https://core.ac.uk/download/pdf/8088427.pdf (accessed on 15th July 2025).
4. Al-Haddad, M., Anand, B. S., Baron, T. H., Berg, D. E., Bhutani, M. S., Bottrell, S. C., & Boyle, M. J. (2014). Clinical evaluation, imaging studies, indications for cytologic study, and preprocedural requirements for duct brushing studies and pancreatic FNA: The Papanicolaou Society of Cytopathology recommendations for pancreatic and biliary cytology. *Diagnostic Cytopathology*. https://deepblue.lib.umich.edu/bitstream/2027.42/106723/1/dc23095.pdf (accessed on 15th July 2025).
5. Alseidi, A., Brasel, K. J., Conroy, P., Glencer, A., O'Neill, S., & Quezada, C. (2021). Unifying the hepatopancreatobiliary surgery fellowship curriculum via Delphi consensus. *HPB*. https://core.ac.uk/download/573393344.pdf (accessed on 15th July 2025).
6. Azzopardi, N. (2014). The great pretender: Autoimmune pancreatitis. *Malta Medical Journal*. https://core.ac.uk/download/46602519.pdf (accessed on 15th July 2025).
7. Baccari, P., Cappabianca, S., D'Andrea, A., Falcone, M., Iacobellis, F., Manetta, R., & Romeo, V. (2016). Pancreatic tumors imaging: An update. *La Radiologic Medica*. https://core.ac.uk/download/98333045.pdf (accessed on 15th July 2025).
8. Balthazar, E. J., Brock, M., Koitka, K., López-Machado, E., Mallick, R., Naguib, N. N., & Taouli, B. (2009). Pancreatic pseudocyst eroding into the splenoportal venous confluence and mimicking an arterial aneurysm. *Emergency Radiology*. https://core.ac.uk/download/14506857.pdf (accessed on 15th July 2025).
9. Bartoș, A., Bartoș, D. M., & Herdean, A. (2017). Gallbladder cancer: Surgical management. https://core.ac.uk/download/322430519.pdf (accessed on 15th July 2025).
10. Bazdulj, E., Hauser, G., Lekic, V., Zelic, M., Petrovic, D., & Filipovic, B. (2018). Biliary tract injuries. https://core.ac.uk/download/322437142.pdf (accessed on 15th July 2025).
11. Bilounga Ndongo, C., Etoundi Mballa, G. A., Hyder, A. A., Juillard, C., Kobusingye, O., & Mock, C. (2010). Patterns of injury and violence in Yaoundé, Cameroon: An analysis of hospital data. *Injury Prevention*. https://core.ac.uk/download/323075033.pdf (accessed on 15th July 2025).

12. Boru, E. C., Guida, A., Iossa, A., Rengo, M., Romeo, V., Tatangelo, F., & Zobel, B. B. (2017). 25th International Congress of the European Association for Endoscopic Surgery (EAES) Frankfurt, Germany, 14–17 June 2017: Oral presentations. *Surgical Endoscopy*. https://core.ac.uk/download/141696623.pdf (accessed on 15th July 2025).
13. Boskoski, I., Crino, S. F., Dhar, J., Facciorusso, A., Fuccio, L., Gkolfakis, P., & Machicado, J. (2025). Diagnostic approach to biliary strictures. *Digestive Endoscopy*. https://core.ac.uk/download/654513733.pdf (accessed on 15th July 2025).
14. Cannavale, A., Catalano, C., Fanelli, F., Fiocca, F., Ginanni, B., Giurazza, F., & Iezzi, R. (2016). Updated management of malignant biliary tract tumors: An illustrative review. *La Radiologic Medica*. https://core.ac.uk/download/98341455.pdf (accessed on 15th July 2025).
15. Cantisani, V., Deganello, A., Dietrich, C. F., Duran, R., Greiner, L., Piscaglia, F., & Sidhu, P. S. (2016). Role of contrast-enhanced ultrasound (CEUS) in pediatric practice: An EFSUMB position statement. *Ultra Schall in der Medizin*. https://core.ac.uk/download/74320188.pdf (accessed on 15th July 2025).
16. Chaube, A., Itoh, A. B., Akosa, A. H., Patel, B. L., Choi, C. D., Anderson, C. D., & Yeo, C. J. (2025). Diagnosis of biliary tract and ampullary carcinomas. *World Journal of Gastroenterology*. https://core.ac.uk/download/pdf/8359865.pdf (accessed on 15th July 2025).
17. Croagh, D., Day, D., McLaren, C. J., & Segelov, E. (2018). Endoscopic ultrasound in pancreatic cancer. https://core.ac.uk/download/322436464.pdf (accessed on 15th July 2025).
18. Czyżowski, J., Juszczak, A., Mazurek, A., Pasternak, A., Piątek, K., Sroczyński, M., & Wróbel, A. (2021). Anatomical variants of coeliac trunk in Polish population using multidetector computed tomography angiography. *Polish Journal of Radiology*. https://core.ac.uk/download/322562432.pdf (accessed on 15th July 2025).
19. Girometti, R., Lorenzin, D., Risaliti, A., Zerial, M., Cereser, L., Como, G., & Bazzocchi, M. (2017). Abdominal cross-sectional imaging of the associating liver partition and portal vein ligation for staged hepatectomy procedure. *Insights into Imaging*. https://core.ac.uk/download/84481950.pdf (accessed on 15th July 2025).
20. Gordon, R. D., & Starzl, T. E. (1988). Changing perspectives on liver transplantation in 1988. *Hepatology*. https://core.ac.uk/download/12204389.pdf (accessed on 15th July 2025).
21. Grazi, G. L. (2007). Liver resections: Complications and survival outcome. *World Journal of Surgery*. https://core.ac.uk/download/11162431.pdf (accessed on 15th July 2025).
22. Hecker, A., Kirkpatrick, A. W., Leppaniemi, A., Pikoulis, E., Mefire, A. C., De Simone, B., & Sakakushev, B. (2019). Duodeno-pancreatic and extrahepatic biliary tree trauma: WSES-AAST guidelines. *World Journal of Emergency Surgery*. https://core.ac.uk/download/288798568.pdf (accessed on 15th July 2025).
23. Illanes, O., Ketzis, J., Köster, L., Rajeev, S., Raverty, S., & Rick, D. (2017). Diagnosis of pancreatic disease in feline platynosomosis. *Veterinary Parasitology*. https://core.ac.uk/download/80696795.pdf (accessed on 15th July 2025).
24. Lamb, K. M., Latona, J. A., Maley, W. R., Pucci, M. J., Tyler, D. S., & Yeo, C. J. (2016). Modified Appleby procedure with arterial reconstruction for locally advanced pancreatic adenocarcinoma: A literature review and report of three unusual cases. https://core.ac.uk/download/46976111.pdf (accessed on 15th July 2025).

25. Lei, J., Lin, W., Wang, Y., Wu, Y., Zhang, X., Wang, J., & Xu, M. (2023). Can GPT-4V(ision) serve medical applications? Case studies on GPT-4V for multimodal medical diagnosis. http://arxiv.org/abs/2310.09909 (accessed on 15th July 2025).

26. Löhr, M., Beuers, U., Vujasinović, M., Alvaro, D., Frøkjær, J. B., Buttgereit, F., Capurso, G., et al. (2020). European guideline on IgG4-related digestive disease–UEG and SGF evidence-based recommendations. *United European Gastroenterology Journal, 8*, 637–666. https://doi.org/10.1177/2050640620934911 (accessed on 15th July 2025).

27. Majaz, H. M. K., Mateen, M. A., Mohan, R., & Muheet, A. (2012). Evaluation of ultrasound-based acoustic radiation force impulse (ARFI) and eSie touch sonoelastography for diagnosis of inflammatory pancreatic diseases. *Journal of Clinical Imaging Science*. https://core.ac.uk/download/619642404.pdf (accessed on 15th July 2025).

28. Miller, J. M., Binnicker, M. J., Campbell, S., Carroll, K. C., Chapin, K. C., Gilligan, P. H., Gonzalez, M. D., et al. (2018). A guide to utilization of the microbiology laboratory for diagnosis of infectious diseases: 2018 update by the Infectious Diseases Society of America and the American Society for Microbiology. *Clinical Infectious Diseases, 67*, e1–e94. https://doi.org/10.1093/cid/ciy381 (accessed on 15th July 2025).

29. N/A (2020). *Diseases of the Abdomen and Pelvis 2018–2021: Diagnostic Imaging–IDKD Book.* https://core.ac.uk/download/478099744.pdf (accessed on 15th July 2025).

30. N/A (2021). *New Techniques in Gastrointestinal Endoscopy*. https://core.ac.uk/download/478120352.pdf (accessed on 15th July 2025).

31. Nydegger, A., Sevilla, A., Gillams, A. R., Gaines, B. A., Colombo, C., Metreweli, C., & Sivit, C. J. (2010). Hepatobiliary and pancreatic imaging in children—Techniques and an overview of non-neoplastic disease entities. *Pediatric Radiology*. https://core.ac.uk/download/pdf/8510110.pdf (accessed on 15th July 2025).

32. Oikarinen, H. (2001). Imaging of biliary carcinoma, fistula and primary sclerosing cholangitis and percutaneous metallic stenting in malignant biliary obstruction. *Acta Radiological*. https://core.ac.uk/download/628862512.pdf (accessed on 15th July 2025).

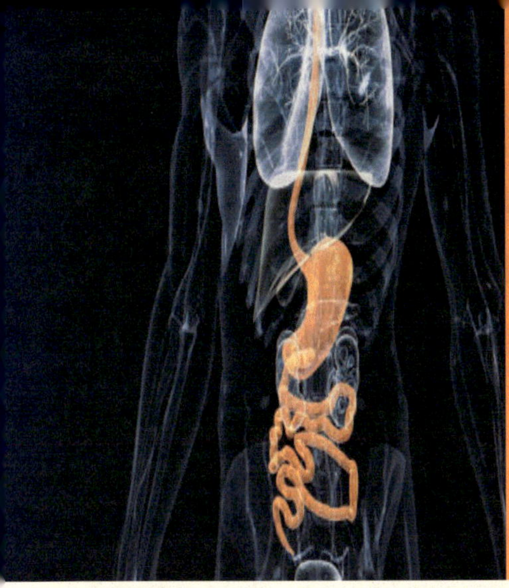

Chapter 7

GASTROINTESTINAL TRACT IMAGING: CT, MRI, AND FLUOROSCOPY

Contents

Introduction

The introduction of imaging of the gastrointestinal tract highlights the evolving role of diagnostic modalities in the optimal evaluation and management of most gastrointestinal diseases. As medical science evolved, modalities such as CT, MRI, and fluoroscopy became an integral part of clinical practice. These modalities not only improve visualization of anatomical landmarks but also enhance visibility of pathological abnormalities. Each modality has unique strengths: CT is renowned for high-speed acquisition of high-resolution data, MRI provides superior soft-tissue contrast, and fluoroscopy is used to dynamically evaluate the movements and functions of the gastrointestinal tract. Awareness of the differences provides the foundation for their application in diagnosing conditions such as Crohn's disease, tumors, and obstructions, thereby further solidifying their position in medical practice today. Different gastrointestinal ailments need respective imaging techniques to increase the diagnostic yield. For instance, CT is most helpful for the quick identification of abdominal abnormalities in acute presentation owing to its speedy and precise nature. MRI, however, is best suited for the evaluation of soft tissue masses and inflammation, with resulting easy differentiation of pathologies without subjecting to ionizing radiation. Fluoroscopy, utilized mostly for monitoring the functioning of the digestive tract, is essential in many procedures such as swallow examinations or contrast examinations of the esophagus and small intestine. As emphasized in the current literature, the concordance of these imaging modalities facilitates the development of an integrated diagnostic strategy for the management of complex diseases, such as the effective evaluation of small bowel Crohn's disease and its extraintestinal manifestations (Albert et al., 2011).

These advances underscore the need for clinicians to enhance imaging selection on a case-by-case basis. Incorporation of advanced imaging techniques into routine practice has a significant influence on outcomes in patients through more timely diagnosis and intervention. Interaction between imaging technology and clinical management is most significant in the context of chronic illnesses like Crohn's disease, where monitoring of disease development is most crucial. Furthermore, imaging evaluation contributes to therapeutic decision-making, both on the medical and surgical sides of management. Sophisticated methods such as capsule endoscopy with MRI enhancement are now essential tools for visualizing the entire small bowel, providing valuable information on disease evolution (Albert et al., 2011). It not only enhances the diagnostic process but also facilitates existing management programs. The introduction of imaging of the gastrointestinal tract, therefore, is not so much a technical summary as it is an essential perspective through which the wider ramifications of care in the patient are appreciated, and how each imaging modality plays the essential roles within the current medical practices.

7.1. Overview of the Gastrointestinal Tract

The GI tract is an intricate arrangement of organs essential for digestion, nutrient absorption, and waste elimination. It begins in the oral cavity, in which mechanical and chemical digestion start with mastication and saliva. The esophagus is a muscular tube by which food travels initially to the stomach, in which gastric juices contribute to additional digestion. Churning of the stomach blends food with enzymes and acid, readying the body for digestion of nutrients. Following is the small intestine, which is the key to digestion, and is sectioned into the three parts of the duodenum, jejunum, and ileum. Here slow absorption of nutrients occurs assisted by villi and microvilli that increase the surface area. The large intestine then processes the waste by reabsorbing water and electrolytes, causing the formation and elimination of feces. Such a sophisticated system emphasizes the requirement of precise imaging procedures for revealing any pathological changes in the GI tract. In the clinical setting, detection of any changes in the gastrointestinal tract is frequently essential for assessing patient outcomes, and thus the use of advanced imaging techniques such as CT, MRI, and fluoroscopy becomes extremely pertinent. Computed tomography (CT) is particularly valuable for its speedy acquisition and high-resolution cross-sectional images, useful for detecting tumors, inflammation, and structural abnormalities. Magnetic Resonance Imaging (MRI) provides better soft tissue differentiation, hence is especially valuable in assessing liver, pancreas, and bile duct pathologies. Fluoroscopy, on the other hand, provides real-time images, particularly valuable for assessing functional disorders such as dysphagia or gastroesophageal reflux. Such techniques are not only important for diagnosis but also for the guidance of therapeutic procedures, such as biopsies. Integration of such imaging technology into routine practice facilitates early, accurate diagnoses and improved management plans, indicating their usefulness in gastrointestinal management. Moreover, advances in imaging technology continue to expand diagnostic potential within the gastrointestinal tract. New advancements, including the utilization of artificial intelligence and machine learning, can make image analysis simpler so that evaluation becomes more sensitive and specific. For instance, AI applications can distinguish between malignant and benign biliary strictures, and this diagnostic process improves (Boskoski et al., 2025). Furthermore, endoscopic ultrasonography (EUS) is a very valuable addition to standard imaging modalities that has significantly improved visualization of submucosal lesions and the harvest of tissue specimens. Combined modalities like these give a multidisciplinary patient management approach that optimizes patient care, deals with indeterminate results, and limits invasive procedures. With the progress of research and technology, the application of high-tech imaging techniques in the management of gastrointestinal diseases remains a crucial element in ensuring proper and timely patient care (N/A, 2006).

7.1.1. Anatomy of the Gastrointestinal Tract

The GI tract is a complex and highly organized system that is responsible for the digestion and absorption of nutrients. It extends from the mouth to the anus and consists of various segments with specific anatomical features and functions. The broad segments comprise the esophagus, stomach, small intestine, large intestine, and accessory organs such as the liver, pancreas, and gallbladder. The food is carried by the esophagus, and the mechanical and chemical digestion happens in the stomach. Then there is the small intestine, which is further divided into the duodenum, jejunum, and ileum, and this is primarily where nutrients are absorbed. Water absorption and the production of feces occur in the large intestine, specifically the cecum, colon, rectum, and anal canal. An understanding of this anatomy is required for appropriate imaging procedures as the morphology of each organ dictates its alterations in disease detectable by imaging modalities (Figure 7.1).

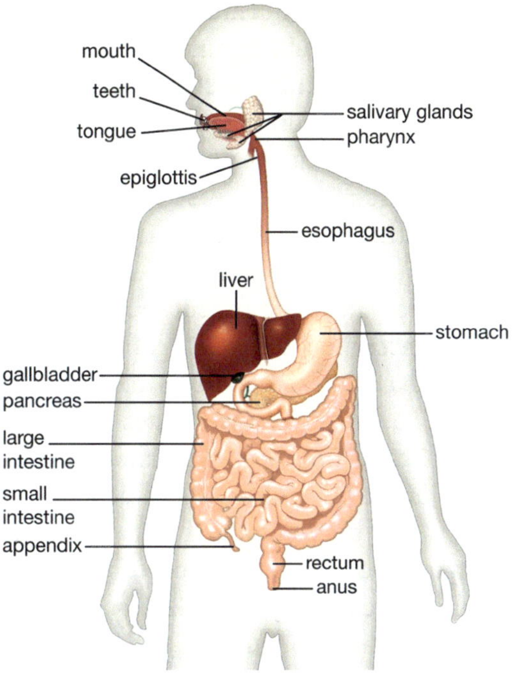

Figure 7.1. An annotated diagram of the entire gastrointestinal tract from the esophagus to the rectum.

Source: https://cdn.britannica.com/39/8039-050-B124FC20/human-digestive-system-front.jpg.

Imaging techniques such as Computed Tomography (CT), Magnetic Resonance Imaging (MRI), and fluoroscopy have a key function in the evaluation of the anatomy of the gastrointestinal tract. CT scanning provides a high-resolution cross-sectional image, enabling soft tissue structures to be seen, mass lesions to be evaluated, and inflammatory conditions such as appendicitis or Crohn's disease to be identified. MRI is particularly effective for visualizing liver and biliary anatomy, providing improved soft-tissue contrast without the need for ionizing radiation. Fluoroscopy, a type of imaging that uses X-rays to visualize, in real-time, the movement of the GI tract, plays a pivotal role in assessing functional abnormalities, such as motility disorders, as well as structural abnormalities like strictures. The strengths and limitations of both modalities are of utmost significance for clinicians in determining the appropriate imaging modality to investigate GI complaints, underpinned by clinical evidence from research comparing gastrointestinal imaging techniques (Hansson et al., 2022). The combination of newer imaging technologies has enhanced the assessment of gastrointestinal disorders and conditions with more accurate diagnosis and treatment planning. For instance, techniques like bimodal ERCP facilitate improved visualization of the anatomy of the biliopancreas, particularly when done under situations like biliary obstruction or complex cholelithiasis (Hansson et al., 2022). These high-technology visualization techniques allow physicians not just to diagnose disease effectively but also to optimize therapeutic maneuvers, such as technique in biliary drainage or stenting. Moreover, radiation exposure should be meticulously considered in gastrointestinal imaging, especially in fluoroscopy and CT scanning, since cumulative doses can be harmful to the patient over time. Thus, knowledge of gastrointestinal anatomy and the use of the most recent imaging modalities provide a paradigm for the best and safest management of gastrointestinal diseases, eventually leading to improved patient outcomes.

7.1.2. Gastrointestinal Disorders

Gastrointestinal disorders are prevalent medical illnesses that not only significantly impact patients' quality of life but also pose problems to effective diagnosis and management. The most common among the gastrointestinal illnesses are Crohn's disease, irritable bowel syndrome (IBS), and diverticulitis, each having unique clinical presentations and management needs. Crohn's disease, for instance, can involve any part of the gastrointestinal tract, often presenting with abdominal pain, diarrhea, and loss of weight. Such advanced imaging modalities as CT and MRI have become indispensable resources in the diagnosis and management of Crohn's disease, providing more precise measurements of intestinal inflammation and complications. Not only does advanced imaging enable detection of disease activity, but it also helps monitor treatment response, underscoring the dynamic role of radiological assessment in gastrointestinal practice (Albert et al., 2011) (Figure 7.2).

Irritable bowel syndrome (IBS), which occurs in a high percentage of the population, is defined by the occurrence of abdominal pain and disordered bowel habits. Unlike Crohn's disease, IBS is a structural gastrointestinal disorder with usual structures that are not apparent on standard imaging. Imaging studies can be used to rule out other diseases with IBS-like symptoms, such as inflammatory bowel disease or structural lesions. Fluoroscopy, in particular, can be employed to evaluate functional characteristics of the gastrointestinal system by measuring motility and identifying structural defects. Imaging thus does not actually diagnose IBS in itself, but is an integral component of the diagnostic process that guides management strategies to enhance patient outcomes within a holistic healthcare setting (Hansson et al., 2022). Diverticulitis is a common gastrointestinal illness characterized by infection or inflammation of diverticula, small sacs in the colon wall. Abdominal tenderness, fever, and changes in bowel habits are typical presenting symptoms in patients. Imaging, most notably CT scanning, has revolutionized the diagnosis and management of diverticulitis by providing definitive visualization of inflamed diverticula and complications such as abscess formation and perforation. Also, imaging assists in choosing the appropriate therapeutic approach, be it conservative therapy or surgery. The application of imaging modalities to treat diverticulitis exemplifies how a multimodal approach to gastrointestinal illnesses is essential for improving care and outcomes for patients through informed decision-making (Albert et al., 2011).

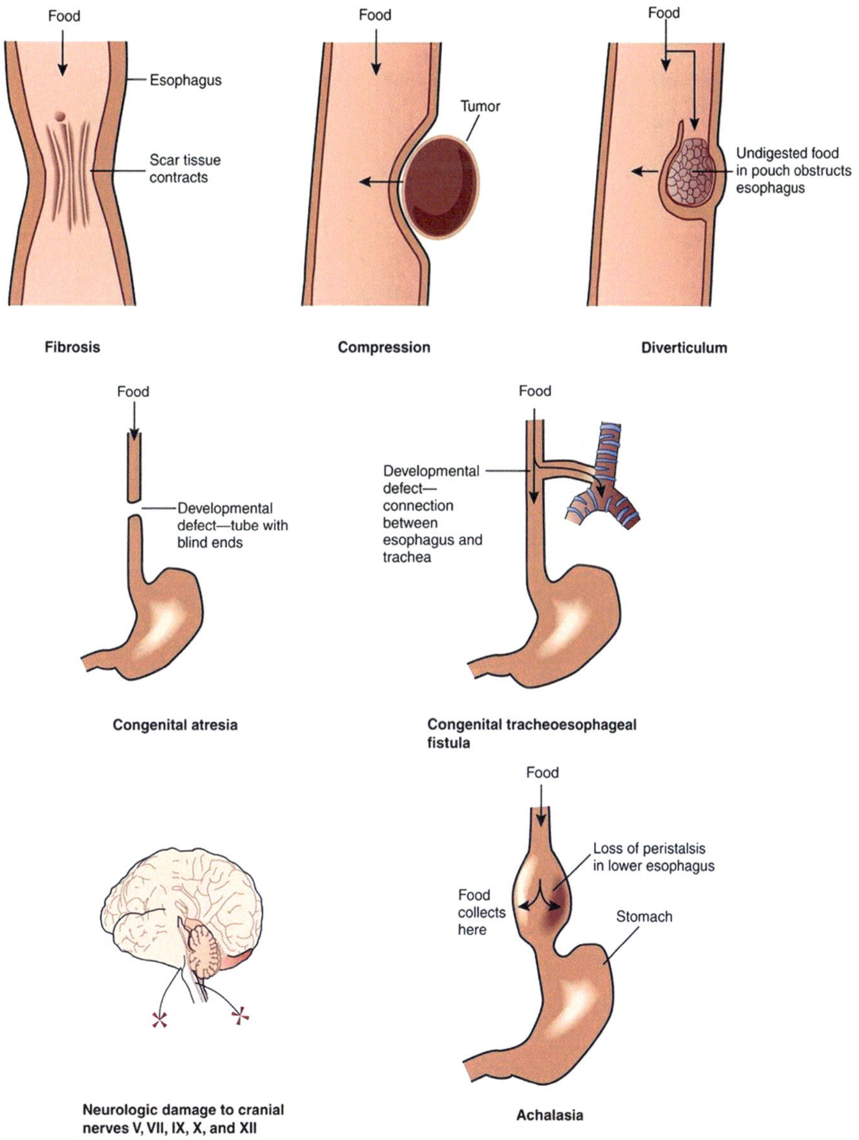

Figure 7.2. Illustration of common gastrointestinal disorders.

Source: https://basicmedicalkey.com/wp-content/uploads/2016/09/F00036Xf36-01-9781455726509.jpg.

7.1.3. Function of Imaging in Gastrointestinal Wellness

To determine gastrointestinal health, imaging methods such as computed tomography (CT), magnetic resonance imaging (MRI), and fluoroscopy are each essential. Physicians utilize these technologies to view the intricate structure of the gastrointestinal (GI) tract, significantly enhancing the accuracy of diagnosis. With cross-sectional imaging, CT scans offer clear pictures of abdominal organs, allowing practitioners to identify conditions such as tumors, inflammation, and structural abnormalities. Additionally, MRI provides superior soft-tissue contrast to CT and is therefore particularly useful in the diagnosis of liver and pancreatic disease (Figure 7.3).

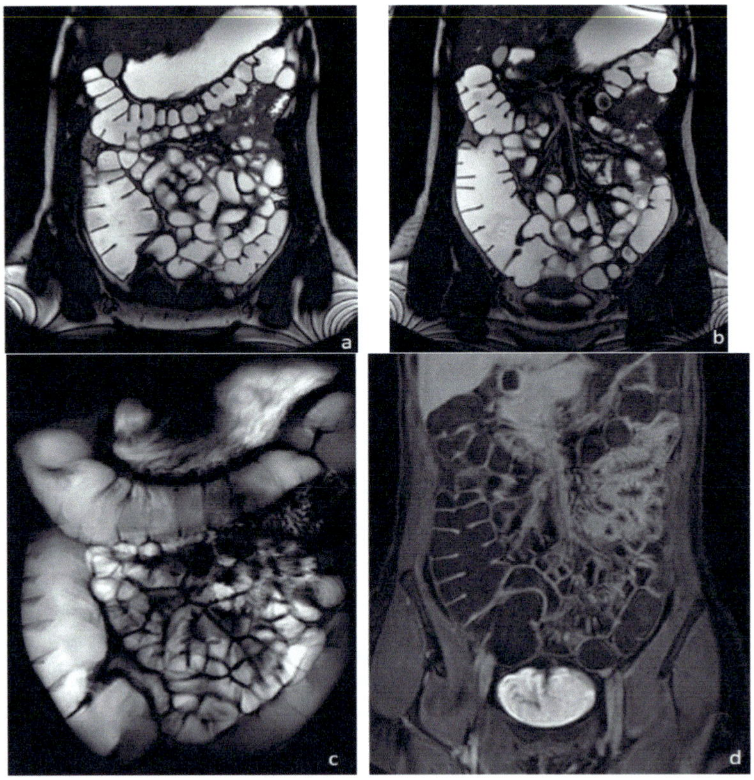

Figure 7.3. Magnetic resonance imaging of the gastrointestinal tract.

Source: https://www.mdpi.com/diagnostics/diagnostics-13-02410/article_deploy/html/images/diagnostics-13-02410-g001.png.

These imaging techniques not only aid diagnosis but also guide therapeutic interventions, thereby improving patient outcomes in gastroenterology. Fluoroscopy, another important imaging technique, facilitates dynamic imaging of gastrointestinal motility and organ function. Employing real-time X-ray imaging, fluoroscopy assists physicians in observing the passage of contrast material through the GI tract and detecting functional disorders such as dysphagia or bowel obstructions. This modality is superior in the evaluation of swallowing dysfunction and diagnosis of gastroesophageal reflux disease (GERD). Also, fluoroscopy plays a central role in the performance of interventional procedures such as biopsies or tube placement. The ability to obtain functional dynamics in real time is a unique advantage of fluoroscopy over static imaging methods, making it a priceless aid in assessing gastrointestinal health. The intersection of newer imaging modalities has also fueled innovations in the minimally invasive procedures in gastrointestinal surgery. Imaging is no longer confined to strictly diagnostic functions but serves a pivotal role in planning and executing robot-assisted procedures that benefit from enhanced visualization and precision. As per recent literature, the combination of imaging modalities with surgical robotics has resulted in radical advances in dexterity and navigation and has become vital during complex procedures. These advances underscore the ongoing evolution of surgical environments and highlight the importance of imaging not just for diagnosis but also for improving surgical procedures and patient outcomes in gastrointestinal interventions (N/A, 1997; Dagnino et al., 2024).

7.2. Computed Tomography (CT) Scanning

Computed Tomography (CT) scans are now a vital diagnostic tool for evaluating gastrointestinal tract diseases, as they can produce high-resolution cross-sectional images. The technique uses advanced X-ray technology combined with computational methods to create detailed images of internal structures, enabling complete visualization of organs such as the liver, pancreas, and intestines. Its great advantage is rapidity and accuracy, which provide crucial information in the diagnosis of diseases like tumors, inflammatory conditions, and obstructions. Also, contrast agents enable better visualization of specific tissues, improving diagnostic accuracy. Despite these benefits, CT image interpretation is highly challenging due to the high heterogeneity of gastrointestinal diseases and requires highly skilled radiologists capable of accurately distinguishing normal anatomy from disease (Bhuiyan et al., 2023).

In recent years, the use of CT imaging in the management of gastrointestinal diseases has come under increasing criticism, particularly due to issues with cumulative radiation exposure. For the frequent imager, such as those with chronic illness, the associated risk of radiation exposure becomes a major concern. Research has indicated that some individuals, most notably those with chronic illness, receive high cumulative effective doses over time, which can raise their risk for injury from radiation. One of these studies, in patients with cystic fibrosis, indicated a significant rise in cumulative effective dose of radiation from CT scanning, which accounted for nearly half of the overall radiation exposure among this population (Eustace et al., 2012). This indicates that radiologists need to weigh the diagnostic benefits of CT against potential risks and practice restraint in imaging. Advancements in technology for CT imaging continue to decrease some of the risks associated with radiation exposure while enhancing image quality. Developments such as iterative reconstruction algorithms and low-dose protocols can potentially reduce radiation dose without compromising diagnostic reliability. Such developments resonate in the scenario of gastrointestinal imaging, where high image quality matters most for detecting subtle abnormalities. Further research into other imaging modalities, such as MRI and ultrasound, reflects the health care community's commitment to minimizing radiation risk while still maintaining effective diagnostic potential. As CT imaging remains a staple of gastrointestinal tract evaluation, regular communication between radiologists, clinicians, and patients is required to optimize imaging strategies and ensure patient safety (Bhuiyan et al., 2023).

7.2.1. Principles of CT Imaging

Principles of computed tomography (CT) imaging play essential roles in the field of gastrointestinal tract imaging, yielding a detailed understanding of internal structures. CT imaging relies on the application of X-rays to produce accurate cross-sectional images of the body, employing a rotating X-ray source and detectors to measure the incoming radiation. These images are built by sophisticated algorithms that convert raw data into high-resolution tissue sections, allowing for improved visualization of organs, vasculature, and disease modifications. In gastrointestinal applications, CT has been extremely useful for evaluating inflammatory bowel disease, tumors, and obstructions. The ease of use of contrast agents also improves the process of diagnosis by providing more information on vascular anatomy and better visualization of lesions. Generally, the regulations constituting CT imaging form the foundation of its pivotal role in the noninvasive diagnostic processes of the gastrointestinal department. Complementing the mechanical processes of image production are the regulations governing the reading and analysis of images in CT imaging. Radiologists have a significant role to play in this process, utilizing their expertise to interpret the resultant images, identify abnormalities, and correlate them with clinical symptomatology. One of the key advantages of CT imaging is that it can stack a number of images together to form a three-dimensional image, allowing easier visualization of complex structures and relationships between different anatomical components. Such 3D reconstruction is particularly valuable in surgical planning since it makes the accuracy of information in the spatial relationship between tumors or lesions to important structures possible, thus informing treatment. In addition, advances in multidetector CT technology have significantly improved image speed and quality, enabling volumetric data to be created that can be evaluated in real time. Such intricacies demonstrate the importance of CT in modern gastrointestinal diagnosis and patient management.

While CT imaging offers many advantages, it also has limitations and risks. While the imaging modality offers better anatomical detail and speed, ionizing radiation exposure remains a primary concern. This is particularly so in gastrointestinal imaging, where several scans may be warranted for diseases that require frequent surveillance, such as cancer management or inflammatory disease. Therefore, the principle of ALARA (As Low As Reasonably Achievable) becomes critical, suggesting that radiation doses be kept as low as reasonably achievable while maximizing diagnostic yield.

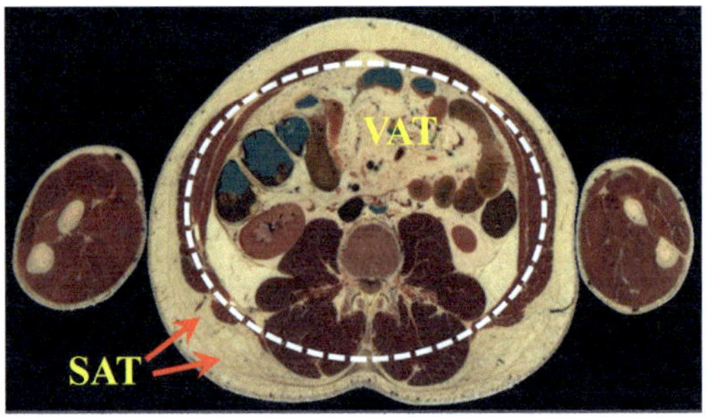

Figure 7.4. Cross-sectional images of the abdomen.

Source: https://www.researchgate.net/profile/Peter-Caracappa/publication/223962904/figure/fig1/AS:341569828868098@1458448001222/A-cross-sectional-image-of-the-abdomen-illustrating-the-division-of-adipose-tissues-into.png.

New technologies, including advanced algorithms and low-dose techniques, are being applied to mitigate these risks without degradation of image quality. Moreover, there is active research into integrating CT imaging with modalities such as single-operator peroral cholangiopancreatoscopy (SOPCP), which may enhance diagnostic yield at lower exposure. These developments are the culmination of the commitment to strengthening the principles of CT imaging in the universal context of gastrointestinal tract evaluation and patient care (N/A, 2006; Hansson et al., 2022) (Figure 7.4).

7.2.2. Advantages of CT in Gastrointestinal Diagnosis

Among the chief advantages of computed tomography (CT) in gastrointestinal diagnosis is its rapid imaging, which significantly enhances patient management in the acute setting. In acute conditions of gastrointestinal emergencies such as perforation or acute pancreatitis, prompt diagnosis is critical in an effort to implement the correct course of intervention. CT scans are rapid to undertake and provide high-resolution imaging, allowing detection of a variety of conditions, including abscesses or collections of fluid. Because detailed cross-sectional images of the abdomen can be obtained easily, clinicians can successfully evaluate the complexity of biliary strictures (Figure 7.5).

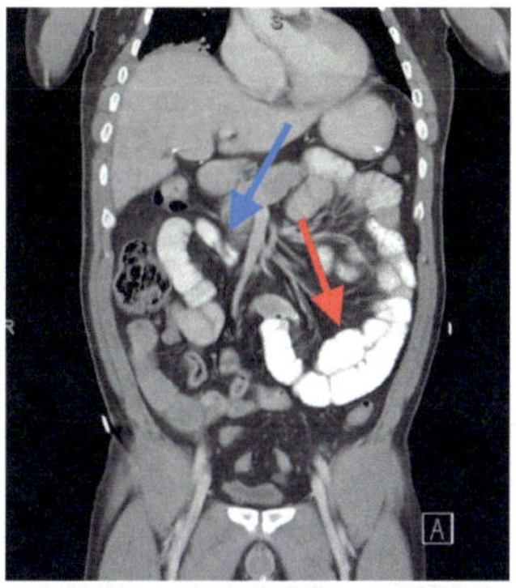

Figure 7.5. A CT scan of the abdomen and pelvis shows small bowel obstruction with contrast within the dilated loops of the small bowel (red arrow), but no contrast noted within the distal decompressed small bowel loops (blue arrow).

Source: https://www.researchgate.net/publication/381657631/figure/fig1/AS:11431281256404446@1719525814496/A-CT-scan-abdomen-pelvis-showing-small-bowel-obstruction-with-contrast-within-the-dilated.png.

This speed and precision underscore the potential of CT as a first-line imaging modality, particularly in critical care applications, where a saved minute matters when life-or-death decisions are being made (Boskoski et al., 2025). A key strength of CT is its ability to image the fine anatomy of the gastrointestinal tract, enabling accurate evaluation of complex disease conditions. Compared with traditional imaging techniques such as ultrasound and fluoroscopy, CT offers greater contrast resolution, which is key to identifying structures and diagnosing anomalies within the abdominal cavity. This is especially advantageous in the detection of most gastrointestinal diseases, such as neoplasms, inflammatory bowel disease, and diverticulitis. Moreover, employment of advanced technologies of CT, such as multidetector CT and CT enterography, increases diagnostic yield significantly through the provision of accurate details regarding the bowel wall and mesenteric structures. Such an ability is paramount in differentiating between benign and malignancy lesions, thus affecting optimal management strategies (Boskoski et al., 2025). Finally, the effectiveness of CT in diagnosing the gastrointestinal system is also testified to by its ability to operate with a variety of contrast agents that have the potential to provide more precise imaging of specific structures and pathology. The provision of oral and intravenous contrast media facilitates full assessment, enabling the detection of low-lying lesions that may go undetected. For instance, the employment of oral contrast can enhance lumen visualization of the bowel, potentially improving the assessment of entities such as small bowel obstructions or ischemic changes. Additionally, with advances such as CT colonography, patients are exposed to less intrusive procedures in colorectal screening and diagnosis. These advances contribute not only to accurate diagnosis but also to improved patient comfort and compliance, further solidifying CT as a cornerstone of gastrointestinal imaging (Boskoski et al., 2025).

7.2.3. CT Imaging Limitations and Risks

The application of computed tomography (CT) scanning in the assessment of the gastrointestinal tract is of enormous advantage, but is not risk-free and without restriction. One of the most remarkable risks is ionizing radiation exposure, which carries a higher risk of cancer, particularly when done repeatedly or in high-risk populations such as children. The cumulative dose from radiation exposure underscores urgent health concerns, making radiologists extremely cautious about the necessity of CT imaging in every clinical situation. Furthermore, while CT scans provide detailed images that enhance diagnostic accuracy, they cannot always distinguish malignant from benign lesions, leading to diagnostic uncertainty. As mentioned in recent studies, excessive reliance on decision-making on CT imaging at times results in misdiagnosis or failure of detection of conditions (Hansson et al., 2022). Another serious limitation of CT imaging is that it cannot provide real-time images, unlike other modalities such as fluoroscopy. This aspect is particularly valuable in dynamic assessments, such as examining biliary strictures or determining the severity of obstructions. Although CT can generate informative static images, its limitations in imaging motion and providing functional data can limit its usefulness in diagnosing certain clinical disorders (Boskoski et al., 2025). Further, contrast agents used during the CT scan, by enhancing the visualization of the organs, may cause adverse reactions. These might range from mild allergic reactions to more serious ones, thereby augmenting the risk profile of the CT scan. Thus, informed consent and pre-screening for potential allergic reactions are integral components of the process of CT imaging. Lastly, economic costs associated with CT imaging might restrict its usage. The costs of CT scans can be a significant burden on health care systems and patients, particularly in regions with limited resources. Moreover, because of the cost of CT technology, medical practitioners may automatically prefer CT scans over less expensive and potentially safer imaging modalities, such as MRI or ultrasound. That preference biases clinical decision-making and directs practitioners to a technology-driven rather than patient-focused model. Taking advantage of the advent of new imaging technologies, such as single-operator peroral cholangiopancreatoscopy (SOPCP) or advanced magnetic resonance modalities, may help offset some of these risks and limitations. Still, the overall approach must remain holistic and sensitive to patient-specific factors (Hansson et al., 2022) (Figure 7.6).

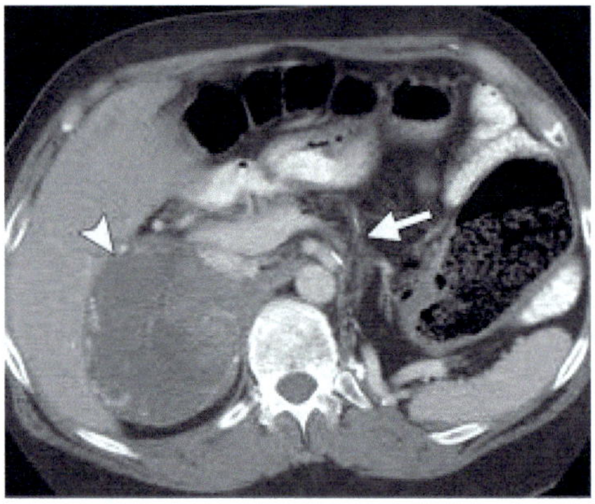

Figure 7.6. Imaging effects of radiation therapy in the abdomen and pelvis.

Source: https://encrypted-tbn0.gstatic.com/images?q=tbn:ANd9GcSC8sXC9rr4lnkw73aQrlIWLgY1LaEU2jZmwQ&s.

7.3. Magnetic Resonance Imaging (MRI)

Magnetic Resonance Imaging (MRI) is increasingly important in the non-surgical assessment of gastrointestinal (GI) tract disease. Unlike computed tomography (CT) and fluoroscopy, MRI employs magnetic fields and radiofrequency waves to produce high-quality images with excellent soft-tissue differentiation. This imaging characteristic is particularly well-suited to image structures that are less well-imaged on other imaging modalities, such as the liver, pancreas, and biliary tract. In evaluating conditions like biliary strictures, MRI is useful in providing accurate information differentiating between benign and malignant causes, which is critical in management. Utilization of MR cholangiopancreatography (MRCP) also maximizes diagnostic potential by imaging bile ducts directly, hence significantly improving treatment planning and minimizing unnecessary invasive procedures. While very valuable, MRI also presents some drawbacks to GI tract imaging. A significant drawback is the greater acquisition time compared to CT scanning, which will pose a problem for claustrophobic patients or those with difficulty maintaining stillness for an extended time. MRI is also less effective in patients with acute hemorrhage or dense calcification, where CT has an advantage due to the speed and availability of CT scanners. However, the advances in techniques such as diffusion-weighted imaging and the use of new contrast media have rendered MRI a more valuable tool in diagnosis with respect to dual evaluation of GI organ anatomy and function. Therefore, awareness of these limitations is necessary while selecting the appropriate imaging modality for proper clinical indications. The use of MRI as part of a multidisciplinary approach is one aspect of a broader trend toward integrated diagnostic methods to the management of gastrointestinal disease. This integration of imaging techniques with biochemical markers and endoscopic techniques allows practitioners to better enhance diagnostic pathways, particularly in the case of complicated biliary strictures. Consistent with recent literature, the integration of MRI with endoscopic retrograde cholangiopancreatography (ERCP) and endoscopic ultrasound (EUS) is pivotal for improving diagnostic precision and therapeutic efficacy by providing comprehensive understanding of biliary pathology (Boskoski et al., 2025). With advances in the field through technological innovations, the role of MRI is only bound to become more pivotal to achieving timely and effective patient management across various gastrointestinal diseases.

7.3.1. Principles of MRI Technology

Magnetic Resonance Imaging (MRI) scans are based on nuclear magnetic resonance, mainly making use of the magnetic properties of hydrogen nuclei in water molecules. MRI excels at imaging soft tissues and is particularly beneficial for imaging the gastrointestinal tract. MRI employs strong magnetic fields and radiofrequency pulses to create images that may reveal anatomical and pathological disease within the gastrointestinal system (Figure 7.7).

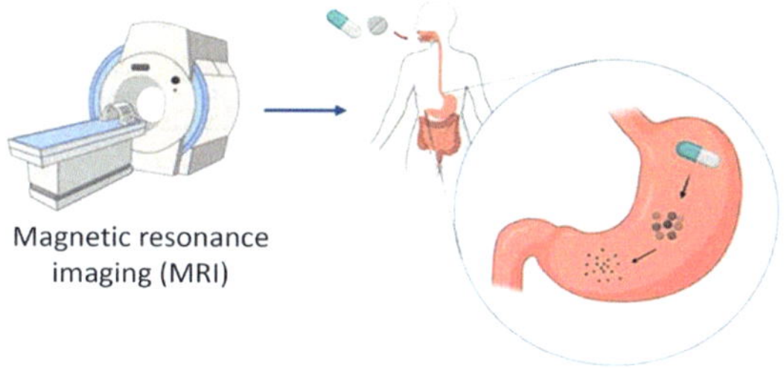

Figure 7.7. Overview of MRI scanner and magnetic field interaction with abdominal tissues.

Source: https://pubs.acs.org/cms/10.1021/acs.molpharmaceut.3c01123/asset/images/medium/mp3c01123_0006.gif.

Unlike CT scans, which use ionizing radiation, MRI is a safer choice because it is especially effective for children and patients who need multiple images. Contrast between different tissues, particularly between water and fat content, allows for MRI to delineate soft tissues with outstanding specificity, achieving maximum diagnostic accuracy while maintaining risks of radiation exposure in imaging at a minimum (N/A, 2006). Furthermore, MRI technology has advanced, with specialist imaging sequences facilitating greater use in the diagnosis of gastrointestinal diseases. Sequences such as diffusion-weighted imaging (DWI), MR cholangiopancreatography (MRCP), and functional MRI (fMRI) have increased the use of traditional MRI. DWI allows cellularity in lesions to be measured, useful in differentiating malignant and benign tumors, while MRCP provides a non-invasive imaging modality for biliary and pancreatic ductal anatomy visualization, essential in the diagnosis of diseases like choledocholithiasis and pancreatitis. Oral and intravenous contrast agents also increase the visibility of gastrointestinal pathology and structures. These developments supplement the role of MRI in clinical settings, enabling whole-body imaging of gastrointestinal pathology without the risks associated with ionizing radiation, thereby reducing safety concerns that plague other imaging modalities (Hansson et al., 2022).

The integration of MRI technology into routine gastrointestinal imaging protocols not only enhances diagnostic capability but also significantly contributes to treatment planning and follow-up. With advancing imaging modalities, the role of MRI in diagnostic workup is gaining significance, particularly in increasingly complex cases where conventional imaging falls short. Such a capability to depict the gastrointestinal tract with an enhanced, more three-dimensional perspective enhances clinicians' ability to deliver better, more enlightened decisions, particularly with treatment response cases or preoperative planning. However, the use of MRI in gastrointestinal imaging is not without issues, including longer testing times and patients' discomfort with small areas in MRI machines. Nevertheless, continued advances in MRI technology—such as the development of open MRI machines—work to eliminate these issues so that this imaging technique can remain an important tool in contemporary gastrointestinal diagnosis (N/A, 2006).

7.3.2. Benefits of MRI for Gastrointestinal Imaging

The application of Magnetic Resonance Imaging (MRI) in imaging the gastrointestinal tract has a number of strengths that provide tremendous advances in diagnostic precision and patient management. Perhaps the greatest strength of MRI is its excellent soft-tissue contrast resolution, which provides clear definition of the complex gastrointestinal anatomy. Whereas CT and fluoroscopy use ionizing radiation, MRI does not; thus, it is safer for patients, especially those requiring multiple follow-up imaging studies. Such is the case in cases of chronic disease, such as inflammatory bowel disease, where repetitive follow-up is a component of management strategies (Figure 7.8).

The ability to acquire detailed images of soft tissues enables clinicians to differentiate between benign and malignant lesions, thereby enabling early and adequate therapeutic interventions (Boskoski et al., 2025). Furthermore, the versatility of MRI lets it to be easily combined with various contrast agents, allowing for adequate visualization of blood vessels and pathological organs within the GI tract. Another significant benefit of MRI in gastrointestinal imaging is its ability to provide functional information alongside structural assessment. Advanced techniques such as diffusion-weighted imaging and dynamic contrast-enhanced MRI can assess tissue properties that indicate disease processes, for example, tumor malignancy or inflammation. Combining these functional data, clinicians can make more informed treatment plan decisions. Furthermore, MRI excels at imaging many liver, pancreas, and biliary tree diseases. For instance, MRI can characterize biliary strictures well, which are typically difficult to assess with other imaging modalities. The integration of advanced imaging techniques yields a more holistic evaluation of the gastrointestinal tract, as thoroughly debated in recent literature on MRI application in biliary obstruction (Gregory et al., 2023). To this, MRI deployment in the imaging of the gastrointestinal system has also been facilitated by technological developments that increase efficiency and patient comfort. Technologies such as faster acquisition time and high-field-strength magnets help reduce scanning time, which reduces discomfort and enables increased levels of patient cooperation during procedures. This is especially crucial for clinical populations with intrinsic mobility limitations or fear of imaging investigations. The increasing application of artificial intelligence in MRI analysis has a vital role in enhancing diagnostic accuracy and workflow efficiency. By assisting radiologists with image interpretation and anomaly detection, AI technology enhances patient outcomes and departmental productivity (Gregory et al., 2023). Consequently, the multifaceted advantages of MRI in gastrointestinal imaging place it at the center stage in modern diagnostic radiology, pushing developments toward improved patient satisfaction and care.

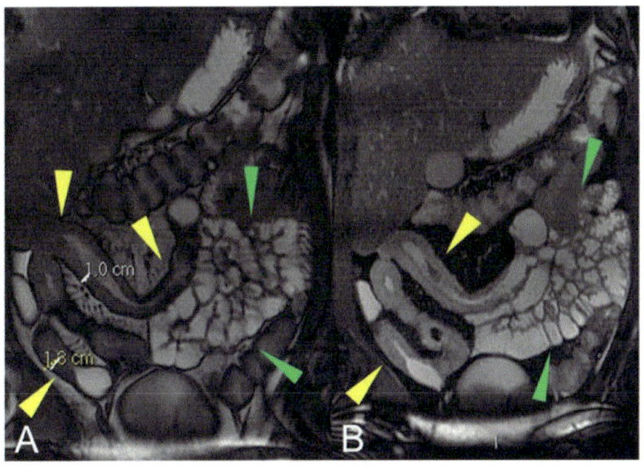

Figure 7.8. Quantification of intestinal strictures. Coronal fast imaging employing steady-state acquisition (FIESTA) images (A, B) show a long segment of the distal ileum affected by pathology (yellow arrowheads). The upstream loops do not show dilatation (green arrowheads) because the pathological loops do not show significant abnormal stiffness or massive luminal reduction. This condition represents a non-functional "stenosis" because the intestinal flow is preserved, so there is no risk of sub-occlusions or intestinal obstruction.

Source: https://www.mdpi.com/life/life-13-01836/article_deploy/html/images/life-13-01836-g002-550.jpg.

7.3.3. MRI Challenges and Contraindications

The use of magnetic resonance imaging (MRI) to image the gastrointestinal tract is hindered by numerous challenges and contraindications that must be addressed to ensure the best results. The major problem is that MRI is very costly, which renders it inaccessible. Many of the centers that offer MRI facilities may not have high-tech equipment for quality gastrointestinal imaging, which would be difficult to apply in everyday practice. In addition, the limited availability of MRI can cause delays in diagnosis, particularly in emergencies where prompt response is critical. Despite such financial challenges, the growing interest in the potential of MRI, especially for evaluating complex bowel disease, underscores the need for more robust infrastructure to enable its use (Busato et al., 2023) (Figure 7.9).

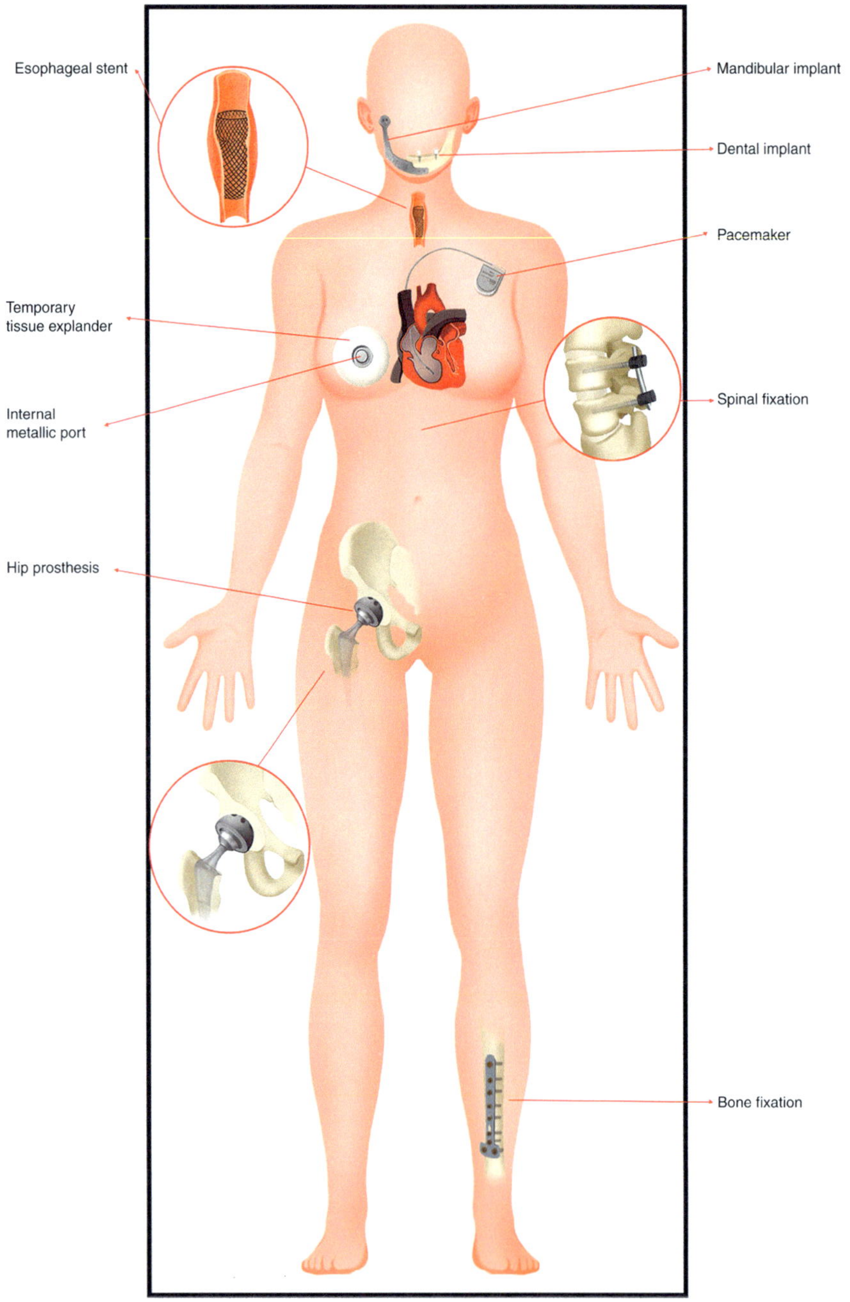

Figure 7.9. Shows a patient with implanted medical devices.

Source: https://www.spandidos-publications.com/article_images/mco/21/4/mco-21-04-02764-g00.jpg.

Another significant challenge is the presence of MRI contraindications inherent to the imaging modality. Implanted devices, such as pacemakers or cochlear implants, pose significant limitations for many patients due to the intense magnetic fields generated during MRI. Furthermore, patients with certain metallic foreign bodies, particularly those implanted within the gastrointestinal tract, risk complications when exposed to MRI. Although technological advances are improving safety, the need for thorough pre-MRI patient screening remains essential to avoid serious adverse effects. Careful individual-by-individual medical history and current health condition assessment is important to manage these contraindications effectively (Brabrand et al., 2015). In addition to patient-related factors, MRI has technical limitations that must also be taken into account. The relatively slow scanning times relative to CT and fluoroscopy can be uncomfortable or even refused, particularly by pediatric and claustrophobic patients. Motion artifacts can further degrade the image quality, impairing accurate diagnosis and assessment. This truth is most critical when evaluating the dynamic processes of the GI tract, where real-time imaging may be unavoidable. Moreover, MRI's vulnerability to bowel gas artifacts may make image interpretation more difficult, being less valuable in certain instances. As more research is conducted, the development of faster sequences and more directed intestinal contrast agents will probably outweigh such technical limitations, eventually increasing the use of MRI in gastrointestinal imaging (Busato et al., 2023).

7.4. Fluoroscopy in Gastrointestinal Imaging

Fluoroscopy is the core of gastrointestinal imaging, providing real-time visualization of the gut. Dynamic evaluation is particularly valuable for the assessment of functional abnormalities, allowing radiologists to observe the motility of various organs, such as the esophagus, stomach, and intestines. Patients may swallow a contrast medium, typically barium, during fluoroscopic procedures. This paint-like material coats the gastrointestinal tract lining and aids in the visualization of normal anatomical structures relative to pathological changes. Fluoroscopy is extensively used in the diagnosis of disorders such as esophageal strictures, gastrointestinal reflux, and obstructions, and also plays an important role in enabling therapeutic interventions such as balloon dilatation or stent delivery. The real-time nature of fluoroscopy enhances the clinician's ability to visualize certain functions, thus providing a full comprehension of gastrointestinal dynamics and priceless insight into patient management. Moreover, fluoroscopy is an essential adjunctive method in other diagnostic tools, such as capsule endoscopy. While capsule endoscopy plays a pivotal role in imaging the small bowel, particularly in diagnosing conditions such as Crohn's disease, it is often supplemented with fluoroscopic techniques to increase diagnostic yield. A case in point is fluoroscopy complementing balloon-assisted enteroscopy, allowing biopsies to be obtained and increasing the overall diagnostic yield in cases of suspected small bowel disease. The blending of these imaging modalities attests to the necessity of multidisciplinary management of complex gastrointestinal diseases. With clinicians resorting to complex imaging modalities more often, understanding how fluoroscopy blends with other strategies is crucial in maximizing patient results, particularly in cases where an acute diagnosis will significantly impact management strategies (Albert et al., 2011). While fluoroscopy offers numerous benefits for gastrointestinal imaging, it is important to assess the potential risks of radiation exposure. The otherwise innocuous procedure involves ionizing radiation and must therefore strike a proper balance between diagnostic usefulness and patient safety. There should be appropriate measures to limit exposure while maintaining image quality, especially in vulnerable populations such as children and pregnant women. Increased education of radiologists and technologists on how to best optimize fluoroscopic methods can help to reduce radiation exposure. In addition, as digital imaging technology continues to advance, more advanced techniques may further reduce exposure without affecting diagnostic quality. While the medical community continues to discuss the safety and efficacy of fluoroscopy within the grand scheme of gastrointestinal imaging, ongoing research and development will play essential roles in shaping the course of practices (N/A, 2006).

7.4.1. Description of Fluoroscopy and Its Function

Fluoroscopy is an imaging technology that provides images of internal structures in real time, which is very useful in the medical field of gastrointestinal (GI) tract imaging. It is done using X-rays projected onto a monitor, forming a continuous series that records the motion of organs and contrast materials as they travel through the GI tract. This modality offers a better understanding of the functional behaviors of the gastrointestinal tract, revealing disorders of motility, obstruction, and abnormality that static imaging equipment, like CT or MRI, may fail to detect.

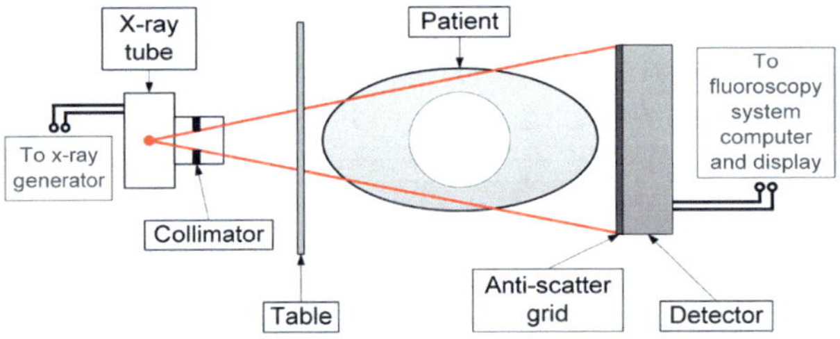

Figure 7.10. Fluoroscopy setup for barium swallow test.

Source: https://www.researchgate.net/publication/353195959/figure/fig3/AS:11431281125975854@1678503733392/Simplified-block-diagram-of-a-fluoroscopy-system-showing-key-components.png.

The real-time feedback provided by fluoroscopic imaging is of significant value in aiding diagnostic and interventional approaches, allowing clinicians to make decisions in a timely manner based on the visual information presented. One of the most significant applications of fluoroscopy in connection with the GI tract is its use in diagnostic imaging, such as barium swallow examinations, upper GI series, and fluoroscopy-assisted treatment. These not only assist in the diagnosis of conditions such as gastroesophageal reflux disease or peptic ulcers but also provide us with details about the structural movements during various stages of digestion. With contrast agents enhancing visibility, fluoroscopy explains complex physiological interactions, thereby increasing diagnostic reliability. Further, newer advances in imaging techniques, such as bimodal ERCP, have demonstrated the potential of fluoroscopy to increase procedural efficiency while greatly reducing radiation exposure, as observed in studies highlighting the fine balance between diagnostic yield and safety (Hansson et al., 2022). While it has numerous positive aspects, fluoroscopy also has limitations. Radiation remains the primary risk factor, especially for patients undergoing multiple fluoroscopic examinations. Efforts to minimize radiation exposure while preserving image quality have led to more sophisticated protocols that lower doses without compromising diagnostic usefulness. For example, cone-beam fluoroscopy is also a developing alternative that can deliver high resolution at lower radiation doses (N/A, 2006). These developments highlight the need for ongoing research and development in fluoroscopy techniques, so that they continue to remain a core part of gastrointestinal tract imaging without undermining patient safety and diagnostic potential (Figure 7.10).

7.4.2. Applications of Fluoroscopy in Gastrointestinal Studies

Fluoroscopy is an important tool in gastrointestinal studies, as it provides real-time imaging to enhance the assessment of many abdominal diseases. The technique employs continuous X-ray imaging, allowing clinicians to see movement in the gastrointestinal tract, including peristalsis and the movement of contrast media. One of the most valuable applications of fluoroscopy is in the study of the upper gastrointestinal tract, such as barium swallows, where it helps diagnose conditions like esophageal strictures, tumors, and motility disorders. With fluoroscopy, medical professionals can acquire dynamic information that static imaging modalities like CT and MRI may not be able to provide. Thus, the ability to visualize the functional features of the gastrointestinal tract makes fluoroscopy a fundamental tool to investigate both structural and functional abnormalities (N/A, 2006). As fluoroscopy continues to advance, it is combined with newer techniques to optimize diagnostic accuracy and therapy. As an example, the development of bimodal endoscopic retrograde cholangiopancreatography (ERCP) offers improved imaging of complex biliopancreatic anatomy. This innovation demonstrates the utility of fluoroscopy in complementing other imaging modalities, such as MRI, which may be limited in real-time applications. Existing research indicates fluoroscopy, together with enhanced imaging modalities, optimizes the treatment of biliary disease, achieving better patient outcomes. Concerns about radiation exposure due to fluoroscopic procedures led to the use of low-dose techniques, maintaining diagnostic quality with decreased risk. Thus, the integration of fluoroscopy into gastrointestinal imaging not only solves clinical needs but also bears witness to a focus on safety for patients (Hansson et al., 2022).

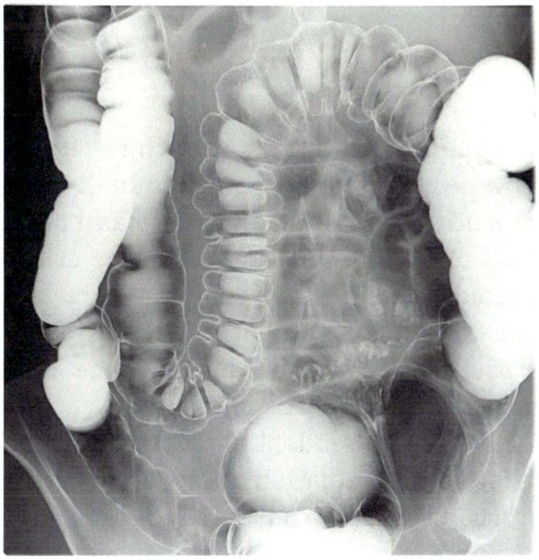

Figure 7.11. Fluoroscopic image from a barium enema procedure.

Source: https://prod-images-static.radiopaedia.org/images/18339436/60003fe5fce5d7cd69059a49dd87b6_big_gallery.jpeg.

Another significant application of fluoroscopy is its function in the guidance of interventional procedures within the gastrointestinal tract. Such procedures include feeding tube placements, stent placements, and biopsies, in which fluoroscopy is used to provide real-time feedback for instrument guidance. The capacity to dynamically image the gastrointestinal lumen is crucial in minimizing complications and optimizing therapeutic outcomes. With technologies such as single-operator peroral cholangiopancreatoscopy, fluoroscopic guidance is increasingly becoming critical in procedures. Research has shown that fluoroscopic guidance is integral to the success of complex biliary interventions, enabling health care providers to make informed decisions in a timely manner. As such, the multi-rational application of fluoroscopy reaffirms its pivotal place in gastrointestinal investigations as a bridging link between treatment and diagnosis effectively (N/A, 2006) (Figure 7.11).

7.4.3. Risks and Limitations of Fluoroscopy

Fluoroscopy, being a real-time imaging technique employing continuous X-ray for visualization of internal anatomy, has a number of risks and limitations that must be critically evaluated. Ionizing radiation exposure is one of the significant concerns associated with fluoroscopy because it increases the risk of cancer with increased duration of exposure, particularly with sequential procedures. Studies have found that radiation dosage from standard fluoroscopic exams can be significant and, in some instances, exceed that of other imaging technologies, such as CT scans. In addition, although adaptations do exist within protocols such as dose reduction measures, meticulous calibration and continuous monitoring are still necessary to ensure patient safety. Thus, operators must weigh the benefit of real-time visualization against potential long-term health consequences of radiation exposure. Another limitation of fluoroscopy is that it depends on the operator's competence and experience. Since the accuracy of the generated images would be a function of the operator's competence, there may be heterogeneity in diagnostic accuracy. Poor image handling or incorrect equipment operation can result in poor visualization, leading to misdiagnosis or missed pathologies. This is particularly acute in complex cases, such as evaluating biliary strictures, where accurate discrimination between benign and malignant etiology is crucial (Hansson et al., 2022). Failure to obtain quality images may interfere with correct treatment decisions and could subject patients to undue interventions or compromise timely critical interventions. Therefore, optimal utilization of fluoroscopy is not only dependent upon technical competence but also on a detailed understanding of the underlying anatomy and pathology by the operating physician. Lastly, fluoroscopy has procedural hazards that can affect patient outcomes, including complications. As an illustration, with fluoroscopically guided procedures like endoscopic retrograde cholangiopancreatography (ERCP), complications like pancreatitis may occur, which adds to patient morbidity and increases hospital stays. There have been recent advances in technology that introduce adjunct approaches to transcend limitations, for example, single-operator peroral cholangiopancreatoscopy (SOPCP), which enhances visualization without increasing the built-in risks of fluoroscopy (Hansson et al., 2022). In addition, although fluoroscopy remains a valuable tool in gastrointestinal imaging, it is necessary to employ a multidisciplinary approach to minimize its risks by introducing other imaging modalities as indicated. This method ensures that patient safety takes precedence in the pursuit of diagnostic accuracy (Figure 7.12).

Type of Procedure	Average Adult Effective Dose (mSv)	Estimated Dose Equivalent (No. of Chest X-rays)
Dental X-ray	0.005-0.01 [6a]	0.25-0.5
Chest X-ray	0.02	1
Mammography	0.4	20
CT	2-16 [6b]	100-800
Nuclear Medicine	0.2-41 [6c]	10-2050
Interventional Fluoroscopy	5-70 [6d]	250-3500

Figure 7.12. Radiation dose chart comparing fluoroscopy with CT.

7.5. Comparison of Imaging Modalities

The advent of newer imaging technologies has, in a significant manner, changed the field of gastrointestinal tract assessment, with several modalities available for studying diseases such as inflammatory bowel disease and malignancies. Of these, the leading choice is computed tomography (CT), which has become prized for its speed and efficacy in disclosing structural flaws. It performs best at diagnosing acute diseases such as appendicitis or diverticulitis due to its ability to produce high-quality images quickly, making it particularly useful in emergency care. Despite its benefits, though, CT is also restricted by exposure to ionizing radiation, which creates problems of cumulative effect, especially with younger patients and those who need to undergo frequent follow-up scans. Thus, while CT is a common procedure, other imaging modalities must be employed to enhance patient safety without compromising diagnostic quality. MRI emerges as a strong candidate to replace CT, particularly for achieving similarly high soft-tissue contrast without ionizing radiation.

This can be particularly beneficial in the management of chronic gastrointestinal conditions, for example, Crohn's disease, where MRI plays a significant role in the assessment of complications and extent of disease. MRI is not only feasible for the assessment of gastrointestinal structures but also of adjacent structures and is therefore valuable for the diagnosis of small bowel as well as extra-intestinal manifestations. Moreover, newer MRI techniques, such as diffusion-weighted imaging and functional MRI, further enhance its diagnostic contribution. Nevertheless, there are some limitations, such as longer acquisition time and contraindication to particular implants or devices, which might affect patient suitability. Thus, the choice between MRI and CT might very well be determined by the specific clinical scenario and patient factors. Fluoroscopy, while less discussed than CT and MRI, is nonetheless an important tool employed in gastrointestinal imaging, but only for functional assessment of the gastrointestinal tract. Barium swallow or barium enema studies are employed to demonstrate motility disorders and structural abnormalities in real time. Dynamic imaging can detect conditions that static imaging with CT or MRI may miss, such as esophageal strictures or dysmotility disorders. Fluoroscopy's capability to assess gastrointestinal function, together with its diagnostic efficacy, makes it particularly valuable in certain clinical settings. However, it has to be noted that fluoroscopy, similar to CT, utilizes ionizing radiation. Therefore, its application must be judiciously weighed against risk in patients in whom frequent imaging becomes required, such as those with chronic gastrointestinal disease (Albert et al., 2011). Finally, a general understanding of these imaging modalities underscores the need for personalized management plans for patients, tailored to their strengths, to optimize diagnostic and therapeutic benefits (N/A, 2006).

7.5.1. Comparative Effectiveness of CT and MRI

In gastrointestinal tract imaging, the use of computed tomography (CT) or magnetic resonance imaging (MRI) is of the highest significance since they each possess unique advantages and disadvantages. CT is typically preferred due to its rapid acquisition time and improved availability, making it particularly helpful in emergency cases where a rapid assessment is critical. It excels especially at imaging acute conditions such as appendicitis and bowel obstruction due to its ability to provide high-resolution images quickly. Naturally, the ionizing radiation of CT and the potential hazards of contrast agents must be taken into account, particularly in vulnerable populations. Therefore, while CT is a first-line diagnostic agent, appropriate regard for patient safety and the specific clinical environment is paramount in determining its effectiveness relative to MRI in gut imaging (Figure 7.13).

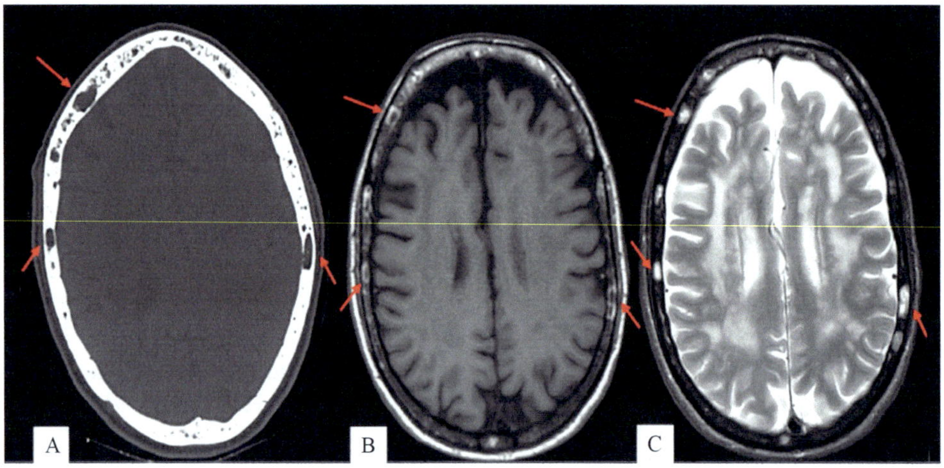

Figure 7.13. Detection of the number of lesions by CT and MRI in a 72-year-old male known case of multiple myeloma (A) CT bone algorithm image shows multiple ill-defined lytic lesions within the diploic space. MRI T1W (B) and T2W (C) images at the same level show multiple lesions appearing hypointense on T1W and hyperintense on T2W image. Both CT and MRI were able to depict various lesions in skull bones.

Source: https://www.researchgate.net/publication/359241365/figure/fig1/AS:11431281101314777@1669422142391/Detection-of-number-of-lesions-by-CT-and-MRI-in-a-72-year-old-male-known-case-of-multiple.png.

Conversely, MRI has superior soft tissue contrast and non-ionizing imaging and would therefore be more appropriate for the evaluation of chronic gastrointestinal illness, especially for complex pathology like liver lesions and biliary strictures. ‘ superior tissue differentiation capability is particularly useful in distinguishing between benign and malignant lesions and thus instrumental in achieving superior diagnostic outcomes. Advances in MRI technology, including MR cholangiopancreatography (MRCP), provide excellent imaging of the biliary tree without the risks associated with invasive methods. This capability is critical in the management of conditions like biliary strictures, where careful characterization is necessary to guide therapeutic interventions. Moreover, MRI not only contributes to diagnosis but also to treatment planning and follow-up, especially in close monitoring, and thus illustrates its role in selected clinical scenarios compared with CT. The use of CT and MRI together in a multi-modality imaging strategy can significantly enhance diagnostic proficiency in the gastrointestinal tract. Both modalities, if utilized effectively, complement and maximize patient outcomes. For instance, while CT may be the imaging procedure of first resort in the acute setting due to its speed and availability, MRI would then be applied for more intricate cases where deep anatomical data is required. Recent literature suggests that a multidisciplinary analysis of both imaging techniques can enhance the distinction of biliary strictures, as emphasized in reviews on the combination of imaging techniques such as CECT, MRI/MRCP, and advanced endoscopy (Boskoski et al., 2025). By taking advantage of each modality's capabilities, healthcare providers can augment diagnostic avenues and offer timely and effective gastrointestinal disease management.

7.5.2. Each Imaging Type Cost Implications

The cost considerations of imaging the gastrointestinal tract play a significant role in selecting diagnostic modalities such as CT, MRI, and fluoroscopy. Computed tomography (CT) is generally preferred in practice due to its short scanning time and relatively lower operating cost. However, the collective expenses of CT increase, particularly for patient preparation, iodinated contrast media administration, and radiation exposure complications. These expenses are augmented by the need for follow-up studies when results are inconclusive, thereby influencing total health expenditure. Hence, while CT provides instant affordability, its cumulative costs need to be aligned with clinical effectiveness to optimize resource utilization in gastrointestinal diagnosis (Figure 7.14).

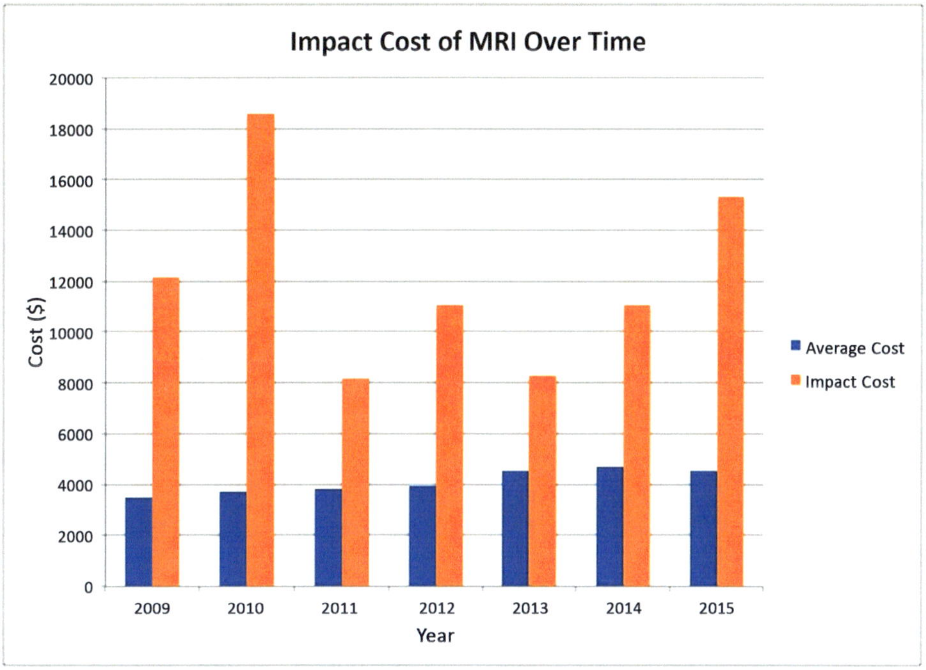

Figure 7.14. Average cost of magnetic resonance imaging (MRI) per year and impact cost of MRI per year, adjusted for inflation and listed in 2009 dollars.

Source: https://www.researchgate.net/profile/Srikanth-Divi-2/publication/338304481/figure/fig2/AS:876301351124997@1585937931911/Average-cost-of-magnetic-resonance-imaging-MRI-per-year-and-impact-cost-of-MRI-per.png.

Magnetic resonance imaging (MRI), though generally more costly than CT, offers several advantages, particularly for examining soft-tissue structures of the gastrointestinal tract. MRI is more costly due to the need for more costly equipment, highly trained personnel, and longer scanning time. Despite all these considerations, MRI is invaluable in some situations, such as in the assessment of liver lesions or inflammatory bowel disease, where its non-ionizing nature exposes to much fewer risks compared to ionizing radiation in CT. In examining cost-effectiveness, it may be justified to use MRI over CT for select patient populations, reducing long-term healthcare costs associated with radiation exposure and potentially avoiding more invasive diagnostic procedures, thereby demonstrating MRI's strategic value within the broader medical economy. Fluoroscopy provides another dimension to cost considerations, as it provides the union of real-time imaging with diagnostic versatility, particularly with functional testing of the gastrointestinal tract with barium swallow or enema study. The flip side of the advantages is that the cost of fluoroscopy is based on a variety of factors: equipment maintenance, use of contrast media, and personnel training. In addition, radiation exposure risks are similar to those of CT. Interestingly, recently developed fluoroscopic techniques have incorporated dose-reduction technologies, but the operational costs to these are within the overall cost. As healthcare systems are increasingly under pressure to optimize resource utilization, it is essential to consider the financial cost of fluoroscopy relative to its clinical usefulness when choosing an imaging modality for gastrointestinal diagnosis.

7.5.3. Patient Safety and Comfort in Imaging Choices

In gastrointestinal imaging, patient safety and comfort are paramount concerns influencing the selection of imaging modalities such as CT, MRI, and fluoroscopy directly. Every technique possesses a distinct array of advantages and disadvantages regarding the patient's experience. CT scans are commonly used with rapid acquisition of high-resolution anatomical information, but ionizing radiation exposure raises an issue with patient safety, especially with sensitive populations such as children and pregnant women. On the other hand, MRI is a radiation-free alternative with improved soft-tissue contrast, but patient comfort must be considered, particularly regarding long scanning times and the narrow MRI bore. Therefore, an educated choice between these imaging modalities not only enhances diagnostic accuracy but also reflects a dedication to patient welfare as a guiding principle in the imaging process. Furthermore, research has begun to elucidate the impact of imaging surfaces on patient comfort and safety, a factor most often overlooked in radiological practice. One study with healthy volunteers, supine on various imaging surfaces, highlighted significant differences in experience, including pain and discomfort. Volunteers reported a noticeable difference in interface pressure across various imaging tables, which revealed new dimensions of patient comfort that need to be prioritized in imaging. The findings highlighted the importance of utilizing appropriate imaging surfaces to prevent pressure-related complications, which can compromise post-procedure patient comfort and recovery. This emerging evidence makes it clear that all aspects of the imaging environment need to be optimized to support patient safety, thereby confirming the necessity for continuous critique and improvement of imaging modalities and their related infrastructure. Lastly, patient contribution to the imaging process is essential to developing experiences that maximize comfort while minimizing discomfort. Health care professionals ought to engage patients in discussions about their concerns and anxieties related to imaging tests. By gaining insight into the psychological aspects of patients' experiences—from fear of radiation hazards to distress with body positioning—medical professionals can intervene to alleviate fears, such as reassuring patients or applying methods to increase comfort during longer tests. This aspect comes into sharp focus in fluoroscopy use, where patient cooperation is required through patient tolerance for real-time imaging. Stressing patient-centered care fosters a compassionate culture that not only addresses medical needs but also individual patient choices, leading to improved outcomes in imaging the gastrointestinal tract (Figure 7.15).

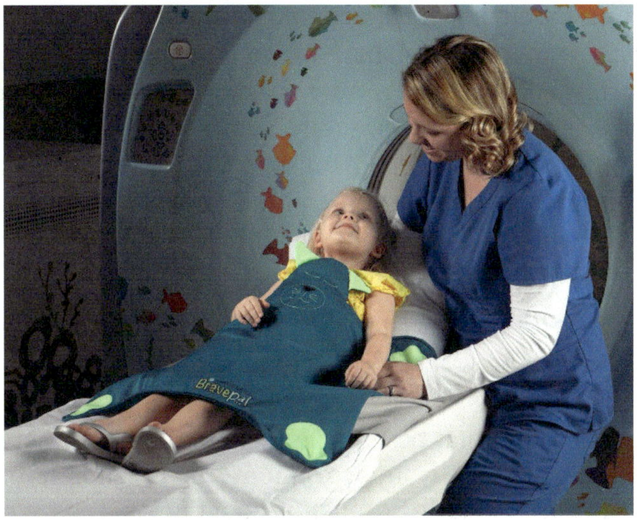

Figure 7.15. Showing patient comfort in CT imaging modality.

Source: https://www.dicardiology.com/sites/default/files/pediatric_ct_patient_safety_best_practices_study.jp.

7.6. Future Trends in Gastrointestinal Imaging

The GI imaging future is filled with great promise for significant improvement driven by new technology and innovative solutions. As the field continues to move toward digital, integration of artificial intelligence (AI) and machine learning will raise diagnostic accuracy and productivity. Such technologies will assist radiologists in interpreting complex imaging data by identifying subtle patterns that the naked eye cannot detect. Imaging technologies will continue to undergo transformational change, such as contrast-enhanced MRI and Electrical Impedance Tomography (EIT), which will improve imaging quality and diagnostic capability and ultimately lead to improved patient outcomes. The aggressive pursuit of the advancement of imaging modalities only underscores the critical necessity for continuous research and development to actually implement such technologies in clinical practice, as well as address concerns in terms of training radiologists to utilize advanced imaging technologies in collaboration (Dagnino et al., 2024).

Beyond technology, the future of gastrointestinal imaging will likely place even greater emphasis on personalized medicine. Customizing imaging protocols to the individual patient's specific anatomical and pathological features will enable more precise evaluation and specific interventions. Personalized imaging protocols may forestall unwarranted procedures and lower exposure of patients to radiation, a crucial factor considering the increased awareness of the possible dangers of over-imaging. Multidisciplinary team-oriented collaborative approaches—coordinating radiologists, gastroenterologists, and oncologists—will become central to deploying customized imaging approaches to optimize diagnostic pathways. While collaborative models are entering routine practice, they will not only enhance patient care but also help unify emerging imaging sciences and improve conformity with the requirements of individual patients (Dagnino et al., 2024). Moreover, the coming years of gastrointestinal imaging will also see innovations in data management and imaging accessibility. Cloud-based imaging technologies will provide access to more images at higher resolutions, thereby enabling specialists to consult irrespective of geographical location. This shift to digital platforms will assure real-time sharing and evaluation of imaging data, thereby facilitating rapid clinical decision-making. Parallelly, adoption of advanced data mining techniques is expected to aid in the analysis of big amounts of image data generated in clinical settings. With the growth of such data analytics capabilities, healthcare experts can extract useful information that aids more precise diagnosis and improved healthcare delivery. Reference to these emerging trends highlights ongoing advances in gastrointestinal imaging and an auspicious revolutionary future with greater accuracy, efficiency, and access (Bhuiyan et al., 2023).

7.6.1. Technological Advancements in Imaging

The field of imaging the gastrointestinal tract has undergone radical change over the past decades and has been technologically driven by improvements in diagnostic efficiency and precision. Computed Tomography (CT) and Magnetic Resonance Imaging (MRI) have evolved to achieve higher resolution and faster acquisition times than traditional approaches. For instance, multidetector CT offers the ability to acquire fast high-resolution images, enabling clinicians to visualize complex anatomical structures of the gastrointestinal tract. In addition, technologies such as dual-energy CT enable discrimination among tissue types and detection of faint pathologies (Figure 7.16).

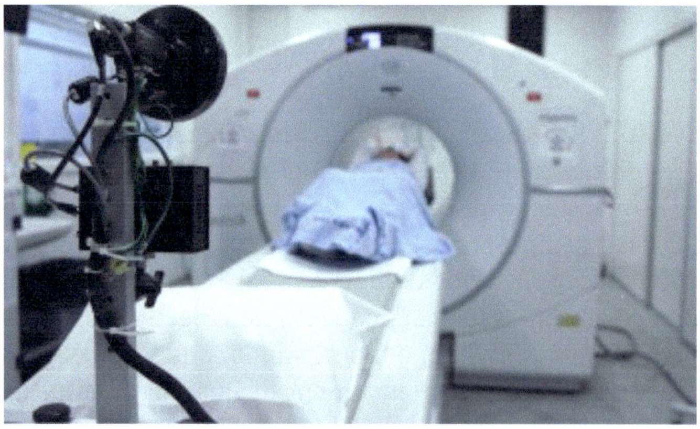

Figure 7.16. AI-assisted detection of intestinal polyps using enhanced CT.

Source: https://cdn.ecancer.org/43483-m.jpg.

These advancements, besides improving the quality of images obtained, also significantly reduce the level of radiation exposure used in such imaging modalities. Such an advancement is particularly important in diseases of the gastrointestinal tract, which require prompt and accurate detection of lesions, as timely treatment tends to be more beneficial for the patient. Other than the advancements in CT and MRI, fluoroscopy also remains a developing technology, making it an even stronger tool for the imaging of the gastrointestinal tract. Digital fluoroscopy provides real-time visualization of the GI tract, which significantly enhances the assessment of motility disorders and structural abnormalities. When used with contrast agents, this technology enables physicians to monitor the movement of substances through the digestive system. Furthermore, advances in imaging processing technologies have enhanced the resolution and quality of the fluoroscopic images, enhancing capabilities in terms of evaluating strictures and lesions, among other medical conditions. Recent technological advances, including the use of fluoroscopy in an interventional context, offer more specific therapies while lowering the need for exploratory invasive procedures. These advances underscore the ongoing utility of fluoroscopy to complete gastrointestinal disease evaluation and encourage interdisciplinary approaches to patient care. Emerging technologies such as artificial intelligence (AI) and machine learning have the potential to further revolutionize imaging practice in the gastrointestinal tract. AI technology can scan imaging data at high speed and high accuracy, helping to detect abnormalities that may go unnoticed by the human eye. As an illustration, the use of AI in image analysis has the ability to increase the diagnostic process efficiency, leading to quicker and more precise results. In addition, current imaging modalities, such as MRCP, facilitate better visualization of biliary anatomy, as noted in conditions such as biliary strictures. Accuracy achieved with MRCP is crucial in distinguishing between malignant and benign strictures, which is normally challenging in consideration of overlapping features. Progress in the field remains centered on a multidisciplinary approach, with the goal of bringing together imaging specialists, gastroenterologists, and oncologists to optimize patient pathways for the management of challenging gastrointestinal disease (Boskoski et al., 2025).

7.6.2. Integration of Artificial Intelligence in Imaging

The application of artificial intelligence (AI) on imaging modalities such as computed tomography (CT), magnetic resonance imaging (MRI), and fluoroscopy is a milestone in gastrointestinal tract diagnosis. AI algorithms, profound learning algorithms, have been shown to hold promise in enhancing image analysis, thereby diagnostic efficiency and accuracy. Such technologies can potentially analyze large datasets quickly, enabling radiologists to catch abnormalities that would otherwise be overlooked. Artificial Intelligence systems can be employed to recognize conditions such as biliary strictures, where distinguishing between benign and malignant etiologies is paramount for appropriate patient management (Figure 7.17).

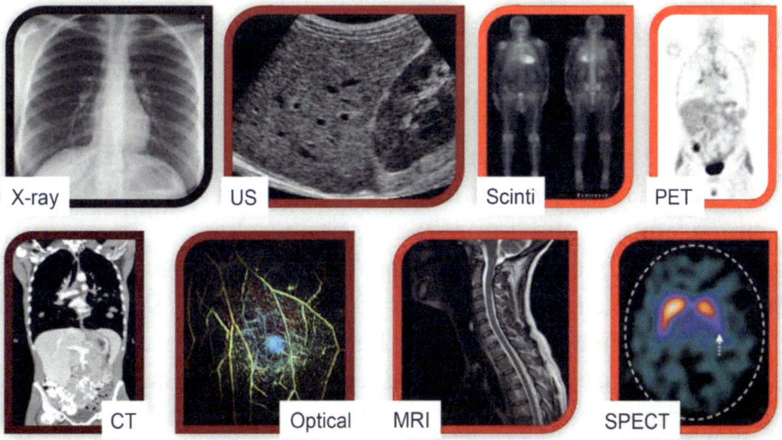

Figure 7.17. Deep learning model interface identifying GI abnormalities on MRI.

Source: https://www.mdpi.com/applsci/applsci-13-10521/article_deploy/html/images/applsci-13-10521-g001.png.

With the ability to process and interpret complex imaging data, AI is a valuable complement to traditional imaging modalities, enabling clinicians to make informed, evidence-based decisions regarding the diagnosis and treatment of gastrointestinal diseases. The incorporation of AI into the diagnostic pipeline has the potential to simplify workflows and reduce the workload for healthcare practitioners. For instance, in fluoroscopy and other imaging modalities, AI can assist in automating routine tasks, such as identifying anatomical patterns and highlighting areas of interest. This not only saves time but also results in better consistency of findings across various radiologists, hence decreasing variability that is inherent in human interpretation. Also, recent advancements have revealed the potential of AI in developing predictive models that estimate outcomes under different conditions based on imaging findings, thereby enabling anticipatory decision-making. In gastrointestinal imaging, these advancements reveal AI's potential to reshape the diagnostic process, both increasing speed and enhancing precision in patient care. Additionally, the combined potential of AI with endoscopic techniques is providing access to more precise interventions. In the context of biliary strictures, for example, AI can be used to integrate advanced imaging modalities to maximize tissue characterization and improve procedural outcomes. ERCP and EUS are some of the methods assisted by analysis from AI, which enhances differentiation between challenging strictures. As suggested in new studies, combining AI with traditional methods can potentially improve diagnostic processes by allowing more patient-specific management methods based on in-depth data analysis. The variety of AI modalities, both imaging and endoscopic, suggests the potential to revolutionize the diagnostic process in gastrointestinal imaging, significantly improving patient outcomes (Boskoski et al., 2025).

7.6.3. Potential for Personalized Imaging Approaches

The evolution of imaging techniques for the gastrointestinal tract has opened the door to individualized imaging approaches that will enable optimization of diagnostic accuracy and treatment planning. Standard imaging modalities such as CT, MRI, and fluoroscopy are highly versatile tools used in the assessment of most gastrointestinal disorders; yet their use is usually by means of fixed protocols that do not consider patient-specific anatomical and physiological variations. Personalized imaging techniques employ advanced technologies, including artificial intelligence and machine learning algorithms, to analyze large volumes of imaging and clinical data (Figure 7.18).

This shift from universal to individualized protocols enables clinicians to take into consideration patient-specific factors such as age, gender, habitus, and medical comorbidities, ultimately leading to more accurate interpretation and improved patient outcomes in gastrointestinal imaging. Additionally, the integration of personalized imaging approaches offers avenues for optimizing patient management, particularly in difficult cases such as biliary strictures. Distinguishing between benign and malignant strictures is difficult because of their similar imaging features. Recent advances, as described in the literature, propose a multidisciplinary assessment that includes biochemical markers, in addition to imaging modalities such as MRI/MRCP and CECT, to improve diagnostic specificity. These combinations have not only the promise of improved image interpretation but perhaps the potential to employ new technologies such as predictive modeling, which could provide the probabilities of disease status given imaging findings. With the prospect of delivering tailored information to healthcare providers, these techniques could substantially reduce unnecessary interventions and expedite appropriate management of biliary tract disorders, thereby enhancing the effectiveness of the healthcare system. Essentially, the possibilities of personalized imaging strategies are not limited to diagnostic purposes; they also extend to therapeutic methodologies tailored to individual patient requirements. Through technological advancements, one can visualize physiological processes in real time, which guides treatment for diverse gastrointestinal diseases. For instance, precision of endoscopic procedures when combined with personalized imaging can be a game-changer for the success of treatments like endoscopic retrograde cholangiopancreatography (ERCP) and endoscopic ultrasound (EUS), as they learn to target specific areas of interest with minimal risk to the patient. As newer endoscopic interventions and AI-driven imaging analysis find their place in the clinic, gastrointestinal imaging diagnosis continues to evolve. This convergence of technology and personalized medicine portends potential improved patient care, ultimately for improved health outcomes in managing the gastrointestinal tract, as highlighted in recent reviews of imaging protocols (Boskoski et al., 2025).

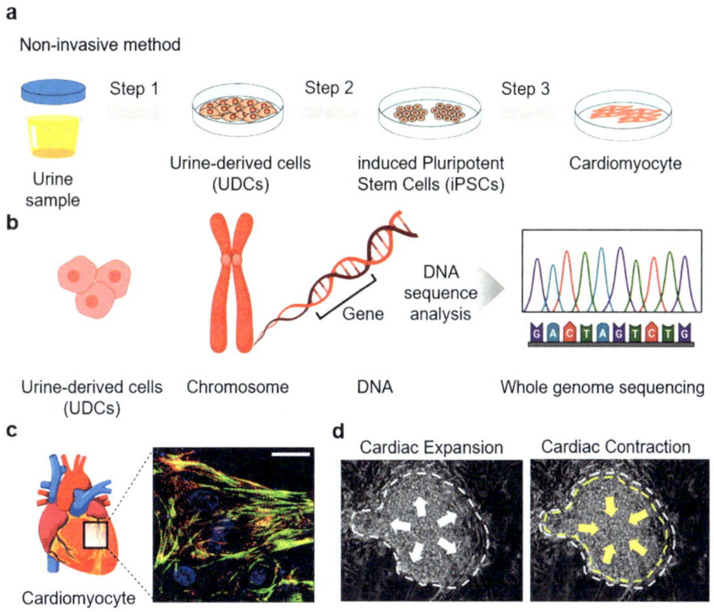

Figure 7.18. Concept illustration of personalized imaging based on genetic and biometric profiles.

Source: https://media.springernature.com/lw685/springer-static/image/art%3A10.1038%2Fs41598-025-02516-8/MediaObjects/41598_2025_2516_Fig2_HTML.png.

SUMMARY

In brief, the advent of high-tech imaging techniques such as CT, MRI, and fluoroscopy has revolutionized the diagnostic setting of gastrointestinal pathology. Each has its respective strengths and weaknesses. For instance, CT is well known for its speed in image acquisition and excellent spatial resolution, which is of utmost importance in the emergency room in cases of appendicitis or bowel obstructions. Conversely, MRI excels at soft-tissue contrast without ionizing radiation and is particularly beneficial for evaluating inflammatory bowel disease and small-bowel disease. Combining these imaging modalities effectively offers a comprehensive evaluation that may be used to guide clinical management and intervention, and emphasizes their strategic importance in contemporary gastroenterology. Imaging techniques are employed not only for diagnosis but also for the ongoing management and follow-up of gastrointestinal disease. Imaging technologies such as capsule endoscopy and balloon-assisted enteroscopy have enabled visualization of the small bowel and the ability to take biopsies, which is essential in the diagnosis of diseases like Crohn's disease. There are newer MRI developments that also provide data on enteral and extra-intestinal involvement, thereby affirming the role of imaging in estimating disease progression and therapeutic outcomes in patients, particularly those who have undergone surgical interventions. Investigators continue to highlight the impact of modern imaging modalities on patient outcomes because they underscore the role of such imaging in disease management strategies (Albert et al., 2011). In addition, integrating computer-aided technology with traditional imaging modalities enhances diagnostic precision and therapeutic planning. For instance, in biliary stricture, the fusion of biochemical markers, high-technology imaging, and endoscopic treatments has enhanced our ability to differentiate between malignant and benign origins of obstruction. The use of MRI/MRCP and other imaging modalities allows clinicians to further delineate complex cases, while advances such as artificial intelligence also have the potential to further increase diagnostic accuracy. This multi-dimensional approach is crucial in curtailing diagnostic difficulties and ensuring timely healthcare provision, ultimately leading to improved patient outcomes in managing gastrointestinal diseases (Boskoski et al., 2025).

CLOSER LOOK

GASTROINTESTINAL TRACT IMAGING

In gastrointestinal tract imaging, modalities such as Computed Tomography (CT), Magnetic Resonance Imaging (MRI), and Fluoroscopy provide critical information for diagnosing a wide range of digestive tract conditions. CT scans, renowned for speed and accuracy, find extensive application in emergency rooms for the diagnosis of acute conditions such as appendicitis and bowel blockage. Its excellent high-resolution images facilitate better identification of masses, inflammations, and other abnormalities, rendering it a valuable tool for clinicians. Further, the advances introduced by CT technology, including multi-slice scanning, have made it more efficient, allowing better assessment of the gastrointestinal tract and, thus, improving diagnostic outcome and patient management. MRI has been a useful alternative, particularly in the evaluation of soft tissue morphology and complex conditions like Crohn's disease. Unlike CT, MRI uses magnetic fields and radio waves, eliminating the use of ionizing radiation, making it highly appropriate for pediatric and pregnant populations. Recent evidence suggests that MRI is beneficial in showing inflammatory changes and complications of inflammatory bowel disease, which has encouraged shifts in the paradigm of diagnosis in gastroenterology. As recognized in previous revisions of diagnostic criteria for pediatric-onset inflammatory bowel disease, MRI has become increasingly recommended on the grounds of being non-invasive and capable of providing comprehensive imaging, thereby justifying its role as a critical component of gastrointestinal imaging (Alexander et al., 2013).

Fluoroscopy occupies a special niche in gastrointestinal imaging due to it providing real-time visualization of the gastrointestinal tract during procedures such as barium swallows or enemas. This capability allows clinicians to diagnose motility and functional disorders accurately. Dynamic imaging of fluoroscopy is quite distinct from the static images of CT and MRI, and hence a necessity for examining the mechanism of swallowing and diagnosing gastroesophageal reflux disease. Additionally, improvements in fluoroscopic methods have improved image quality and reduced radiation exposure, enhancing patient safety. In the advancement of medical imaging, the fusion of these modalities will generate an upgraded understanding of gastrointestinal diseases, ultimately resulting in improved diagnostic accuracy and patient care (Lei et al., 2023).

The selection of an appropriate imaging modality is essential for the diagnosis and treatment of gastrointestinal tract disease. Each imaging technique—computed tomography (CT), magnetic resonance imaging (MRI), or fluoroscopy—has inherent strengths that can be a lifesaver. For instance, CT scans are often the first choice due to its rapid acquisition of high-quality cross-sectional images, which enable clinicians to assess acute conditions such as appendicitis or bowel obstruction quickly. Conversely, MRI is very useful for assessing soft tissues, and the tool of preference when one is testing some cancers and inflammatory conditions of the gastrointestinal tract. Fluoroscopy, with its preeminence for real-time imaging, is of most importance when conducting functional examinations like swallowing tests or gastrointestinal motility assessment. The choice between these modalities affects not only diagnostic clarity but also radiation exposure, contrast risk, and overall patient comfort, and as such, demands careful consideration by health care providers. Furthermore, the evolving state of medical imaging technology once again highlights the need for a proper modality. One such advancement is digital imaging along with artificial intelligence, which has revolutionized radiology, improving the quality of images as well as the pace of interpretations. As noted, digital imaging enables immediate reviewability and reduces patient radiation exposure through sophisticated automatic exposure controls (Gregory et al., 2023). Additionally, innovations like three-dimensional reconstructions and maximum intensity projections (MIP) enhance the visualization of anatomical structures, thereby enhancing pre-surgical planning and evaluation of complex cases. This trend emphasizes the importance of clinicians and radiologists staying abreast of technological advancements so they can choose the most appropriate imaging modality for each individual's condition, ultimately leading to improved diagnostic precision and patient outcomes. Lastly, the outcomes of a proper imaging modality extend beyond the urgency of diagnostic benefit; they have long-term effects on patient care and treatment algorithms. The consequences of delayed or inaccurate diagnosis can be grave, particularly in conditions such as gastrointestinal cancers, where early detection is the most significant factor. The correct imaging device not only facilitates timely interventions but can also avoid unnecessary tests that can arise from misreads. With the healthcare environment increasingly focused on patients, the consequences of use and limitations of each imaging device should be familiar to practitioners so they can make informed choices. This widening emphasis on specialized imaging solutions is one component of a general commitment to improving patient outcomes and safety, further attesting to the overriding significance of choosing the right modality for imaging the gastrointestinal tract (N/A, 1985).

REFERENCES

1. Hausmann, J., & Albert, J. G. (2011). Detecting and managing small bowel Crohn's disease – capsule endoscopy becoming a first line diagnostic method? *Journal of Gastrointestinal & Digestive System*, *07*(04). https://doi.org/10.4172/2161-069x.s1-002Alexander, A., Barth, B., Bartunkova, T., Bernstein, C., Bousvaros, A., Boyce, T., et al. (2013). ESPGHAN Revised Porto Criteria for the diagnosis of inflammatory bowel disease in children and adolescents. https://core.ac.uk/download/83095760.pdf (accessed on 15th July 2025).
2. Bhuiyan, M. M. H., Gupta, K. D., Hossain, I., Islam, M. S., Jahan, N., Rahman, A., et al. (2023). Introduction of medical imaging modalities. http://arxiv.org/abs/2306.01022 (accessed on 15th July 2025).
3. Boskoski, I., & Spada, C. (2025). Diagnostic approach to biliary strictures. https://core.ac.uk/download/655042175.pdf (accessed on 15th July 2025).
4. Boskoski, I., Crino, S. F., Dhar, J., Facciorusso, A., Fuccio, L., Gkolfakis, P., Machicado, J., et al. (2025). Diagnostic approach to biliary strictures. https://core.ac.uk/download/654513733.pdf (accessed on 15th July 2025).
5. Brabrand, K., Cantisani, V., Correas, J. M., Cui, X. W., Dietrich, C. F., Dong, Y., & Xu, J. M., et al. (2015). EFSUMB guidelines on interventional ultrasound (INVUS), Part II: Diagnostic ultrasound-guided interventional procedures (Long Version). https://core.ac.uk/download/480425559.pdf (accessed on 15th July 2025).
6. Busato, L., Cardaccio, S., Catalano, C., Longhi, F., Manfrin, M., Priola, A. M., & Vitale, G. (2023). Magnetic resonance imaging of the gastrointestinal tract: Current role, recent advancements and future prospectives. https://core.ac.uk/download/621401868.pdf (accessed on 15th July 2025).
7. Dagnino, G., & Kundrat, D. (2024). Robot-assistive minimally invasive surgery: Trends and future directions. https://core.ac.uk/download/613613924.pdf (accessed on 15th July 2025).
8. Gregory, D. (2023). Innovations of radiology. https://core.ac.uk/download/619747458.pdf (accessed on 15th July 2025).
9. Lehigh Valley Health Network. (2009). Healthy you. https://core.ac.uk/download/267869826.pdf (accessed on 15th July 2025).
10. Lei, J., Lin, W., Wang, Y., Wu, Y., Zhang, X., Wang, J., & Xu, M. (2023). Can GPT-4V(ision) serve medical applications? Case studies on GPT-4V for multimodal medical diagnosis. http://arxiv.org/abs/2310.09909 (accessed on 15th July 2025).
11. N/A (1985). *Focal Spot, Spring/Summer 1985.* https://core.ac.uk/download/129069249.pdf (accessed on 15th July 2025).
12. N/A (1997). *Focal Spot, Fall/Winter 1997.* https://core.ac.uk/download/129069309.pdf (accessed on 15th July 2025).
13. N/A (2006). *Focal Spot, Spring 2006.* https://core.ac.uk/download/129069350.pdf (accessed on 15th July 2025).
14. N/A (2007). *Focal Spot, Winter 2006/2007.* https://core.ac.uk/download/129069354.pdf (accessed on 15th July 2025).

15. N/A (n.d.). Radiologic imaging in cystic fibrosis: Cumulative effective dose and changing trends over 2 decades. https://core.ac.uk/download/160477137.pdf (accessed on 15th July 2025).
16. Reuterwall Hansson, M. (2022). New technologies for the further advancement of ERCP. https://core.ac.uk/download/516463912.pdf (accessed on 15th July 2025).
17. Rogers, C. (2015). Radiological perspective of the formation of pressure ulcers - A comparison of pressure and experience on two imaging surfaces. https://core.ac.uk/download/603206223.pdf (accessed on 15th July 2025).

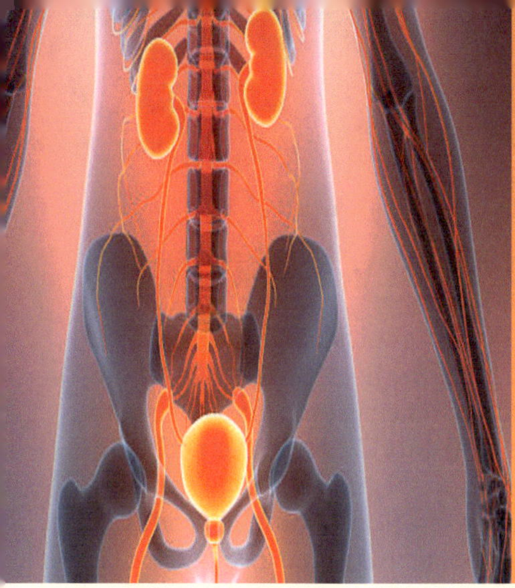

Chapter 8

GENITOURINARY IMAGING: KIDNEYS, BLADDER, AND PROSTATE

Contents

Introduction

Of all the systems in the realm of medical imaging, the genitourinary system stands out not only for its anatomical complexity but also for its clinician-generating complexities. The kidneys, bladder, and prostate are critical structures that are involved in many of our physiological processes, such as excretion of waste and endocrine balance. With advances in imaging technology, so has our understanding of diseases and disorders related to these organs. Accurate imaging techniques such as ultrasound, computed tomography (CT), and magnetic resonance imaging (MRI) allow the clinician to visualize anatomical structures and assess pathological conditions well. This capability is of the most significant importance in the planning of efficacious treatment strategies for kidney stones, bladder cancer, and prostatic diseases. Greater awareness of the pitfalls of genitourinary pathologies again emphasizes the importance of good diagnostic imaging protocols in practice. Understanding the effects of genitourinary disease extends beyond the confines of physiological presentation; it also involves overall determinants of an individual's quality of life, including sexual health and emotional status. Prostatic disorders, for instance, can have profoundly important effects on sexual function and satisfaction. Sexual health is a paramount consideration when addressing urological imaging, as it traverses biological, physiological, and societal features of human sexuality. Imaging techniques like single photon emission computed tomography (SPECT) and positron emission tomography (PET) can describe the integrity of male sex organs at a physiological level, which improves our comprehension of male sexuality as well as the potential disorders of it. These results not only have value for improving clinical strategies but also for aiding patients in managing their treatment, thereby strengthening the pivotal role of imaging in contemporary urological practice (Adenilson et al., 2008).

The integration of newer imaging techniques in evaluating genitourinary illness provides a twofold benefit: improved diagnostic precision and help in the differentiation of benign from malignant tumors. For instance, prostatic inflammatory myofibroblast tumors diagnosis can be particularly challenging since such unusual conditions typically imitate more aggressive malignancies. Distinguishing between malignant tumors and benign alternatives for proper management schemes is essential.

The case of a 44-year-old man who came to the clinic with gross hematuria shows how important it is to use comprehensive imaging studies and lab work to make an accurate diagnosis. This fine balance between clinical presentation and imaging diagnostics underscores the necessity for continuous research and development in these areas, since these developments are crucial to advancing patient outcomes and guiding appropriate interventions for genitourinary conditions (Kundargi et al., 2024).

8.1. Anatomy of the Genitourinary System

The anatomy of the genitourinary system is intricate and critical to the maintenance of the body's homeostasis. The system consists of the kidney, bladder, prostate, and allied structures, and it functions to regulate fluid balance, electrolytes, and excretion of waste products. The function of the kidneys as the prime filtering organs is critical, as they undergo nephrons that filter blood to eliminate waste products while reabsorbing essential substances. The bladder is a reservoir that uses muscular contractions to expel urine, whereas the prostate gland is involved in reproductive function by secreting seminal fluid. Knowledge of these anatomic details is crucial for the proper use of imaging modalities, which are helpful to comprehend the pathologies of these organs. Imaging methods such as ultrasound, computed tomography (CT), and magnetic resonance imaging (MRI) are used to evaluate the genitourinary systems organs and identify abnormalities. Each method offers a unique benefit, enabling clinicians to visualize soft tissues, monitor blood flow, and identify tumors or cysts in detail. For instance, ultrasound is able to provide real-time images of the kidneys and bladder, aiding in the diagnosis of hydronephrosis and bladder stones. Alternatively, cross-sectional images obtained with CT scans enhance detection of renal masses or metastatic disease, whereas MRI offers better soft-tissue contrast, which is important in the assessment of prostatic disease. Selection of the optimal imaging modality is often based on the clinical context and the specific structures to be examined. In addition to the structures of the anatomical genitourinary system, it is also necessary to know about the physiological implications of imaging findings. The correlation of anatomical features with their corresponding functions could account for some clinical diseases. For instance, imaging procedures not only aid in diagnosing anatomical abnormalities but also provide insights into the physiological processes involved in diseases such as prostate hypertrophy or bladder failure. The use of advanced imaging methodologies such as single-photon emission computed tomography (SPECT) and positron emission tomography (PET) provides additional information about tissue metabolic activity. This combined consideration of anatomy and physiology is essential to devising effective therapy plans that account for not only the structural but also the functional aspects of genitourinary pathology, as advocated by Adenilson et al. (2008). Also, the inclusion of this information could yield more effective therapeutic strategies and improved patient results.

8.1.1. Structure and Function of the Kidneys

The kidneys are vital organs of the body with the primary role of filtration and excretion in the genitourinary system. Each kidney is structurally an outer cortex and inner medulla, and nephrons, which are functional units, are embedded within. A nephron comprises a glomerulus, where filtration of blood occurs, and a renal tubule that reabsorbs vital substances and secretes waste. This intricate structure enables the kidneys to regulate water, electrolytes, and acids, thereby maintaining homeostasis. Filtration begins in the glomerulus, where waste and excess substances are removed from the blood into the renal tubule, where selective reabsorption of necessary nutrients occurs, demonstrating that the kidneys serve a dual purpose: excretion and conservation of necessary nutrients. In addition to their architectural complexity, the functional dynamics of the kidneys are a crucial aspect in understanding their role within the genitourinary system. They are responsible for regulating blood pressure, electrolyte homeostasis, and acid-base balance. Hormonal stimulation, such as that of the renin-angiotensin-aldosterone system, significantly affects renal function by dictating sodium and water reabsorption, further regulating blood volume and pressure. In addition, the kidneys produce erythropoietin, a hormone responsible for red blood cell production, indicating their involvement in systemic physiologic functions beyond mere filtration. The comingling of structure and function in the kidneys shows that the kidneys play a vital role in overall health, hence their assessment is pertinent in the case of genitourinary imaging, while not losing focus on the impact of neighboring organs. The effects of treatments on surrounding organs, such as the prostate, can affect the kidneys. Cancer treatments of the prostate, such as radiotherapy, have treatment constraints due to the proximity of the kidney and bladder to the target region. According to existing research, the dosimetry of such treatments can have adverse effects on surrounding structures, and therefore side effects such as incontinence or impairment that compromise renal functions.

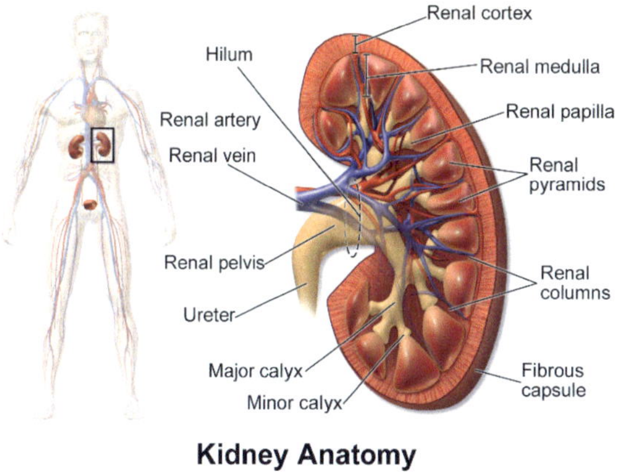

Figure 8.1. Cross-sectional anatomy of the kidneys showing cortex, medulla, and renal pelvis.

Source: https://upload.wikimedia.org/wikipedia/commons/d/d6/Blausen_0592_KidneyAnatomy_01.png.

Identification of these correlations is crucial since radiation dose-dependent side effects are capable of altering patients' quality of life during treatment for genitourinary disease. Therefore, effective imaging protocols that accurately measure kidney structure and function are pivotal to optimizing treatment strategies and patients' well-being (Schaake et al., 2020). Further, ongoing developments in imaging modalities are imperative for evaluating such interactions, thereby improving patient care (N/A, 2007) (Figure 8.1).

8.1.2. Anatomy of the Bladder

The anatomy of the bladder is a part of the study of the genitourinary system, particularly when supported by imaging techniques that identify and assess its structures. The muscular bag in the pelvic region, the bladder, acts as a reservoir for urine and plays a key role in its storage and expulsion. Its wall has several layers, such as the mucosa, submucosa, and detrusor muscle, which allow the bladder to stretch and contract during filling and emptying. The trigone area, which is limited by the openings of the ureters and the urethra, is part of bladder anatomy since it provides stability to the bladder and allows precise urination. Understanding this complex anatomy is critical for health professionals, especially radiologists, while evaluating imaging modalities that quantify bladder function and integrity. Imaging techniques are used to diagnose bladder pathology and are directly involved in clinical decision-making (Figure 8.2).

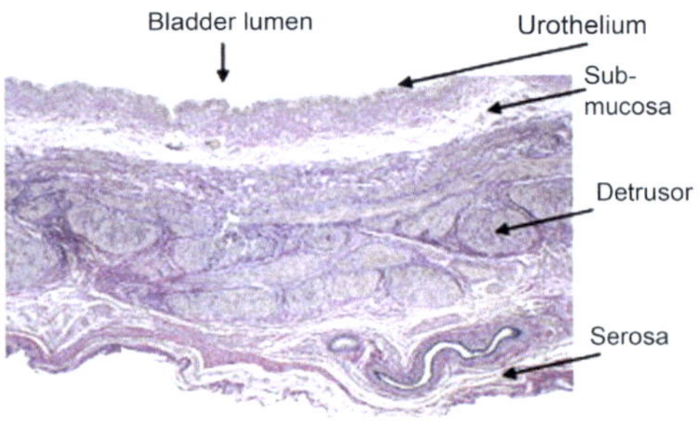

Figure 8.2. An overview of bladder wall structure.

Source: https://ars.els-cdn.com/content/image/1-s2.0-S1472029909000654-gr1.jpg.

Routine modalities such as ultrasound, computed tomography (CT), and magnetic resonance imaging (MRI) provide good visualization of bladder anatomy and pathologies that may develop in it. For instance, ultrasound can provide precise measurements of bladder wall thickness and detect diverticula or tumors, which can profoundly affect a patient's management. CT scans, which offer cross-sectional images, allow comprehensive assessment of neighboring tissues and potential metastasis, underscoring the importance of precise anatomical understanding in imaging. The coincidence of these imaging modalities underscores the necessity of accurate anatomical knowledge for effective treatment of genitourinary disease. In addition, bladder anatomy's significance is not just in the organ but also in the extent to which it relates to other structures in the vicinity, such as the prostate and ureters. This relatedness has implications on the interpretation of imaging studies. In men, for instance, the anatomical proximity of the prostate to the bladder may complicate pathologies such as benign prostatic hyperplasia or prostate cancer by influencing bladder function and filling patterns. Detailed comprehension of such correlations enables radiologists to distinguish between disease and morphologically normal anatomical variations. With advancing imaging technology on the horizon, the subtleties of bladder anatomy are the biggest contributors to insights that improve diagnostic results and the management of genitourinary conditions, thereby improving patient outcomes in urology (Burity et al., 2014; Plotnikov et al., 2017).

8.1.3. Overview of the Prostate Gland

The prostate gland, a vital component of the male reproductive system, has functions beyond hormone secretion. Located under the bladder and encircling the urethra, the walnut-sized prostate gland is solely dedicated to the production of seminal fluid, which nourishes and transports sperm during ejaculation. Anatomically distinct, the prostate comprises several zones, including the peripheral, central, and transition zones, each with unique histological features and clinical significance. The peripheral zone is significant in that it is susceptible to prostate cancer; thus, imaging this is of extreme importance in early diagnosis and treatment planning. A thorough understanding of the anatomical position and functional roles of the prostate is important, particularly in the process of investigating related conditions such as benign prostatic hyperplasia (BPH) and prostate cancer, where genitourinary imaging plays a vital role in assessment and treatment, as highlighted in the context of LUTS (Chandrasekar et al., 2020) (Figure 8.3).

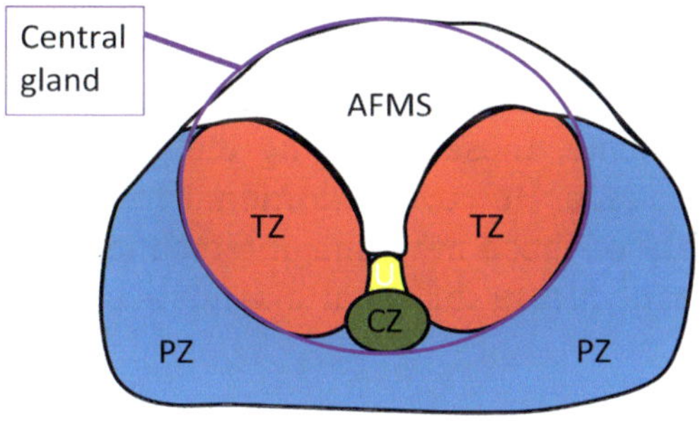

Figure 8.3. Prostate gland anatomical zones on axial MRI.

Source: https://www.researchgate.net/profile/Francisco-La-Rosa/publication/264054821/figure/fig1/AS:601809144000512@1520493889095/llustration-of-anatomic-zones-of-the-prostate-gland-on-axial-slice-through-the-mid-gland.png.

Notably, the prostate gland's pathophysiology is closely linked to a range of urological conditions, most of which fall under lower urinary tract symptoms (LUTS). Such symptoms can have multiple etiologies, such as BPH, bladder outlet obstruction (BOO), and changes related to prostate cancer, each having unique diagnostic challenges. For instance, storage symptoms tend to manifest as frequency, urgency, or nocturia, while voiding symptoms tend to manifest as straining during micturition or a poor stream. The identification of these symptom domains is critical for successful imaging decisions and the resulting management plan. Genitourinary imaging, including ultrasound and MRI, is critical for assessing the underlying prostate pathology and morphology, thereby guiding clinical decisions on treatment selection and intervention timing (Das et al., 2024). Furthermore, advances in imaging technologies have revolutionized the diagnosis and treatment of prostate disease. Modalities such as multiparametric MRI are increasingly being used to assess suspected prostate cancer with precise anatomical localization and characterization of the tumors. This imaging modality not only enhances the diagnostic accuracy but also in differentiation between malignant lesions and benign processes such as BPH. With the growing exposure of proton beam therapy as a treatment method, data from imaging examinations help create customized treatment regimens. The integration of advanced imaging with conventional assessment provides a comprehensive picture of prostate health, making treatment approaches specific to the individual clinical presentation of the patient and enhancing overall results in urotherapy, as reviewed under the implications on cancer treatment models (Das et al., 2024).

8.2. Imaging Techniques for the Kidneys

The application of imaging modalities to assess renal function is at the heart of modern urology.

Renal imaging helps visualize anatomical and pathological abnormalities, and hence affects clinical management. The most well-proven technique is ultrasound, and it is a first-line imaging tool since it is a non-invasive and non-ionizing radiation-based method. It is beneficial for the diagnosis of renal cysts, hydronephrosis, and other structural pathologies. Following ultrasound, computed tomography (CT) has become a critical modality for renal stone and tumor diagnosis. Owing to its sensitivity and ability to provide high-definition cross-sectional images, CT significantly improves the diagnostic accuracy of renal pathologies. Furthermore, with technological advancements, CT urography has been implemented, incorporating a range of imaging techniques to provide multi-aspect analysis of the kidneys and urinary tract (Halpern et al., 2018). Magnetic resonance imaging (MRI) is also a valuable imaging modality for evaluating kidney diseases, particularly for differentiating benign from malignant tumors. MRI also has superior soft-tissue contrast compared to CT, which is very helpful for characterizing renal masses and identifying the extent of tumor invasion. This is particularly helpful for evaluating complicated renal lesions or in patients who are contraindicated for CT contrast agents. MRI is crucial for characterizing cancer type and the extension of adjacent structures, thereby aiding staging. While MRI has a number of benefits, higher cost and increased acquisition time may limit its use in specific clinical settings, rendering it as a whole less accessible than CT in acute situations. But MRIs' broad imaging capabilities remain necessary for patient management and preoperative planning (Plotnikov et al., 2017). As the art of renal imaging advances, it is being supplemented by new imaging technologies that enhance diagnostic performance compared to traditional methods. For instance, the fusion of positron emission tomography (PET) with CT and MRI is gaining popularity, marrying metabolic information with anatomy. This hybrid approach is particularly pertinent in oncology, as it enables identification and evaluation of renal malignancy and metastatic disease. Additionally, the progress in molecular imaging technologies that use targeted biomarker signals early and accurate diagnosis of kidney disease. By combining imaging with individualized medicine, these emerging technologies can transform the face of renal imaging and improve patient care. However, additional research and testing are needed to demonstrate the efficacy and safety of these new imaging technologies for application in routine clinical practice, proposing a vibrant future for renal diagnostics (Halpern et al., 2018).

8.2.1. Renal Assessment Using Ultrasound Imaging

Ultrasound scanning is presently a useful tool for renal assessment, with critical information regarding kidney architecture and function being derived without the use of ionizing radiation. This non-invasive technique uses sound waves to create real-time images of the kidneys, facilitating the evaluation of a variety of conditions, such as hydronephrosis, renal neoplasms, and kidney stones. One of the significant advantages of ultrasound is its ability to provide dynamic imaging, thereby enhancing the clinician's ability to assess the kidneys under various physiological conditions. Moreover, the portability of the ultrasounds also enables bedside evaluation, making it especially useful in the acute setting, where rapid evaluation can influence immediate clinical care (Figure 8.4).

Therefore, ultrasound is the imaging modality of first choice, supplementing other approaches and being an essential element of an integrated diagnostic approach to renal disease. The application of ultrasound in renal assessment extends beyond mere anatomical imaging; it is also an extremely effective method for guiding interventions. For instance, ultrasound is usually employed in renal biopsies to target pathology with minimal blind technique-related complications. In addition, ultrasound is utilized in the drainage of abscesses or hydronephrosis, whereby access enhanced by ultrasound provides increased precision. Most significantly, in children, where radiation exposure is minimized, ultrasound is particularly helpful. It offers a safe and effective alternative to more invasive imaging methods, such as CT scans, and therefore adheres to best practice standards aimed at optimizing patient safety. All these factors together accentuate the role of ultrasound as a valuable asset to the renal imaging repertoire. Within the grand paradigm of genitourinary imaging, the role of ultrasound in renal assessment not only serves the clinician in managing acute urological conditions but also in monitoring chronic kidney disease. Time-based visualization of alterations enables sound decisions regarding treatment modalities and potential interventions. Moreover, the cost-effectiveness of ultrasounds compared to other imaging methods, such as CT and MRI, lends itself to its use in extremely diverse healthcare environments, particularly in resource-limited environments. While its sensitivity and specificity may not be superior to other cutting-edge imaging techniques, its inclusion in standard renal assessment protocols can maximize outcomes in patients. Looking ahead to further advancements in imaging technology, ultrasound remains a cornerstone in the assessment and treatment of renal health, as evidenced by the growing body of research demonstrating its effectiveness and relevance in practice (Halpern et al., 2018; Catena et al., 2019).

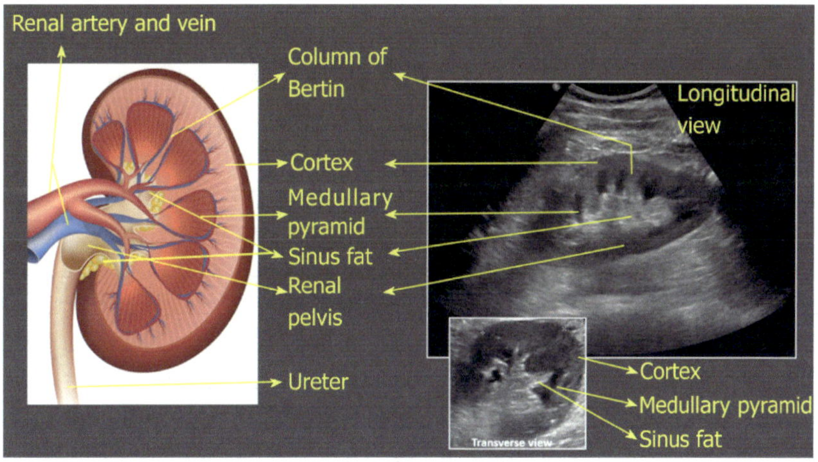

Figure 8.4. Renal ultrasound.

Source: https://f6publishing.blob.core.windows.net/aa5b2b52-5962-410a-b948-688733172771/WJN-8-44-g008.png.

8.2.2. CT Scans and Their Use in the Assessment of Kidneys

In the field of genitourinary imaging, one of the critical components is the computed tomography (CT) scan, which is an essential tool for the evaluation of kidney disease. With their ability to create detailed cross-sectional images of renal anatomy, accurate diagnosis of varied pathologies like tumors, stones, and cystic structures becomes possible. CT scan is handy in mass characterization of the kidney, providing diagnostic information regarding size, shape, and density that is essential for diagnosis and management. Further, CT imaging enhances the detection of renal blood flow abnormalities and vascular lesions, thus supplementing traditional imaging methods. The quantitative assessment provided by CT scans aids in distinguishing benign from malignant lesions, cementing their place in current renal evaluation and treatment algorithms (Plotnikov et al., 2017) (Figure 8.5).

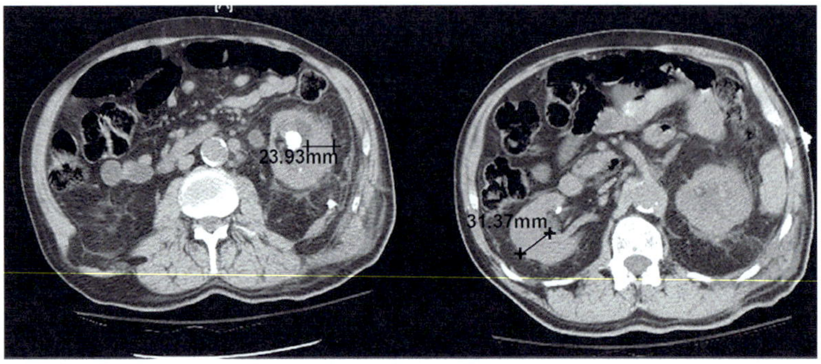

Figure 8.5. Measurement of renal parenchyma thickness for obstructed renal unit (A) and non-obstructed renal unit (B).

Source: https://www.researchgate.net/profile/George-Haleblian/publication/24170804/figure/fig1/AS:601762226528285@1520482703811/Measurement-of-renal-parenchyma-thickness-for-obstructed-renal-unit-A-and.png.

The contribution of CT scan in the diagnosis of urolithiasis, which refers to kidney stones, cannot be overstated. A non-contrast CT scan is far and away the gold standard for stone detection due to its excellent sensitivity and specificity. The imaging of the kidneys, ureters, and bladder simultaneously allows practitioners to assess the size and location of stones, which directly informs management. In addition, CT provides information regarding potential kidney stone complications, such as hydronephrosis or renal trauma. These findings are important, especially when considering disease progression or surgical intervention. As kidney stones are so prevalent, the use of CT to facilitate timely treatment should be underscored even more, further supporting its application in urological practice (N/A, 1987). Aside from its use in diagnostics, CT scans are also an effective method in the evaluation of kidney transplant procedures and posttransplant assessment. Imaging enables the detection of complications like fluid collections, vascular thromboembolism, or graft rejection. CT scans on follow-up in transplant patients can detect significant changes in renal perfusion and function that may warrant treatment. In addition, more advanced imaging modalities, such as multiphasic CT scans, permit better visualization of the renal vasculature and adjacent tissues to enable a complete post-transplant evaluation. Therefore, the application of CT scan technology for the assessment of kidneys is a part not only of preoperative evaluation but also of follow-up care of patients who undergo kidney transplantation, hence of immense relevance to the practice of genitourinary imaging (Plotnikov et al., 2017).

8.2.3. Applications of MRI in Kidney Imaging

Magnetic Resonance Imaging (MRI) has emerged as a revolutionary imaging modality for assessing renal pathologies, enhancing diagnostic sensitivity across an array of kidney diseases. This imaging technique provides enhanced soft tissue contrast compared to the traditional imaging techniques of ultrasound and computed tomography scans, and hence is of great value for the characterization of complex renal masses. MRI can differentiate between malignant and benign masses based on the unique signal characteristics of the renal tissues, and thus, treatment decisions can be made in a better manner. Additionally, advanced techniques such as diffusion-weighted imaging (DWI) and functional MRI allow evaluation of renal blood flow and tissue perfusion and provide information on the pathologic processes of renal disease and disorders such as acute kidney injury and chronic kidney disease (Figure 8.6).

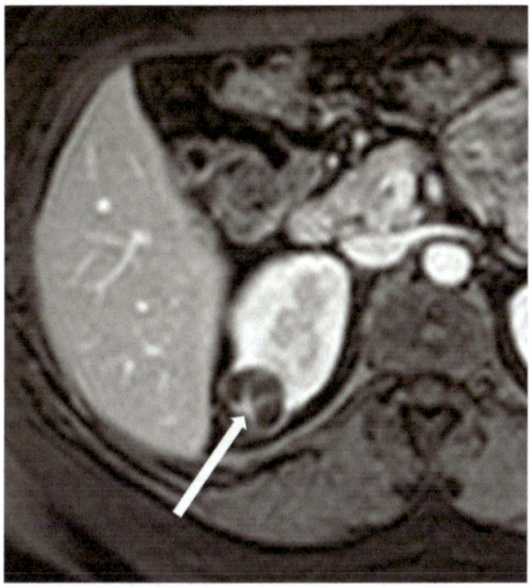

Figure 8.6. CT and MR imaging of cystic renal lesions.

Source: https://media.springernature.com/lw685/springer-static/image/art%3A10.1186%2Fs13244-019-0826-3/MediaObjects/13244_2019_826_Fig8_HTML.png.

Apart from its use in diagnosis, MRI plays a significant role in the preoperative planning and postoperative assessment of kidney procedures. For instance, in renal neoplasms, MRI not only helps in tumor localization and definition but also in assessing the extent of infiltration into surrounding structures. This is useful for planning surgical methods and approaches, particularly with nephron-sparing procedures. Furthermore, the non-invasive modality of MRI allows repeated imaging studies, useful for follow-up measurements of disease activity or response to treatment, without exposing patients to harmful ionizing radiation. With continued advancement in genitourinary imaging, MRI is specifically distinctive for the complete assessment of renal anatomy and pathology. Although it has advantages, the application of MRI in renal imaging also has some disadvantages, largely in terms of accessibility, cost, and operational speed. The need for specialized equipment as well as staff may delay implementation in clinical settings, particularly where resources are inadequate. The reality that MRI, unlike other imaging technologies, possesses longer scan times may, however, be discomforting to patients and less efficient in high-throughput centers. However, ongoing technological advancement, such as high-speed acquisition sequences and improved magnet design, holds the potential to overcome such difficulties and enhance the feasibility of MRI for urological use. Emphasis on these advances is essential because the integration of MRI into the standard assessment of renal disease has the potential to dramatically improve patient outcomes, underscoring the need for concerted action to overcome existing obstacles to its implementation and utilization.

8.3. Imaging Techniques of the Bladder

In genitourinary imaging, the bladder is a pivotal organ, particularly in the early diagnosis of tumors such as bladder cancer. Cystoscopy remains the gold standard for diagnosing bladder tumors because it allows direct inspection and biopsy of suspected tumors. It plays a key role in patients presenting with hematuria, a common symptom in bladder cancer. Despite its advantages, there are some shortcomings of cystoscopy, such as its failure to adequately detect carcinoma *in situ* (CIS) and distinguish between malignant and benign masses. Such shortcomings underscore the significance of other imaging techniques that enhance diagnostic accuracy and staging choices in bladder pathology and provide room for more effective therapeutic protocols for affected patients (Halpern et al., 2018).

Computed tomography (CT) is presently an up-to-date modality for evaluating bladder disease, but most significantly in the staging of bladder cancer. It may be performed in two modes: conventional CT and computed tomographic urography (CTU). While both modalities provide valuable information on tumor location and size, they fail to distinguish T1 and T2 bladder cancers. Additionally, they tend to find nodal staging challenging, which is vital to consider when establishing the extent of disease and planning therapy. In contrast, magnetic resonance imaging (MRI) has proved to be a better option for evaluating muscle-invasive bladder carcinoma (MIBC) than non-muscle-invasive bladder carcinoma (NMIBC), thereby informing therapeutic decisions. But like CT, MRI is not flawless for nodal staging, and there is a gap that needs to be bridged by investigating emerging imaging technologies (Halpern et al., 2018).

Emerging imaging technologies, such as positron emission tomography (PET) and hybrid systems like PET/CT and PET/MRI, can potentially improve the diagnostic landscape for bladder cancer. PET/CT is particularly favored for nodal staging due to its enhanced sensitivity and ability to detect metastatic disease more precisely. PET/MRI is the next generation and further offers better discrimination between pathological and normal structures. While these new imaging technologies have great potential, there is more to be done to unravel the complexities of bladder cancer management. None of the existing imaging modalities preserve all the characterization and staging dimensions needed for optimal patient care, underscoring an imperative need to continue research into targeted imaging approaches that use biomarkers to enable early, accurate, and complete assessment of bladder cancer (Halpern et al., 2018).

8.3.1. Cystography and Its Importance

Cystography, a radiological imaging test that images the bladder, is a core modality in the diagnosis of urologic diseases. Cystography is performed by injecting a contrast medium into the bladder and obtaining sharp, accurate images with X-ray or fluoroscopy.

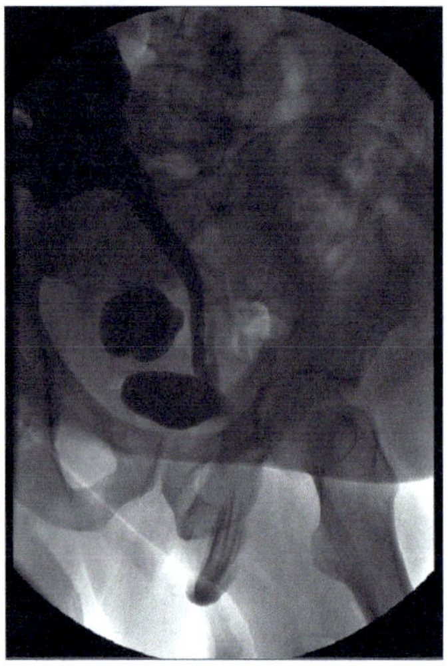

Figure 8.7. Retrograde cystogram (following percutaneous nephrostogram) indicating bladder herniation into the left hemiscrotum, incorporating the right-sided ureteroneocystostomy and distal transplant ureter into the hernia.

Source: https://www.researchgate.net/profile/Tinus-Du-Toit/publication/308340828/figure/fig2/AS:567553365901315@1512326675713/Retrograde-cystogram-following-percutaneous-nephrostogram-indicating-bladder-herniation.png.

Cystography is significant because it can reveal structural abnormalities, such as bladder diverticula, tumors, or vesicoureteral reflux, which can lead to recurrent urinary tract infections or renal damage. Additionally, the non-invasive nature of cystography, coupled with its application in assessing the function and morphology of the bladder, highlights its significance in both the acute and chronic states. For instance, in patients presenting with clear signs of trauma, cystography is useful to evaluate suspected injury of the genitourinary tract, providing key information for therapy planning. This capacity to support clinical decision-making underscores the utility of cystography within the broader realm of genitourinary imaging. The function of cystography extends beyond mere anatomical visualization; it is crucial in guiding clinical management strategies to urologic trauma (Figure 8.7).

Renal and urogenital system injuries, which occur in approximately 10-20% of abdominal trauma, require a balanced management strategy considering anatomical injury versus hemodynamic stability. Cystography may help determine the extent of bladder injury, thereby influencing operative versus non-operative treatment. The American Association for the Surgery of Trauma (AAST) guidelines suggest that an interprofessional team of urologists, interventional radiologists, and trauma surgeons is needed in treating such injuries successfully. By facilitating easy assessment of bladder integrity, cystography makes a final contribution to improved patient outcomes by helping provide the timely intervention necessary for traumatic injury of the genitourinary system (Catena et al., 2019). Apart from diagnosis, cystography also plays a role in evaluating bladder conditions and further consolidates its position in clinical practice. For example, cystography for detection and assessment of interstitial cystitis or neurogenic bladder disease may enable targeted therapy. In addition, advances in imaging technology and technique are now allowing progressively refined information about bladder pathophysiology. Textbooks on modern techniques in medical imaging emphasize the importance of developing systematic training materials to ensure a high level of learning among students. With the introduction of these elements of learning into practical applications, cystography will remain an important tool for future generations of medical professionals (Barannik et al., 2020). Therefore, its applicability in the context of genitourinary imaging remains solid and relevant, necessitating ongoing research and optimization of techniques to achieve optimal patient care.

8.3.2. Ultrasound Imaging of the Bladder

In genitourinary imaging, ultrasound has been a cornerstone in the evaluation of bladder pathology. This is an office-based technique that is highly valuable because it offers real-time imaging with no ionizing radiation, making it the first mode of choice in many clinical scenarios. Bladder volume and wall thickness can be accurately measured by ultrasound, which are extremely critical for diagnosing conditions such as bladder cancer and bladder dysfunction. It also enables detection of urinary retention and can be used to identify bladder lesions, thereby enabling early intervention. Its role in guiding biopsies or interventions is another bonus to its clinical relevance in bladder management (Figure 8.8).

As ultrasound technology continues to advance, its integration with other imaging modalities will likely yield even more comprehensive assessments of bladder pathologies and underscore its paramount contribution to genitourinary imaging. Moreover, the use of ultrasound in evaluating bladder cancer has been of interest because other imaging modalities are challenging. While cystoscopy remains the gold standard for initial diagnosis, it is not without flaws when it comes to detecting carcinoma *in situ* (CIS) or distinguishing benign from malignant masses. In contrast, non-invasive ultrasound offers a complementary technology that can help increase diagnostic confidence, particularly in the presence of suspected malignancy. The modality's ability to visualize the bladder wall enables detection of abnormalities requiring further assessment. In addition, a study highlighted that even though conventional imaging methods like CT and MRI are commonly used, ultrasound provides a complementary perspective, especially in patients with hematuria. This prudent use of ultrasound can thus enhance early detection of bladder cancer and overall treatment planning, providing a more comprehensive and extended view of patient health (Halpern et al., 2018).

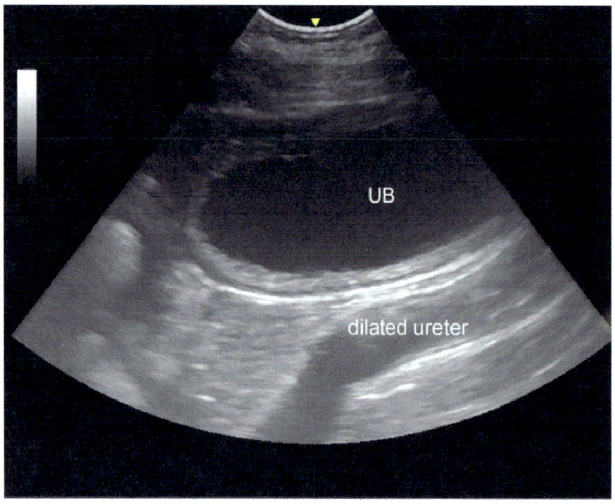

Figure 8.8. Ultrasonography of the urinary bladder.

Source: https://www.imv-imaging.com/media/9112/image-9-dilated-ureter.jpg.

The use of ultrasound in the diagnosis of urogenital tuberculosis (UGTB) is yet another validation of its value as a diagnostic tool in the case of bladder imaging. UGTB can involve the urinary bladder, and if not diagnosed at an early stage, can result in severe complications. Ultrasound has proved very effective for diagnosing bladder involvement by showing thickened bladder walls or disease-like lesions.

This method is consistent with the differential diagnosis requirement, particularly in populations with known risk factors such as endemic exposure. Early ultrasound diagnosis may enable early medical treatment, with the benefit of better patient prognosis and the prevention of end-stage complications of untreated UGTB. With a greater understanding of bladder pathology, the use of ultrasound in clinical practice is likely to increase, further establishing its vital role in genitourinary imaging (Kearns et al., 2022).

8.3.3. CT and MRI in Bladder Pathology

Bladder pathology is highly aided by advanced imaging modalities such as CT and MRI. Both modalities possess unique strengths in depicting the anatomical detail and pathological changes in the urinary bladder to improve diagnostic accuracy. CT scanning is beneficial for the identification of bladder neoplasms, stones, and inflammatory conditions. CT can quickly scan and generate accurate cross-sectional images to detect abnormal wall thickening or mass lesions.

Additionally, contrast agents on CT can further outline bladder lesions, providing valuable staging information for cancer and for therapy. This powerful imaging tool, despite its radiation exposure, remains the first option in emergencies and for assessing complicated bladder disease (N/A, 2007). On the other hand, MRI has some advantages, particularly in assessing soft-tissue bladder disease and differentiating benign from malignant lesions (Figure 8.9).

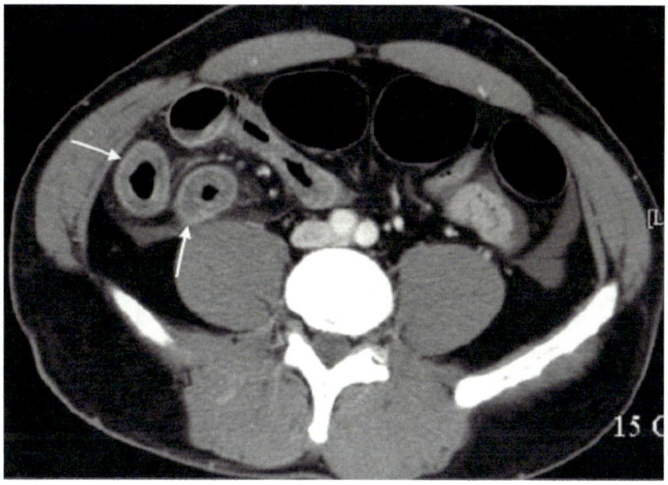

Figure 8.9. Contrast-enhanced CT scan showing a bladder mass with wall thickening.

Source: https://www.researchgate.net/profile/Eun-Lee-7/publication/44632738/figure/fig1/AS:277033583169544@1443061361719/Case-three-a-A-contrast-enhanced-CT-scan-shows-that-the-bladder-wall-thickening-is.png.

Due to its higher contrast resolution and the absence of ionizing radiation, MRI is a useful tool for evaluating the integrity of the bladder wall and surrounding structures. MRI is also good at demonstrating tumor infiltration into surrounding organs, useful in preoperative planning. MRI is also used to evaluate other genitourinary structures, enabling detailed evaluation in cases of complex pathology. T2-weighted sequences are particularly beneficial for revealing bladder wall layers and any resulting lymphadenopathy, thereby enhancing bladder cancer staging and appropriate management (Sudhakar et al., 2013). Using both CT and MRI in combination allows clinicians to optimize diagnostic protocols for patients with bladder pathology. Both modalities are complementary; CT provides rapid, broad-spectrum evaluation without radiation risks, and MRI provides accurate characterization of soft tissues without radiation risks. This synergistic blend is highly useful in challenging cases, where treatment decisions are based on precise anatomical details. With advances in imaging technology, the future in using CT and MRI in bladder disease is sure to be even better, with detection at an earlier stage, better characterization, and better results for the patient. Thus, a multidisciplinary genitourinary imaging strategy not only enhances diagnostic acuity but also promotes individualized treatment approaches tailored to patients' specific needs (N/A, 2007; Sudhakar et al., 2013).

8.4. Imaging Modalities of the Prostate

Technological developments in imaging modalities have substantially enhanced the detection and diagnosis of prostate diseases, both benign and malignant. Among the principal modalities employed are transrectal ultrasound (TRUS), magnetic resonance imaging (MRI), and computed tomography (CT). TRUS is an essential component in the assessment of prostate pathology and is commonly utilized to guide biopsies and visualize tissue architecture. MRI, particularly with the evolution of multi-parametric imaging, provides better soft-tissue contrast, thereby enabling tumor staging and concurrently providing information about adjacent anatomical structures. In addition to this, CT scans find sole application in the treatment plan and metastatic disease evaluation. Together, these modalities enhance diagnostic accuracy and facilitate the development of tailored therapeutic interventions. The utility of multi-parametric MRI for prostate imaging is particularly important because it combines multiple sequences to provide a comprehensive assessment of the gland.

It employs T2-weighted imaging, diffusion-weighted imaging, and dynamic contrast-enhanced imaging, each providing unique information regarding prostate lesions. For instance, diffusion-weighted imaging allows distinction between benign and malignant tissue based on cellular density, a concern given the rising rates of prostate cancer. Further, the American College of Radiology encouraged standardized reporting through the Prostate Imaging Reporting and Data System (PI-RADS), encouraging uniform MRI interpretation among practitioners. Such protocols also enhance patient management pathways with resultant better clinical outcomes. Optimizing the imaging pathway for prostate health also requires clinicians to consider patient-specific factors that inform the best choice of technique. For example, men with elevated levels of prostate-specific antigen (PSA) may be best served by initial screening via TRUS, while those with imaging suspicious findings may be in need of a follow-up MRI for characterization prior to any invasive evaluation. Moreover, the addition of functional imaging modalities, such as positron emission tomography (PET) using new tracers, is emerging as an adjunct tool to identify recurrent disease and guide salvage therapy. As these imaging tools evolve, they will further influence the landscape of prostate diagnostics and therapy, underscoring the need for ongoing research and clinical validation (Iles et al., 2013; Plotnikov et al., 2017).

8.4.1. Transrectal Ultrasound in Prostate Assessment

Transrectal ultrasonography (TRUS) has become a mainstay imaging modality for the evaluation of the prostate, particularly in the detection of prostate cancer and in the guidance of biopsy. TRUS is a type of imaging procedure that uses high-frequency ultrasound waves to produce an intense two-dimensional image of the prostate gland. One of the greatest advantages of TRUS is its ability to provide real-time imaging, which enables accurate needle placement during biopsy. The facility provided by dynamic evaluation allows urologists to optimize diagnostic yield and bring tissue samples from the most suspicious areas, thereby increasing the likelihood of finding malignancies. As a result, TRUS has not only facilitated the diagnosis of prostate cancer at an early stage but has also immensely aided in assessing tumor behavior and staging, which are crucial for effective patient management and treatment planning. Additionally, TRUS is essential in the assessment of patients with lower urinary tract symptoms, typically combining anatomical and functional evaluation (Figure 8.10).

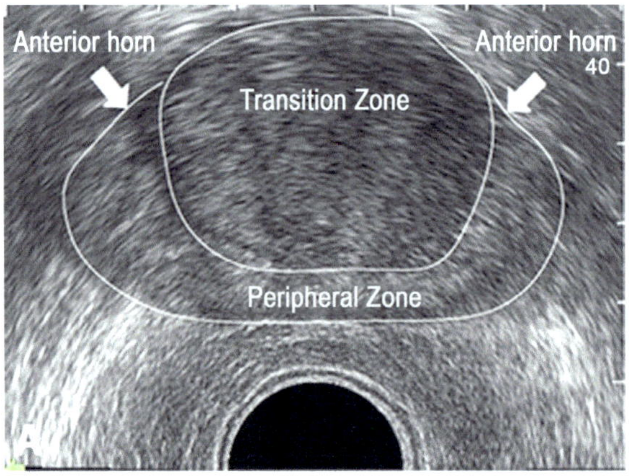

Figure 8.10. Ultrasound for prostate biopsy.

Source: https://radiologykey.com/wp-content/uploads/2017/09/A145750_2_En_11_Fig5_HTML.gif.

The imaging process is used in the diagnosis of several conditions like benign prostatic hyperplasia and prostatitis, enabling doctors to differentiate between pathological states. By demarcating the anatomy of the prostate and any pathology, TRUS aids caregivers in choosing proper treatment methods. The modality's versatility is not only for diagnostic purposes; it also facilitates therapeutic interventions such as transurethral needle ablation and brachytherapy. These uses demonstrate the full scope of TRUS in modern urology, as it provides useful adjuncts to other diagnostic methods and augmentation of general patient care. Over the past decade, advances in imaging technology have further increased the utility of TRUS for prostate assessment. More advanced imaging modalities, such as combining TRUS with elastography, have recently appeared that improve the evaluation of tissue stiffness, which can be associated with cancer. Furthermore, integration of MRI and targeted biopsy techniques has enhanced the diagnostic algorithm for prostate cancer to allow a better evaluation of the degree of disease and potential metastasis. As illustrated by evidence detailing TRUS's effectiveness when used in tandem with emerging imaging technology, the modality has a decisive influence on patient outcomes and therapeutic decision-making. In the future, ongoing developments and research hold great potential for the optimal exploitation of TRUS utility in prostate evaluation, eventually enhancing the diagnostic workup in genitourinary imaging (Adenilson et al., 2008; Anttinen et al., 2021).

8.4.2. MRI for Prostate Cancer Detection

The application of magnetic resonance imaging (MRI) for the diagnosis of prostate cancer has revolutionized the process of urological diagnosis. Traditionally, PSA testing and digital rectal examination have been used as the primary initial screening tools; however, both tend to raise false negatives and positives, leading to unnecessary biopsies or false reassurance on the absence of cancer in cases of false-negative results. MRI, particularly multiparametric MRI (mpMRI), provides improved soft-tissue contrast and enables more accurate localization of suspect lesions. This skill is crucial for the discrimination between significant prostate cancer requiring treatment and indolent tumors that can be safely monitored. Current evidence supports mpMRI as an adjunct to the diagnostic process, enhancing biopsy and treatment planning while limiting complications of overdiagnosis (Halpern et al., 2018). Furthermore, MRI is now an invaluable tool in prostate cancer staging, providing critical information upon which to base treatment. Accurate determination of tumor size and extent, and of nodal involvement, is crucial and can significantly impact the therapeutic regimen, particularly whether a patient is eligible for localized therapies such as surgery or radiation vs systemic therapies (Figure 8.11).

MRI's precision in delineating the prostate margins and any prostatic extension is invaluable for staging. Assessment of response to therapy and recurrence following therapy can also be performed with MRI and is thus a valuable component of the cancer treatment cascade. With advances in imaging techniques, integrating advanced MRI protocols with clinical data will further personalize patient care and outcomes (N/A, 2007). Though it has its benefits, the widespread use of MRI for prostate cancer detection does come with challenges. Access to high-quality MRI and the need for experienced radiologists to read the pictures will deter its application in some healthcare settings. Furthermore, the financial cost of MRI is substantial, with implications for patient access and health equity. There remains a pressing need for uniform protocols and quality assurance processes to ensure consistent accuracy across sites. Further research into the integration of MRI with other imaging modalities, for example, molecular imaging agents targeting specific biomarkers, could further refine diagnostic accuracy and patient outcomes. With advancements in the field of genitourinary imaging, MRI's potential contribution to the detection and treatment of prostate cancer will continue to increase, making it important to attract attention from practitioners as well as researchers (Halpern et al., 2018).

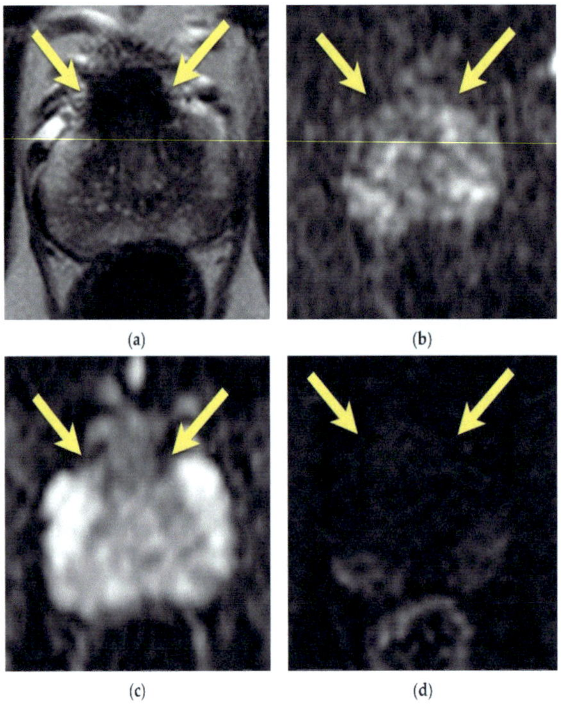

Figure 8.11. Prostate cancer and its mimics—A pictorial overview.

Source: https://pub.mdpi-res.com/cancers/cancers-15-03682/article_deploy/html/images/cancers-15-03682-g001a.png?1690457126.

8.4.3. PET Scan Role in Imaging of Prostate

The role of PET scans in the imaging of the prostate has become increasingly significant with advances in technology and imaging modalities. Prostate cancer management necessitates accurate diagnosis followed by follow-up, and PET scans make it possible through their ability to provide functional imaging beyond the usual anatomical assessment. The technique employs radiotracers with specificity for certain biological events, hence providing a more discriminating image of the tumor's activity and progression. As the biological behavior of prostate cancers becomes better understood, PET imaging offers the potential to identify metastatic disease with greater precision, thereby improving treatment and patient care decisions (Hricak et al., 2008). More particularly, the use of alpha- and beta-emitting tracers in PET scans is a milestone in prostate cancer imaging. The application of tracers such as ^68Ga-PSMA (prostate-specific membrane antigen) has been a notable advancement in the detection of prostate cancer, especially for biochemical recurrence (Figure 8.12).

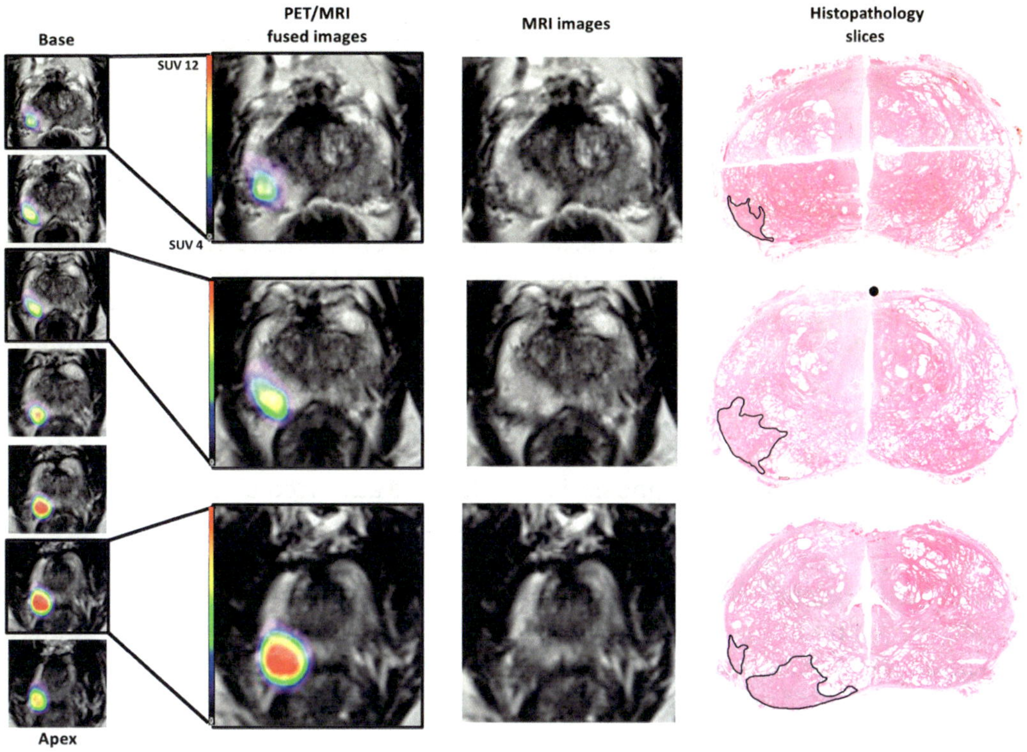

Figure 8.12. PET/MRI fused images qualitatively compared to T2WI axial slices of MRI and digitally recreated histopathology slices for a patient from the MRI−/PET+ group. Note the similar localization of the tumur: right posterior from base to apex. The histology slices are digitally recreated from multiple histology slides, and the tumor outlines (black) were performed by an experienced uro-pathologist. Note the spacing between the fused images is 3 mm, whereas the histopathology slides are approximately 10 mm.

Source: https://www.mdpi.com/jcm/jcm-13-07384/article_deploy/html/images/jcm-13-07384-g001-550.jpg.

These targeted imaging modalities not only improve tumor localization but also measure the extent of disease spread, enabling more individualized treatment plans. Therefore, the use of PET scans in the imaging arsenal furnishes oncologists with critical information about the biology of tumors and enables them to design precision medicine strategies tailored for an individual, such that overall therapeutic efficacy is enhanced (N/A, 2003). Moreover, the function of PET scans is not merely diagnostic but also serves an important role in monitoring treatment response and follow-up. With therapy modalities evolving continuously, it becomes a necessity to understand how tumors react to treatment. PET imaging is also a critical modality applied in the evaluation of the metabolic response of prostate cancer cells to treatment such as hormone therapy or radiation, hence playing a role in the assessment of treatment effectiveness. In addition, by detecting residual cancer or recurrence before other modalities, PET scans have emerged as the cornerstone of optimal surveillance protocols and can influence long-term outcomes for prostate cancer patients, highlighting their role in the sustained management of genitourinary cancers (Hricak et al., 2008).

8.5. Conditions Found Commonly Using Imaging

Imaging techniques are essential for diagnosing common genitourinary tract disorders, particularly of the kidneys, bladder, and prostate. Ultrasound, CT scanning, and MRI are techniques that provide good-quality images to help detect abnormalities. For instance, renal calculi, which are generally asymptomatic until they cause obstruction, can be easily detected with non-contrast CT, so speedy diagnosis is ensured, and treatment can be planned. In addition, the use of ultrasound in bladder pathology evaluation, i.e., urinary retention or bladder tumor, proves its utility in giving real-time feedback on the function of the urinary tracts. The non-invasive nature of these imaging modalities contributes significantly towards patient management, allowing clinicians to design interventions promptly based on precise anatomical and pathological information. Among the many conditions imaged, tumors and urinary tract infections (UTIs) are significant urological issues. Although UTI is typically diagnosed clinically, imaging is warranted in the presence of frequent recurrences or complications. Anatomic abnormalities, such as hydronephrosis or renal abscesses, which put a patient at risk for recurrent infection, can be best assessed by ultrasound and CT scan. The occurrence of tumors, including transitional cell carcinoma of the bladder or renal cell carcinoma, often relies on imaging modalities to assess the size, extent, and metastatic potential. Imaging findings are of utmost importance in planning subsequent interventions, including surgical planning or cancer treatments, and determining prognostic outcomes. The incorporation of imaging information enhances the overall management of complex genitourinary disease. Among the less commonly reported but equally important conditions, urinary tract tuberculosis (UTTB) is a vital entity commonly diagnosed by imaging modalities. This occult disease presents with nonspecific constitutional symptoms that can lead to a delay in accurate diagnosis, leading to severe renal damage if untreated. Imaging modalities such as CT and MRI are important for visualizing the extent of renal disease and its often encountered complications, and for understanding the pathophysiology of these conditions. UTTB is typically found in association with genital tuberculosis, and so genitourinary tuberculosis versus other forms of disease manifestation needs to be differentiated because the presentation is highly variable. Because advanced UTTB can lead to loss of renal function, early diagnosis based on imaging is essential to institute proper treatment regimens to prevent serious morbidity associated with this condition (Aguirre-Avalos et al., 2018).

8.5.1. Kidney Stones and Their Imaging Characteristics

Imaging of the characteristics of kidney stones is imperative to arrive at an accurate diagnosis and effectively treat the disease. A variety of imaging modalities is employed in renal calculi evaluation, with ultrasound and computed tomography (CT) scans being the most common methods employed. Ultrasound is a nonpainful process utilizing sound waves to visualize the kidneys and urinary tract and is particularly useful in pregnant women or patients who do not want to be irradiated (Figure 8.13).

However, ultrasound may lack the ability to view small stones or those found in difficult-to-image sites, such as the distal ureter, resulting in false negatives. CT scans, particularly non-contrast helical CT, have improved sensitivity for stone detection because they can identify calcified structures within surrounding soft tissue, allowing proper stone localization and assessment of stone size and composition, which are important for the formulation of the appropriate treatment plan. The radiologic appearance of kidney stones also provides clues to their composition and the potential cause of stone formation. Stones vary in radiopacity, depending on their chemical makeup; that is, calcium oxalate stones are typically well-visible on CT, while uric acid stones may be less apparent due to their lower density. Composition will typically direct both the risk of spontaneous passage as well as the intervention requirement.

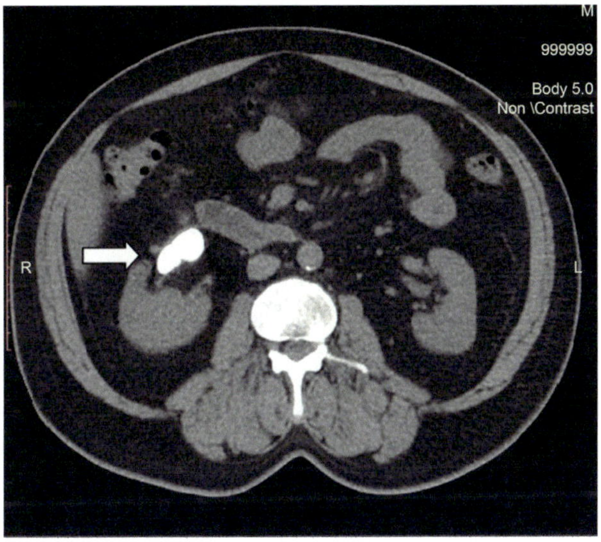

Figure 8.13. Non-contrast CT image of a kidney stone located at the ureteropelvic junction.

Source: https://www.researchgate.net/profile/Alamin-Musa/publication/267328735/figure/fig1/AS:616384530743310@1523968932669/Non-contrast-axial-CT-image-showing-renal-stone.png.

Additionally, imaging can reveal secondary effects of stone formation, such as hydronephrosis or associated infection, that must be treated concomitantly. Appreciation of these imaging nuances not only facilitates modification of treatment plans but also patient education in the prevention strategies to reduce recurrence through diet and lifestyle changes tailored to each patient's stone type. Interventional imaging procedures also have a vital role in the treatment of kidney stones, especially when conservative treatment fails. Techniques such as ureteroscopy, guided by fluoroscopic or ultrasonographic imaging, allow direct visualization and removal of urinary tract stones.

For larger or more intricate stones, percutaneous nephrolithotomy (PCNL) is used, requiring advanced imaging to enable accurate renal access and stone fragmentation. Imaging may assist with the delineation of stone burdens and perioperative planning to guarantee a successful result with minimal complications. Importantly, the integration of imaging modalities enhances the safety and effectiveness of therapy for the patient through real-time assessment during such interventional procedures. Ongoing enhancement of clinical understanding of kidney stone imaging characteristics makes cross-sectional collaboration between imaging specialists and urologists instrumental to the delivery of optimal patient care and improved clinical outcomes in managing renal calculi. Further research in developing effective imaging features are still needed.

8.5.2. Urinary Bladder Infections and Tumors

Bladder infections, or cystitis, are a serious condition that may affect anyone of any age, particularly women. Bladder infections are generally characterized by the infection of the bladder by bacteria and resulting in dysuria, frequency, and urgency. Bladder infections are typically diagnosed through imaging studies, particularly in cases of recurrent infections and atypical symptoms.

Genitourinary imaging modalities such as ultrasound and computed tomography (CT) play a central role in assessing bladder anatomy, ruling out complications, and identifying structural abnormalities that predispose to recurrent infections. As the prevalence of outpatient and inpatient care for bladder infection rises, efficient imaging techniques have become important in guiding clinical decisions, ultimately influencing patient outcomes (Plotnikov et al., 2017) (Figure 8.14).

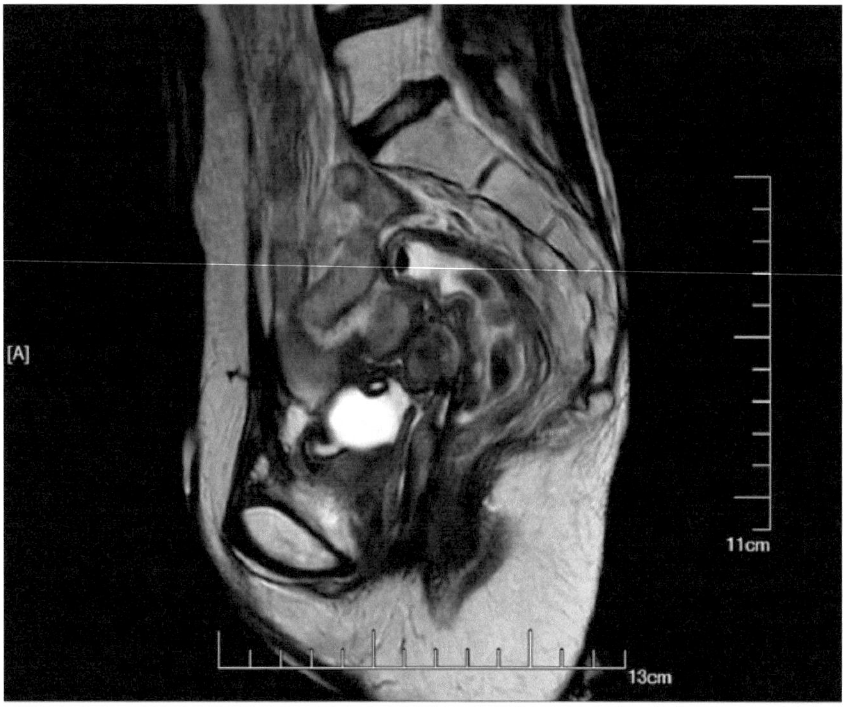

Figure 8.14. The MRI imaging revealed bladder wall thickening, which may extend to the left ureter. The enhancement of the vaginal stump appeared irregular, with indistinct separation from the bladder, suggesting the possibility of urine fluid leakage.

Source: https://www.researchgate.net/publication/381749604/figure/fig3/AS:11431281257411989@1719661101870/The-MRI-imaging-revealed-bladder-wall-thickening-which-may-extend-to-the-left-ureter.png.

Whereas bladder infections are a less serious and complicated issue in the same organ system, bladder tumors are a more serious and complex issue. Bladder cancer remains a prevalent malignancy worldwide, and diagnosis often occurs after symptomatic presentation, including hematuria. Imaging plays a very critical role in bladder tumor diagnosis, and imaging modalities like CT urograms (CTU) provide a detailed evaluation of the urinary tract. The sensitivity and specificity of CT scanning also assist specifically in tumor stage evaluation and the status of any lymphadenopathy or distant metastasis. Notably, combined interdisciplinary approaches in urology and imaging enhance early diagnosis, which can significantly influence treatment modalities and outcomes for patients. Further, technical developments in imaging modalities continue to enhance the detection of malignancies, with direct implications for survival (Agha et al., 2018). The relationship between bladder infection and tumor requires a complex approach to identifying both conditions in clinical practice. In most instances, a pattern of repeated bladder infections will raise suspicion for underlying malignancy in the event of atypical or unresponsive presentation to routine therapy. The use of imaging tests by clinicians, therefore, becomes instrumental in determining whether additional diagnostic evaluation, such as cystoscopy or biopsy, is warranted. In addition, about an understanding of malignancy as a potential in chronic infection patients, imaging becomes not only a diagnostic tool but a focal aspect of chronic patient management. Thus, the role of genitourinary imaging extends beyond simple diagnosis and becomes an integral component of the treatment of both straightforward and complex bladder conditions, encouraging a holistic healthcare practice (Plotnikov et al., 2017; Agha et al., 2018).

8.5.3. Detection of Prostate Enlargement and Cancer

Prostatic enlargement, or benign prostatic hyperplasia (BPH), is a common condition in older men, characterized by prostatic tissue growth. While BPH is not cancerous, its presentations are the same as prostate cancer, so sensitive evaluation and distinction must be undertaken. Symptoms such as frequency, urgency, and nocturia can significantly affect quality of life. Medical practitioners should undertake thorough assessments, such as patient history, physical examination, and laboratory investigations, to establish if an enlargement is due to a benign or malignant condition. The implications of establishing a distinction between BPH and cancer of the prostate are far-reaching; inappropriate treatments for one will exacerbate conditions associated with the other. A well-informed diagnostic approach is thus crucial in the efficient management of these urological conditions and improving patient outcomes. Imaging modalities play a key role in the diagnosis and treatment of benign prostatic enlargement and potential malignancy. Transrectal ultrasonography (TRUS) and magnetic resonance imaging (MRI) have emerged as crucial modalities for assessing the prostate gland. TRUS is not only employed in prostate volume measurement but also in the direction of biopsy in case of suspicion of malignancy. MRI, particularly multiparametric MRI, enables high-definition imaging that permits characterization of prostatic lesions and thus improves diagnostic specificity (Figure 8.15).

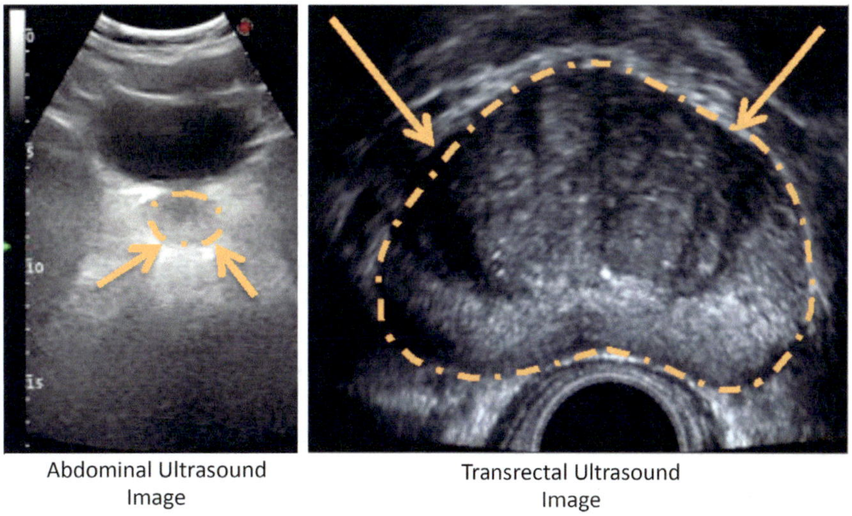

Figure 8.15. Ultrasound of enlarged prostate.

Source: https://www.mdpi.com/applsci/applsci-12-01390/article_deploy/html/images/applsci-12-01390-g001.png.

These imaging techniques allow for early detection, a factor critical to the success of the treatment. Imaging also provides for monitoring disease progression and surgical planning. Inclusion of these new modalities in the armamentarium of urologic diagnostics underscores their importance and their contribution to optimizing patient management protocols. The importance of incorporating evidence-based care in the detection of prostate cancer has been a point of interest in the last few years. Current guidelines emphasize the use of both imaging and clinical assessments to improve diagnostic accuracy. Plotnikov et al. (2017) suggest that the use of systematic protocols in the application of various imaging modalities can contribute significantly to the identification of clinically significant prostate cancer. Similarly, Barannik et al. (2020) explain modern procedures in educational models with a view to creating experiential abilities in medical experts in detecting prostate disorders effectively. Since the health profession is in continuous evolution, ongoing education and adherence to best practices in imaging will be most vital in enhancing diagnostic methods, ultimately leading to better management of prostate enlargement and cancer detection. All this coordination of education, imaging technology, and practice will enable better treatment of patients with such problems.

8.6. Advances in Genitourinary Imaging

Modern innovations in genitourinary imaging have revolutionized diagnostics, particularly for diseases of the kidneys, bladder, and prostate. The traditional imaging modalities of ultrasound, computed tomography (CT), and magnetic resonance imaging (MRI) have been employed extensively to assess and follow these organs. Newer image acquisition devices introduced in the recent past, however, promise greater accuracy and specificity. For instance, modalities such as PET/CT and emerging PET/MRI are revolutionizing our ability to stage malignancies earlier. These new imaging modalities enable visualization of tumor metabolic activity, possibly even detecting problems not otherwise detected with conventional imaging techniques. As such, clinicians can make more informed decisions regarding patient management and treatment options and hence improve patient outcomes in genitourinary oncology. In the diagnosis of bladder cancer, recent literature describes the evolution of imaging modalities into more accurate and reliable ones. Historically, cystoscopy has been used as the gold standard for initial diagnosis, but it has the drawback of not accurately identifying carcinoma in situ (CIS) or differentiating benign from malignant lesions. Recent studies suggest that integration of imaging modalities like CT urography and MRI will increase diagnostic precision. Literature points out that MRI is extremely helpful in discriminating between muscle-invasive bladder carcinoma (MIBC) and non-muscle-invasive bladder carcinoma (NMIBC), while PET/CT is also indispensable in nodal staging by helping to identify metastases that may not be identifiable with the use of standard imaging modalities. Even with these advances, the cumulative evidence underscores the ongoing need for novel imaging modalities targeting unique biomarkers to enhance early detection and staging of bladder cancer, thereby bridging existing modality gaps (Halpern et al., 2018). Beyond that, genitourinary imaging advancements to the diagnosis and management of prostate cancer are a realm increasingly reliant on precision imaging technology. Multiparametric MRI is a key imaging modality that allows precise characterization of prostate lesions that can be indicative of malignancy. Apart from improving detection rates for clinically significant prostate cancers, the imaging method also facilitates precise tumor localization, which guides biopsies and treatment planning. Integration of functional imaging techniques, such as diffusion-weighted imaging and dynamic contrast-enhanced MRI, also increases the ability to assess the aggressiveness of the tumor and potential spread. Concurrent with advances in cellular imaging, novel radiopharmaceuticals are being developed, offering improved targeted imaging techniques. By employing these technological innovations, medical practitioners can leverage their diagnostic capabilities and maximize therapeutic interventions for prostate cancer, ultimately revolutionizing patient management in the genitourinary arena (Plotnikov et al., 2017).

8.6.1. Technological Innovations in Imaging Techniques

New technological advancements in imaging have significantly enhanced diagnostic capabilities, particularly for the prostate, bladder, and kidneys. High-field MRI is now an important tool in evaluating prostate cancer by providing accurate anatomical information as well as functional information without exposing patients to radiation. Methods such as mpMRI combine multiple imaging sequences to provide detailed evaluation of prostate morphology and pathology. In addition, the integration of artificial intelligence algorithms into mpMRI image analysis is revolutionizing the identification of clinically relevant tumors, hence improving patient outcomes and refining targeted and less invasive therapy plans. Apart from MRI, ultrasound technology has also advanced significantly (Figure 8.16).

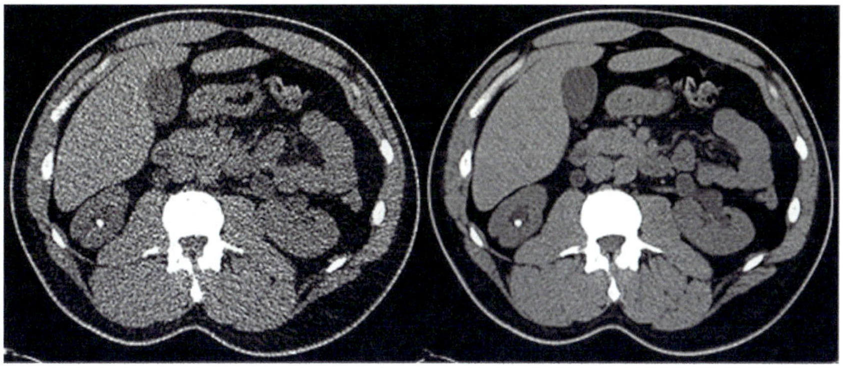

Figure 8.16. Low-resolution versus high-resolution renal imaging using updated CT technology.

Source: https://www.researchgate.net/profile/Ibraheem-Malkawi/publication/289489655/figure/fig1/AS:614259327250447@1523462244302/Both-low-dose-left-and-high-dose-right-scans-showed-a-positive-finding-of-right-renal.png.

The development of contrast-enhanced ultrasound (CEUS) offers increased sensitivity in the detection and characterization of renal and bladder lesions. CEUS uses microbubble contrast agents, which increase the echogenicity of tumor blood flow and are visible in real-time, with vascular properties analyzed. This technique is particularly valuable for evaluating renal masses, where discrimination between benign and malignant lesions is critical. With these innovations incorporated, clinicians can enhance diagnostic precision, leading to more informed decision-making regarding the management of genitourinary pathology. Furthermore, the advent of 3D imaging modalities transformed genitourinary imaging. Three-dimensional imaging techniques such as 3D CT and 3D MRI provide enhanced visualization of anatomical structures, thereby enabling improved surgical planning and intervention strategies. These techniques allow precise reconstructions of the prostate, bladder, and kidneys, allowing for improved understanding of spatial relationships between organs and tissues. With advances in imaging technologies, future applications in preoperative simulations may help surgeons see their specific anatomy prior to actual procedures being performed. The cross-examination and integration of these technologies not only enhance diagnostic accuracy but also bring to the forefront the promise of innovations that could revolutionize clinical practices in genitourinary imaging.

8.6.2. The Role of Artificial Intelligence in Imaging

The application of artificial intelligence (AI) in imaging has revolutionized the way genitourinary illnesses, especially those of the prostate, bladder, and kidneys, are managed. Traditional diagnostic methods require more time and effort, leading to delays in patient care. AI-assisted imaging, particularly with technologies such as computed tomography urography (CTU), enables rapid analysis and interpretation. In a recent study, AI models were reported to possess high sensitivity and negative predictive values, indicating their potential to automate work and reduce the burden on radiologists. For instance, AI diagnosis of CTU not only increases diagnostic accuracy but also improves the detection of urinary bladder cancer in patients with macroscopic hematuria, ultimately leading to early treatment and improved patient outcomes (Abuhasanein et al., 2024). The benefits of AI imaging extend beyond accuracy and include economic and logistical advantages to healthcare systems (Figure 8.17).

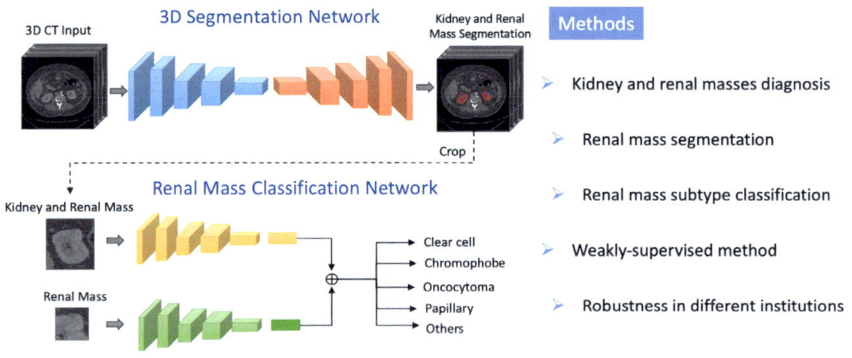

Figure 8.17. AI-driven robust kidney and renal mass segmentation and classification on 3D CT images.

Source: https://pub.mdpi-res.com/bioengineering/bioengineering-10-00116/article_deploy/html/images/bioengineering-10-00116-ag.png?1674090517.

With increasing demands on healthcare professionals, AI technologies can streamline resource planning by reducing the need for invasive interventions such as cystoscopy. In research on the use of AI in CTU scanning, results indicated that as many as 57% of patients could potentially avoid cystoscopy altogether, thus reducing unnecessary healthcare costs and patient discomfort. Moreover, the investment in AI-driven diagnostic tools not only conserves resources but also enables clinicians to handle more complex cases, thereby improving the quality of care (N/A, 2016). Further,

AI's contribution to the world of genitourinary imaging is evidenced in its capability to make new diagnostic modalities possible. New urine tests for cancer markers, along with AI interpretation, have been described in recent studies to enhance the early diagnosis of urinary bladder cancer. For example, the GeneXpert BC test has been shown to be highly sensitive and to have a negative predictive value for excluding malignancy, indicating a possible reduction in primary investigations in a subset of patients. The synergistic benefits of AI with such novel tests signal a paradigm shift in the management of genitourinary disease, as it not only improves diagnostic processes but also ensures patient safety and satisfaction by reducing procedural invasiveness and expediting diagnosis (Abuhasanein et al., 2024) (Figure 8.18).

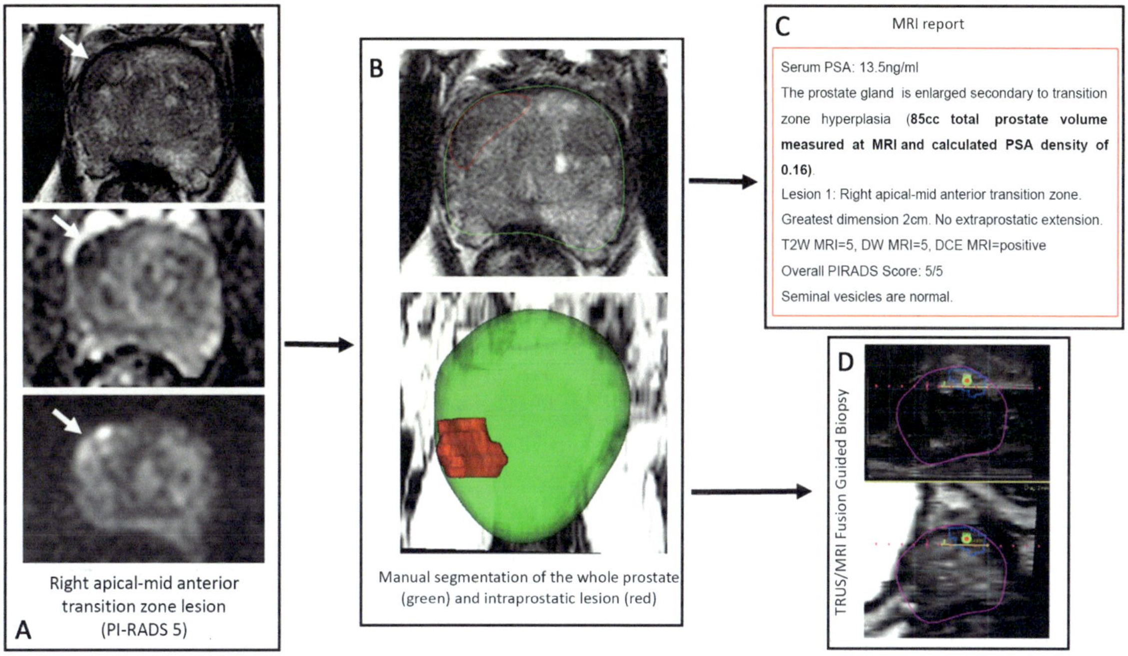

Figure 8.18. Illustration of AI-driven segmentation of prostate zones on MR images.

Source: https://media.springernature.com/lw1200/springer-static/image/art%3A10.1186%2Fs41747-022-00287-9/MediaObjects/41747_2022_287_Fig2_HTML.png.

8.6.3. Future Trends in Genitourinary Imaging

The genitourinary imaging domain is poised for significant expansion, predominantly driven by technological advancements and the integration of artificial intelligence (AI) into imaging modalities. These changes are expected to enhance diagnostic accuracy and improve patient outcomes. For instance, the application of machine learning algorithms for interpreting imaging information can lead to improved detection and characterization of abnormalities in the kidney, bladder, and prostate. Also, AI can help radiologists interpret complex MRI and CT scans more effectively, thereby unloading the workload and reducing the potential for error. As these technologies evolve, there is a strong likelihood that they will be adopted as standard features in clinical procedures and practices, transforming how healthcare practitioners address genitourinary conditions. More specifically, the evolution of targeted therapy in the treatment of prostate cancer is revolutionizing the imaging role in patient management. Prostate-specific membrane antigen positron emission tomography-computed tomography (PSMA PET-CT) and magnetic resonance imaging (MRI) are revolutionizing the diagnosis and treatment planning of localized prostate cancer. In a precise measurement of tumor localization and biological activity, these imaging modalities enable personalized treatment approaches (Figure 8.19).

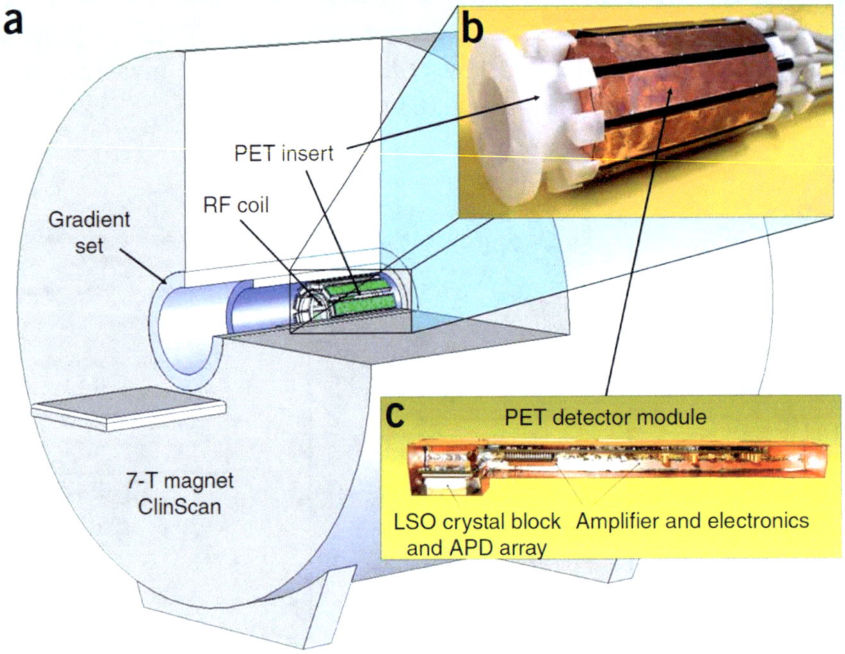

Figure 8.19. Integration of the multislice PET scanner into a 7-T MRI apparatus.(a) Drawing of PET-MRI combination showing the PET insert placed inside the MRI scanner, matching the centers of both fields of view. (b) Photograph of the MRI-compatible PET insert consisting of 10 radially arranged detector modules. (c) Single PET detector module showing the LSO scintillator block, APD array, and preamplifier built into a MRI-compatible copper shielding.*Source:* https://www.researchgate.net/profile/Martin-Judenhofer/publication/5477011/figure/fig1/AS:267284061093889@1440736894422/ntegration-of-the-multislice-PET-scanner-into-a-7-T-MRI-apparatusa-Drawing-of-PET-MRI.png.

Directions in the future call for greater reliance on MRI-guided procedures, such as MRI-guided transurethral ultrasound ablation (TULSA), as it offers a minimally invasive option while preserving oncologic control. These advancements promise not only optimal results but also minimizing side effects typically associated with traditional therapy, as evidenced by early reports that have been shown to effectively utilize TULSA in local control of prostate cancer (Anttinen et al., 2021).

In the future, genitourinary imaging will also place greater emphasis on combining multimodal imaging methods to better understand disease states. Integration of modalities, such as MRI with ultrasound or nuclear medicine imaging, improves characterization of genitourinary pathology and increases diagnostic yield. It may be truly helpful in managing complex cases, such as those with multifocal disease or overlapping signs of multiple genitourinary diseases. Additionally, ongoing research to enhance radiotracers for PET imaging will further improve the performance of current imaging modalities, enabling greater specificity and sensitivity in cancer detection. With more and more collaborative work among radiologists, oncologists, and technologists, the incorporation of these novel techniques will definitely streamline diagnostic protocols and treatment modalities in genitourinary imaging, ensuring that patient care remains at the forefront of clinical innovation (Burity et al., 2014) (Figure 8.20).

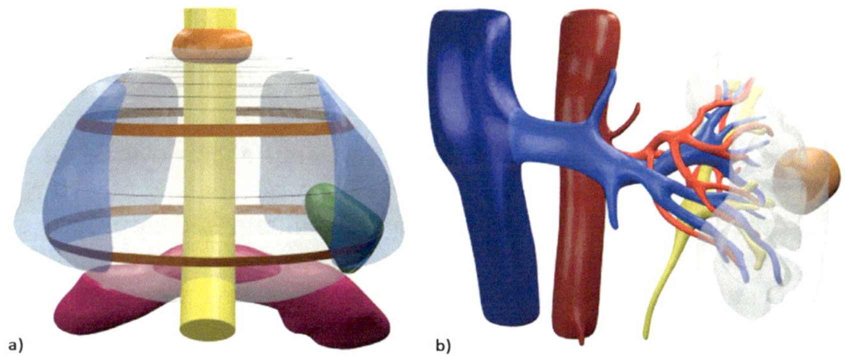

Figure 8.20. Visual extended reality tools in image-guided surgery in urology.

Source: https://media.springernature.com/lw685/springer-static/image/art%3A10.1007%2Fs00259-024-06699-6/MediaObjects/259_2024_6699_Fig1_HTML.png.

SUMMARY

In conclusion, the genitourinary imaging subspecialty is an important aspect of treating kidney, bladder, and prostate diseases. With advances in diagnostic imaging technology, clinicians can employ various modalities, including ultrasound, CT, and MRI, to enhance diagnostic accuracy. Each imaging modality has definite strengths and limitations that influence clinical practice and outcome. As an illustration, ultrasound is often favored because it is easy to use and safe for initial investigation, especially for hematuria, while CT may provide accurate information on complex pathologies. Using these modalities patients, enabling optimal patient management, guiding intervention, and monitoring the long-term evolution of the disease. Moreover, imaging results have consequences far beyond diagnosis; they provide insights into the pathophysiology of genitourinary disease. With accurate imaging, medical professionals can diagnose congenital anomalies, such as those of the seminal vesicles, which can complicate fertility and urogenital health overall (Akata et al., 2019). Awareness of these anomalies is necessary because they may accompany other urinary and genital disorders, worsening the clinical picture. Accordingly, an integrated approach to genitourinary imaging enables a proper understanding of patients' needs and helps formulate individualized treatment protocols. Lastly, integrating data from multiple imaging modalities maximizes clinical judgment and significantly improves patient outcomes in genitourinary medicine. Previous studies demonstrate the usefulness of unobtrusive imaging approaches for evaluating conditions such as hematuria, in which ultrasonography was superior to intravenous urography (Momeni et al., 2009). This will require a paradigm shift in diagnostic practice, with preference for an initial focus on ultrasonography as the first-line imaging modality. With ongoing development, ongoing research, and technical innovation, these imaging modalities are likely to be further refined, ultimately to better diagnose and treat patients.

CLOSER LOOK

GENITOURINARY IMAGING

The increase in prostate cancer (PCa) incidence has also led to the need to find new imaging techniques and therapies. Traditional therapies, such as whole-gland surgery and radiation, are accompanied by side effects, which have triggered the demand to identify less invasive techniques. Advances in imaging modalities, such as magnetic resonance imaging (MRI) and positron emission tomography-computed tomography (PET-CT) using prostate-specific membrane antigen (PSMA), have significantly enhanced PCa detection, localization, and characterization. The imaging modalities support image-guided therapies with targeted functions that are likely to achieve the best balance of disease control and preservation of urinary and sexual function, thus revolutionizing the practice of PCa treatment. The emergence of techniques such as MRI-guided transurethral ultrasound ablation (TULSA) represents a paradigm in the treatment of localized prostate cancers using effective, reduced-complication treatment (Anttinen et al., 2021).

In addition to imaging and treatment developments, understanding the biological mechanisms of prostate change throughout aging is crucial in the design of successful interventions. Aging is one of the key risk factors for the majority of cancers, including PCa, and investigations have unveiled the role of the microenvironment in prostatic aging. Recent studies have also shown that T and B lymphocytes increase significantly in the mouse prostate between 6 and 12 months, suggesting that immune processes are behind chronic inflammation, or so-called "inflammaging." In addition, similar inflammatory processes were detected within the bladder, suggesting an interrelationship among the urogenital apparatus during aging. This information provides a fundamental basis for exploring preventive interventions to manage age-related changes, ultimately contributing to reduced cancer risk and improved patient outcomes (Fox et al., 2020).

Moreover, the integration of advanced imaging modalities like MRI and PSMA PET-CT is crucial not only for diagnosis but also for determining the success of treatment. As recent studies have illustrated, these imaging techniques play a key role in assessing the extent of localized disease pre-intervention, such as with TULSA, and in tracking patient response post-treatment. PSMA PET-CT's sensitivity for metastatic disease detection enables clinicians to tailor treatment strategies. With improving research, the focus is placed on optimizing the use of these imaging modalities in treatment plans, with the ultimate goal of achieving superior oncologic control and limiting unwanted side effects. In so doing, such an integrated framework underscores the importance of incorporating imaging technology into the clinical practice of genitourinary health to prioritize patient-centered care over treatment plans (Anttinen et al., 2021).

Accurate imaging techniques are the hallmark of treatment planning in genitourinary medicine, especially for diseases affecting the kidneys, bladder, and prostate. As urological pathology becomes increasingly complicated, one cannot overestimate the requirement for precise anatomical visualization. Techniques such as magnetic resonance imaging (MRI) and computed tomography (CT) provide the clinician with detailed information on the anatomy and physiology of the organs. This form of imaging enables tumor size, stage, and location to be assessed, and is most critical to the planning of an optimal surgical intervention or other treatment. Through delivering accurate imaging, health care professionals can create more individualized treatment plans, taking into consideration each patient's unique aspects of his/her condition, minimizing the risk of complications because of incorrect or insufficient treatment, and enhancing patient outcomes. Furthermore, imaging with advanced modalities, particularly those that provide three-dimensional (3D) imaging, illustrates how accurate imaging is crucial for treatment planning. 3D printing, based on imaging data, to create high-fidelity anatomical models, is a novel method for preoperative planning and patient education. As highlighted by recent literature, the utilization of 3D-printed models allows for enhanced visualization of intricate anatomy and pathology and, significantly, facilitates the visualizing capacity of the surgeon before the intervention (Sheikh et al., 2018). Visualization before surgery allows for the anticipation of possible complications and more optimal surgical techniques, which in turn result in better surgical outcomes. The ability of such models to be tailored to the patient's anatomical landscape underscores the transformative potential of accurate imaging to enhance procedural success in urology. The consequences of faulty imaging to treatment planning can be catastrophic, potentially resulting in misdiagnosis, improper therapy, and adverse outcomes for the patient. For genitourinary pathology, this results in direct emotional and physical sequelae for patients. Therefore, stringent imaging protocols and the employment of newer technologies are necessary. Medical practitioners need to remember the limitations and potential variations across imaging modalities. Imaging studies training and education are routinely a requirement for healthcare professionals so that they are brought up to date with the correct way of interpreting imaging results and making proper treatment decisions. Thus, establishing a culture of precision and accuracy in imaging not only enhances clinical efficacy but also builds patient trust in the health care system, mirroring the greater responsibility health care providers have to deliver optimal patient care.

REFERENCES

1. McGeady, J. B., & Breyer, B. N. (2013). Current Epidemiology of genitourinary Trauma. *Urologic Clinics of North America, 40*(3), 323–334. https://doi.org/10.1016/j.ucl.2013.04.001Abuhasanein, S. (2024). Optimizing the early diagnosis process of urinary bladder cancer: On standardized care pathway, computed tomography, artificial intelligence, and a newly developed urine-based cancer marker. https://core.ac.uk/download/620664460.pdf (accessed on 15th July 2025).
2. Agha, M., & Eid, A. F. (2018). 64 MS-CTU: Review of techniques and spectrum of the ureteric diseases. https://core.ac.uk/download/478436807.pdf (accessed on 15th July 2025).
3. Aguirre-Avalos, G., & Amaya-Tapia, G. (2018). Urinary tract tuberculosis. https://core.ac.uk/download/322436565.pdf (accessed on 15th July 2025).
4. Akata, D., Karaosmanoglu, A. D., Karcaaltıncaba, M., Ocal, O., et al. (2019). Imaging findings of congenital anomalies of seminal vesicles. https://core.ac.uk/download/187426624.pdf (accessed on 15th July 2025).
5. Anttinen, M. H. J. (2021). Novel imaging and image-guided therapy of prostate cancer. https://core.ac.uk/download/475143092.pdf (accessed on 15th July 2025).
6. Barannik, K. S., Havva, N. V., Krijanovskaya, E. U., Moiseyenko, D. A., et al. (2020). *Urology (Methodical Elaborations of Practical Classes for Students): Textbook Edition, Second Edition, Supplemented and Redone.* https://core.ac.uk/download/346618549.pdf (accessed on 15th July 2025).
7. Beheshti, M., Bomanji, J., Calais, J., Ceci, F., Cho, S. Y., Eiber, M., Fanti, S., et al. (2023). PSMA PET/CT: Joint EANM procedure guideline/SNMMI procedure standard for prostate cancer imaging 2.0. https://core.ac.uk/download/611901511.pdf (accessed on 15th July 2025).
8. Boumelhem, B. B. (2017). The *in vitro* differentiation of prostate epithelial cells and gonadal adipocytes from mouse embryonic stem cells. https://core.ac.uk/download/212692412.pdf (accessed on 15th July 2025).
9. Burity, J., Fonte, I. B. da, & Melo, P. B. de. (2014). Radiological Society of North America (RSNA) 3D printing Special Interest Group (SIG): Guidelines for medical 3D printing and appropriateness for clinical scenarios. https://core.ac.uk/download/212867900.pdf (accessed on 15th July 2025).
10. Catena, F., Coccolini, F., Kluger, Y., Leppäniemi, A., et al. (2019). Kidney and uro-trauma: WSES-AAST guidelines. https://core.ac.uk/download/286810613.pdf (accessed on 15th July 2025).
11. Chandrasekar, M. D. T. (2020). Male LUTS–Introduction and overview. https://core.ac.uk/download/288847009.pdf (accessed on 15th July 2025).
12. Das, I. J., Davis, B. J., Deville, C., Frank, S. J., et al. (2024). ACR-ARS practice parameter for the performance of proton beam therapy. https://core.ac.uk/download/620954484.pdf (accessed on 15th July 2025).
13. de Souza da Fonseca, A., Bernardo-Filho, M., Beutel, M. E., Bouchelouche, K., Chaffanjon, P. C., Choe, W., Dennerstein, L., et al. (2008). Nuclear medicine procedures and the evaluation of male sexual organs: A short review. https://core.ac.uk/download/82923336.pdf (accessed on 15th July 2025).

14. Fox, J. J., Garcia, A. J., Goldstein, A. S., Hashimoto, T., et al. (2020). Highly multiplexed immune profiling throughout adulthood reveals kinetics of lymphocyte infiltration in the aging mouse prostate. https://core.ac.uk/download/334985042.pdf (accessed on 15th July 2025).

15. Halpern, E. J., Kim, S., Salmanoglu, E., Thakur, M., et al. (2018). A glance at imaging bladder cancer. https://core.ac.uk/download/227055407.pdf (accessed on 15th July 2025).

16. Han, D. S., Jang, H., Kim, J. O., & Yuk, S. M. (2013). A rare case of primary malignant small cell carcinoma combined with urothelial cell carcinoma in the ureter. https://core.ac.uk/download/pdf/81794899.pdf (accessed on 15th July 2025).

17. Hricak, H., & Hudolin, T. (2008). Genitourinarni karcinomi: Potencijalna uloga oslikavanja. https://core.ac.uk/download/532569622.pdf (accessed on 15th July 2025).

18. Iles, K., & Zammit, D. (2013). Posterior fossa craniectomy and C1/C2 laminectomy for Arnold-Chiari II decompression of syrinx. https://core.ac.uk/download/46603963.pdf (accessed on 15th July 2025).

19. Kearns, D., Kemp, B., Kundasamy, P., Lyon, S., et al. (2022). A rare case of disseminated genitourinary tract tuberculosis complicated by emphysematous prostatitis and seminal vesicle abscess. https://core.ac.uk/download/616662409.pdf (accessed on 15th July 2025).

20. Kundargi, V. S., Patil, S. R., Patil, S. B., Shukla, A., et al. (2024). A rare prostatic tumor masquerading clinically as benign prostatic hyperplasia. https://core.ac.uk/download/613230021.pdf (accessed on 15th July 2025).

21. Momeni, A., & Rajaie Esfahani, M. (2009). Comparison of ultrasonography and intravenous urography in the screening and diagnosis of hematuria causes. https://core.ac.uk/download/143846651.pdf (accessed on 15th July 2025).

22. N/A (1987). Focal Spot, Spring 1987. https://core.ac.uk/download/129069259.pdf (accessed on 15th July 2025).

23. N/A (2003). Focal Spot, Fall/Winter 2003/2004. https://core.ac.uk/download/129069889.pdf (accessed on 15th July 2025).

24. N/A (2007). *Focal Spot, Winter 2006/2007*. https://core.ac.uk/download/129069354.pdf (accessed on 15th July 2025).

25. N/A (2016). The Bulletin: Sidney Kimmel Medical College at Thomas Jefferson University, Volume 65, Issue 4, Fall 2016. https://core.ac.uk/download/83049488.pdf (accessed on 15th July 2025).

26. Plotnikov, P. V., & Zebentaev, A. A. (2017). *Urology*. https://core.ac.uk/download/80152221.pdf (accessed on 15th July 2025).

27. Schaake, W. (2020). Radiation-induced toxicity in prostate cancer: Prediction and impact on quality of life. https://core.ac.uk/download/286186020.pdf (accessed on 15th July 2025).

28. Sheikh, A., Christensen, A., Gupta, A., Ionita, C. N., Ballard, D. H., Mitsouras, D., Arribas, E., et al. (2018). Radiological Society of North America (RSNA) 3D printing Special Interest Group (SIG): Guidelines for medical 3D printing and appropriateness for clinical scenarios. https://core.ac.uk/download/323073690.pdf (accessed on 15th July 2025).

29. Sleman, A. A. H. (2023). CAD system for early diagnosis of diabetic retinopathy based on 3D extracted imaging markers. https://core.ac.uk/download/588595911.pdf (accessed on 15th July 2025).

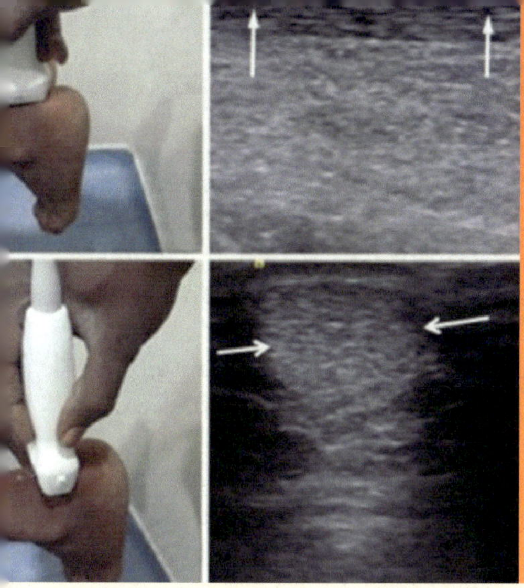

Chapter 9

MUSCULOSKELETAL IMAGING: BONE AND SOFT TISSUE

Contents

Introduction

The musculoskeletal imaging specialty has gained increasing prominence in recent times, reflecting the growing demand for advanced diagnostic modalities amid a booming population and escalating lifestyle-related musculoskeletal disorders. Rising cases of musculoskeletal ailments not only demand early detection but also proper assessment to enable timely intervention. Traditional imaging modalities, namely X-rays and computed tomography (CT), have long dominated the depiction of bone structures; however, these modalities are now supplemented by newer techniques such as magnetic resonance imaging (MRI) and ultrasonography. These advances enable medical professionals to provide a comprehensive assessment of bone as well as soft tissue pathologies, which ultimately lead to improved patient outcomes through enhanced clinical decision-making. As the landscape of musculoskeletal disorders evolves, integrating biomarkers with imaging has become an important strategy for maximizing diagnostic accuracy and monitoring disease progression. Biomarkers can uncover the underlying biological mechanisms of osteoarthritis and osteoporosis and facilitate early diagnosis, enabling tailored therapeutic interventions. For instance, biochemical markers of inflammation and bone remodeling significantly contribute to the diagnostic utility of imaging examinations, allowing for the detection of disease, as well as the evaluation of the success of treatment. In this capacity, imaging complements biomarkers, providing a global overview of patient management from both visual and molecular data. It is this confluence of information that holds the key to enhancing orthopedic treatments and facilitating greater clinical success. Emerging technologies are also revolutionizing musculoskeletal imaging, introducing enhanced accuracy and personalized medicine. Technologies such as artificial intelligence, 4D computed tomography (4DCT), and 3D printing for implants can transform diagnostics. These newer modalities not only increase the accuracy of imaging results but also enable tailored treatment plans that account for a patient's unique anatomical and physiological characteristics. With all that, getting such technologies to work, though, is never easy, with integration into current clinical processes and technology adoption still areas for concern. Overcoming them is key to realizing the full potential of advanced musculoskeletal imaging to optimize patient outcomes and care in the specialty (N/A, 2002; Adamczyk et al., 2025).

9.1. Bone Imaging Modalities

The selection of appropriate imaging modalities is an essential factor in the assessment of bone and soft tissue pathology because it significantly affects diagnosis and also treatment planning. Among the numerous imaging modalities available, Cone Beam Computed Tomography (CBCT) has emerged as a leading modality for musculoskeletal imaging. Initially intended for dental imaging, CBCT is now recognized as having the capability of producing high-resolution images of bone and joint anatomy, further enhanced by the comparatively low cost and reduced doses of radiation compared to traditional methods. The ability of CBCT to resolve fine anatomical detail makes it particularly sensitive for detecting and characterizing musculoskeletal disorders, from fractures to degenerative disease. Furthermore, the use of CBCT with arthrography has been noted to enhance the detection of cartilage lesions, further entrenching it as a valuable imaging modality in the diagnostic armamentarium. With respect to CBCT, other advanced imaging modalities such as MRI and MDCT also play major roles in the investigation of musculoskeletal disorders.

MRI excels due to its ability to provide excellent soft-tissue contrast, which is invaluable for evaluating marrow edema, soft-tissue trauma, and ligamentous integrity. Such a technique is beneficial when one is assessing for conditions such as osteomyelitis or tumors, where the importance of considering the soft tissue prevails. MDCT, however, is highly sensitive, provides rapid acquisition times, and is well-suited for the detection of complex fractures and internal trauma. Because both modalities are complementary, incorporating MRI and MDCT into the imaging protocol allows for comprehensive evaluation, enabling clinicians to formulate accurate diagnoses and personalized treatment plans based on a complete understanding of bone and soft-tissue involvement (Audenaert et al., 2010). Advanced imaging modalities also extend beyond mere visualization, serving key functions in surgical planning and outcomes. Modalities such as CBCT have enabled precise anatomical mapping, which is essential for orthopedic surgical planning. The three-dimensional reconstructions generated via high-end imaging can assist surgeons in understanding patient-specific anatomical variations, thereby enabling tailored intervention strategies (Audenaert et al., 2010). This advanced imaging method becomes significantly crucial in complex interventions of soft tissue configurations and osseous structures, where conventional imaging may fall short. With new advances in the field of musculoskeletal imaging, integration of these technologies is all set to enhance diagnostic accuracy, enhance the efficiency of surgery, and ultimately improve patient outcomes through the responsiveness to the nuances of bone as well as soft tissue disease.

9.1.1. Indications for Bone Imaging

The requirement for bone imaging arises from a wide variety of clinical indications, both therapeutic and diagnostic in nature. One of the primary indications is assessment of traumatic injury, where imaging can confirm fractures, measure their severity, and guide therapy. As an example, cross-sectional imaging modalities like CT are particularly valuable for imaging complex fractures that are not apparent on plain radiographs. In addition, the diagnosis of malignant or benign bone tumors requires sophisticated imaging modalities that can provide not only anatomic but also functional data on tumor metabolism. Imaging of the bone is essential in staging and follow-up of malignancies so that clinicians can plan appropriate therapeutic maneuvers. With the help of sophisticated imaging techniques, healthcare providers can efficiently diagnose and manage a wide range of bone-related conditions. Apart from trauma and neoplastic disorders, bone imaging is indicated in inflammatory and metabolic disorders of the musculoskeletal system. Inflammatory conditions such as osteomyelitis, rheumatoid arthritis, and osteoporosis require careful imaging for accurate diagnosis and therapy. For example, in suspected osteomyelitis, MRI is the modality of choice due to its superior ability to image bone marrow edema and soft tissue alterations, thereby enabling earlier diagnosis and possibly quicker therapeutic intervention. The assessment of metabolic bone disease also includes quantitative imaging techniques to measure bone structure and density, which aid in diagnosing conditions like osteoporosis. High-resolution imaging of these conditions is essential as it determines the management plan directly, for example, the requirement for medical treatment or surgery. Emerging bone imaging modalities, such as dual-energy CT and photon-counting detectors (PCDs), are enhancing diagnostic performance in this context. Dual-energy CT enhances material differentiation—for example, bone and various types of calcifications—by applying various energy levels to improve contrast.

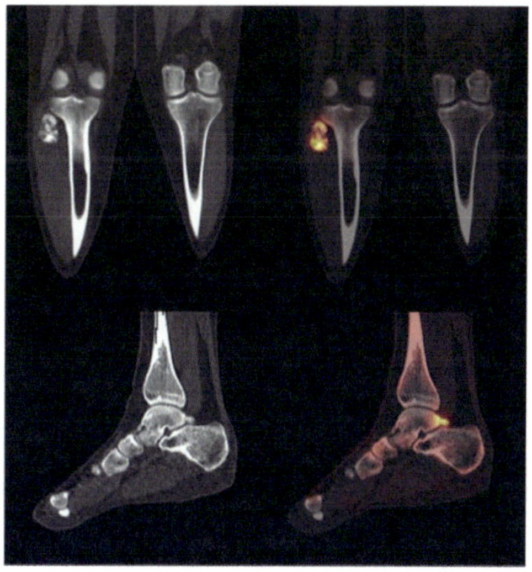

Figure 9.1. Indications for bone imaging.

Source: https://media.springernature.com/lw685/springer-static/image/art%3A10.1186%2Fs41824-019-0054-6/MediaObjects/41824_2019_54_Fig6_HTML.png.

This capacity is particularly valuable for detecting crystalline deposits in bone, which occur in some anatomical conditions referred to as specific arthropathies. Similarly, PCDs offer greater advantages in spatial resolution and noise rejection, which increase the quality of images obtained during scans. This refinement can improve the visibility of complex structures and facilitate the characterization of pathology in bone imaging, such as the evaluation of surgical implants or osseous lesions (Becce et al., 2024). This innovation speaks to the ever-evolving nature of this discipline and the necessity for continual research to ensure that the clinical uses for these technologies are optimized (Becce et al., 2024) (Figure 9.1).

9.1.2. Advantages and Limitations of X-Rays

The use of X-rays for musculoskeletal imaging is beneficial in many respects, particularly when used to investigate bone injury and fractures. X-rays are good diagnostic agents because they provide quick, straightforward imaging of bone architecture, making them the imaging agent of preference for trauma. Their wide availability, in addition to their relatively low cost compared with other tests, adds to their utility in the clinic.

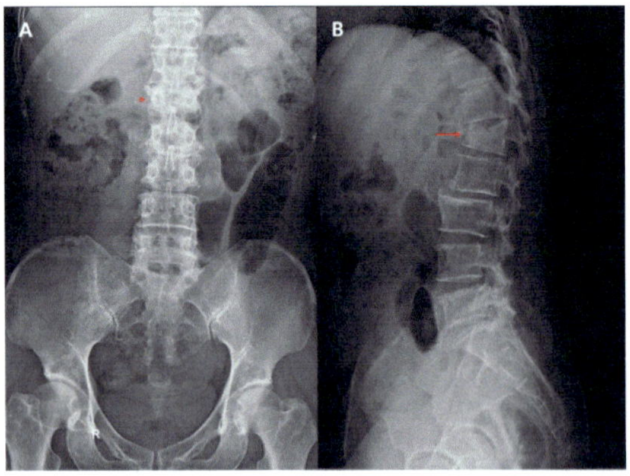

Figure 9.2. X-ray image displaying osteoporotic changes in the vertebral column.

Source: https://www.researchgate.net/publication/385908515/figure/fig1/AS:11431281291205119@1731949239408/Typical-X-ray-images-of-osteoporotic-vertebral-compression-fracture-The-AP-image-A.png.

Additionally, technology has increased the quality of X-ray images to a level where minor fracture and bone pathology can be visualized better. Also, X-ray imaging is non-invasive and carries a low radiation exposure compared to advanced imaging modalities, making it an ideal first choice among clinicians when evaluating musculoskeletal pathology for the first time. Therefore, in diseases such as fractures, dislocations, and some tumors, X-rays are a foundation for efficient treatment regimens. However, despite their major benefits, X-rays do have certain limitations that must be understood. One of them is that they are not very good at viewing soft tissue, thus some injuries are partially examined (Figure 9.2).

For example, while fractures can be well identified on X-rays, they also fail to diagnose ligament or muscle strains, a detail that requires more advanced imaging such as MRI or ultrasound. In addition, X-ray sensitivity can be unpredictable, potentially missing minor fractures or subtle pathologies. Lastly, although exposure to ionizing radiation is low, it will accumulate and become a concern, especially for patients who require multiple tests. Therefore, although X-rays are a key element of musculoskeletal imaging, clinicians must consider their limitations and the potential use of other imaging modalities when necessary. To circumvent the limitations of X-rays, especially in complex disorders such as osteomyelitis, clinicians prefer more sophisticated imaging techniques. For instance, MRI has been shown in studies to provide improved soft tissue contrast and is therefore far better at detecting early bone marrow changes due to infection than X-rays, which may not detect bone marrow involvement until late stages (Buchanan et al., 2016). Also, CT scans, with their higher radiation dose than X-rays, can provide high-resolution cross-sectional images that delineate intricate bony anatomy and disease, making them beneficial for pre-surgical planning (Kalová et al., 2019). A combination of information from two imaging modalities would enable detailed evaluation of musculoskeletal disorders, thereby enhancing diagnostic yield. Lastly, one must be able to understand both the advantages and the disadvantages of X-rays for complementary imaging technology in order to optimize patient care in musculoskeletal imaging.

9.1.3. Role of CT in Bone Assessment

The application of computed tomography (CT) in bone evaluation is changing at lightning speed and hence is a priceless asset in musculoskeletal imaging. With conventional imaging methods like X-rays and MRI being limited in various settings, the accuracy and resolution provided by CT become a major advantage for assessing bony structures. One of the greatest strengths of CT is that it can produce high-resolution images that illustrate fine bone architectural details and thus diagnose fractures, tumors, and metabolic bone disease. Furthermore, CTs' cross-sectional imaging capability allows for three-dimensional reconstructions, which enable enhanced visualization of complex anatomical relationships. These features are especially beneficial for surgical planning and treatment evaluation, enabling clinicians to create informed decisions based on extensive and correct imaging information (Figure 9.3).

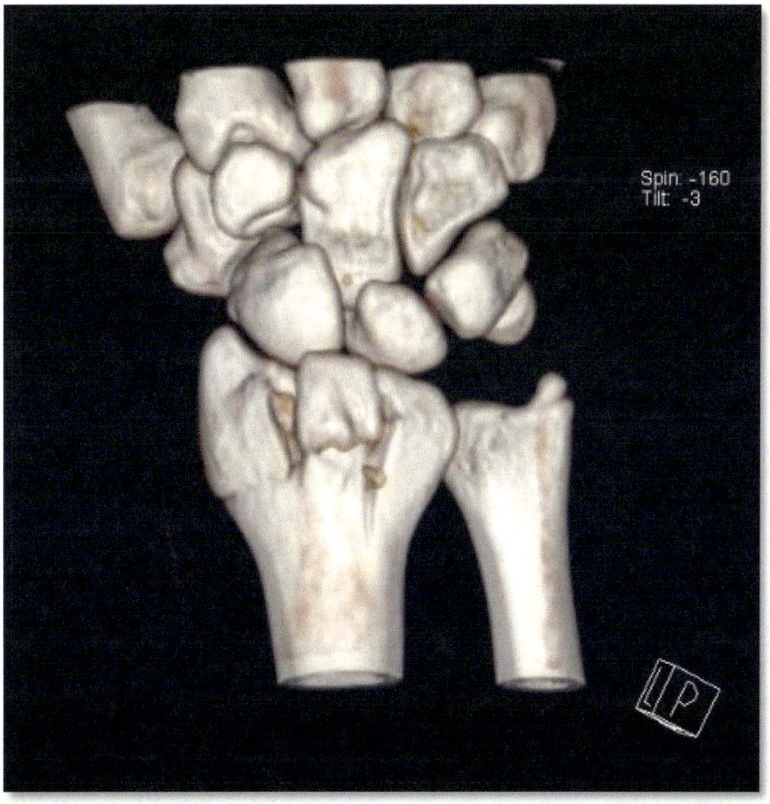

Figure 9.3. 3D reconstructed CT scan of the wrist highlighting fracture pattern.

Source: https://www.researchgate.net/publication/363729703/figure/fig4/AS:11431281087955824@1664901202901/D-reconstructed-CT-wrist-showing-the-fractures.ppm.

With increasing research, CT use in clinical practice is less overt and forms part of advanced bone evaluation strategies (Adamczyk et al., 2025). Sophisticated CT approaches are now being developed to address specific clinical issues in bone evaluation. For instance, four-dimensional computed tomography (4DCT) has shown promise in defining dynamic changes in joints, which are crucial for diagnosing pathology such as patellofemoral instability and ligamentous injury. This imaging technique allows one to assess biomechanical modifications across various joint positions, thereby facilitating improved understanding of joint mechanics and potential pathologies. Furthermore, CBCT offers advantages for imaging the peripheral joints in weight-bearing positions, providing essential information about disease processes that may be masked by traditional imaging techniques. DECT also permits visual and quantitative assessment of certain conditions, such as gout, by differentiating among multiple tissue types based on variations in material properties. These novel CT modalities offer a revolutionary advantage in clinical outcomes by enabling early and accurate diagnosis (Carrino et al., 2022). Implementation of these new CT modalities in routine clinical practice comes with advantages and limitations. Improved diagnostic imaging benefits are very apparent, but the logistical limitations in the roll-out of new technologies present a hindrance to their extensive use. For example, the need for sophisticated equipment and expert training to perform more complicated CT scans can be a limitation in some hospitals. Additionally, radiation exposure can be mitigated, particularly for those who must undergo repeated imaging examinations. As musculoskeletal imaging has advanced, studies should consistently provide protocols that maximize the benefits of CT while minimizing harm. By exploring avenues for the implementation of artificial intelligence and automated review, professionals can harness CT's capabilities to not only improve accuracy in bone assessment but also maximize patient outcomes through individualized therapy plans (Adamczyk et al., 2025).

9.2. Imaging Methods of Soft Tissue

Evaluation of soft tissues in the musculoskeletal system is now feasible with advanced imaging modalities that can distinguish among various tissue types. Magnetic Resonance Imaging (MRI) is regarded by the majority as the gold standard for imaging soft tissues due to its excellent ability to outline muscles, tendons, ligaments, and other non-osseous tissue without the use of ionizing radiation. This function is especially helpful in diagnosing conditions such as tendon tears, muscle strain, and soft tissue tumors. Also, with the aid of advanced MRI sequences, image definition can be enhanced, allowing assessment of minimal pathologies that may not be apparent on other imaging modalities. With the rapid advances in health care, the use of techniques that provide three-dimensional anatomical and geometric delineation of soft tissues is becoming increasingly popular, providing clinicians with improved information for surgical planning and intervention (Audenaert et al., 2010). MRI, apart from its application, has other imaging techniques, such as ultrasound and Cone Beam Computed Tomography (CBCT), that are also employed to assess soft tissues. Ultrasound is an invasive real-time imaging modality ideal for evaluation of superficial structures and musculoskeletal dynamic function. It serves as an excellent tool for guiding interventions, like injections or aspirations, with instantaneous feedback and is thus extremely useful in sports medicine. CBCT has proven to be a useful imaging modality in musculoskeletal imaging due to its provision of low radiation exposure and excellent spatial resolution. Though in the past it has been utilized in dental imaging, its application has now been expanded to the assessment of fractures, dislocations, and cartilage lesions, particularly in osteochondral injury in the small joints. The ability of CBCT to image fine anatomical details is complementary to MRI and ultrasound, thereby enabling more extensive assessment of soft tissue status (Desimpel et al., 2018). Diagnostic accuracy and musculoskeletal disease treatment planning are significantly enhanced through multimodal imaging techniques. The integration of MRI, ultrasound, and CBCT can aid in a fuller understanding of soft tissue pathology, leading to better patient outcomes through more enlightened intervention. Furthermore, advances in imaging technology, such as three-dimensional reconstruction and improved software algorithms, have revolutionized the visualization of soft tissues, hence aiding education and clinical practice. As the musculoskeletal imaging field continues to expand, comparative effectiveness studies of these imaging modalities will be essential. It will help identify the unique strengths and weaknesses of each modality and foster interprofessional collaboration among orthopedic surgeons and radiologists to optimize patient care for soft-tissue management (Audenaert et al., 2010; Desimpel et al., 2018).

9.2.1. MRI's Superiority in Soft Tissue Evaluation

In musculoskeletal imaging, magnetic resonance imaging (MRI) stands out for its unparalleled assessment of soft tissue structure compared to standard imaging techniques such as X-rays and CT scans. One of MRI's key advantages is the high contrast resolution, enabling more precise visualization of muscle, tendons, ligaments, and cartilage. This is particularly significant in diagnosing musculoskeletal disorders such as tears, strains, and inflammation that directly engage soft tissues. Unlike X-rays, which only reflect bone, MRI provides complete information about the underlying soft tissue diseases that could be causing musculoskeletal symptoms and, therefore, facilitates a more accurate diagnosis and consequent treatment plan. Moreover, the non-invasive nature of MRIs and the lack of ionizing radiation make it a safer method for patients, especially those requiring repeated imaging, such as athletes with recurring injuries. Since MRIs have the ability to utilize varying imaging sequences, they can take detailed pictures in multiple planes, which makes the diagnosis more accurate. MRI has been shown by research to be particularly helpful in the diagnosis of sports injuries, including those that are in accordance with the new nomenclature of inguinal disruption, as it picks up on minor soft tissue pathology in the area of the groin (de Beaux et al., 2014). Such precision is crucial in creating targeted treatment strategies, which ultimately lead to more standardized outcomes for patients.

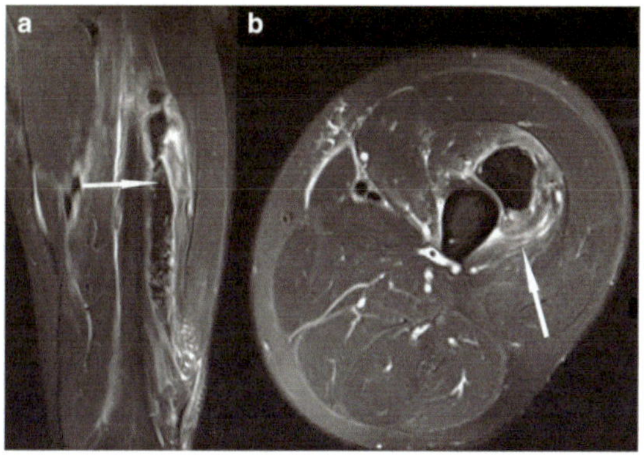

Figure 9.4. Imaging of hip and thigh muscle injury.

Source: https://media.springernature.com/lw685/springer-static/image/art%3A10.1186%2Fs13244-019-0702-1/MediaObjects/13244_2019_702_Fig1_HTML.png.

Furthermore, MRI is an essential component of managing complex conditions such as diabetic foot infections, where accurate imaging is paramount. Evidence-based recommendations indicate that MRI is often the initial advanced imaging modality, particularly for assessing the depth of infection in the foot (Chakravartty et al., 2024). It allows clinicians to visualize not only the bones but also the surrounding soft tissues, facilitating thorough evaluations of complications such as osteomyelitis or Charcot neuro-osteoarthropathy. These instances underscore MRI's capacity to provide critical information that may alter treatment approaches, highlighting its role as a cornerstone in soft-tissue assessment within musculoskeletal imaging (Figure 9.4).

9.2.2. Ultrasound Applications in Soft Tissue Imaging

The use of ultrasound for imaging soft tissues is a groundbreaking development in the history of musculoskeletal diagnostics. As a real-time, non-invasive imaging tool, ultrasound clearly delineates soft tissues such as muscles, tendons, ligaments, and synovial structures. Based on its own properties, it enables dynamic evaluation to observe musculoskeletal structures in motion and visualize their anatomy and function (Figure 9.5).

Unlike other imaging techniques, ultrasound does not use ionizing radiation, making it less harmful to patients, particularly in pediatric patients and those requiring multiple follow-up studies. With a mixture of frequencies, ultrasound can provide high-resolution images and identify small pathologies, allowing early diagnosis and treatment of conditions such as tendinitis, tears, and bursitis. This skill enhances the efficacy of patient management regimens and underscores the importance of ultrasound in contemporary musculoskeletal imaging protocols. Beyond diagnosis, ultrasound has become a critical tool for guiding therapeutic interventions in musculoskeletal medicine. A case in point is ultrasound-guided injections, which have gained widespread use as a reliable method of delivering drugs to affected joints or soft tissues, thereby optimizing outcomes.

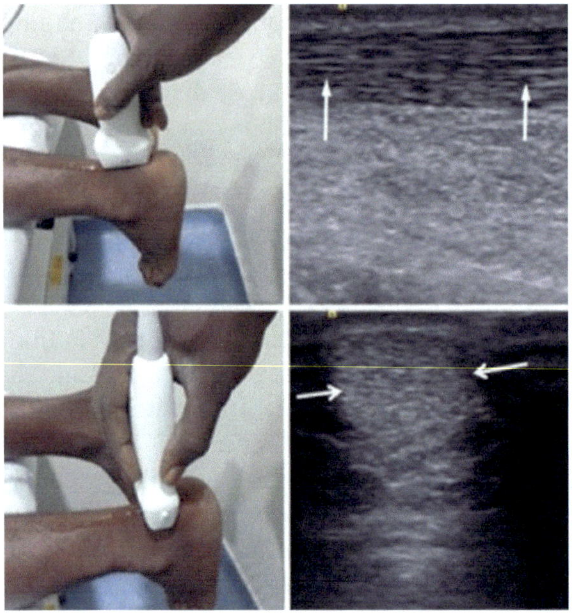

Figure 9.5. Ultrasonography of a normal Achilles tendon (arrows) showing the transducer position and equivalent sonographic image in longitudinal/long-axis view (A, B) and transverse/short-axis view (C, D).

Source: https://www.researchgate.net/profile/Bukunmi-Idowu/publication/347810751/figure/fig1/AS:983508092715008@1611498010229/Ultrasonography-of-a-normal-Achilles-tendon-arrows-showing-the-transducer-position-and.jpg.

This accuracy reduces the risk of blind injection complications and improves the efficacy of procedures such as corticosteroid or hyaluronic acid injections. Additionally, improved ultrasound technology, such as three-dimensional imaging and elastography, gives greater insight into tissue qualities and pathology. These developments, coupled with more incorporation of ultrasound into interventional frameworks, put it at the forefront of musculoskeletal disorder treatment, particularly for disorders that become refractory to conventional therapy. New technologies such as MRI-guided focused ultrasound surgery (MRgFUS) further establish the role of ultrasound in imaging and intervention of soft tissues. This technique, which combines therapeutic ultrasound with high-resolution imaging, enables practitioners to deliver focused, specific therapy for musculoskeletal disorders while monitoring treatment efficacy in real time. Integrating MR imaging with targeted ultrasound not only sheds greater light on ultrasound interactions with biological tissue but also expands the reach of treatable diseases, providing new avenues for non-invasive therapies.

In addition, advances in computer-assisted orthopedic surgery (CAOS) systems offer opportunities to enhance the effectiveness and precision of ultrasound applications. By using modalities such as ultrasound for surgical planning, in addition to navigation, CAOS systems demonstrate the convergence of technology and clinical practice and the potential to create significant improvements in the treatment of musculoskeletal disorders (Albisinni et al., 2015; Kalová et al., 2019).

9.2.3. Limitations of X-Ray in Soft Tissue Analysis

The use of X-ray imaging in the diagnosis of musculoskeletal disorders is widely recognized for its ability to image bone structures. However, the limitations of X-ray for soft-tissue imaging are significant. X-ray technology primarily depends on differences in tissue density to create images, and hence soft tissues like muscles, ligaments, and cartilage become unspecific and can merge into the adjacent tissues effortlessly. This absence of contrast significantly limits the diagnostic abilities of X-rays when dealing with conditions presenting in the form of soft tissue damage or illness. In addition, abnormalities such as inflammation or minute tears may fail to appear prominently on X-ray films and thus may result in misdiagnosis or failure to detect important pathology (Figure 9.6).

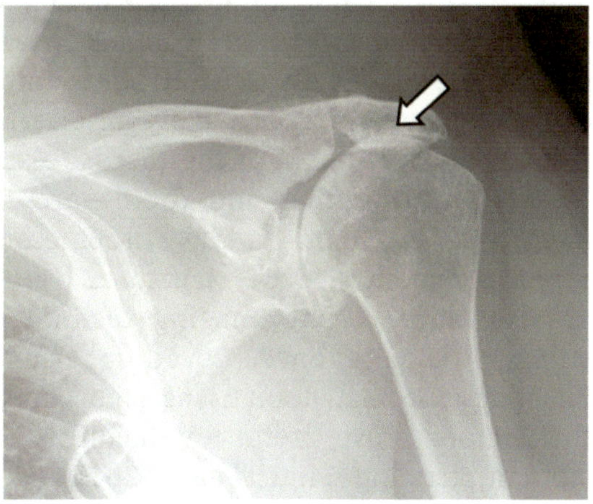

Figure 9.6. X-ray of the shoulder failing to capture soft tissue detail.

Source: https://www.mdpi.com/jcm/jcm-12-02946/article_deploy/html/images/jcm-12-02946-g004-550.jpg.

Therefore, although X-ray is a main imaging modality in orthopedic practice, it cannot provide a comprehensive evaluation of soft tissue, underscoring the need for additional imaging techniques. Another important limitation of X-ray for the analysis of soft tissues arises from the technique's exposure to ionizing radiation. If recurrent imaging is warranted, as is often the case in the follow-up of patients with chronic soft tissue complications, the suggested risk of cumulative radiation exposure is of concern. Beyond suggested carcinogenic effects, recurrent radiation exposure can result in tissue injury or exacerbate underlying diseases in susceptible subjects. This is of particular concern in pediatric or chronic populations, where recurrent imaging sessions may be necessary. Thus, clinicians are commonly compelled to seek imaging alternatives that minimize radiation exposure while still providing the information needed for diagnosis. Novel modalities, such as magnetic resonance imaging (MRI) and ultrasound, provide non-ionizing imaging with good soft-tissue visualization, thereby improving patient safety and care quality. Finally, the inability of X-rays to provide accurate anatomical information about soft tissues commonly leads to inadequate clinical assessment. For example, gout requires widespread imaging for effective treatment, as symptoms of the disease—such as soft tissue swelling and tophi—are not evident on X-ray. Although X-ray will sometimes show involvement of bone structures in joint illnesses, more recent imaging techniques, such as ultrasound, have proved superior in delineating gout-related soft tissue abnormalities and therefore prove useful for diagnosis and treatment planning (Finucci et al., 2015). More importantly, emerging technologies such as MRI-guided focused ultrasound surgery (MRgFUS) indicate a development of further sophisticated imaging technologies that combine diagnostic precision with therapeutic capabilities (Albisinni et al., 2015). Such developments prepare for the subtleties of musculoskeletal disease, thereby maximizing patient outcomes and remedying the inherent limitations of conventional X-ray imaging effectively.

9.3. Common Conditions Diagnosed

Among the numerous musculoskeletal disorders diagnosed with imaging modalities, Medial Tibial Stress Syndrome (MTSS) is a prevalent condition, particularly among athletes and physically active individuals. MTSS is characterized by tibial pain resulting from cumulative lower limb stress, which leads to inflammatory changes around the tibia. The inherent complexity of this condition is also augmented by the fact that there is no single causative factor, thus preventing prevention and effective treatment strategies. Imaging, particularly with high-technology modalities such as MRI, is a critical component in making the diagnosis and ruling out associated injuries. Due to the colossal effect of MTSS on sporting performance, the emphasis on prophylactic interventions is increasingly important, underscoring the need for further research into both traditional and new therapeutic techniques for the successful management of this condition (Yamasaki et al., 2019).

Another widespread musculoskeletal disorder is gout. This is an inflammatory disorder resulting from crystallization of monosodium urate in soft tissue and joints. The history of gout is often separated into distinct phases, from asymptomatic hyperuricemia to chronic tophaceous gout, each with unique clinical presentations. Musculoskeletal imaging, particularly with ultrasound, has emerged as an important aid in diagnosing and managing gout in the long term. The imaging technique allows visualization of the affected joint with structural changes consistent with gout that would perhaps not be visible on plain X-rays. With the progression of the disease, progression may be monitored and treatment efficacy evaluated using ultrasound, emphasizing the growing importance of tailored management protocols for individuals affected by this disabling condition (Finucci et al., 2015).

The interplay between disorders such as MTSS and gout on musculoskeletal imaging exemplifies the broad spectrum of pathologies that may be addressed with appropriate imaging techniques. Effective diagnosis with advanced imaging modalities enables clinicians to design focused treatment plans tailored to individual patient needs. For example, recognition of the characteristic imaging features of MTSS can guide rehabilitation with a focus on strengthening and flexibility, and, in the case of gout, imaging findings can guide dietary therapy and pharmacotherapy. This advanced strategy is the best way to highlight the unifying role of musculoskeletal imaging, not only in diagnosis but also in directing holistic pathways of care that ultimately aim to optimize patient quality of life without unduly accelerating relapse from such omnipresent but interloping disorders. The need for ongoing research and development of imaging technologies remains imperative to optimizing the management of such a pervasive musculoskeletal disease.

9.3.1. Fractures and Their Radiological Appearance

Fracture evaluation necessitates a lucid understanding of its imaging characteristics, as the latter plays a crucial role in both diagnosis and therapeutic planning. Traditional imaging methods, such as plain radiography, have been the cornerstone of fracture assessment; however, their limitations can hinder the identification of complex injury patterns. For instance, overlapping anatomical structures of fractures may hinder easy visual identification, vitiating diagnostic precision (Figure 9.7).

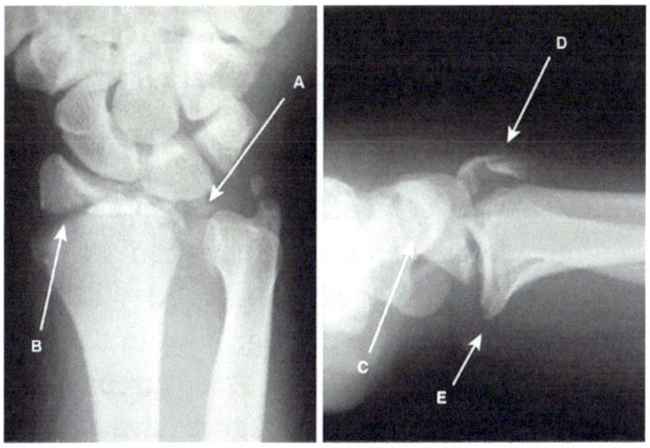

Figure 9.7. X-ray of a distal radius fracture with clear cortical disruption.

Source: https://clinicalgate.com/wp-content/uploads/2015/03/B9781416040835000056_f003-021-9781416040835.jpg.

The development of new imaging modalities, such as Cone Beam Computed Tomography (CBCT), offers a promising solution. CBCT enhances the detection of subtle fractures and other musculoskeletal pathologies due to its increased spatial resolution and ability to generate three-dimensional reformations. This achievement highlights the necessity of precise imaging in the creation of effective intervention policies and in follow-up studies (Desimpel et al., 2018). Differentiating fracture types and their imaging characteristics is important for supporting clinical decision-making. Fractures are classified into many subgroups, including open, closed, displaced, and non-displaced, with different imaging signatures for each. Open fractures expose bone to the outside world and require immediate treatment to prevent infection, whereas closed fractures do not necessarily present with any noticeable external findings. The varying degrees of displacement in fractures also affect treatment; for example, a displaced fracture is commonly treated by surgical reduction. Furthermore, high-tech imaging modalities are essential for assessing the complexity of associated soft-tissue injury with fractures. Understanding these characteristics enhances clinicians' abilities to minimize complications and achieve maximum patient outcomes (Kalová et al., 2019). In addition to conventional imaging, computer-aided orthopedic surgery (CAOS) systems are increasingly becoming well-liked in the assessment and treatment of fractures. CAOS systems use three-dimensional CT or MRI views to enable precise surgical planning and execution, improving outcomes for complex fractures. The integration of real-time navigation with mechanical devices enables highly precise interventions, minimizing surgical errors and ensuring maximum precision. Moreover, CAOS systems provide for anatomical patient variation, offering tailored solutions to fractures that pre-existing conditions might complicate. As musculoskeletal imaging evolves, the future use of CAOS systems in conjunction with traditional modalities is expected to increase, both in diagnostic accuracy and therapeutic options for fracture and associated musculoskeletal disorders. The interplay of these emerging technologies with the traditional imaging continues to redefine standards for orthopedic therapy (Kalová et al., 2019).

9.3.2. Tumors and Lesions in Bone and Soft Tissue

Correctly diagnosing tumors and lesions of bone and soft tissue is a vital function of musculoskeletal imaging, as these lesions can pose complex problems for clinicians. Imaging modalities, including radiography, CT, and MR imaging, are important tools for detecting and characterizing such lesions. While plain radiographs remain the standard of reference for initial evaluation, CT and MR imaging provide precious information about the nature, size, and potential impact of the lesions on the surrounding structures. For example, the signs assessed by these newer imaging techniques can differentiate benign from malignant lesions, which is crucial for planning appropriate management (Ladd et al., 2017) (Figure 9.8).

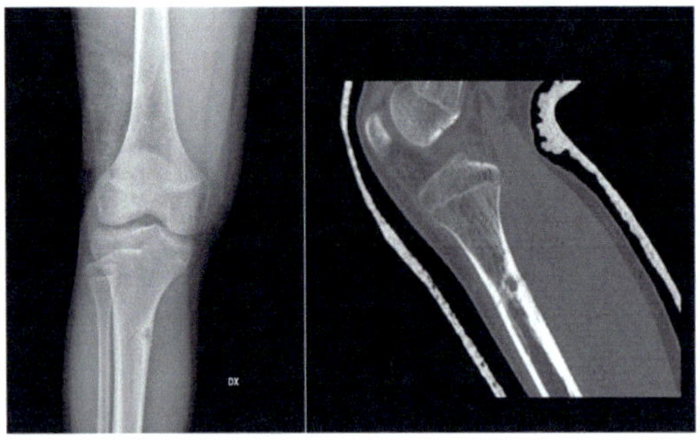

Figure 9.8. MRI showing a benign bone tumor in the proximal tibia.

Source: https://www.mdpi.com/jcm/jcm-11-00699/article_deploy/html/images/jcm-11-00699-g001.png.

Thus, the overall approach to imaging not only improves the yield but also guides therapeutic decision-making and prognostic evaluation in patients with musculoskeletal tumors. In recent years, the use of dynamic imaging techniques, particularly dynamic F-18 fluorodeoxyglucose (FDG) positron emission tomography/computed tomography (PET/CT), has transformed diagnostic practice for musculoskeletal lesions. This technique allows one to assess lesion metabolic activity and distinguish between benign and malignant tumors. Research has indicated that there are general differences in SUVmax values across various musculoskeletal lesions and that these differences provide useful information for differential diagnosis. For instance, dynamic scans show an increase in SUVmax over time in malignant lesions, in contrast to a relatively constant SUVmax in benign lesions (Bando et al., 2023). The ability to assess lesion characteristics dynamically not only enhances imaging examination specificity but also improves patient management through proper staging and treatment planning. Furthermore, understanding the imaging features about specific tumors and lesions is required for appropriate diagnosis and management. Benign lesions such as osteochondromas and enchondromas typically have sharp borders and characteristic appearances on imaging, and can most often be diagnosed with high certainty using simple radiography. In contrast, malignant tumors such as osteosarcoma and Ewing sarcoma have more aggressive imaging features, such as permeative destruction of bone or soft tissue spread. High-level imaging modalities, such as MRI, are extremely helpful in assessing tumor extent and involvement of adjacent structures, particularly in challenging cases (Ladd et al., 2017). By integrating accurate imaging results with clinical information, practitioners can obtain a more comprehensive image of musculoskeletal tumors and lesions, thereby leading to better patient outcomes.

9.3.3. Inflammatory Conditions and Their Imaging Findings

Inflammatory conditions within the musculoskeletal system pose a unique challenge for diagnosis and management, as their imaging findings can often overlap with those of other diseases, including neoplastic processes. A notable example is isolated iliac bone tuberculosis, a rare presentation that can initially mimic various inflammatory disorders. A case study highlights the diagnostic journey of a patient who presented with low back pain and swelling, where initial imaging with plain radiography revealed minimal changes, primarily slight sclerosis of the iliac side of the sacroiliac joint (Figure 9.9).

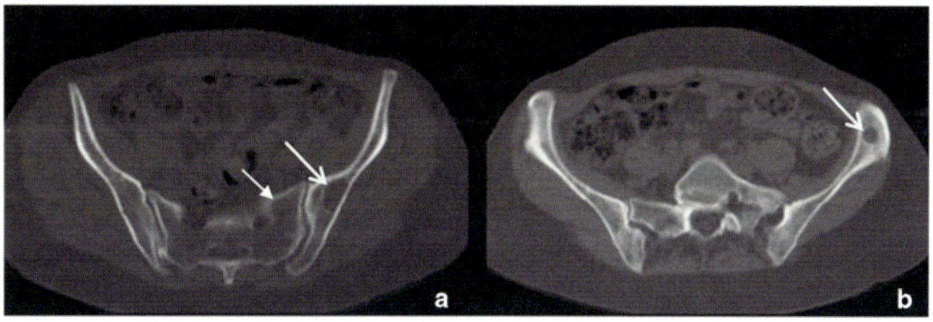

Figure 9.9. CT image illustrating lytic lesions in inflammatory arthritis.

Source: https://www.researchgate.net/publication/340810191/figure/fig3/AS:960050994634771@1605905402801/Axial-CT-scan-images-of-pelvis-showing-a-focal-lytic-lesion-in-right-part-of-sacrum.jpg.

The follow-up MRI was far more indicative, revealing low T1, high T2 signal appearance in association with the bony lesion and soft tissue components, demonstrating the importance of advanced imaging modalities in arriving at a definitive diagnosis and guiding beneficial treatment interventions—highlighting the importance of seeking the non-specificity of such lesions on imaging reports (Ismail et al., 2009). One other common inflammatory disease is gout, which arises secondary to the deposition of monosodium urate crystals in joints and surrounding soft tissues and results in acute inflammatory reactions. Imaging manifestations of gout are crucial in differentiating it from other forms of arthritis. Musculoskeletal ultrasonography is an essential modality for diagnosing gout, effectively imaging abnormalities such as synovial inflammation, erosions, and tophi, which are disease features. The four phases of gout—symptomatic hyperuricemia, acute gout attacks, intercritical periods, and chronic tophaceous gout—may be assessed using ultrasound, which provides extensive information on disease development. Not only is imaging useful for the diagnosis but also for the treatment of gout, as early and accurate detection of crystalline deposits may enable more effective intervention (Finucci et al., 2015). Beyond tuberculosis and gout, a wide variety of other inflammatory conditions cast a heterogeneous array of imaging appearances. Rheumatoid arthritis, psoriatic arthritis, and ankylosing spondylitis are among the more notable examples of diseases that also require precise imaging evaluation to characterize disease course and assess treatment response. Techniques such as MRI and ultrasound are particularly well-suited to the detection of joint effusion, synovitis, and bone erosion. Each has important therapeutic planning and patient education implications. Inflammatory illnesses, due to their complexity, call for a multifaceted imaging approach that is responsive to technical progress yet tethered to clinical context. Enhanced understanding of the radiologic characteristics of such inflammatory illnesses consequently enhances diagnostic accuracy and encourages more customized patient care within musculoskeletal imaging practice (Ismail et al., 2009; Finucci et al., 2015).

9.4. Advances in Musculoskeletal Imaging

The musculoskeletal imaging area has seen significant advances in diagnostic and therapeutic applications for bones and soft tissues. Three-dimensional (3D) imaging technologies have been a milestone in imaging complex anatomical structures. High-resolution computer tomography has been made possible by scientists' techniques that allow muscle and neurovascular structures to be segmented accurately and geographically represented. This 3D reconstruction enables detailed understanding of musculoskeletal biomechanics and provides essential information for orthopedic surgical interventions. Additionally, these anatomical models benefit from dual use, enabling quantitative analyses that can be applied across multiple disciplines, such as minimally invasive procedures and robotic interventions, thereby enhancing the effectiveness of therapeutic interventions in orthopedics and rehabilitation (Audenaert et al., 2010). The other significant development in musculoskeletal imaging is the inclusion of MRI-guided focused ultrasound surgery (MRgFUS), a revolutionary new move into non-surgical treatments. This leading-edge technology combines therapeutic ultrasound with MRI guidance, allowing real-time imaging and precise targeting of musculoskeletal disorders. The non-ionizing nature of both imaging and therapeutic elements reduces patient exposure to harmful radiation, making MRgFUS an attractive method for the treatment of numerous pathologies, ranging from joint disease to soft-tissue injuries. Notably, MRgFUS illustrates how collaborative scientific studies incorporating ultrasound physics and biological tissue responses can lead to innovative therapeutic approaches. As the clinical applications of MRgFUS continue to grow, it will transform conventional treatment models in musculoskeletal medicine (Albisinni et al., 2015). The arrival of advanced imaging technologies has not only improved the diagnostic accuracy but also paved the way towards personalized treatment plans according to individual patients' needs. With medicine moving toward personalized medicine, musculoskeletal imaging plays an increasingly vital role in developing targeted interventions by precise anatomical and functional evaluations. Artificial intelligence and machine learning algorithms' utilization in imaging analysis further enhances the detection rate of subtle pathological changes that could be missed in traditional imaging evaluation. As they continue to evolve, such technologies have the potential to redefine the role of musculoskeletal imaging in therapy and diagnosis, with far-reaching implications for future orthopedic and rehabilitation practice. The ongoing evolution of imaging modalities is thus necessary to advance knowledge and treatment of musculoskeletal disorders.

9.4.1. Technological Innovations in Imaging

The musculoskeletal imaging profile has undergone a revolutionary transformation due to significant technological developments that have markedly enhanced diagnostic capabilities and treatment planning. Among technological advancements, magnetic resonance imaging (MRI) has become a pillar for imaging bone and soft tissue diseases. Advances in MRI technology, such as higher magnetic field strengths and advanced pulse sequence techniques, have led to higher image resolution and shorter acquisition times. Such advances allow radiologists to detect subtle alterations in soft tissue and cortical bone that were otherwise undetectable, thereby enabling early diagnosis of complex musculoskeletal pathologies (Figure 9.10).

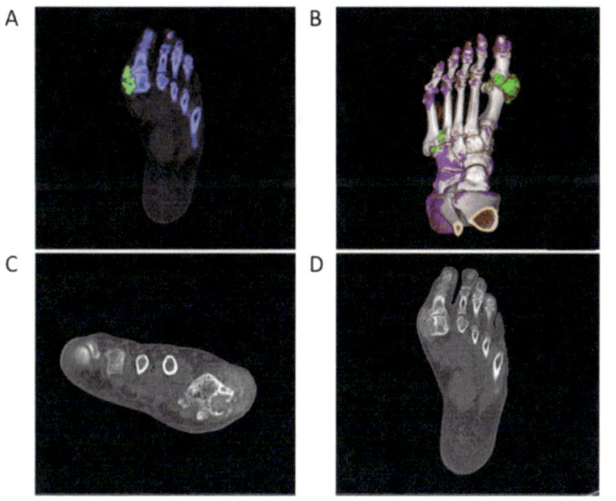

Figure 9.10. Dual-energy CT (DECT) scan showing urate crystal deposition in gout.

Source: https://www.researchgate.net/publication/352845087/figure/fig1/AS:1040422264651777@1625067406750/Dual-energy-computed-tomography-DECT-images-A-Color-mapping-showing-uric-acid.png.

Moreover, improvements in functional MRI and diffusion tensor imaging also provide an in-depth understanding of musculoskeletal disorders by enabling assessment of tissue integrity and biomechanical properties, thereby improving patient management. Apart from MRI innovation, the technological development of computed tomography (CT) has also significantly impacted musculoskeletal imaging. Such advances, such as dual-energy CT and iterative reconstruction algorithms, have provided radiologists with tools to enhance image quality while reducing radiation dose. Dual-energy CT, for instance, allows differentiation of materials by atomic number, thereby permitting bone and soft-tissue lesions to be defined in greater detail. Furthermore, the introduction of portable CT scanners has revolutionized imaging, enabling point-of-care assessment that accelerates diagnosis and treatment. These technologies are particularly critical in emergencies, where timely decision-making is paramount, and demonstrate how technology further increases the flexibility and timeliness of musculoskeletal imaging in practice. Nuclear medicine applications, particularly the evolution of single photon emission computed tomography (SPECT) and SPECT/CT, have given dynamic insight into musculoskeletal imaging. Developments such as the transition from bulky photomultiplier tubes to new detectors have enhanced spatial resolution and detection efficiency, which have made SPECT a valuable tool in evaluating complex musculoskeletal disorders. Contemporary SPECT technologies with custom collimators and semiconductor detectors, such as cadmium-zinc-telluride (CZT), demonstrate how technology facilitates shorter scanning times and greater patient comfort. Additionally, the adoption of iterative reconstruction methods has alleviated the general limitations of quantitative imaging, ultimately verifying the utility of SPECT/CT in the diagnosis and monitoring of musculoskeletal disorders. This convergence of technology underscores the need for multi-faceted imaging approaches to most effectively maximize patient outcomes and enhance care quality in musculoskeletal medicine (N/A, 2002; AlSaadi et al., 2024).

9.4.2. The Role of Artificial Intelligence in Interpretation

The use of artificial intelligence (AI) in interpreting musculoskeletal imaging has proven to be a revolutionary development in radiology. With advances in machine learning and deep learning, radiologists are increasingly using AI to enhance diagnostic effectiveness and precision. The technologies enable automated image analysis, significantly impacting the interpretation of intricate musculoskeletal conditions. As AI algorithms become smarter and more advanced, they can provide valuable information about imaging outcomes that would otherwise be missed (Figure 9.11).

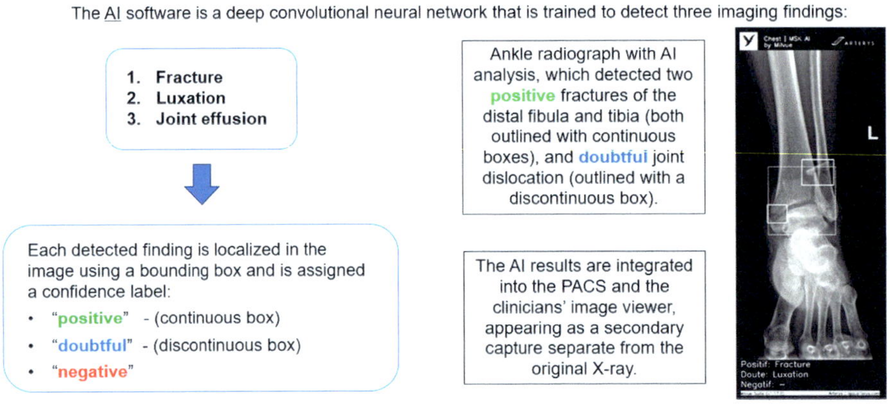

Figure 9.11. AI-powered radiology software interpreting musculoskeletal X-rays.

Source: https://pub.mdpi-res.com/diagnostics/diagnostics-15-00491/article_deploy/html/images/diagnostics-15-00491-g009.png?1739859025.

This shift not only improves diagnostic speed but also supports radiologists in managing higher volumes of cases. Ultimately, the integration of AI into the workflow of musculoskeletal imaging aims to augment the decision-making process rather than replace human expertise (Akkaya et al., 2025). Deep learning-based approaches represent a particularly promising subset of AI applications in musculoskeletal radiology. Recent studies have demonstrated that these algorithms can effectively diagnose internal joint derangements, including anterior cruciate ligament tears and rotator cuff disorders. Beyond simply identifying pathologies, more advanced deep learning frameworks begin to characterize these conditions and assess their severity. For instance, algorithms have been developed to evaluate Achilles tendon tears and predict recurrence in musculoskeletal neoplasms, showcasing a broad spectrum of applicability. The ability of AI to perform at levels comparable to experienced radiologists in identifying abnormalities is a noteworthy development, making it a valuable tool in clinical settings (Fritz et al., 2022). However, an essential aspect of this advancement is the necessity for ongoing validation in real-world clinical environments. Despite AI's potential, gaps remain in our understanding of how these technologies can be effectively implemented in routine practice. Studies comparing the performance of radiologists interpreting musculoskeletal MRI with and without AI assistance are limited, raising questions about the practical benefits of AI integration. Additionally, conversations about the generalizability and clinical applicability of AI algorithms highlight a need for empirical data in this field. Although some studies have shown that AI can match or surpass human diagnostic performance, there remains widespread skepticism about its readiness for widespread clinical use. For AI to truly transform musculoskeletal imaging, robust evidence demonstrating its clinical utility in everyday practice is required. Therefore, the future of AI in this domain hinges on continued research and development, ultimately fostering an environment where human expertise and AI capabilities coexist harmoniously (Fritz et al., 2022).

9.4.3. Future Trends in Musculoskeletal Imaging

The evolution of musculoskeletal imaging is shifting rapidly towards advanced technological integration, especially with the rise of computer-assisted orthopedic surgery (CAOS) systems. These systems represent a pivotal advancement in clinical orthopedics, enabling precise treatment strategies for a range of musculoskeletal disorders. CAOS encompasses a range of tools that use volumetric images from modalities such as computed tomography (CT) and magnetic resonance imaging (MRI), as well as 2D and 3D fluoroscopic images. The integration of these imaging modalities facilitates improved surgical planning and navigation, enhancing the accuracy of orthopedic interventions (Figure 9.12).

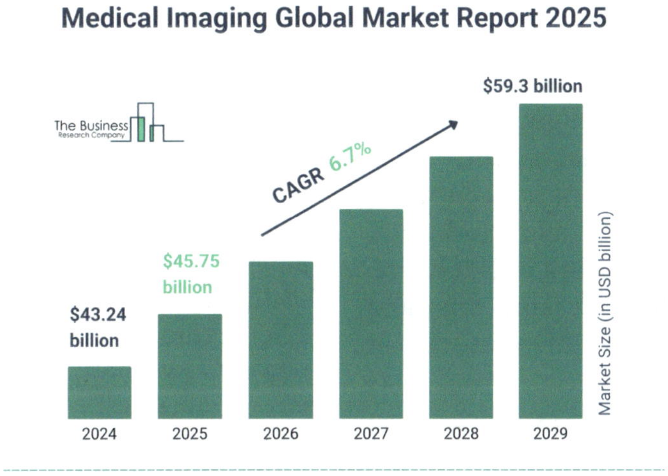

Figure 9.12. Conceptual graph of future trends in musculoskeletal imaging technology.

Source: https://www.thebusinessresearchcompany.com/graphimages/Medical_Imaging_Market_2025_Graph.webp.

Furthermore, the incorporation of kinetic information about joints deepens the complexity and efficacy of surgical procedures. As the field progresses, the close interplay between imaging technologies and surgical applications will likely yield superior outcomes for patients with bone and soft-tissue ailments, fundamentally transforming the landscape of musculoskeletal treatment (Kalová et al., 2019). In addition to technological advancements, the role of ultrasound imaging (USI) in musculoskeletal diagnostics is becoming increasingly prominent. Particularly in regions like New Zealand, the utilization of USI by physiotherapists highlights a burgeoning trend toward non-invasive imaging approaches among healthcare professionals. This trend is not merely an adaptation of existing practices; it marks a pivotal shift in the way musculoskeletal conditions are diagnosed and managed. Evidence shows that physiotherapists employing USI can use the technique for various purposes, ranging from diagnostic applications to rehabilitative measures such as biofeedback, thereby expanding their scope of practice. However, barriers to widespread adoption, such as training disparities and equipment accessibility, remain significant challenges. Addressing these barriers will likely enhance the integration of USI into standard clinical practices, broadening the diagnostic capabilities available within the musculoskeletal domain (University A of Technology et al., 2018). The future of musculoskeletal imaging is poised to witness further evolutionary leaps as artificial intelligence (AI) and machine learning (ML) become integral components. By leveraging AI-driven algorithms, imaging modalities can automate the analysis of complex datasets, thus increasing diagnostic accuracy and efficiency. These technologies can aid in identifying subtle changes in imaging studies that may be overlooked by human interpretation, thereby improving disease detection rates. Moreover, AI can streamline the workflow in imaging centers, enabling faster turnaround times for patients and clinicians. As AI continues to develop, the landscape of musculoskeletal imaging will likely become more collaborative, with radiologists, orthopedic surgeons, and physiotherapists engaging in interprofessional teams enhanced by these technologies. This progressive integration signifies a promising future, not only in improving patient outcomes but also in fostering an environment conducive to continuous advancement in musculoskeletal health management.

9.5. Clinical Applications and Case Studies

Clinical applications of musculoskeletal imaging have expanded significantly with the adoption of advanced techniques such as Cone Beam Computed Tomography (CBCT). Initially utilized predominantly for dental imaging, CBCT has gained traction in the musculoskeletal domain due to its capacity to deliver high-resolution images with lower radiation exposure compared to traditional methods. This imaging modality is particularly beneficial for diagnosing fractures and dislocations of small bones and joints. Notably, CBCT combined with arthrography has emerged as a potent tool for detecting cartilage lesions in small joints, demonstrating its ability to outperform conventional radiography in settings where anatomical overlap complicates visual assessment. This shift not only enhances diagnostic accuracy but also facilitates more precise treatment plans tailored to individual patient needs, highlighting the evolving landscape of musculoskeletal imaging in clinical practice (Desimpel et al., 2018). In addition to CBCT, MRI-guided focused ultrasound surgery (MRgFUS) represents a significant advancement in the treatment of musculoskeletal disorders. This minimally invasive technique uses MRI for precise guidance, enabling real-time monitoring of treatment progress. MRgFUS operates without ionizing radiation, making it an appealing alternative for various conditions, including tendon injuries and osteoarthritis. The method's effectiveness stems from its non-invasive nature and the ability to focus energy on specific problem areas, minimizing damage to surrounding tissue. Clinical case studies illustrate the versatility of MRgFUS in achieving pain relief and promoting healing in patients who have not responded well to traditional interventions. As a testament to its potential, ongoing research continues to explore its applications, which may revolutionize the treatment landscape for musculoskeletal disorders (Albisinni et al., 2015). Moreover, both CBCT and MRgFUS embody the trend toward integrating sophisticated imaging technologies into therapeutic strategies for musculoskeletal disorders. A growing body of clinical evidence supports their efficacy, demonstrating marked improvements in patient outcomes when these modalities are employed. Case studies highlight instances in which CBCT has accurately staged complex injuries or characterized bone lesions that might otherwise have remained undiagnosed. Similarly, MRgFUS has shown promising results in clinical settings, particularly for individuals suffering from chronic pain conditions. The convergence of imaging and treatment technology not only enhances diagnostic precision but also paves the way for personalized medicine approaches in musculoskeletal care. As these innovations continue to be refined, they signal a transformative shift in how practitioners diagnose and manage musculoskeletal diseases, ultimately improving patient satisfaction and quality of life (Albisinni et al., 2015; Desimpel et al., 2018).

9.5.1. Case Study: Imaging in Sports Injuries

The efficacy of imaging in diagnosing sports injuries is paramount, as athletes are prone to a range of musculoskeletal injuries that can impede their performance.

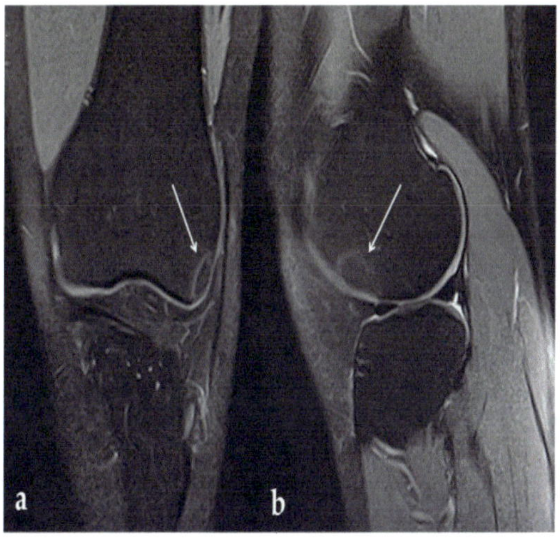

Figure 9.13. MRI bone abnormality of the knee following ultrasound therapy.

Source: https://www.mdpi.com/ijerph/ijerph-19-14202/article_deploy/html/images/ijerph-19-14202-g001.png.

Advanced imaging techniques, such as magnetic resonance imaging (MRI) and ultrasonography, play a crucial role in evaluating both bone and soft tissue damage. These modalities provide detailed visualization, allowing for the identification of stress fractures, tendon tears, and contusions with greater accuracy. Moreover, MRI is particularly beneficial because it can assess soft-tissue injuries without the risks associated with ionizing radiation. Integrating imaging findings into clinical assessments helps healthcare providers determine appropriate management strategies for athletes, which is essential for their recovery and return to play (Figure 9.13).

The ability to pinpoint the exact location and nature of an injury not only facilitates timely treatment but also helps in preventing future occurrences of similar injuries. In the context of sports injuries, imaging extends beyond diagnosis; it also plays a vital role in monitoring the healing process. Regular imaging evaluations can assess whether a specified treatment plan is effective or if modifications are necessary. For instance, in cases of stress fractures, periodic imaging can help determine whether continued rest is needed or weight-bearing activities can be initiated. This iterative process between diagnosis, treatment, and follow-up imaging is crucial for optimizing recovery timelines for athletes, who often face immense pressure to return to competition swiftly. Furthermore, understanding the progression of an injury through imaging aids in educating athletes about their conditions, which is vital for adherence to rehabilitation protocols. Such an informed approach minimizes the risk of exacerbating the injury and fosters a proactive mindset toward long-term musculoskeletal health. Ultimately, the integration of imaging techniques in the management of sports injuries exemplifies a multidisciplinary approach that is becoming increasingly essential in contemporary sports medicine. This approach underscores the collaboration between radiologists, orthopedic specialists, and physiotherapists to ensure holistic care for athletes. Each imaging modality contributes unique insights that enhance the clinical decision-making process, allowing for tailored treatment plans that address not just the injury but the athlete's overall well-being. Additionally, implementing preventive strategies informed by imaging findings can mitigate future injury risk, a critical consideration in sports medicine. As research continues to evolve, enhancing imaging technologies and techniques will likely further revolutionize the landscape of sports injury management, providing athletes with more effective pathways to recovery and performance optimization.

9.5.2. Case Study: Imaging for Arthritis Diagnosis

The case study on imaging for arthritis diagnosis highlights the evolving landscape of musculoskeletal imaging technologies that accurately identify various forms of arthritis. Traditional imaging modalities, such as X-rays, have long been used to diagnose arthritis because they effectively reveal bone deformities and joint space narrowing. However, the limitations of X-rays in assessing soft tissue structures underscore the necessity for advanced imaging techniques (Figure 9.14).

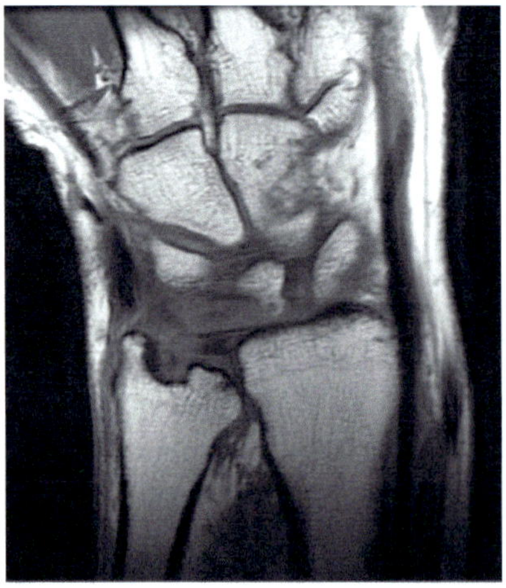

Figure 9.14. MR imaging of rheumatoid arthritis.

Source: https://radsource.us/wp-content/uploads/2016/05/1a.jpg.

Magnetic resonance imaging (MRI) and ultrasound have now taken an important place here, with improved visualization of the soft tissues, joint effusions, and inflammatory changes. These techniques enhance diagnostic sensitivity, enabling clinicians to differentiate between arthritic conditions, such as gout and rheumatoid arthritis, which have specific imaging findings vital for appropriate therapy. In gout, for instance, musculoskeletal ultrasound has proved particularly beneficial for diagnosing pathologies such as monosodium urate crystal deposition and hypertrophy of the synovium. Ultrasound allows clinicians to visualize abnormalities not readily apparent on X-ray, hence facilitating early diagnosis and intervention. According to the literature, ultrasound can detect all gout-related changes and transform the methods of monitoring the progression of disease and the response to therapies by clinicians. The application of such imaging tools not only helps track clinical outcomes but also enhances patient care through on-time, targeted treatment strategies. As the incidence of arthritis increases—partly due to aging populations and lifestyle—and given the role of these sophisticated imaging modalities in establishing overall arthritis management, their importance cannot be overstressed (Finucci et al., 2015). Imaging modalities also have use in biomarker use, which adds another layer to diagnostic capability. Biomarkers are helpful imaging adjuncts because they offer a glimpse into arthritic disease biology that complements the anatomy provided by imaging modalities. Improved and earlier diagnosis is facilitated by this complementary method, with interventions offered at the right time that can significantly influence the disease course. As highlighted by current research, technological innovations in imaging, such as 4DCT and artificial intelligence, have the potential to revolutionize our understanding and treatment of musculoskeletal diseases. The integration of advanced imaging technology with biomarkers is an anticipatory strategy that ensures accurate diagnosis and improves patient outcomes in the treatment of arthritis (Adamczyk et al., 2025).

9.5.3. Case Study: Imaging in Trauma Cases

In trauma, successful imaging plays a crucial role in the diagnosis and treatment of musculoskeletal trauma. Prompt and precise evaluation of fractures, dislocations, and soft tissue abnormalities is essential for administering early treatment and achieving optimal results for the patient. Among various available imaging devices, Cone Beam Computed Tomography (CBCT) is a powerful imaging modality with low-dose radiation and high resolution. This technology offers improved visualization of complex structures, particularly of small bones and joints, where plain radiography can offer inconclusive findings.

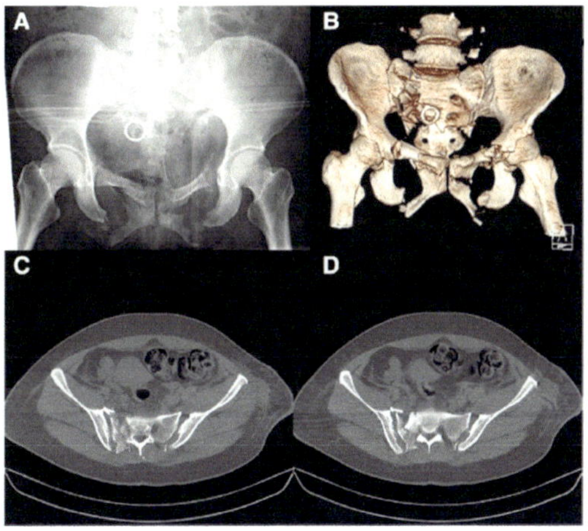

Figure 9.15. CT reconstruction of pelvic fractures from a blunt trauma case.

Source: https://www.researchgate.net/publication/330645342/figure/fig1/AS:719148074151936@1548469670150/a-d-AP-view-and-CT-3D-reconstruction-of-pelvic-fracture-showed-type-C3-Tile.png.

Furthermore, CBCT is superior in assessing degenerative joint disease and cartilage lesions, easily overlooked by plain radiologic methods. Therefore, the inclusion of CBCT in trauma imaging protocols can enhance diagnostic sensitivity and inform surgical planning and thereby lead to improved patient outcomes in musculoskeletal trauma scenarios (Desimpel et al., 2018). Computer-assisted orthopedic surgery (CAOS) systems also stand out because of the way they can increase the accuracy of surgery for the management of traumatic musculoskeletal disease (Figure 9.15).

With the integration of imaging modalities such as CT and MRI with advanced navigation and planning systems, CAOS enables surgeons to visualize anatomical structures with clarity which was not possible before. Not only does this new technology facilitate accurate positioning of orthopedic implants, but it also lessens soft tissue damage, a problem essential even in trauma cases, where the adjacent structures will be at risk. The integration of volumetric and kinetic information into the surgical procedure has led to better results, reducing the incidence of complications and facilitating faster recovery. With technology progressing in musculoskeletal imaging, the application of CAOS systems in trauma care continues to represent an important milestone towards more personalized and efficient surgeries (Kalová et al., 2019). In addition to these newer imaging modalities, close interdisciplinary cooperation between orthopedic surgeons, radiologists, and trauma specialists is essential to treat musculoskeletal trauma successfully. This integrated approach aims to incorporate imaging information into the clinical presentation so that the specific situation of the individual patient is accounted for. For instance, while imaging provides important information regarding the severity of injury and associated soft tissue injury, clinical examination allows us to evaluate patient function and pain as a comprehensive unit. Hence, integrating diagnostic imaging and clinical evaluation can lead to personalized treatment plans that meet the short- and long-term needs of trauma patients. This integration model supports the establishment of trauma care, highlighting the significant role of imaging in improving patient outcomes for the treatment of musculoskeletal injury (Desimpel et al., 2018; Kalová et al., 2019).

SUMMARY

In the evolving landscape of musculoskeletal imaging, the significance of newer imaging technologies cannot be overstated. The ability to discriminate among various conditions affecting bone and soft-tissue structures is significant, especially since misdiagnosis can lead to complicated situations. Newer imaging modalities, such as MRI and CT, have been immensely beneficial for making precise observations of pathologies that may present with nonspecific clinical appearances. For example, isolated iliac bone tuberculosis illustrates the need for appropriate imaging—initial misinterpretation can lead to delays in therapy and suboptimal patient outcomes. This reinforces that, while imaging results can be subtle, incorporating patient history and advances in techniques can enhance diagnostic accuracy, ultimately resulting in effective clinical management (Ismail et al., 2009). The advent of Cone Beam Computed Tomography (CBCT) heralds a paradigm shift in imaging musculoskeletal conditions, particularly of smaller joints and bones. The superior spatial resolution of CBCT enables more accurate evaluation of conditions such as cartilage lesions and degenerative joint disease. Its advantages over conventional radiography are particularly important where adjacent bony structures prevent clear definition—the diagnosis and monitoring of the progression of musculoskeletal disease are easily feasible. The relatively low cost and low radiation exposure of CBCT also underpin its widespread clinical application. With advances in imaging, the role of CBCT becomes even more relevant, especially when integrated with other modalities such as MRI and conventional CT to provide comprehensive assessments (Desimpel et al., 2018).

Generally, future musculoskeletal imaging requires a multi-faceted approach that embraces new technologies alongside conventional methods. With the introduction of imaging technologies such as CBCT and the prudent use of MRI, healthcare professionals can treat musculoskeletal conditions more effectively. Practitioners need to keep up with these technological advancements to achieve optimal diagnostic yield and patient outcomes. Furthermore, studies into the applications and limitations of various imaging technologies will continue to shape best practice within the specialty. Lastly, the addition of these diagnostic technologies will not only enhance our understanding of musculoskeletal pathologies but also improve patient care for those dealing with these complex conditions (Ismail et al., 2009; Desimpel et al., 2018).

CLOSER LOOK

MUSCULOSKELETAL IMAGING

In the field of musculoskeletal imaging, several relevant points emerge that highlight the interdependence between imaging technologies and their application to understanding bone and soft-tissue structure. Advanced imaging modalities such as magnetic resonance imaging (MRI) and computed tomography (CT) provide extremely valuable information regarding the subtle aspects of musculoskeletal anatomy. Not only do these technological devices function to enhance diagnostic precision, but also to facilitate pre-surgical planning and post-surgical assessment. By viewing complex anatomical relationships, radiologists and orthopedic surgeons can better visualize the pathophysiology of musculoskeletal diseases, enabling individualized treatment plans that account for the unique characteristics of each case. Another distinguishing characteristic of musculoskeletal imaging is its ability to evaluate developmental and degenerative changes in bone and soft tissue. For instance, biomechanical influences of fetal movement, as argued in the contemporary literature, highlight their impact on bone development. Abnormalities in fetal movement have been associated with most musculoskeletal diseases; hence, the need to attach greater significance to the early recognition of mechanical forces (Nowlan et al., 2015). This insight not only aids in the diagnosis of congenital diseases but also offers new hope for prenatal therapies, potentially enhancing the destiny of afflicted children and infants. Furthermore, the emergence of computer-aided orthopedic surgery (CAOS) systems constitutes a revolutionary breakthrough in musculoskeletal therapies. By integrating imaging data with surgical navigation technology, CAOS enables surgeons to perform precise, minimally invasive surgery, expediting recovery while avoiding complications. The systems utilize a variety of imaging modalities, including 2D and 3D fluoroscopic images, to create highly detailed surgical plans tailored to individual anatomical variations (Kalová et al., 2019). The technology is a step towards more personalized medicine in orthopedics, as it allows clinicians to more effectively chart complex anatomical landscapes, which are crucial to successful surgical outcomes and overall musculoskeletal health development.

Accurate imaging is at the core of musculoskeletal disease treatment planning, as it directly contributes to clinical decision-making and patient outcomes. High-resolution imaging techniques, such as magnetic resonance imaging (MRI) and computed tomography (CT), provide superior anatomical visualization that is crucial to defining the precise location and extent of musculoskeletal diseases, including bone fractures and soft tissue lesions. Inaccurate or inadequate imaging may result in misdiagnosis and inappropriate treatment, leading to complications including delayed healing or unfavorable surgical results. As such, medical practitioners increasingly turn to precise imaging methods to guide their approach, individualize interventions, and deliver focused therapy for their patients, thereby improving the quality of care at musculoskeletal treatment centers. The advent of computer-assisted orthopedic surgery (CAOS) systems is revolutionizing the function of accurate imaging in treatment planning. Through the integration of volumetric images from CT or MRI into the surgical procedure, CAOS facilitates greater accuracy in orthopedic procedures. These devices not only enable precise localization of pathologies but also assist surgeons in planning potential surgical outcomes, thereby enhancing intraoperative decision-making. The union of superior imaging technologies with mechanical devices underscores the role played by precision in imaging as it is on this that successful surgical procedures are developed. Such a blending of imaging and surgical planning best illustrates how accurate technological advances in imaging can translate into better procedural success and improved patient satisfaction in treating musculoskeletal disorders, reinforcing the role of precision in imaging methods (Kalová et al., 2019). New methods such as MRI-guided focused ultrasound surgery (MRgFUS) also underscore the transformative nature of treatment protocols, highlighting the critical role of imaging in developing less invasive procedures. MRgFUS improves diagnostic information and enables real-time monitoring of therapeutic procedures, making it specifically applicable to musculoskeletal use. This upper-level imaging technique is programmed to provide adequate real-time visualization during the intervention, allowing clinicians to adjust their strategies based on imaging feedback. With the increased use of new technologies by practitioners, the reliance on appropriate imaging becomes even more significant, as real-time visualization and monitoring of the intervention render interventions safer and more successful. Finally, as clinical practice and research both continue to advance, the emphasis on accurate imaging will only remain at the forefront of optimizing outcomes in musculoskeletal patients and thus become an integral part of current treatment planning (Albisinni et al., 2015).

REFERENCES

1. Trestka, G., Domino, W., Zelik, U., Przygoda, M., Śnieżna, J., Stępień, K., Adamczyk, S., Florczak, W., Włodyka, J., Dziewic, J., & Dzwonnik, K. (2025). Imaging diagnostics, biomarkers, and emerging trends in orthopedic research and treatment. *Quality in Sport*, *37*, 57103. https://doi.org/10.12775/qs.2025.37.57103Akkaya, Z., Bhattacharjee, R., Majumdar, S., Tong, Q., et al. (2025). Artificial intelligence in musculoskeletal applications: A primer for radiologists. https://core.ac.uk/download/647989534.pdf (accessed on 15th July 2025).
2. Albisinni, U., Battista, G., Bazzocchi, A., Catalano, C., et al. (2015). MRI-guided focused ultrasound surgery in musculoskeletal diseases: The hot topics. https://core.ac.uk/download/98341478.pdf (accessed on 15th July 2025).
3. AlSaadi, A., Jain, A., Al-Jabri, A., Delanerolle, G., Zabah, J., Shi, J. Q., Phiri, P., et al. (2024). Technological advances in SPECT and SPECT/CT imaging. https://core.ac.uk/download/613741130.pdf (accessed on 15th July 2025).
4. Auckland University of Technology, Forrest, G., Jedrzejczak, A., Leech, M., McKiernan, M., Ministry of Health, New Zealand Medical Radiation Technologists Board, et al. (2018). Exploring the clinical use of ultrasound imaging: A survey of physiotherapists in New Zealand. https://core.ac.uk/download/155776972.pdf (accessed on 15th July 2025).
5. Audenaert, E., Mahieu, P., Pattyn, C., Van Hoof, T., et al. (2010). Soft tissue structure modelling for use in orthopaedic applications and musculoskeletal biomechanics. https://core.ac.uk/download/55761253.pdf (accessed on 15th July 2025).
6. Bando, Y., Beuthien-Baumann, B., Harada, M., Irahara, S., et al. (2023). Dynamic FDG PET/CT in MSLs. https://core.ac.uk/download/477750521.pdf (accessed on 15th July 2025).
7. Baur, A., Baur, A., Baur, A., Baur-Melnyk, A., Mahnken, A. H., Groves, A. M., Baur-Melnyk, A., et al. (2007). Whole-body imaging of the musculoskeletal system: The value of MR imaging. https://core.ac.uk/download/pdf/7752049.pdf (accessed on 15th July 2025).
8. Becce, F., Booij, R., Gallego Manzano, L., Mourad, A., et al. (2024). Chances and challenges of photon-counting CT in musculoskeletal imaging. https://core.ac.uk/download/610639100.pdf (accessed on 15th July 2025).
9. Buchanan, M. D., Shuler, F. D., et al. (2016). A comparison of imaging modalities for the diagnosis of osteomyelitis. https://core.ac.uk/download/232729304.pdf (accessed on 15th July 2025).
10. Calvert, G., Hanrahan, C. J., Jones, K. B., Li, X., et al. (2014). Coccidiomycosis infection of the patella mimicking a neoplasm: Two case reports. https://core.ac.uk/download/323070868.pdf (accessed on 15th July 2025).
11. Carrino, J. A., de Cesar Netto, C., Demehri, S., Ibad, A., et al. (2022). Computed tomography: State-of-the-art advancements in musculoskeletal imaging. https://core.ac.uk/download/622991659.pdf (accessed on 15th July 2025).
12. Chakravartty, R. M., Gheysens, O., Glaudemans, A. W. J. M., Kwee, T. C., et al. (2024). Diagnostic imaging of the diabetic foot: An EANM evidence-based guidance. https://core.ac.uk/download/612336516.pdf (accessed on 15th July 2025).
13. Chimbo, N. de J. P., Dávila, D. A. D., Montero, F. G. S., Valdés, R. L., et al. (2024). 3D imaging techniques for the diagnosis and surgical planning of complex limb fractures: A systematic review. https://core.ac.uk/download/635339063.pdf (accessed on 15th July 2025).

14. de Beaux, A., Kingsnorth, A., Sheen, A. J., Akermark, B., Stephenson, B. M., Beatty, B., Brennan, B., et al. (2014). 'Treatment of the sportsman's groin': British Hernia Society's 2014 position statement based on the Manchester Consensus Conference. https://core.ac.uk/download/9362135.pdf (accessed on 15th July 2025).

15. Desimpel, J., Posadzy, M., & Vanhoenacker, F. (2018). Cone beam CT of the musculoskeletal system: Clinical applications. https://core.ac.uk/download/147045015.pdf (accessed on 15th July 2025).

16. El-Tallawy, S. N., Nalamasu, R., Salem, G. I., LeQuang, J. A., Pergolizzi, J. V., & Christo, P. J. (2021). Management of musculoskeletal pain: An update with emphasis on chronic musculoskeletal pain. *Pain and Therapy, 10*, 181–209. https://doi.org/10.1007/s40122-021-00235-2 (accessed on 15th July 2025).

17. Finucci, A., Iagnocco, A., Rutigliano, I. M., Scirocco, G., et al. (2015). Musculoskeletal ultrasonography in gout. https://core.ac.uk/download/74318651.pdf (accessed on 15th July 2025).

18. Fritz, B., & Fritz, J. (2022). Artificial intelligence for MRI diagnosis of joints: A scoping review of the current state-of-the-art of deep learning-based approaches. https://www.zora.uzh.ch/id/eprint/221318/1/ZORA_s00256_021_03830_8.pdf (accessed on 15th July 2025).

19. Ismail, M., Sinha, N. R., & Szmigielski, W. (2009). Isolated iliac bone tuberculosis: A case report. https://core.ac.uk/download/161629239.pdf (accessed on 15th July 2025).

20. Kalová, M., Kubíček, J., Oczka, D., Tomanec, O., et al. (2019). Recent trends, technical concepts and components of computer-assisted orthopedic surgery systems: A comprehensive review. https://core.ac.uk/download/287649034.pdf (accessed on 15th July 2025).

21. Ladd, L. M., & Roth, T. D. (2017). Computed tomography and magnetic resonance imaging of bone tumors. https://core.ac.uk/download/84831211.pdf (accessed on 15th July 2025).

22. LeBoff, M. S., Greenspan, S. L., Insogna, K., Lewiecki, E. M., Saag, K. G., Singer, A., & Siris, E. S. (2022). The clinician's guide to prevention and treatment of osteoporosis. *Osteoporosis International, 33*, 2049–2102. https://doi.org/10.1007/s00198-021-05900-y (accessed on 15th July 2025).

23. N/A. (2002). *Focal Spot, Summer 2002*. https://core.ac.uk/download/129069324.pdf (accessed on 15th July 2025).

24. Nowlan, N. C. (2015). Biomechanics of fetal movement. https://core.ac.uk/download/76995826.pdf (accessed on 15th July 2025).

25. Yamasaki, S. (2019). A review of the treatment and prevention options for medial tibial stress syndrome. https://core.ac.uk/download/213464302.pdf (accessed on 15th July 2025).

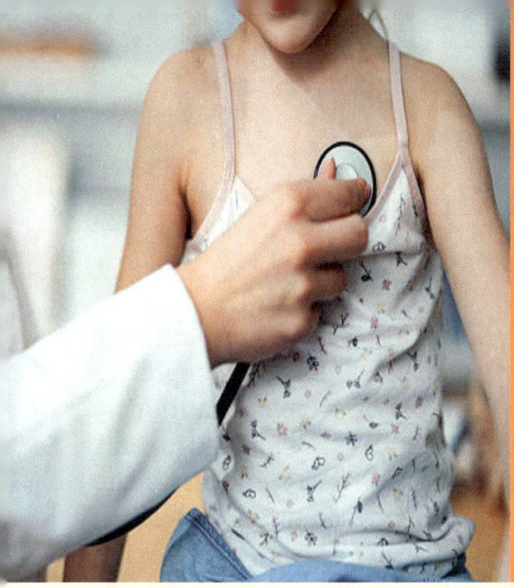

Chapter 10

PEDIATRIC DIAGNOSTIC IMAGING PRINCIPLES

Contents

Introduction

Pediatric imaging diagnostics is responsible for quite several approaches that attempt to accurately determine medical conditions in children with the least possible risks, particularly those posed by exposure to radiation. Given the increasing reliance on medical imaging, it is essential that parents and doctors be in possession of a proper understanding of the underlying principles driving its use. This information not only enlightens about wise decision-making but also ensures that imaging advantages consistently surpass inherent threats, especially in vulnerable populations such as children. It is important to recognize children's greater sensitivity to radiation than adults, necessitating a tailored approach that ensures their safety while providing clinically relevant data. By exploring the principles of diagnostic imaging specific to children, this chapter aims to offer a balanced contribution to the understanding of the risks, benefits, and highest standards in pediatric imaging. One of the most significant areas of discussion in pediatric imaging is the potential health impact of ionizing radiation. Literature has shown that, more than adults, children are at a greater risk of acquiring diseases resulting from radiation in the long run, due primarily to their ever-dividing cells and longer lifespan post-exposure. As outlined by recent studies, the requirement for effective communication of these risks cannot be overstated. Educating parents and guardians about radiation exposure helps relieve their apprehensions and enhances their confidence in radiographic examinations. For instance, a teaching pamphlet was found to significantly increase parental awareness and knowledge regarding the risks and benefits associated with dental radiographs, ultimately fostering increased comfort in allowing their children to undergo such imaging (Hwang et al., 2017).

This emphasizes healthcare professionals' need to engage in open communication with patients' families. In addition to highlighting the significance of effective communication of risks, application of guidelines based on well-established principles in pediatric imaging is crucial to ensure patient safety and optimize healthcare outcomes. The ALARA principle is well-established as a cornerstone for minimizing radiation exposure in pediatric patients. This principle demands that imaging be performed only when absolutely required and with the minimum effective dose. Imaging modality decisions are crucially in the hands of healthcare professionals who must interpret these guidelines and exercise wise judgments regarding imaging modalities.

Further, the integration of the developments made in imaging technology, such as ultrasound and magnetic resonance imaging, can promote safer alternatives that avoid ionizing radiation altogether (N/A, 2011). Therefore, a thorough understanding of pediatric diagnostic imaging principles is crucial for creating a culture of safety in clinical practice.

10.1. Safety Considerations

In compliance with protection in pediatric diagnostic imaging, the risk posed by exposure to radiation per se must be weighed cautiously against the gain in diagnosis. Children's developing bodies are more susceptible to the harmful effects of ionizing radiation; therefore, minimizing exposure is extremely crucial. Because radiation can cause late morbidity in the form of cancer, the principle of "as low as reasonably achievable" (ALARA) assumes a particular significance in children. This regulation requires medical professionals to use the smallest radiation dose necessary while still achieving the diagnostic detail required. An assessment of the risk/benefit ratio forms a fundamental component of this decision-making process since it requires an explicit appreciation of the likely benefit of the imaging examination and the short-term and long-term risk posed by radiation exposure in young patients (Donya et al., 2014). In addition to dose optimization, the use of appropriate imaging modalities is also crucial for making diagnostic procedures in children safer. Alternative non-ionizing imaging techniques, such as ultrasound and magnetic resonance imaging (MRI), should often be the initial option in cases where they can provide sufficient diagnostic information. For instance, MRI is particularly valuable because it is ionizing radiation-free, and therefore it can be used more safely in children, particularly for monitoring certain diseases or injuries. However, the availability, cost, and procedure time for each imaging modality are also factors that govern their use. By properly selecting the most suitable imaging modality for the child's needs, clinicians can easily minimize the potential risks associated with pediatric diagnosis (N/A, 1993). Training of staff and continuous education on pediatric imaging is essential in shaping a safety culture. Radiographers and radiologists must possess strong knowledge of pediatric anatomy, how children differ in their response to radiation, and current safety practices. Ongoing updating of knowledge and skills ensures that practitioners are competent in using the most efficient safety measures and maintaining ethical practice in care. Moreover, engagement in multidisciplinary discussion is essential because inter-professional collaboration can lead to institutional policies that prioritize patient safety. Adoption of comprehensive training programs establishes a culture in which safety measures are not only recognized but directly integrated into every aspect of pediatric imaging practices, thereby enhancing the results among the youthful patients (Donya et al., 2014).

10.1.1. Radiation Exposure in Pediatric Patients

The issue of exposure to radiation in children has drawn significant attention due to the potential long-term health effects associated with ionizing radiation. Children are the most vulnerable group exposed to radiation, considering that their cells are exponentially dividing and their bodies are growing. The lifelong risk of developing cancer from radiation exposure is much higher for pediatric patients compared to adults.

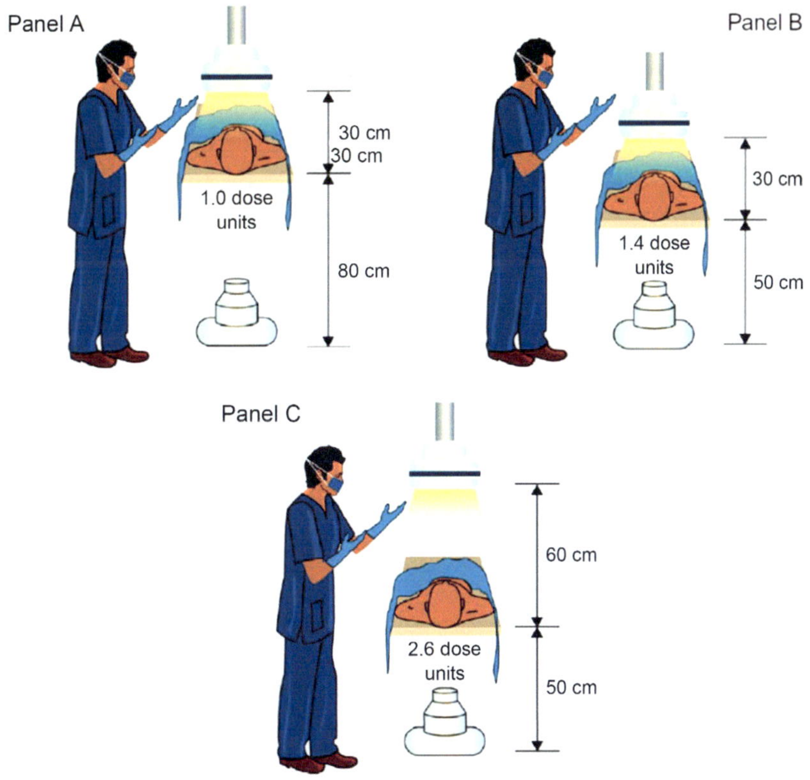

Figure 10.1. Pediatric patient positioned for low-dose chest X-ray with shielding in place.

Source: https://www.researchgate.net/profile/Georgios-Christakopoulos/publication/283975887/figure/fig1/AS:296599436709904@1447726224530/Example-of-optimal-table-positioning-to-minimize-patient-dose-The-patient-should-be.png.

According to the World Health Organization, diagnostic imaging not only plays a crucial role in diagnosis and treatment, but also it is the responsibility of medical professionals to assess imaging procedure-related risks carefully. Informed discussions about risks can help medical professionals and caregivers make balanced choices between diagnostic needs and radiation exposure minimization requirements (Hwang et al., 2017). Communication between the care provider and patient is important in radiation hazard management. Previous studies have indicated that parents and guardians are less informed about the effects of exposure to radiation by medical imaging. Research at the Boston University Pediatric Oral Healthcare Center revealed that the distribution of an educational brochure improved parents' knowledge of the risks and benefits of dental radiographs. Before education, few parents were confident in allowing their children to undergo imaging tests. Following education, an increased level of confidence was observed, showing the importance of good and correct communication about radiation risk to enhance parents trust in medical decisions for their children (Hwang et al., 2017). This suggests growing acknowledgment of the value of patient and caregiver education as a major component of pediatric care. Methods to reduce radiation exposure in pediatric imaging are paramount to safeguarding the health of younger patients. One of the most common methods is the use of optimized imaging protocols that minimize radiation dose without compromising diagnostic dependability. Improvements in imaging technology, including digital radiography and reduced-dose computed tomography, also help to reduce exposure. In addition, the institution of guidelines for minimizing the overuse of imaging tests ensures that radiation is used only when it is clinically necessary. According to the words in global talks, appreciation of the risk/benefit ratio in medical practice is important, as it has a direct effect on patient outcomes. Therefore, establishing a culture of safety in pediatric diagnostic imaging clinics is crucial, as children undergo necessary care without increased radiation exposure (Figures 10.1; 10.2).

Diagnostic Procedure	*Typical Effective Dose (mSv)*[a]	*Number of Chest X-rays for Equivalent Effective Dose*	*Number of Days of Background Radiation for Equivalent Effective Dose*
Chest x-ray (PA)	0.02	1	72
Skull x-ray	0.07	3.5	255
Lumbar spine	1.3	65	159
Upper GI	3	150	366
Barium enema	7	350	852
Head CT	≤2	≤100	243
Chest CT	≤3	≤150	366
Abdomen CT	≤5	≤250	609

Figure 10.2. Radiation dosage across common pediatric imaging modalities.

Source: https://i0.wp.com/obgynkey.com/wp-content/uploads/2021/08/pg135_1.jpg?w=960.

10.1.2. Use of Contrast Agents

The use of contrast agents in pediatric diagnostic imaging is integral to enhancing the clarity and diagnostic efficacy of various imaging modalities, such as X-ray, MRI, and CT scans. Pediatric patients often present unique challenges due to their smaller body sizes and varying physiological responses to imaging procedures. Contrast agents help distinguish between normal and pathological tissues, allowing for more precise assessments of conditions such as tumors or organ dysfunction. Their effectiveness, however, depends on selecting the appropriate type and dosage, tailored to the child's age, weight, and clinical indication. For instance, the use of iodine-based contrast media in CT scans is well-established in pediatric imaging, offering effective visualization while necessitating careful risk-benefit assessments concerning potential allergic reactions and nephrotoxicity (Figure 10.3).

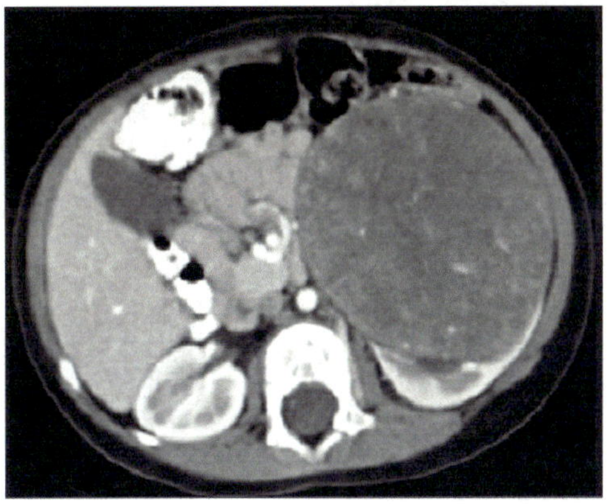

Figure 10.3. Sample contrast-enhanced abdominal CT scan in a pediatric case.

Source: https://www.researchgate.net/profile/Fredric-Hoffer-2/publication/233798579/figure/fig1/AS:484791125581825@1492594619659/Contrast-enhanced-CT-scan-of-abdomen-in-2-year-old-patient-with-palpable-abdominal-mass.png.

The selection of contrast agents must weigh the potential risks, particularly in pediatric populations. Children are more susceptible to harmful reactions due to the maturation of their organs and systems; therefore, considerable care must be taken in selecting contrast protocols. As an example, even though gadolinium is relatively safe for use in MRI, it has sounded an alarm for nephrogenic systemic fibrosis in compromised renal patients. In children, in whom the incidence of such complications remains low, standards and guidelines must take these into account for optimal safety.

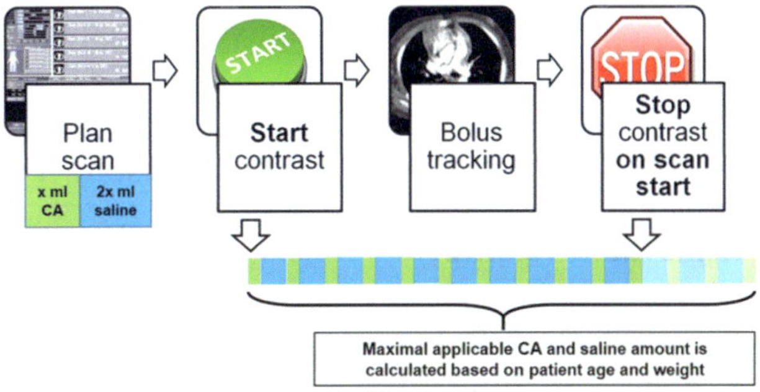

Figure 10.4. Poster displaying pediatric contrast agent protocols and allergy alerts.

Due to variability in response among individuals, clinicians must also take care to identify potential toxic effects of contrast media, as highlighted by one recent study comparing the toxic effects of treatments for diseases such as acute lymphoblastic leukemia (Attarbashi et al., 2016). New evidence continues to refine existing knowledge regarding the use of contrast agents in pediatric diagnostic imaging.

New compounds and other drugs are under investigation to minimize side effects and maximize patient safety. For example, advancements in non-iodinated contrast agents aim to reduce the risk of allergic reactions while maintaining diagnostic performance and capability. Furthermore, artificial intelligence used during imaging procedures improves the interpretability of contrast scans, enabling radiologists to make more informed decisions while incorporating patient-specific data. With advances in pediatric imaging, upholding agreed-upon strategies and inter-disciplinary communication are required to optimize patient outcomes. This inter-disciplinary communication will allow for ongoing refinement of imaging practices and ensure that the diagnosis needs a patient safety balance is struck consistently, hence serving as a barometer for future developments in the field (N/A, 1999).

10.1.3. Guidelines for Minimizing Risks

Pediatric diagnostic imaging has several challenges, the biggest being the potential risks of radiation exposure. The guidelines for minimizing the risks center on adhering to the As Low As Reasonably Achievable (ALARA) principle. It encourages doctors to use the minimum amount of radiation necessary to obtain diagnostic-quality images. Pediatric patients, having a greater sensitivity to radiation, require special attention to ensure that they remain safe. Monitoring radiation exposure and routine audits of imaging practice will go a long way in ensuring conformity with ALARA. Alternative imaging modalities, for example, ultrasound or magnetic resonance imaging, should be considered where feasible to avoid ionizing radiation, further reducing risk factors associated with pediatric diagnostic imaging (Figure 10.5).

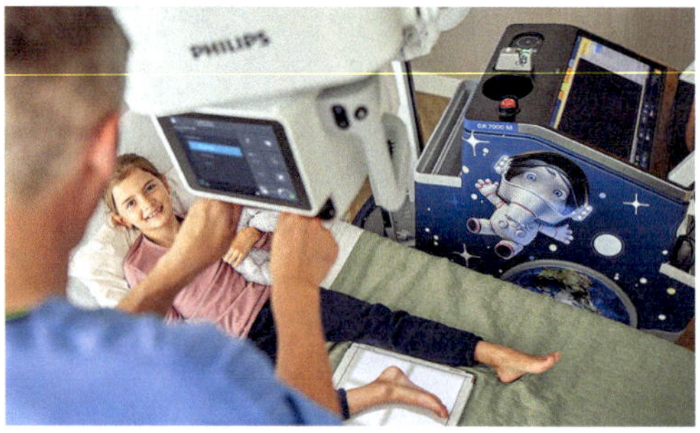

Figure 10.5. Checklist used by technologists to ensure imaging safety in pediatric patients.

Source: https://www.philips.com/c-dam/corporate/newscenter/global/standard/resources/healthcare/2024/q-and-a-with-atul-gupta-md/dr-7000-m-application-tech-pediatric-eth.jpg.

Finally, establishing and following these guidelines ensures a cautious approach towards managing radiation exposure among pediatric patients while providing essential medical care (Donya et al., 2014). Educational programs also play a significant role in minimizing risk during pediatric imaging diagnostics. Physicians must communicate effectively with legal guardians and parents regarding the rationale for recommending specific imaging examinations. Studies have shown that informed appreciation of radiation risks can be beneficial in achieving the desired parental comfort level regarding children's exposure to diagnostic imaging. For instance, the use of information brochures, as demonstrated in trials conducted in pediatric oral health clinics, has resulted in increased parental awareness of the risks and benefits of ionizing radiation. By ensuring caregivers are properly informed, healthcare practitioners not only increase patient trust but also enable more informed decision-making regarding the need for imaging. Involving caregivers through detailed discussions allows caregivers' anxieties to be removed, eventually being part of a concerted action to prioritize patient safety in diagnostic testing (Hwang et al., 2017).

In addition to addressing the need for improved communication, the development of uniform pediatric imaging protocols can introduce uniform practice within healthcare facilities. Age-specific adjustments to imaging techniques and dosages should be part of protocols without compromising diagnostic value, while emphasizing patient safety. Imaging departments should use age-specific charts to determine exposures appropriate to the child's developmental age. Intensive training of radiologists and technologists in pediatric-specific protocols is crucial in achieving the best outcome. Coordination among the oncology, pediatrics, and radiology departments also helps streamline these protocols in accordance with the latest research on fetal and childhood risks from radiation exposure. By fostering collaboration and standardizing pediatric imaging protocols, healthcare systems can reduce risks efficiently while providing children with the diagnostic care they need (Donya et al., 2014).

10.2. Developmental Considerations

The complex interplay between developmental stages and pediatric imaging diagnostics underscores the need for personalized methodology in imaging modalities. Varying anatomy and physiology between children and adults are essential in interpreting imaging results. With increasing age, body composition, fat distribution, and organ maturation change, which may affect the efficacy and safety of certain imaging methods. For instance, equipment sensitivity, such as MRI or CT scans, can result in heterogeneity of results, and therefore, radiologists must understand these differences in development. Understanding the developmental milestones profoundly enables proper diagnosis and follow-up, so that opportunities of misinterpretation based on adult-oriented imaging methodologies are eliminated (Figure 10.6).

Further, advances in imaging technologies, such as diffusion imaging techniques like diffusion tensor imaging (DTI) and high angular resolution diffusion imaging (HARDI), provide critical data on brain development in pediatric populations. Using these modalities, clinicians can image white matter microstructure and interrogate developmental disorder-associated neuroanatomical diversity, including congenital brain malformations. The results from the use of DTI and HARDI are a clear pointer towards how abnormal connectivity in developing brains will develop into gross clinical presentations. As such, the inclusion of advanced imaging in pediatric diagnosis not only enhances diagnostic accuracy but also enables focused intervention for developmental disorders, thereby improving patient outcomes.

The availability of specialized imaging tests points to the growing complexity of pediatric radiology focused on developmental issues. The implications of developmental factors for imaging extend beyond mere anatomical variations, including psychological and emotional maturity. The child's perceptual and cognitive capacities significantly contribute to their ability to comply with imaging protocols. The emotional context of the pediatric patient needs to be considered in the development of effective imaging protocols and in improving the overall experience. Age-related issues, developmental milestones, and previous healthcare experience may all determine a child's response to diagnostic imaging. Radiologists and healthcare providers must, therefore, adopt child-centered approaches, communicate effectively, and hold preparatory sessions to avoid discomfort and anxiety. Highlighting these psychosocial considerations underscores the multidisciplinary context of pediatric imaging, which involves meeting both physical and emotional needs during diagnosis.

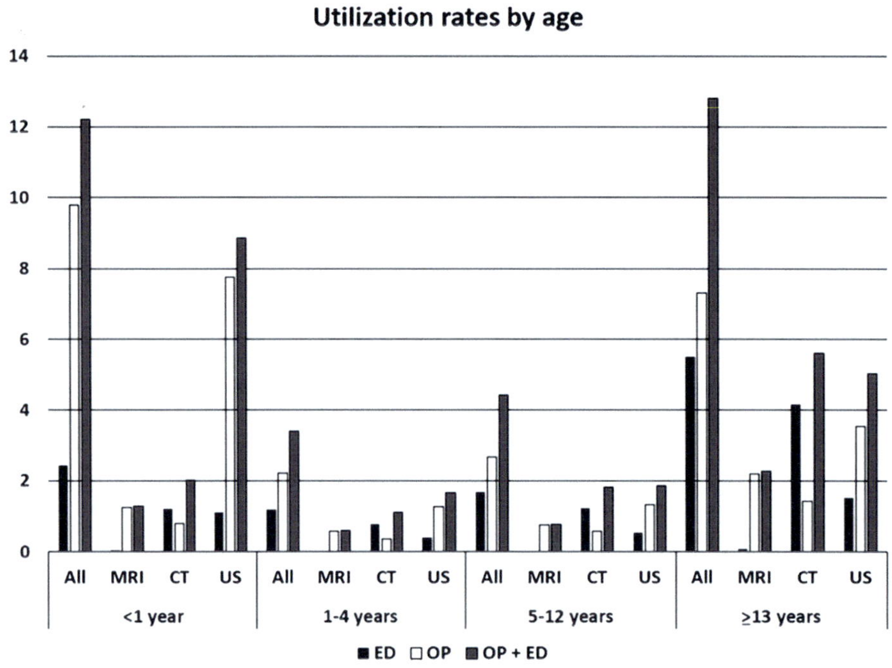

Figure 10.6. Timeline diagram showing age-specific imaging modality preferences.

Source: https://www.researchgate.net/publication/354666972/figure/fig2/AS:1069253553819649@1631941321109/Graph-shows-imaging-utilization-rates-for-different-imaging-modalities-according-to-age.png.

10.2.1. Age-Related Imaging Modalities

Age-based imaging protocols are crucial in pediatric imaging to obtain accurate diagnoses while minimizing potential risks. Children are not miniature adults; they are anatomically and physiologically different, which requires a tailored imaging plan. For example, neonates and infants require special versions of imaging modalities due to their unique body composition and developmental stages. Techniques such as ultrasound are generally preferred in younger patients due to their safety profile and lack of ionizing radiation, which makes them especially important given the vulnerability of tissues in development. Further, the psychological load imposed by imaging tests must also be considered, as younger children can become anxious under test conditions (Figure 10.7).

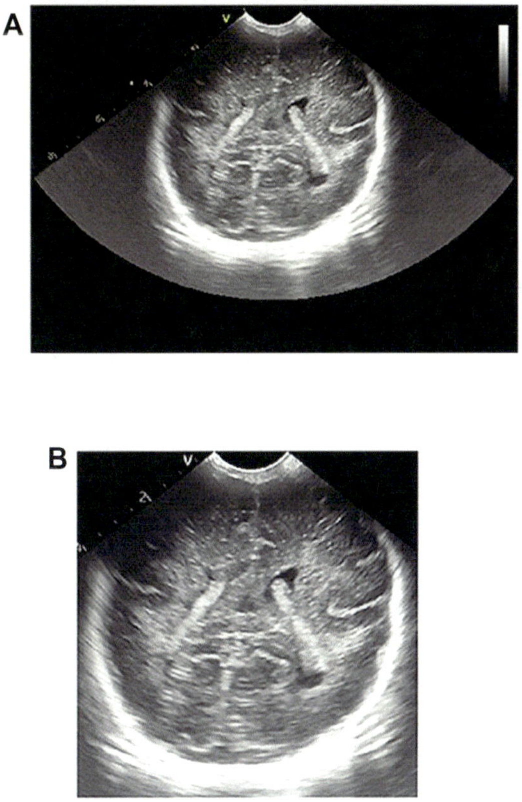

Figure 10.7. Analysis of cranial ultrasound images for newborn.

Source: https://www.frontiersin.org/files/Articles/1090275/fneur-13-1090275-HTML/image_m/fneur-13-1090275-g001.jpg.

An environment that accommodates these age-specific requirements not only improves the quality of imaging but also enhances the quality of the patient experience, which is key to cooperation during procedures. As children mature, their imaging needs evolve, necessitating adjustments in technique and technology. For instance, increasing the accuracy and safety of magnetic resonance imaging (MRI) has made it a vogue choice in adolescents. MRIs non-invasiveness and ability to image soft tissues with high resolution enable physicians to investigate a broad range of conditions, from neurological disorders to musculoskeletal injuries, with the assurance of not exposing patients to ionizing radiation. Further, advances in imaging technology offer scan time reduction and greater tolerance for motion, applicable particularly for this age group that may find it more challenging to remain still. The application of sedation in particular cases, though closely monitored, can help to achieve necessary imaging with minimal discomfort or stress to the adolescent patient. A proper understanding of age-specific imaging is thus needed to provide effective and safe diagnostic therapy relevant to the developing child. Moreover, the transition from pediatric to adult imaging protocols poses additional challenges. With increasing age, clinicians must consider the psychosocial aspect of imaging since adolescents are prone to body image and autonomy issues. These issues are addressed by engaging adolescents in their own treatment and bringing them in as active participants in decision-making regarding diagnostic imaging. The choice of imaging modality must not only take into account diagnostic efficacy but also enable the patient to feel relaxed and in control. More and more, technologists and radiologists are being trained in age-decipherable communication, allowing explanations in language the patient understands, which alleviates fears and stimulates cooperation. This emphasis on individualized approaches through various developmental stages makes the utmost priority of age-specific approaches in pediatric diagnostic imaging the guarantor of pediatric patients' emotional and physical well-being (N/A, 1989; N/A, 1992).

10.2.2. Psychological Impact on Children

The psychological impact of pediatric imaging on children is a significant issue that must be handled sensitively. Children undergoing imaging procedures, such as X-rays and MRIs, become more anxious due to unfamiliar environments and equipment. Phobia of the unknown may increase stress levels even higher so that health professionals must implement effective ways of minimizing emotional distress. For instance, preparing children for imaging through demonstrations and explanations appropriate to their age has been shown to enhance control and understanding (Figure 10.8).

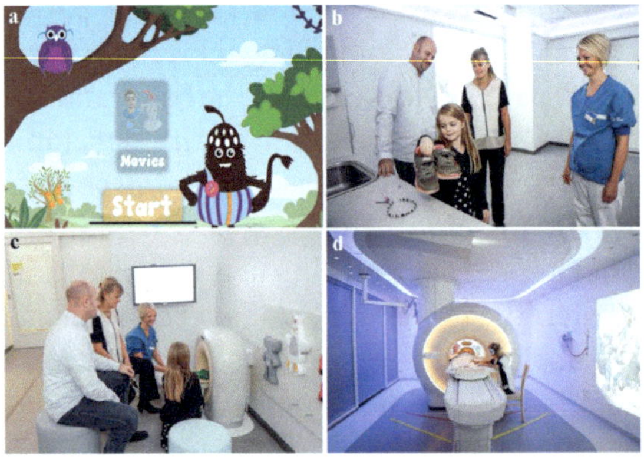

Figure 10.8. Photograph of a radiology room designed for children with visual distractions.

Source: https://media.springernature.com/lw685/springer-static/image/art%3A10.1007%2Fs00247-024-06111-3/MediaObjects/247_2024_6111_Fig2_HTML.jpg.

Furthermore, the potential consequences of imaging results, whether positive or negative, can create an atmosphere of anxiety that persists beyond the procedure itself. Therefore, addressing the psychological ramifications of diagnostic imaging is paramount to ensuring a holistic approach to pediatric healthcare. In addition to immediate anxiety, the long-term psychological effects of repeated imaging exposure may also be significant. Studies indicate that children who routinely undergo medical procedures may develop maladaptive coping mechanisms or chronic anxiety related to healthcare encounters. These outcomes are further complicated by the potential stigma associated with needing imaging, as children may perceive they are different from their peers. Therefore, healthcare providers must recognize that the implications of diagnostic imaging extend beyond physical health; they can also influence emotional well-being and social development. Implementing supportive measures, such as involving child life specialists, can help create a more positive experience, reducing psychological distress and fostering resilience. Moreover, the implications of imaging procedures can also intersect with familial concerns, as parents often grapple with the potential impact on their child's health.

The stress parents experience can inadvertently affect the child's emotional state, as children are highly attuned to their caregivers' emotions. This dyadic relationship highlights the importance of a supportive and communicative environment that encompasses both the child and their family. It is essential to inform parents about the imaging process and alleviate their concerns, translating this information into reassurances for the child. By addressing both the children's and parents' psychological needs, healthcare professionals can create a more comprehensive approach to pediatric diagnostic imaging. This approach not only alleviates anxiety but also promotes an atmosphere of trust and understanding, ensuring the child's psychological well-being throughout the diagnostic journey (Figure 10.9).

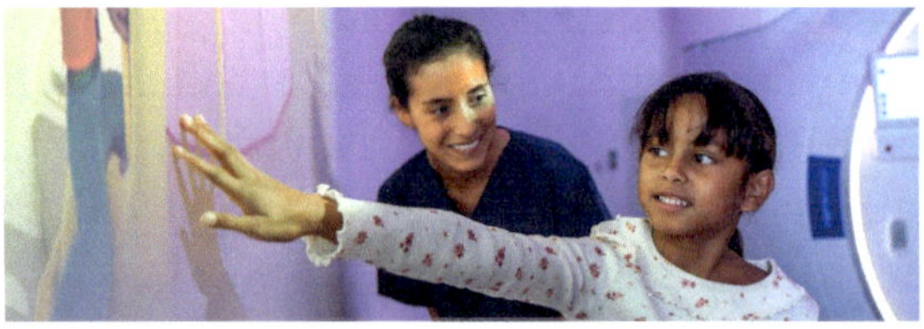

Figure 10.9. Showing stress-reducing techniques during pediatric MRI scans.

Source: https://images.philips.com/is/image/philipsconsumer/ae21f964fc374a838122af4300f42aae?extend=0,-1197,0,-591&wid=1922&hei=641&fit=stretch,1&$jpglarge$.

10.2.3. Parental Involvement in Imaging Procedures

Effective parental involvement in pediatric imaging procedures is vital in preventing anxiety and bringing about positive outcomes. Kids are likely to endure severe anxiety when undergoing diagnostic imaging due to unfamiliar surroundings and procedures that tend to disrupt cooperation. Research reveals that active parental involvement can neutralize such anxieties, making children's experiences better. For instance, pre-procedure counseling, particularly through electronic methods, has been shown to provide children and their families with substantial information about the imaging procedure. Such counseling, aside from reducing anxiety, increases knowledge and satisfaction with the procedure, as indicated by research pointing to enhanced patient-centered outcomes and imaging effectiveness (Kaakinen et al., 2022).

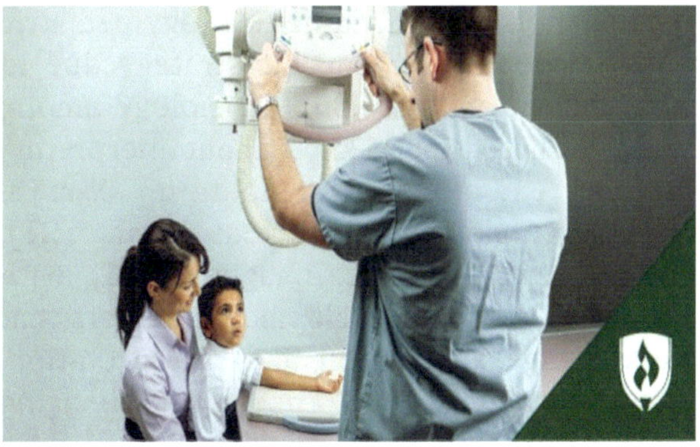

Figure 10.10. A radiologic technologist engaging a parent in a pre-imaging explanation.

Source: https://www.rasmussen.edu/images/rasmussenlibraries/blogs/working-in-pediatric-radiology-.jpg.

By educating parents and teaching them coping mechanisms, health professionals may help create a less stressful environment, eventually making imaging sessions smoother for children. Beyond anxiety management, parent involvement contributes to better patient outcomes. In line with advances in pediatric neuroimaging, parents often hold a therapeutic misconception that imaging studies provide an immediate benefit to their child's well-being. This misconception can complicate informed consent processes, where parents may not fully understand the diagnostic nature of research and imaging studies (D\u27Arcy et al., 2008). To counteract these misconceptions, healthcare professionals must engage parents in open and honest discussions about the reasons for imaging and its potential implications (Figure 10.10).

Efforts to facilitate transparency and provide educational materials can help parents understand the intent and nature of the procedures, thereby fostering cooperation. Greater understanding, leading to increased parental support through imaging, can be an outcome of this, which is crucial for the child's emotional comfort and compliance. Apart from the immediate procedural benefits, parental involvement can also form long-term alliances with healthcare providers, facilitating trust and communication. Parents who are involved in the imaging process are also likely to advocate for their child's needs in future medical encounters. Such advocacy is essential in the instance of long-term or chronic illness, when children may require numerous imaging tests over the course of years. Long-term working relationships between parents and healthcare providers can lead to adequate care and improved diagnostic outcomes, according to best practices in pediatrics. As empowered parents become more informed and experienced, the resulting dynamic has the potential to significantly reduce the aggregate stress associated with pediatric imaging procedures, thereby helping achieve better health outcomes in children (Kaakinen et al., 2022).

10.3. Interpretation of Imaging Results

Interpretation of imaging results in pediatric diagnostic imaging is a critical component that underscores accuracy and proficiency in medical practice. Owing to children's unique anatomical and physiological characteristics, radiologists and physicians must be aware of these differences during image interpretation. For instance, the interpretation of child brain structures differs significantly from that of adults because the brain develops progressively during childhood. This convergence makes pediatric imaging a technical science that requires professionals to excel in the detection of age-related differences. Furthermore, the application of advanced imaging techniques enhances the validity of interpretations, enabling earlier and more accurate diagnoses that significantly impact young patients' treatment. To obtain valid imaging results, it is crucial to incorporate advanced techniques to assist in interpretation. One of the promising techniques is resting state functional magnetic resonance imaging (fMRI), which is particularly valuable for pediatric patients. Resting state fMRI is a non-invasive technique that is capable of elucidating resting state networks without requiring the necessity of asking patients to perform elaborate tasks, hence accommodating young or mentally retarded patients. Evidence demonstrates that resting-state fMRI can successfully localize sensorimotor networks, an improvement over traditional approaches such as direct electrocortical stimulation. As shown in studies comparing these modalities, resting state fMRI can achieve similar localization results with less discomfort and injury to children patients (Hacker et al., 2019).

Finally, there is also a requirement for multidisciplinary collaboration among radiologists, neurologists, and other clinicians to confirm that imaging results are interpreted within the proper clinical context. This is a cooperative process that not only improves the diagnostic process but also permits a more accurate appreciation of the implications of imaging findings. It is, for instance, quite possible to identify abnormal structures or networks in the brain, and this requires integrating the patient's clinical history and imaging results. As stressed in the literature, effective communication among specialists can enhance the reliability of the diagnosis and ultimately influence treatment strategies tailored to the specific needs of pediatric patients (N/A, 2000). In all, accurate analysis of imaging findings, backed up by collective expertise and state-of-the-art methodologies, is an essential role in the realm of pediatric diagnostic imaging.

10.3.1. Role of Pediatric Radiologists

The pediatric radiologists' position is at the center of medical imaging in a child-oriented world. Compared with adult radiology, pediatric radiology requires a specific strategy due to variations in anatomy and physiology among children. These experts know about interpreting imaging examinations, including X-rays, ultrasonography, computed tomography (CT), and magnetic resonance imaging (MRI), with a keen sense of the developmental factors that shape image acquisition and interpretation. They are trained in the proper use of imaging modalities that balance diagnostic yield with the need to minimize radiation exposure—a decidedly important factor in pediatric care, where sensitivity to ionizing radiation is likely to be greatly increased. Further, they engage proactively with pediatricians and other caregivers to ensure that the imaging pathway of choice is considered and thoughtful, thereby optimally maximizing the efficacy and efficiency of pediatric diagnosis. Along with technical expertise, pediatric radiologists have a most significant role as advocates for patients, prioritizing the psychological comfort of infant patients during imaging. The unique demands of imaging children call not just for technical expertise in medical technology but also for extremely high-level communication skills. Radiologists often work closely with patients and families to explain procedures in child-friendly language, creating a climate of comfort and trust in potentially daunting circumstances. By adapting communication styles and applying child-sensitive techniques, pediatric radiologists decrease anxiety and increase compliance with imaging. Emotional empathy with patients is very important, and this not only enhances the overall diagnostic process in the form of quality images but also by handling patients' behavior efficiently. Such comprehensive interaction creates positive experiences, culminating in diagnostic outcomes and the overall health experience in children. In addition, pediatric radiologists' roles extend beyond such direct clinical responsibilities and encompass assistance in research and education in pediatric imaging. These experts remain current with ongoing education, hence conscious of evolving technology and imaging modalities that continue to advance diagnostic methods. Through clinical investigations, pediatric radiologists contribute to the development of evidence-based guidelines, hence enhancing the standards of practice that govern pediatric imaging practice. They also educate other radiologists and healthcare providers through their practice by providing educational materials on child-specific radiation safety principles and pediatric image interpretation. Their commitment to sharing information ensures that best practices are adopted in every healthcare facility, reinforcing pediatric diagnostic imaging principles and improving patient care in diverse healthcare settings (N/A, 1994; 2007) (Figure 10.11).

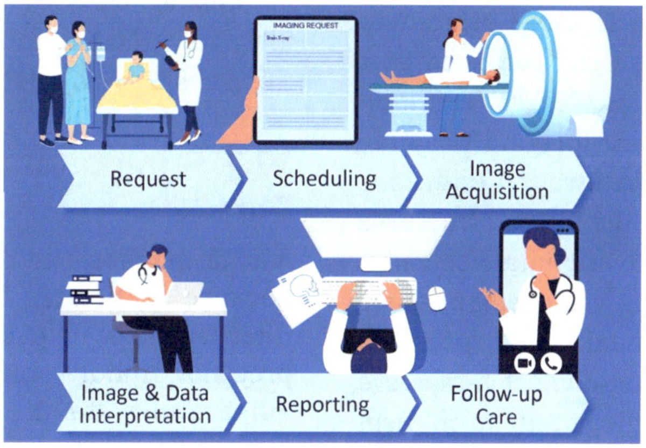

Figure 10.11. Workflow of pediatric imaging interpretation by a subspecialist radiologist.

Source: https://enlitic.com/wp-content/uploads/MicrosoftTeams-image-97.jpg.

10.3.2. Common Pediatric Conditions Diagnosed

Familiarity with common disorders such as acute lymphoblastic leukemia (ALL) is necessary in pediatric diagnostic imaging. ALL is a malignancy of hematologic origin that is one of the most notable indications of cancer diagnosis in children and demands immediate and accurate detection by imaging techniques. The diagnosis of ALL is difficult because of its heterogeneous presentation, and frequently requires differentiation from other childhood illnesses. Medical imaging techniques such as ultrasound, computed tomography (CT), and magnetic resonance imaging (MRI) are important for evaluating children with presumed leukemic infiltration or disease complications (Figure 10.12).

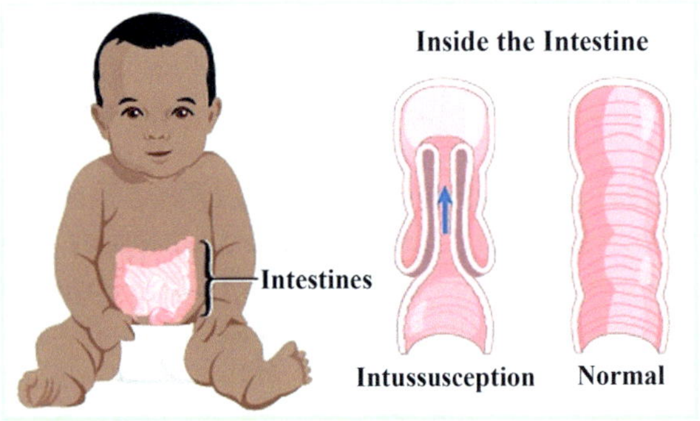

Figure 10.12. Image showing a diagnosis of intussusception in a child.

Source: https://kidshealth.org/content/dam/patientinstructions/en/images/intussusception_a_enIL.jpg.

Practical imaging not only aids in initial diagnosis but also in assessing treatment response and identifying potential toxic effects of therapies, such as those related to chemotherapy, which can significantly impact long-term patient outcomes. Several common pediatric conditions require imaging to guide diagnosis and treatment pathways. Conditions such as pneumonia, appendicitis, and fractures are routinely encountered in clinical settings, each with unique imaging requirements. For instance, pediatric pneumonia often presents with respiratory distress, and chest X-rays are typically the first-line imaging study to confirm the diagnosis and assess the extent of lung involvement. Conversely, acute appendicitis in children may require both ultrasound and CT scans to elucidate the diagnosis, particularly in complicated cases where atypical presentations occur. Similarly, when evaluating trauma in young patients, identifying fractures through X-ray imaging ensures proper management and can play a critical role in preventing complications. The efficiency and accuracy of imaging modalities are vital in ensuring that pediatric patients receive timely and effective care. Lastly, pediatric diagnostic imaging must consider potential risks, including radiation exposure, particularly when repeated imaging assessments are performed. The field has seen a gradual shift towards employing lower-radiation techniques and alternative imaging modalities that mitigate such risks.

For conditions like ALL, where long-term survival rates are improving, the increased awareness of treatment-associated toxicities highlights the importance of careful imaging management. Research initiatives have focused on creating consensus definitions for the effects of chemotherapy and the requisite imaging follow-ups, promoting standardization around how diagnostic imaging impacts treatment evaluation and patient safety. By embracing less invasive imaging strategies and continually refining protocols, healthcare providers can enhance the accuracy of diagnoses while minimizing potential harms to pediatric patients, ultimately leading to better health outcomes in this sensitive population.

10.3.3. Importance of Accurate Diagnosis

A true diagnosis is most critical in pediatrics because it dictates follow-up treatment and interventions. In pediatric imaging, however, precision is more crucial given the population's vulnerability to disease and the impact of diagnostic interventions. Misleading imaging results will lead to misdiagnosis, and this can result in inappropriate intervention and extended suffering. utilize advanced imaging modalities properly, taking full advantage of their ability to reveal concealed pathologies that are, in some instances, not readily diagnosable with standard examination procedures. This need for caution is reinforced by the growing application of artificial intelligence (AI) in imaging diagnostics, aimed at enhancing the accuracy of diagnosis and overcoming pediatric-specific challenges related to patients with special physiological and psychological characteristics (Figure 10.13).

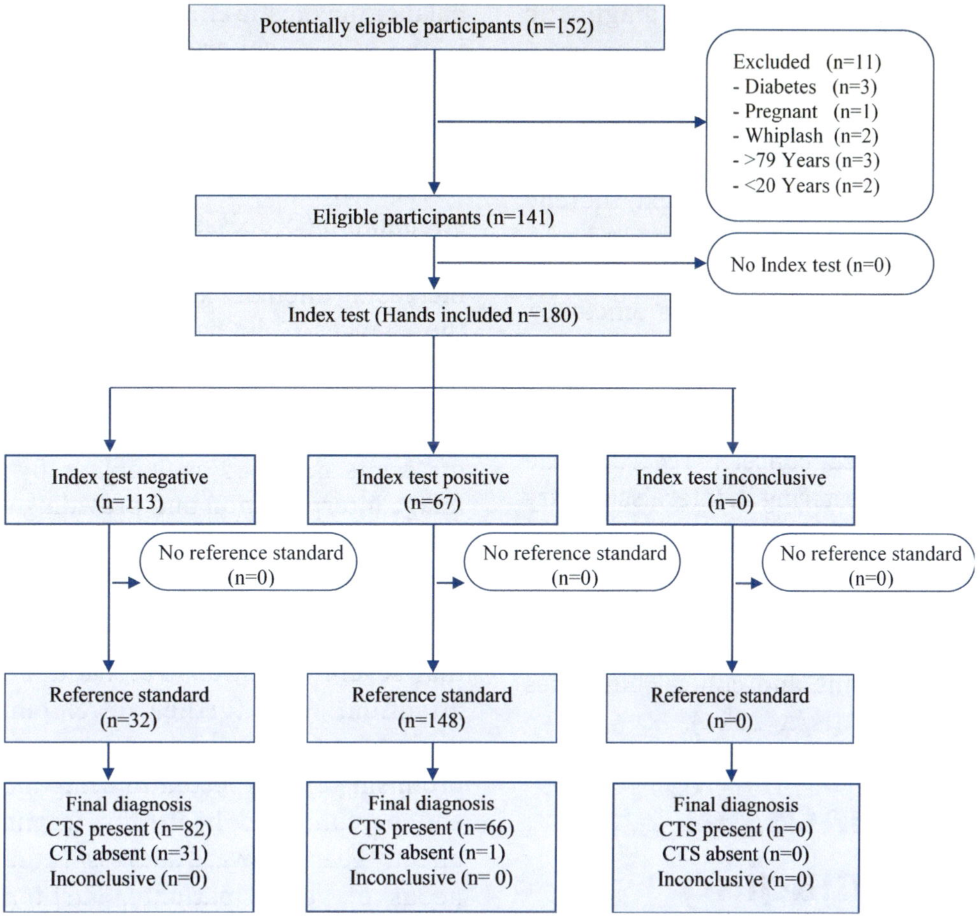

Figure 10.13. Flowchart of the diagnostic accuracy study. The Reference standard was the Nerve Conduction Studies (NCS), while the Index test was the clinical battery composed of the Functional Dexterity Test (FDT), Phalen's test and Tinel's sign. In this chart, the FDT net scores threshold was set at >84th percentile of the normative values.

Source: https://www.researchgate.net/publication/346218881/figure/fig3/AS:962810959908883@1606563429740/Flowchart-of-the-diagnostic-accuracy-study-The-Reference-standard-was-the-Nerve.png.

AI applications in child imaging are a dynamic frontier reshaping diagnostic protocols. AI technologies, including deep learning methods and convolutional neural networks, have proved to have tremendous potential to improve image quality and remove artifacts, which are imperative for delivering accurate analyses. These enhancements to imaging processes provide practitioners with the opportunity to make more reliable decisions regarding patient care. Also, the use of AI makes low-dose imaging protocols possible that reduce radiation exposure, a critical factor in pediatric care due to the long-term hazards posed by prolonged radiation exposure. By focusing on imaging accuracy and patient safety, healthcare systems can find a balance that enables effective diagnosis without compromising the well-being of young patients, promoting the use of AI-assisted methods in routine practice to increase diagnostic confidence and reliability (Adeleke et al., 2025).

The use of AI in pediatric diagnostic imaging aligns with the need to develop accurate diagnostic protocols tailored to individual patients' needs. This tailoring can improve outcomes by enabling directed imaging tailored to an individual child's clinical context, thereby preventing unwarranted repositioning and scan repetition. This not only enhances diagnostic accuracy but also radiology process efficiency, enabling doctors to optimally allocate resources. Besides, amid the evolving trend in pediatric diagnostics, it is essential to address regulatory restrictions and ethical concerns regarding the application of AI. By fostering an interdisciplinary environment among radiologists, pediatricians, and technologists, healthcare organizations can leverage the benefits of AI-based imaging modalities, ultimately leading to improved diagnostic mechanisms and clinical outcomes in pediatric patients (N/A, 2011).

10.4. Advances in Pediatric Imaging

Recent advances in pediatric imaging have revolutionized the diagnostic landscape in pediatrics, leading to better outcomes and earlier intervention. Advances in technologies such as high-resolution ultrasound, advanced magnetic resonance imaging (MRI), and advanced computed tomography (CT) have significantly improved the resolution and specificity of imaging results. Unlike traditional methods that expose children to higher doses of radiation, current methods prioritize safety using methods like low-dose CT scans and MRI that are based on non-ionizing radiation. Not only does such a shift decrease health risks, but it also addresses pediatric patients' unique susceptibilities whose tissues are still developing and hence more susceptible to the effects of radiation. The evolution of these imaging techniques illustrates an attempt to balance diagnostic efficiency with patient safety in the care of children, ultimately forming an enabling framework for accurate diagnosis and tailored treatment regimes. The integration of artificial intelligence (AI) in pediatric imaging has also increased diagnostic efficiency while streamlining processes. AI software can rapidly review large amounts of imaging data, thereby increasing anomaly identification and reducing the chances of human error. This software is particularly valuable in children, in whom there are multifaceted anatomical variations and overlapping ages, and the interpretation of results becomes challenging. By enhancing image interpretation and providing differential diagnoses, AI programs are functioning as rich complements to radiologists' skills.

They also help in sorting the cases so that severe conditions receive due immediate attention. With further development of AI, its applications in pediatric imaging are also promising and expected to bring more precise and personalized healthcare regimens more directly geared toward addressing the individual needs of young patients. Furthermore, the study of the psychological effects of imaging procedures on young patients has also emerged as an important field of study, with new developments aimed at maximizing the patient experience. Having noted that kids often develop heightened states of anxiety when they receive imaging exams, such advanced technologies as distraction techniques and virtual reality (VR) are coming into play in soothing and mitigating discomfort. By utilizing deep virtual environments that are calming or absorbing distractions, care providers can inhibit stress and promote cooperation for image studies. This combined approach not only benefits better imaging outcomes but also encourages a more favorable patient and family experience. In understanding the psychological elements of pediatric care, developments in imaging are moving toward incorporating compassion and empathy into the mix, exemplifying a commitment to healing the whole child rather than just their medical conditions.

10.4.1. Technological Innovations

The landscape of pediatric imaging diagnosis has been revolutionized by advances in technology, the kernel of which is to enhance the precision and security of tests. Sophisticated imaging technologies such as magnetic resonance imaging (MRI) and computed tomography (CT) rely on advanced algorithms and software to enable high-fidelity image acquisition and processing. These technologies not only increase the resolution of images obtained but also reduce procedure time, exposing young patients to less radiation. Additionally, the integration of artificial intelligence into imaging technologies enables automated image analysis, accelerating diagnosis and helping radiologists detect abnormalities (Figure 10.14).

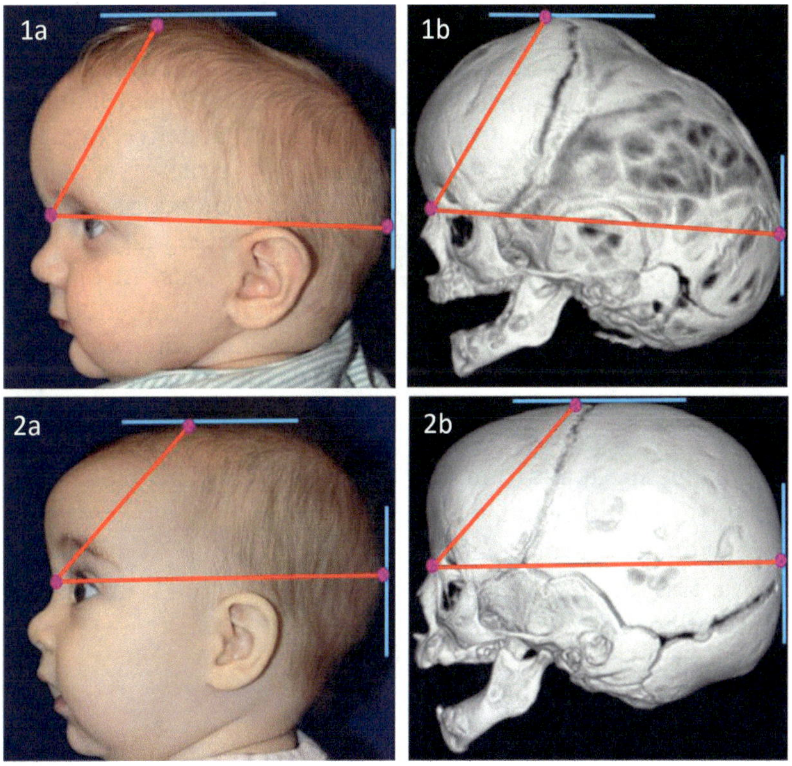

Figure 10.14. Side-by-side preoperative clinical photographs and 3D reconstructed CT images of one actual sagittal patient (image 1a, 1b) with a VNO angle of 62°, and one presumed sagittal patient (image 2a, 2b) with a VNO angle of 48°. The presumed sagittal patient was referred to our craniofacial team due to reported worsening scaphocephaly with a cranial index of 0.68 noted on our initial evaluation. Note the height and relative anterior position of the vertex in the actual sagittal patient compared to the presumed sagittal patient.

Source: https://www.researchgate.net/publication/360068251/figure/fig2/AS:1172127390679040@1656468355377/Side-by-side-preoperative-clinical-photographs-and-3D-reconstructed-CT-images-of-one-true.jpg.

As imaging technology continues to advance, medical professionals are better placed to make accurate diagnoses, particularly in children, where prompt treatment has a direct impact on patient outcomes. Beyond that, the introduction of mobile imaging devices has revolutionized care in pediatrics, making diagnostic imaging methods more accessible and mobile. Traditional imaging requires patient transport to radiology departments, and this can be challenging for young children in terms of anxiety or physical limitations. Portable ultrasound devices, for instance, may be transported to the patient's bedside and enable immediate assessment in a comfortable environment. This not only enhances patient satisfaction but also enhances workflow efficiency within healthcare facilities. Technological progress in wireless transmission and image compression has enabled pediatricians and radiologists to have real-time consultations, enabling decision-making at the earliest from readily available information. The ability to make a speedy diagnosis and correct one within the child's own environment is the best testimony to the relentless push to improve pediatric care through technology. Finally, the application of 3D printing technology in combination with pediatric diagnostic imaging is a revolutionary breakthrough in the area. This technology allows doctors to create patient-specific anatomical models based on imaging data, which can aid preoperative planning and patient education. As an example, surgeons can visualize complex congenital anomalies with the use of these models to improve intraoperative expectations. Additionally, 3D-printed models empower children and families to better understand medical conditions by providing a tangible representation of their unique anatomical setup. Such developments serve to underscore the key role of technological innovations in bridging the gap between advanced medical concepts and patient comprehension, ultimately towards a more integrated pediatric healthcare paradigm. As such technologies advance further, the future of pediatric diagnostic imaging holds promise of even better diagnostic capabilities and improved patient experience.

10.4.2. Role of Artificial Intelligence

The integration of artificial intelligence (AI) into pediatric diagnostic imaging represents a historic leap in medical practice, particularly given the unique challenges of imaging children. The very frailty of the pediatric patient necessitates an emphasis on patient safety, yet it must be achieved without sacrificing diagnostic integrity. AI technologies have been instrumental in developing low-dose imaging protocols that deliver higher image quality while reducing the risk of ionizing radiation exposure, an essential concern in radiology. With the help of deep learning algorithms and convolutional neural networks, AI applications have shown vast potential in reducing noise, eliminating artifacts, and fine-tuning imaging parameters in modalities such as computed tomography and X-ray (Figure 10.15).

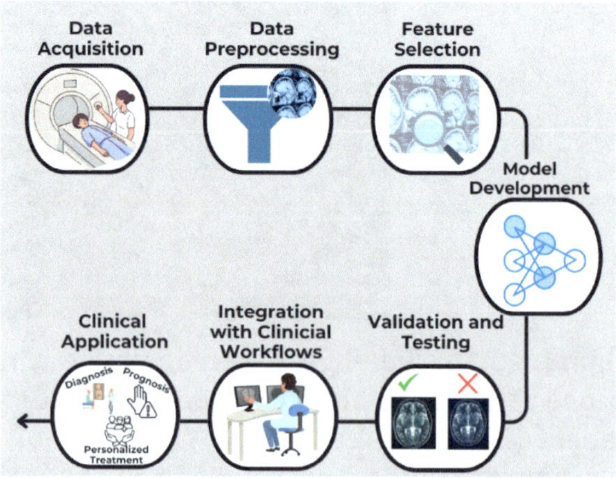

Figure 10.15. Side-by-side comparison of traditional X-ray and AI-enhanced image.

Source: https://pub.mdpi-res.com/cancers/cancers-17-00622/article_deploy/html/images/cancers-17-00622-g003.png?1739440971.

These innovations facilitate high-grade imaging for accurate assessments and respond to the primary aim of minimizing potential health risks to pediatric patients, thereby transforming the practice of pediatric radiology and making working conditions safer for susceptible groups (Adeleke et al., 2025).

Beyond radiation protection, AI provides services to transform radiology workflows, particularly during heightened demands on pediatric radiologists. The specialty is confronted with a twofold challenge of expanding patient volume and persistent shortages of personnel, making slow procedures more challenging. AI-based solutions can accelerate processes such as image reading and interpretation and enhance efficiency, freeing radiologists to focus on higher-level evaluative functions. By allowing repetitive tasks to be dispensed with, such technologies enhance the productivity of operations and also balance the playing field in accessing specialist wisdom. Pediatric radiologists can therefore make effective use of their time, resulting in improved patient care and diagnostic turnaround times. The potential of AIs in this context underscores the imperative to adopt these technologies to correct labor shortages and enhance clinical service delivery in pediatric imaging (Arthurs et al., 2021).

The revolutionary potential of AI in pediatric diagnostic imaging is unquestionable, but there are issues with the adoption of these technologies that must be addressed with care. Maintaining the transparency and reproducibility of AI research findings is necessary for clinical adoption, particularly in consideration of the heterogeneity of initial reporting. Pediatric radiology stakeholders need to implement AI-specific reporting standards to improve the usability and clarity of their findings, thereby increasing clinicians' confidence in AI-based tools. Further, as pediatric radiologists get more engaged in AI research, their contribution to developing good, standardized guidelines will be an important contribution to the field. By addressing regulatory, ethical, and computational challenges, the pediatric radiology community can realize the full potential of AI, leading to better diagnostic outcomes and stronger health systems (Arthurs et al., 2021).

10.4.3. Future Trends in Pediatric Imaging

With continued advances in pediatric imaging diagnostics, technology is central to determining future directions. One promising direction is the integration of artificial intelligence (AI) with traditional imaging modalities. AI instruments enhance image interpretation and diagnostic capabilities by applying machine learning algorithms to analyze large datasets. This is particularly crucial in pediatrics, where accurate and timely diagnosis is necessary. The application of AI is able to reduce the burden of work on radiologists, which leads to a more efficient workflow and timely management of the patient. Moreover, the further development of imaging modalities, such as ultra-low-dose CT and MRI, indicates a harmonized community effort aimed at reducing the risk of ionizing radiation exposure in children, with safety and efficiency remaining the primary focus in imaging protocols (N/A, 2008) (Figure 10.16).

Another essential trend in pediatric imaging is the increasing emphasis on patient-centered care, in which the specific needs and fears of children and parents are prioritized. This paradigm shift aims to create less intimidating and more pleasant imaging environments for children, which can lead to enhanced cooperation and more accurate imaging results. Technologies such as child-centered imaging and the development of mobile imaging units will simplify imaging, enabling healthcare practitioners to reach a larger population of patients, especially in scattered communities.

Additionally, enhancing education facilities for families and healthcare practitioners on the need and procedure of pediatric imaging will develop an interlocking treatment model. Through these efforts, the practice will maximize diagnostic capability while improving patient experience and overall outcomes in pediatric imaging (Goldblatt et al., 2019).

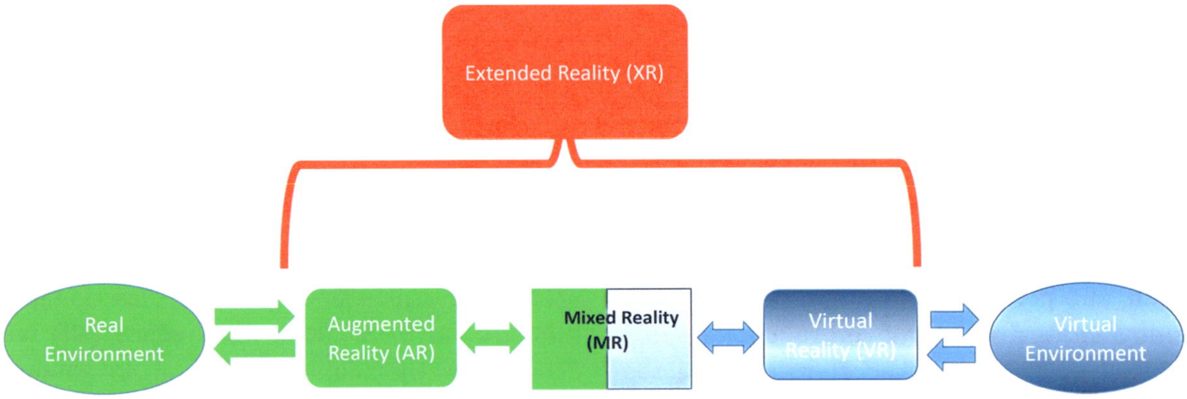

Figure 10.16. Conceptual rendering of future pediatric imaging suite using virtual reality.

Source: https://pub.mdpi-res.com/robotics/robotics-13-00069/article_deploy/html/images/robotics-13-00069-g001.png?1715070442.

Finally, the future of pediatric imaging will be transformed through greater collaboration between global health organizations to manage rare diseases. Developments in technology and data-sharing have registered significant advances in the diagnosis and understanding of such conditions. The creation of global consortia highlights the establishment of harmonized protocols and model consent language for research into rare diseases. These collaborations result in the enrollment of heterogeneous populations and enhance the utility of diagnostic imaging to enable the understanding of complex conditions. As pediatric imaging increasingly adopts such collaborative patterns of practice, the world will better understand pediatric disease, ultimately enhancing clinical practice and the treatment of children with atypical and difficult medical conditions (N/A, 2008).

10.5. Ethical and Legal Issues

The balance between ethical and legal considerations is most significant in pediatric diagnostic imaging, particularly due to the unique vulnerabilities of child patients. Pediatricians and radiologists must navigate the fine line between protecting patients and ensuring accurate diagnoses. The danger of misinterpretation of imaging results, such as in instances of suspected child abuse, underscores the need for adherence to ethical practices. For example, in the case of shaken baby syndrome, clinicians are faced with the task of separating abuse from accidental trauma. This dilemma necessitates an ethical obligation to approach each case with fastidiousness and objectivity, minimizing harm while being transparent with caregivers and legal authorities. Maintaining both medical ethics and applicable law in diagnostic practice is important for safeguarding pediatric patients and the clinicians who care for them. In pediatric imaging diagnosis, informed consent is the most important ethical standard, but it poses special challenges due to the inherent communication hurdles in dealing with cases involving children. Legal policy typically requires guardians to sign off on medical treatment, but ethical standards encourage healthcare professionals to involve young patients in the decision-making process whenever appropriate. This introduces a complex debate about children's rights and agency within health settings. As an example, pediatricians need to work to help parents understand the risk-versus-benefit balance of imaging tests while, at the same time, carefully conveying information appropriately graded for the child's developmental level.

By fostering a culture of trust and open communication, health professionals can honor the ethical imperatives of agency and child respect, ensuring that legal mechanisms of consent are not merely procedural but rooted in true patient advocacy. Furthermore, the limits of privacy and confidentiality are a critical legal consideration that must be scrupulously adhered to in pediatric diagnostic imaging. Given that medical imaging often reveals sensitive information about a child's health status, the safety of such data is paramount. Ethical considerations compel healthcare providers to use rigorous measures to prevent patient data from ending up in the wrong hands, thus complying with laws such as the Health Insurance Portability and Accountability Act (HIPAA). Solicitations of these privacy codes can lead to extreme legal repercussions and the disintegration of trust among families and healthcare providers. Furthermore, the incorporation of digital imaging and electronic health records has rendered the ethical requirement of confidentiality even more complex. Practitioners must be vigilant in ensuring that all imaging information is used only for intended medical purposes, thereby protecting the integrity and confidentiality of pediatric patients' medical information in an evolving technological environment.

10.5.1. Informed Consent in Pediatric Imaging

Pediatric imaging informed consent is a critical component of ethical medical care, particularly given the vulnerabilities of children. Children, unlike adults, cannot provide informed consent on their own; instead, it falls on parents or guardians. Such a relationship necessitates that health care providers clearly communicate the rationale, risks, and benefits of various imaging tests, thereby ensuring that caregivers are adequately aware. Misconceptions about radiation exposure risk, for instance, will potentially cause unnecessary parental anxiety, which can damage the decision process regarding their child's care. Meta-analyses indicate that educational materials are likely to greatly enhance knowledge, highlighting the benefits of full communication as part of the consent process in pediatric settings (Hwang et al., 2017). The subtleties of informed consent are also compounded by the variations in pediatric imaging technologies such as computed tomography (CT) and magnetic resonance imaging (MRI), which have inherently diverse risk profiles (Figure 10.17).

Children are susceptible to radiation; therefore, a greater emphasis on educating parents regarding these risks is essential. Literature indicates that parents are largely not well-educated regarding the long-term effects of exposure to ionizing radiation in tests like CT scans. Aids such as educational leaflets can minimize these disparities and encourage parental comfort levels and preparedness to sign consent for mandatory imaging, as indicated by studies that demonstrate enhanced understanding following educational intervention (Hwang et al., 2017). Ideally, the purpose of informed consent is not just to meet legal requirements but to encourage a participatory practice in which caregivers feel at ease making informed choices about imaging for their children. Also, ethical concerns of informed consent in pediatric imaging are extended to issues of data privacy and family participation, similar to more general medical research ethical concerns. Organizations developing model consent provisions emphasize the significance of the explanation of information on the use of data, particularly in the context of rare disease research studies where imaging may be critical. These model clauses outline specific aspects such as imaging data collection and storage, and implications of family participation in research settings. By incorporating transparency and ethical practices, healthcare workers can build trust with families, leading to enhanced patient-centered care in pediatric imaging cases. Thus, informed consent is not a professional nicety but rather a foundation of ethical practice to ensure that parents, patients, and practitioners are united in efforts to achieve healthier outcomes for children.

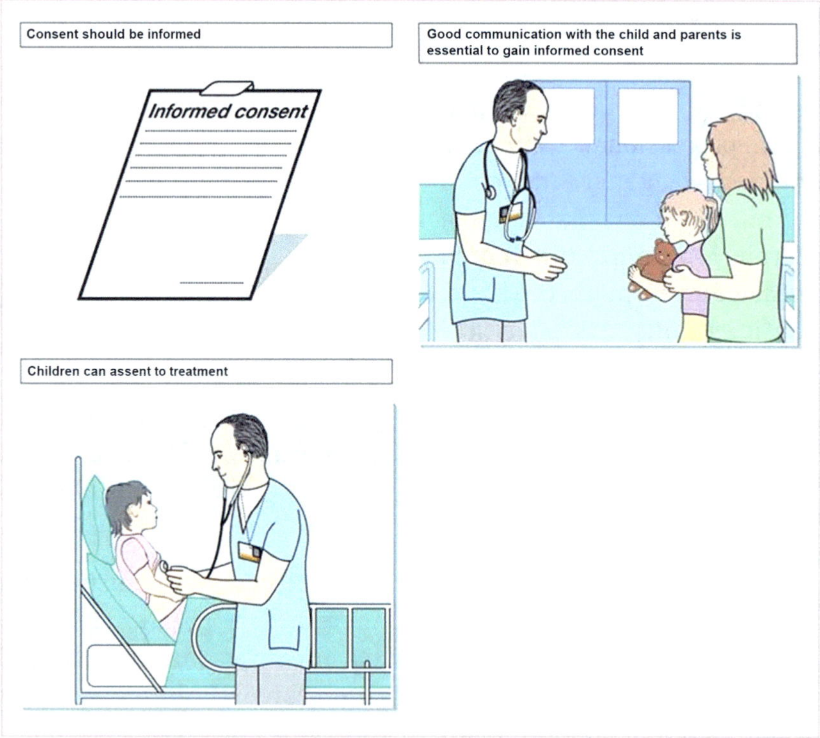

Figure 10.17. Informed consent for pediatric imaging.

Source: https://i0.wp.com/nursekey.com/wp-content/uploads/2018/10/c06f001.jpg?w=960.

10.5.2. Privacy and Confidentiality Issues

In pediatric imaging for diagnosis, confidentiality and privacy issues are at the forefront because of the sensitive information involved. The ethical management of children's medical records warrants the most serious consideration, especially with advancing technologies and increasingly more information in electronic form. Health care providers must be well-educated on how to understand and deal with the complexities of maintaining the confidentiality of pediatric patients, such as adherence to laws like the Health Insurance Portability and Accountability Act (HIPAA) (Figure 10.18).

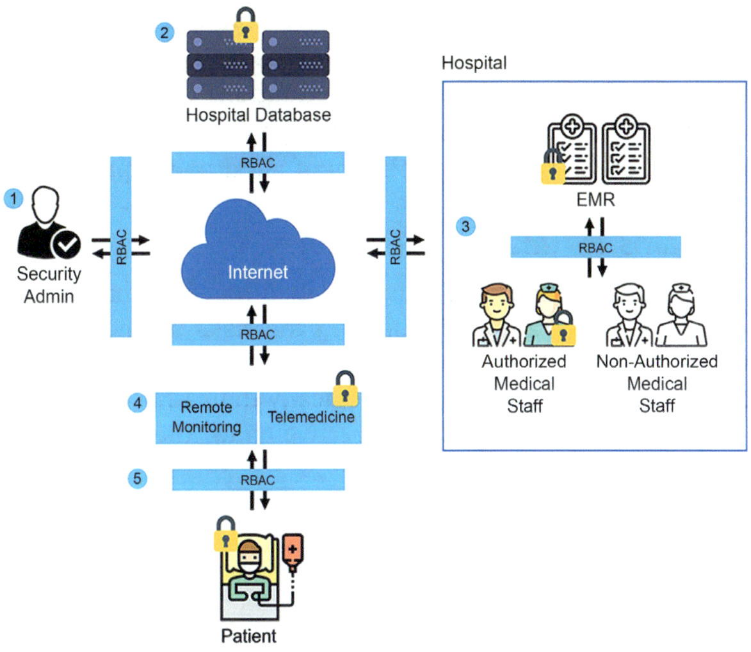

Figure 10.18. Medical data protection access control model.

Source: https://www.researchgate.net/figure/Medical-data-protection-access-control-model_fig2_335981739.

This legal corpus aims to protect individual health information, but the truth is that unauthorized disclosure, whether inadvertent or intentional, can severely erode trust between healthcare professionals and patients. The presence of a strict patient information handling protocol is the first step toward retaining these standards, particularly within imaging centers where precise and intimate health information is easily generated and disseminated across different stakeholders. Moreover, the application of artificial intelligence (AI) in pediatric healthcare also brings its own set of privacy and confidentiality challenges. As much as diagnostic capabilities are enhanced by AI, health care use of AI systems does raise ethical issues regarding data usage, especially with children's health. At present, no in-depth set of policies addresses these ethical issues in pediatric settings compared to adult medicine, where such frameworks exist more clearly. This is particularly concerning because it may lead to decisions not made with adequate consideration of the ethical ramifications. Resolution of these issues requires the development of child-centered ethical guidelines given in documents like the Pediatrics Ethical Recommendations List for AI (PEARL-AI) to guide clinicians, along with AI developers, towards the delivery of child-friendly AI-powered systems, thus fostering a healthier setting overall (Cheng et al., 2025). In collaborative research work, particularly in pediatric specialties such as rheumatology, privacy is a critical concern, especially where regional regulatory settings are significantly disparate. The absence of a unifying European Union (EU) regulation complicates the case since the researcher must deal with the variation of laws and ethical standards on pediatric information. SHARE project, to develop evidence-based recommendations for collaborative pediatric research, stresses ethics committees and advisory opinions to simplify these guidelines. The approach underscores the importance of valid processes of ensuring informed consent, data sharing, and management of pediatric databanks and biobanks in maintaining confidentiality. The following recommendations from these efforts not only reduce the risk of privacy breaches but also enhance the integrity of pediatric studies through ethical practices that account for the unique susceptibilities of child participants (Anton et al., 2017).

10.5.3. Ethical Problems in Imaging Decisions

Ethical dilemmas occur relatively frequently in pediatric imaging diagnosis due to the delicate balance between the need for accurate diagnosis and the risks of imaging procedures. The most critical problem is exposure to radiation in children, particularly with modalities like CT scans. Because children's tissues are more sensitive radiologically than adult tissues, medical practitioners have to assess the necessity for imaging with care, weighing the benefits against the potential long-term consequences (Figure 10.19).

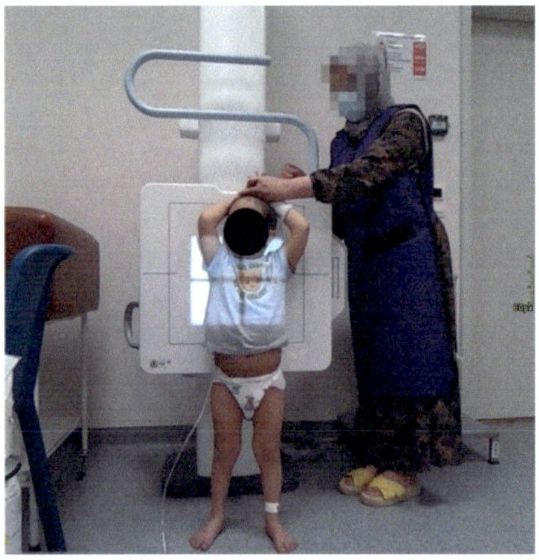

Figure 10.19. Pediatric critical care ethics.

Source: https://media.springernature.com/lw685/springer-static/image/art%3A10.1007%2Fs00247-023-05671-0/MediaObjects/247_2023_5671_Fig1_HTML.png.

Parent expectations compound this because parents might have a therapeutic misconception that advanced imaging will lead to authoritative diagnostics and therapies for the illness of their children. Physicians are subsequently tasked with ensuring informed consent and educating parents about the inherent risks and limitations of imaging techniques, thereby fostering a shared decision-making process that respects the family's autonomy while prioritizing child safety. A second ethical challenge is the use of imaging in the context of research studies, especially in pediatric neuroimaging. As noted in more recent literature, therapeutic misconception can quite seriously interfere with the informed consent process when parents refer their children in as research participants, either as ill subjects with neurological disease or healthy controls. Parents may not explicitly understand the distinction between research and clinical care and, hence, may believe that participation would likely help their child directly. Thus, their judgment would become clouded. This misperception poses deep ethical issues concerning the consent obtained in such circumstances. It also poses problems for IRBs to evaluate the ethical merit of pediatric neuroimaging research. These problems must be addressed through a combination approach that enhances communication and enhances ethical standards while not losing sight of the fact that parents are adequately educated about the aims of the study as well as potential impacts on their children (Figure 10.20).

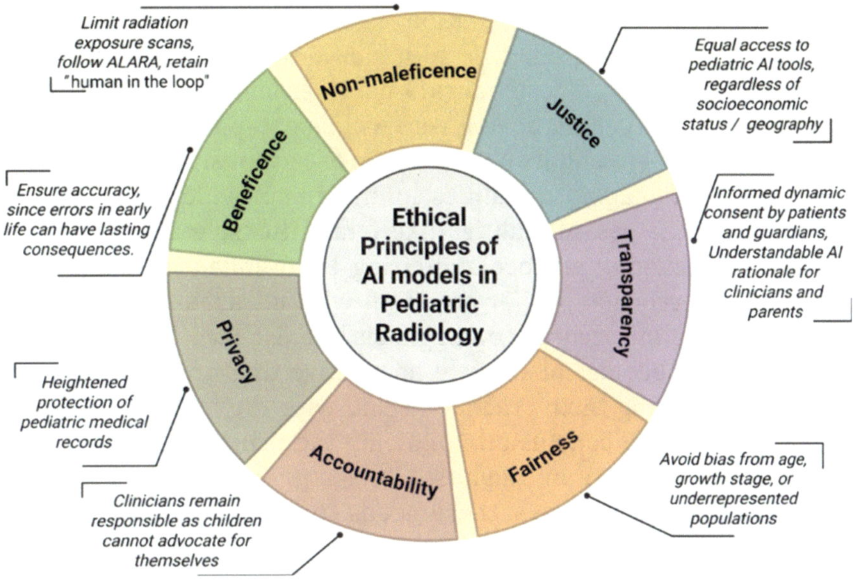

Figure 10.20. Interdisciplinary meeting for pediatric imaging ethical case review.

Source: https://media.springernature.com/lw1200/springer-static/image/art%3A10.1007%2Fs00247-025-06497-8/MediaObjects/247_2025_6497_Fig2_HTML.png

Lastly, management of disorders such as XY gonadal dysgenesis illustrates the ethical subtleties involved in pediatric imaging decisions. Imaging in these instances would be useful to gauge the paucity of gonadal development and risk of malignancy. Without universal criteria for clinical management, ethical concerns arise, particularly about the timing and necessity of invasive measures like gonadectomy. Healthcare professionals must navigate the complicated landscape of medical ethics, considering not just the urgent imaging demand but also the potential psychological and emotional impact on patients and their families. The call for personalized care in these instances demands mutual understanding between healthcare professionals and families to ensure decisions are made based on current evidence and ethical principles. This involves an understanding of imaging concepts and hazards, so that families can be adequately informed to make decisions that are consistent with their values and in the best interests of their child.

SUMMARY

In summary, the principles of pediatric diagnostic imaging emphasize the delicate balance between gaining needed clinical information and limiting potential harm, especially radiation exposure. The increasing reliance on imaging technology puts greater emphasis on well-informed caregiver and health care provider decision-making. Notably, the provision of informational pamphlets has been shown to enhance parental knowledge of radiation risks and benefits significantly, and ultimately lead to increased comfort in allowing children to undergo needed imaging exams, as attested by the findings of Hwang et al. (2017). These educational interventions are important in addressing issues of diagnostic imaging safety in that caregivers will be equipped with the knowledge required to take stands on behalf of their children's health in a responsible manner. Furthermore, the technological advancements of imaging modalities continue to provide clearer and more informative evaluations of children's sicknesses. Modalities like fetal MRI have also recently become crucial adjuncts to the traditional imaging protocols, offering even enhanced diagnostic capabilities to conditions that may not be accorded proper attention with ultrasound alone, as in Stafrace et al. (2008). They not only improve the accuracy of diagnosis but also facilitate an anticipatory approach to pediatric care. As such, it becomes absolutely imperative that professionals remain up-to-date with such advancements, bringing their practice in line with the latest evidence-based principles of diagnostic imaging. Finally, the conclusion, following the principles, sets out a commitment to pediatric patients' safety and welfare in diagnostic imaging. As healthcare workers deal with the challenge offered by imaging technologies, there needs to be constant dialogue with families, an open and trusting culture. Placing education and patient-centeredness at the forefront, healthcare workers can reduce anxiety about the imaging process while battling for the best outcome for patients. By definition, through the unification of practice and knowledge, adherence to these principles will further shape the future of pediatric diagnostic imaging, rendering the children safe and effective care.

CLOSER LOOK

PEDIATRIC DIAGNOSTIC IMAGING PRINCIPLES

There are several principal issues that dictate the imaging and treatment of children in pediatric diagnostic imaging. Children are more sensitive to radiography than adults, and as such, low-dose imaging examinations must be employed wherever it is possible. This is especially necessary in the diagnosis of conditions like acute lymphoblastic leukemia, where diagnostic imaging must be balanced against radiation exposure's long-term effects. When practitioners consider imaging modalities, including ultrasound, MRI, and computed tomography (CT), the choice must reflect both clinical necessity and a commitment to minimizing harm, as an effective protocol prioritizes patient safety without compromising diagnostic accuracy. Moreover, standardization of imaging protocols significantly contributes to reliable results and improves patient care. The inconsistency in definitions and assessments of toxic effects, as seen in the body of evidence on acute lymphoblastic leukemia protocols, identifies the dangers in pediatric imaging. Protocols varied extensively in handling acute toxic effects and their definitions, with none adequately covering all potential risks inherent to treatment (Attarbaschi et al., 2016). This inconsistency invokes a concerted effort that informs schools of pediatric oncologists and radiologists how to apply consensus definitions, ultimately resulting in improved communication among medical practitioners. The formulation of standardized procedures facilitates adequate comparison of the efficacy and safety of treatment, as well as averts the sabotage of the critical management of the entire pediatric patient. Lastly, interphase incorporation is essential in improving pediatric diagnostic imaging results. Interdisciplinary collaboration ensures mutual coordination between various medical experts, for example, radiologists, pediatricians, and oncologists, in trying to offer patient-focused treatment. Collaborative effort like this is complemented by counsel from international study groups advocating for the integration of consensus definitions of adverse effects experienced by pediatric patients being subjected to imaging (N/A, 1985). Such collaboration not only streamlines treatment protocols but also enables the sharing of best practices and imaging technology innovations, ultimately benefiting children who are to be diagnosed with dangerous diseases. By encouraging a spirit of teamwork, healthcare providers are able to enhance the accuracy of diagnosis while, at the same time, addressing the special susceptibility and needs of pediatrics.

REFERENCES

1. David-Olawade, A. C., Olawade, D. B., Vanderbloemen, L., Rotifa, O. B., Fidelis, S. C., Egbon, E., Akpan, A. O., Adeleke, S., Ghose, A., & Boussios, S. (2025). AI-Driven Advances in Low-Dose Imaging and Enhancement—A Review. *Diagnostics*, *15*(6), 689. https://doi.org/10.3390/diagnostics15060689Anton, J., Avcin, T., Benseler, S. M., Beresford, M. W., et al. (2017). Recommendations for collaborative paediatric research including biobanking in Europe: A Single Hub and Access point for Paediatric Rheumatology in Europe (SHARE) initiative. https://core.ac.uk/download/146488032.pdf (accessed on 15th July 2025).
2. Apostol, I., Belis, V., Calota, R. G., Duncea, A., et al. (2017). Forensic and clinical diagnosis in shaken baby syndrome, between child abuse and iatrogenic abuse. https://core.ac.uk/download/144553178.pdf (accessed on 15th July 2025).
3. Arthurs, O. J., Dos Santos, D. P., Meshaka, R., Sebire, N. J., et al. (2021). Artificial intelligence reporting guidelines: What the pediatric radiologist needs to know. https://core.ac.uk/download/477687828.pdf (accessed on 15th July 2025).
4. Attarbaschi, A., Barzilai, S., Escherich, G., Frandsen, T. L., et al. (2016). Consensus definitions of 14 severe acute toxic effects for childhood lymphoblastic leukemia treatment: A Delphi consensus. https://core.ac.uk/download/42370388.pdf (accessed on 15th July 2025).
5. Barkovich, A. J., Mukherjee, P., & Wahl, M. (2010). Diffusion imaging and tractography of congenital brain malformations. https://core.ac.uk/download/323074405.pdf (accessed on 15th July 2025).
6. Bastarrika, G., De Cecco, C. N., Geyer, L. L., Laghi, A., et al. (2015). State of the art: Iterative CT reconstruction techniques. https://core.ac.uk/download/54522078.pdf (accessed on 15th July 2025).
7. Cheng, L. T. E., Chng, S. Y., Chong, Y. S., Eriksson, M., et al. (2025). Ethical considerations in AI for child health and recommendations for child-centered medical AI. https://core.ac.uk/download/646847577.pdf (accessed on 15th July 2025).
8. D'Arcy, R., Downie, J., Hadskis, M., Kenny, R., et al. (2008). The therapeutic misconception: A threat to valid parental consent for pediatric neuroimaging research. https://core.ac.uk/download/568216503.pdf (accessed on 15th July 2025).
9. Donya, M., ElGuindy, A., Firmin, D., Radford, M., et al. (2014). Radiation in medicine: Origins, risks and aspirations. https://core.ac.uk/download/77008838.pdf (accessed on 15th July 2025).
10. Goldblatt, J., Isasi, R., Jagut, M., Jonker, A. H., et al. (2019). Model consent clauses for rare disease research. https://core.ac.uk/download/237010883.pdf (accessed on 15th July 2025).
11. Hacker, C. D., Leuthardt, E. C., Limbrick, D. D., Roland, J. L., et al. (2019). A comparison of resting state functional magnetic resonance imaging to invasive electrocortical stimulation for sensorimotor mapping in pediatric patients. https://core.ac.uk/download/225001086.pdf (accessed on 15th July 2025).
12. Hwang, H. (2017). Knowledge, attitude and perception on radiation imaging among children's caregivers in the pediatric dental clinic. https://open.bu.edu/bitstream/2144/23797/5/Hwang_bu_0017N_12842.pdf (accessed on 15th July 2025).

13. Kaakinen, P., Kekäläinen, S., Kääriäinen, M., Oikarinen, H., et al. (2022). Effectiveness of digital counseling before pediatric diagnostic imaging. https://core.ac.uk/download/628870139.pdf (accessed on 15th July 2025).

14. McCann-Crosby, B., Schlomer, B., Macias, C. G., Roth, D. R., Austin, E. G., Dietrich, J. E., McCullough, L. B., et al. (2014). State of the art review in gonadal dysgenesis: Challenges in diagnosis and management. https://ijpeonline.biomedcentral.com/track/pdf/10.1186/1687-9856-2014-4?site=ijpeonline.biomedcentral.com (accessed on 15th July 2025).

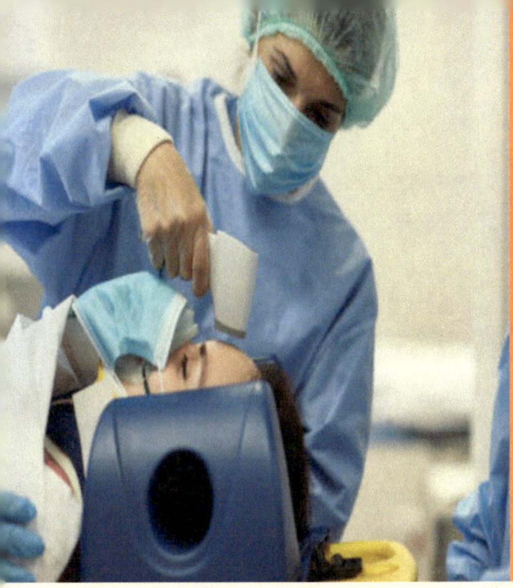

Chapter 11

EMERGENCY AND TRAUMA IMAGING PROTOCOLS

Contents

Introduction

In emergency care, imaging algorithms play a vital role in the rapid assessment and treatment of traumatized patients. With the incorporation of new imaging modalities, healthcare providers can make life-or-death decisions promptly, which in most instances have direct ramifications on patient outcomes. Knowledge of the emergency and trauma imaging algorithms is required because of the variability and intricacy of trauma cases. These protocols are not merely guidelines; they are evidence-based practices that have evolved as new research becomes available and technology advances. Learning about these protocols allows practitioners to better manage the needs of novel clinical presentations and use resources more effectively. This compilation of emergency imaging protocols highlights the utility of systematic protocols to enhance patient care and operational efficiency within high-stakes environments. Underlying the success of imaging protocols in the emergency setting is continual research network creation that is focused on improving clinical practice and outcomes.

Some examples include networks such as the Pediatric Emergency Care Applied Research Network (PECARN), which illustrate how design-organized research agendas can drive innovations in children's emergency care. Their well-organized infrastructures and collaborative research efforts ensure that new evidence is rigorously implemented into practice, thereby enhancing the quality of care young patients experience in emergencies (Kim et al., 2014).

Use of findings from such research networks not only standardizes imaging protocols across institutions but also ensures that healthcare professionals are educated to make full use of advancing technologies and methodologies. Hence, the development of evidence-based protocols is key to strengthening diagnostic accuracy and clinical management in the setting of trauma. Additionally, the relevance of good imaging protocols is even more significant in the context of the scarcity of resources and unequal access to healthcare. As highlighted by ongoing research and funding initiatives, such as Highlands & Islands Enterprise and other funding initiatives, the sustenance of enhanced research and practice is pivotal in the establishment of emergency response capacity (Eadie et al., 2016).

The initiatives highlight long-term sustainability within productive imaging practices through ongoing adaptation and learning. In addition to facilitating better diagnosis and, therefore, hastening treatment, adherence to such protocols can also make operational workflows simpler, enabling medical teams to handle large volumes of patients effectively. Finally, the research and implementation of emergency imaging protocols systematically are an important component of modern trauma care, which makes it possible for patients to receive timely and appropriate interventions (Figure 11.1).

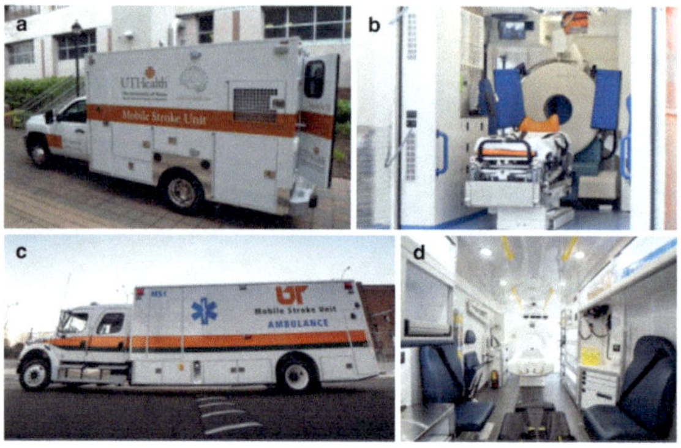

Figure 11.1. Triage area of an emergency department equipped with mobile imaging units.

Source: https://media.springernature.com/lw685/springer-static/image/chp%3A10.1007%2F978-3-319-99016-3_35/MediaObjects/430405_1_En_35_Fig1_HTML.png.

11.1. Indications for Imaging in Emergency Situations

In the acute care medical setting, imaging is crucial in the expedient assessment of patients with acute disease. The protocol for selecting an image relies on a variety of factors, including the patient's clinical history, presentation, and suspected illness or trauma.

For instance, during cases of potential neurological compromise, immediate imaging such as CT or MRI is vital to detect hemorrhages, lesions, or other urgent interventions as detailed in Dhoot et al. (2024). Imaging tests are also important to efficiently triage patients, facilitating speedy decision-making to improve outcomes. Adherence to established procedures enables medical professionals to effectively diagnose and treat patients, mitigating delays that may lead to deteriorating conditions or complications. Not only is emergent imaging necessitated by the necessity for immediate diagnostics, but it also entails continuous monitoring of patient responses to treatments. For example, in trauma patients with anticipated intracranial or intra-abdominal trauma, imaging can provide immediate feedback regarding the success of interventions, thus guiding future treatment. The use of high-level imaging modalities, such as ultrasound, has become fashionable in emergency settings as well, particularly for bedside evaluation capable of decreasing patient transport times. This can be particularly useful in hospitals with limited resources or for patients in remote or prehospital settings, where standard imaging may not be immediately available, as shown in (Barlas et al., 2018). Thus, the utilization of diverse imaging modalities is crucial for international emergency care.

Imaging protocols must also consider patient safety and the optimization of resources in emergency departments. The hazards of unwarranted radiation exposure, especially in vulnerable populations such as children, call for a considered policy regarding imaging selection. Clinical decision support technology may help practitioners choose the most appropriate imaging method based on the presenting clinical condition and align with best-practice recommendations. Through critical evaluation of each imaging study's necessity, healthcare professionals can weigh the required diagnosis with minimum risks and thus enhance patient care during emergencies. Effective use of such protocols is also a key factor contributing to the general performance of emergency and trauma imaging because it enables timely and appropriate decisions for the patient's health and well-being.

11.1.1. Evaluation of Fractures and Dislocations

Dislocation and fracture evaluation is an important component of guidelines for emergency and trauma imaging. Timely and correct diagnosis can potentially influence patient outcome and treatment, in addition to overall management of trauma. In practice, the initial impression is most commonly started by clinical assessment, which includes examination of the mechanism of injury, visual inspection of physical deformity, and identification of concomitant signs and symptoms such as swelling and pain. This initial evaluation is important, as it can inform the choice of imaging modalities, ranging from plain radiography to advanced techniques such as computed tomography (CT) or magnetic resonance imaging (MRI). Correct imaging protocol not only reveals the extent and nature of injury but also is important for preventing complications arising from misdiagnosis or delayed treatment.

Radiographs remain the imaging modality of choice for the examination of suspected dislocations and fractures due to their accessibility, speed, and low cost. However, certain fractures pose diagnostic challenges, particularly those such as suspected scaphoid fractures. Evidence has shown that actual fractures are uncommon among suspected cases, reducing the likelihood that a positive imaging finding is related to an actual fracture and making it even harder to achieve diagnostic accuracy (Doornberg et al., 2021). In the presence of such uncertainty, clinicians should incorporate clinical prediction rules that use demographic and clinical factors to narrow the diagnostic process. In this way, doctors can appropriately stratify patients for secondary imaging, thereby maximizing the pretest probability of a true fracture and optimizing the interpretative value of more sophisticated imaging modalities (Figure 11.2).

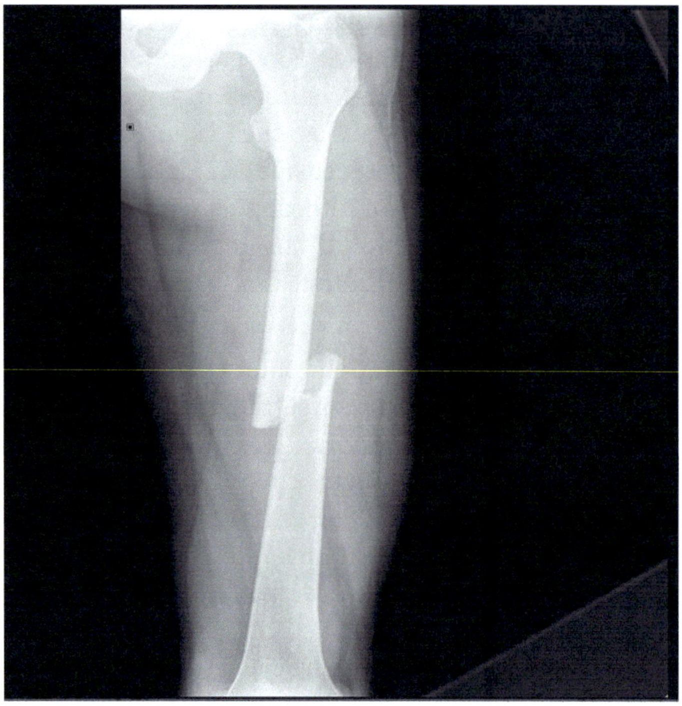

Figure 11.2. X-ray image showing a mid-shaft femoral fracture with displacement.

Source: https://prod-images-static.radiopaedia.org/images/3030426/6d91c93a6a565320a67ff78ad8b240_big_gallery.JPEG.

With the rapidly expanding specialty of emergency medicine, the integration of artificial intelligence (AI) has begun to transform the way dislocations and fractures are analyzed. Technologies such as convolutional neural networks (CNNs) have the potential to improve the detection of scaphoid fractures on radiographs. Although past research suggests that these AI-driven models have not yet outperformed diagnoses by seasoned clinicians for complex cases, they are promising for future use (Doornberg et al., 2021). The ability to employ machine-learning algorithms has the potential to improve risk stratification and diagnostic performance and learn from new data over the long term. This emerging paradigm represents an exciting new frontier in emergency and trauma imaging protocols that unite clinical expertise with leading-edge technology to increase patient care and success with therapy.

11.1.2. Assessment of Internal Injury

In the critical evaluation of internal trauma, imaging protocols are the most crucial aspect of swift triage and trauma resuscitation of injured patients. Computed tomography (CT) scans and ultrasound are the preferred advanced imaging modalities for identifying organ injury that may be occult on physical examination. These modalities offer doctors a non-destructive imaging method for difficult areas of anatomy, making them indispensable in emergency cases where timing is not on their side (Figure 11.3). For instance, CT scans are best at detecting hemorrhagic events, visceral injury, or fractures, which allow medical professionals to strategize intervention quickly.

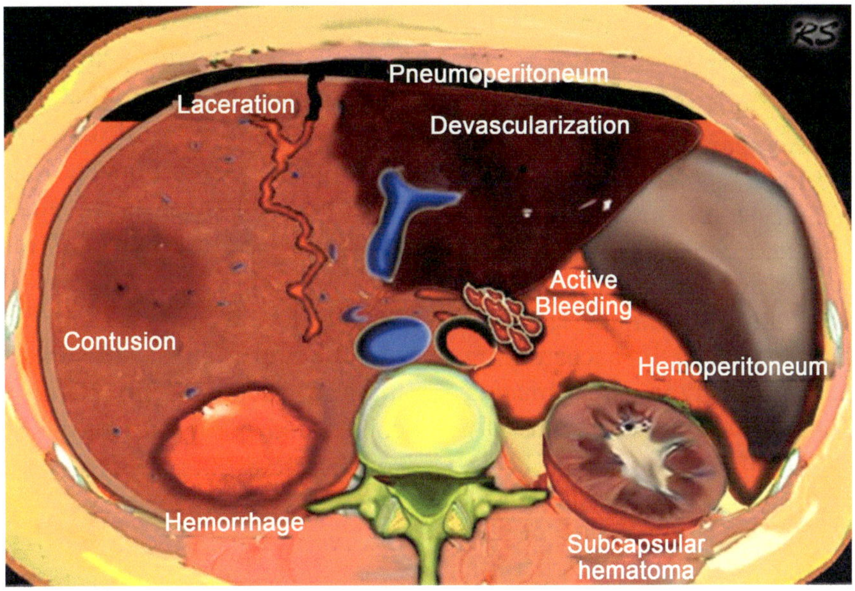

Figure 11.3. CT scan demonstrating liver laceration from blunt abdominal trauma.

Source: https://radiologyassistant.nl/img/containers/main/acute-abdomen-role-of-ct-in-trauma/a5097977b370e9_TEK-lever-trauma.jpg/63936aa1a0162cdc8a1962c57d9b3ca9.jpg.

Therefore, the use of standard imaging algorithms can significantly enhance the diagnostic accuracy, reduce unnecessary exploratory procedures, and improve patient outcomes in trauma settings. For pediatric polytrauma patients, evaluation of internal trauma requires an even more specialized effort due to their characteristic physiological response and anatomical differences from adults. Given the specialized nature of caring for children, emergency departments must have equipment and protocols explicitly tailored to their age group to properly evaluate. Educating personnel on the importance of expeditious diagnosis in this high-risk population is also critical, as delays can be disastrous. Research stresses the importance of following a systematic approach in pediatric trauma cases, with improved outcomes being a result of faster identification of internal injuries, which quite prominently leads to early treatment initiation (As et al., 2014). Hence, the application of advances in imaging technologies coupled with a complete understanding of pediatric anatomy and pathology is crucial in effective emergency trauma management. Also of importance is focus on the conditions that are specifically arising from internal injuries, as witnessed by the complications that have developed in burn patients who have been exposed to traumatic situations. Existing research indicates that exposure to severe thermal injuries can initiate simultaneously occurring heart injuries, which have a significant impact on patient prognosis. Evaluation of such complications demands an integrated strategy that not only examines surface trauma but also watches for subtle internal injury by echocardiography and other cardiac imaging modalities. Recognition of myocardial thickening and thrombi, as illustrated in involved cat patients, shows that complete evaluations should be reflective of multisystem involvement in trauma (Epstein et al., 2020). This three-dimensional analysis of injury evaluation is essential, not only for acute management, but also for directing long-term care and rehabilitation planning for trauma patients.

11.1.3. Identification of Neurological Disorders

Neurological disorder identification in emergency settings is of paramount importance, especially considering the high prevalence of traumatic brain injury (TBI) among patients who come for treatment. Since TBIs contribute significantly to all traumatic cases, clinical practitioners are required to employ rigorous diagnostic imaging methods in ascertaining the extent of damage and type. New imaging technologies, such as computed tomography (CT) and magnetic resonance imaging (MRI), are now standard modalities in this effort. These modalities enable clinicians to obtain critical information about the brain's structural integrity and distinguish between mild and severe patterns of injury. This function is essential not only for immediate treatment but also for long-term management plans aimed at addressing potential complications, such as chronic headache, cognitive deficits, and other neurological dysfunction that may arise after injury (Figure 11.4).

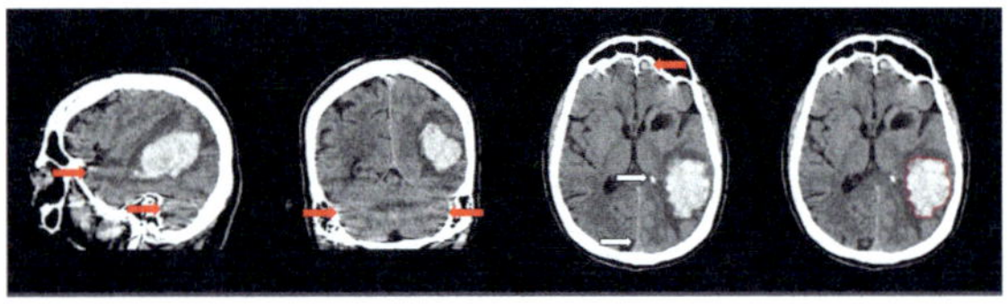

Figure 11.4. Non-contrast head CT highlighting acute intracerebral hemorrhage.

Source: https://media.springernature.com/full/springer-static/image/art%3A10.1038%2Fs41598-019-54491-6/MediaObjects/41598_2019_54491_Fig1_HTML.png.

Therefore, robust imaging protocols are of paramount significance to enhancing patient outcomes in emergency situations. Given the heterogeneity and complexity of neurologic diseases, particularly with neurotrauma in the picture, developing specific biomarkers is the most hopeful area for diagnostics. Current methods rely primarily on behaviorally expressed symptoms that are perceived as being subjective and inadequate for early diagnosis. As emphasized in state-of-the-art research, there is an emergent need for reliable chemical markers in biofluids that would serve as effective diagnostic tools for invisible injuries, enabling the identification of TBIs and their severity modulations. Brain injuries exist with complexities that must be considered highly carefully, particularly since concussive events are typically unrecognizable by means of standard imaging only. Thus, new interventions based on proteomics and the assessment of neurological markers hold the promise for enhancing diagnostic precision and patient care by enabling clinicians to follow injury trajectories and predict outcomes with greater specificity (Loo et al., 2014).

The incorporation of rigorous biomarker testing with imaging protocols has the potential to revolutionize emergency treatment of patients with neurological disease. The application of quantitative mass spectrometry techniques enables effective analysis of specific neurotrauma markers, thereby enhancing the potential for identifying candidate clinical assays. These advances overcome significant challenges of TBI diagnostics since prevailing shortcomings of standardized biofluid tests restrict short-term clinical decision-making. Validation of neurotrauma markers will enable timely interventions and avoid serial concussive exposures that can lead to irreversible neurological impairments. Thus, adding advanced imaging and biomarker analysis to emergency protocols not only meets contemporary scientific requirements but also advances the overall objective of optimizing patient safety and long-term outcomes in trauma (Loo et al., 2014).

11.2. Imaging Protocols for Specific Injuries

Imaging protocols play a critical role in the rapid assessment of specific injuries in traumatic and emergency settings. For instance, fractures in the thoracolumbar spine are prevalent in patients with high-energy trauma. Prompt diagnosis and optimal imaging of these injuries are crucial because they can produce significant morbidity and even death if not handled appropriately. High-technology imaging modalities, such as computed tomography (CT) or magnetic resonance imaging (MRI), are typically employed to assess the size of the fracture and associated neurological damage. As explained in current studies, a stepwise model of emergency thoracolumbar trauma care, including proper imaging protocols, can be a key factor in patient outcomes. The use of known classification systems also individualizes case management strategies, leading to optimized intervention results and ultimately improved patient survival rates (Bloemers et al., 2024).

In children, the employment of standardized imaging protocols is equally crucial, particularly in blunt trauma. Literature shows that the effectiveness in acquiring images correlates with the time to definitive care, which translates into morbidity and mortality rates. Effective trauma response will reduce the time from emergency department arrival to imaging tests, as seen in recent literature wherein adoption of specific guidelines resulted in significantly reduced time for CT scanning and focused assessment with sonography for trauma (FAST) examinations. This rapid imaging acquisition plays a central role in accurate diagnoses of injuries and delineation of appropriate interventions, thereby facilitating expedited patient care (Cross et al., 2019). Enhanced efficiency in imaging protocols underpins faster clinical decisions, ultimately improving patient outcomes in emergencies.

Moreover, the implementation of personalized imaging protocols should be adapted to the unique anatomical and physiological differences of different age groups, most notably children. The pediatric patient also has its own response patterns to trauma, and therefore it must be addressed with specially adapted imaging techniques and analysis. Because traumatic injury in children often occurs in the context of high-energy events, imaging must provide not just accurate information regarding injuries but also needs to take into account developmental parameters that could influence treatment pathways. By fine-tuning these protocols with improved adherence to pediatric management, clinicians can limit unnecessary radiation exposure while maximizing recognition of significant injuries. The development of evidence-based practices, as evidenced by improved imaging efficiencies in more recent studies, is important in further advancing trauma care protocols and the overall delivery of care for injured children (Cross et al., 2019).

11.2.1. Head Trauma Protocols

Effective handling of head trauma in the emergency setting is of greatest significance, given the potential of ensuing significant morbidity and mortality due to delayed treatment. The establishment of effective protocols detailing the imaging process is central to achieving timely diagnosis and treatment. For instance, it has been shown that the introduction of an optimized trauma team strategy can reduce the time from ED arrival to CT acquisition, as evidenced by a statistically significant reduction in intervention times following system change (Cross et al., 2019) (Figure 11.5).

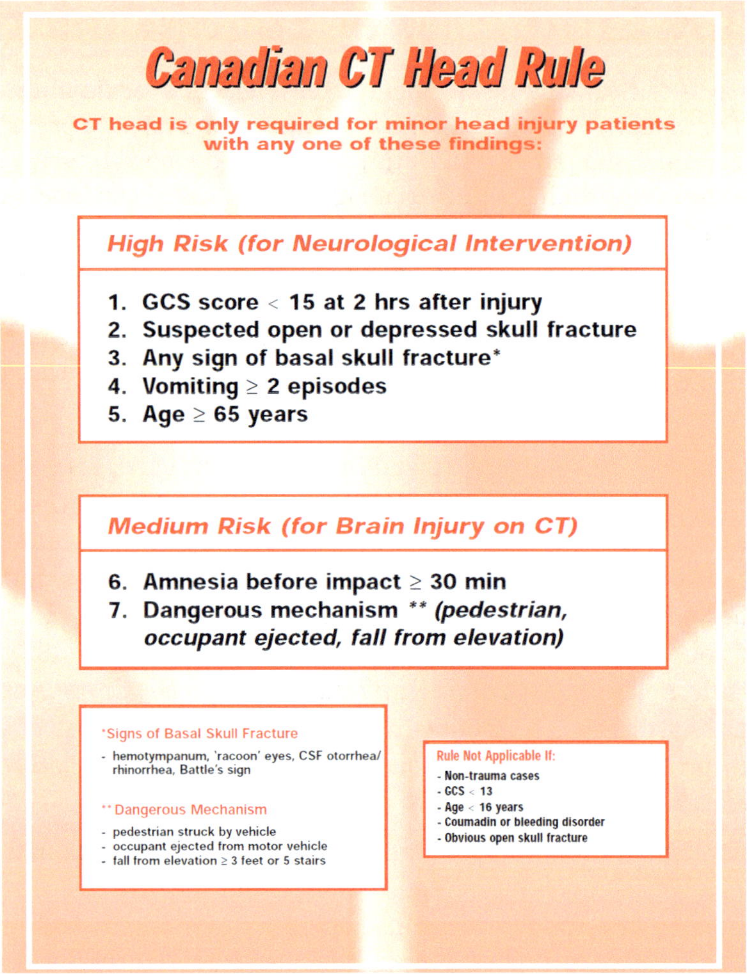

Figure 11.5. Emergency head CT protocol flowchart including decision criteria and imaging sequences.

Source: https://www.researchgate.net/publication/339019405/figure/fig2/AS:854855547633667@1580824853834/Canadian-CT-head-rule-poster-as-published-by-Stiell-et-al-5-reproduced-with-permission.png.

AgrRapid imaging not only aids in the diagnosis of injuries but also optimizes the entire disposition of patients and, thus, avoids complications associated with delayed evaluation and management. These efficiencies highlight the need to abide by set protocols to optimize patient outcomes in head trauma. The development of guidelines such as those of the Pediatric Emergency Care Applied Research Network (PECARN) has also further improved pediatric head trauma examination protocols. The adherence to the PECARN guidelines has been examined in one study, where it was discovered that the proportion of patients requiring CT scans decreased when introducing the guidelines (Bingham et al., 2020). This decrease means that adherence to some imaging guidelines, including mechanisms of injury or clinical signs, can decrease unwanted radiation with the added confidence that patients who need imaging will receive it promptly. Interestingly, even when

CT was warranted, incidental findings created issues in patient management and anxiety, and underscore the value of a careful approach to the decision for imaging. Initiation of such protocols not only aids optimal injury assessment but also encourages a quality improvement culture within emergency departments. By continually evaluating how existing protocols function, hospitals can pinpoint areas for improvement, particularly regarding the appropriateness and timeliness of imaging referrals. For example, findings from various studies highlight the importance of continuous training and quality assurance processes to refine imaging practices in pediatric populations (Cross et al., 2019; Bingham et al., 2020). With further efforts towards minimizing delays in trauma management by healthcare systems, constant review and optimization of imaging protocols will be critical in providing the best outcome for head trauma patients.

11.2.2. Chest Injury Protocols

Protocols for chest trauma in the context of emergency and trauma imaging are essential for early diagnosis and treatment. The protocols aim to suitably screen for life-threatening pathology, such as pneumothorax, hemothorax, and rib fractures, that are typically present with chest trauma. Strategic use of imaging modalities such as chest X-ray and CT scans is essential in such situations. An evidence-based approach to imaging prioritization with clinical markers enables healthcare providers to promptly identify significant injuries, direct rapid management, and reduce the risk of adverse outcomes. Such protocols then center on an evaluation of the patient's hemodynamic status and level of consciousness to determine the optimal imaging modality, thus offering patients tailored care aligning with their unique context and circumstances (Figure 11.6).

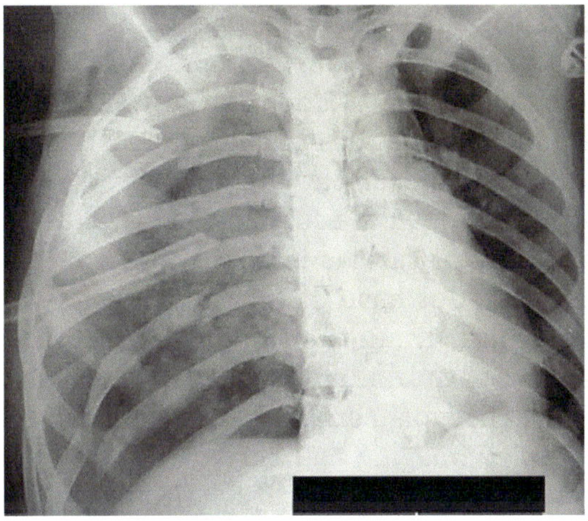

Figure 11.6. Chest X-ray of a patient with flail chest and rib fractures following trauma.

Source: https://www.researchgate.net/profile/Nick-Theakos/publication/42975001/figure/fig1/AS:636441298227201@1528750838381/Chest-X-ray-showing-a-flail-chest-of-the-right-haemithorax-with-two-chest-tubes-in-place.png.

The use of whole-body multidetector computed tomography (MDCT) is becoming more prominent in the field of trauma protocols among patients who are presenting with chest trauma. Studies confirm that MDCT can uncover extensive injuries in patients who appear stable at presentation, demonstrating its potential to maximize patient outcomes. For instance, a study investigated 81 patients with dangerous trauma mechanisms and found that 34.4% possessed critically important injuries as identified by MDCT, which emphasizes the need for such thorough investigations in suspected chest trauma. However, whole-body imaging has its limitations, including safety problems of exposure to radiation, particularly in the young, and its repeated usage. Therefore, developing better triage techniques and studying low-dose approaches are essential in finding a balance between the diagnostic benefit of MDCT and decreasing the threats from radiation exposure, maintaining protocols that are both safe and effective for patients (Blaz et al., 2009). Moreover, the prevalence of substance abuse, such as cocaine, complicates patients' assessment protocols for chest pain within trauma settings. Understanding the relationship between cocaine use and presentations of chest injury is crucial to clinical management and imaging strategies. Cocaine can lead to acute coronary syndromes or other fatal cardiac illnesses that appear as chest pain but have distinct diagnostic issues from typical traumatic injury. For instance, a diagnosis of cocaine abuse in those patients who visit for chest pain can initiate referral for more aggressive imaging and cardiovascular testing to rule out acute severe conditions. Reports from emergency departments indicate that there exists a variety of cocaine prevalence among these patient groups that necessitates imaging and treatment protocol modification to be able to give proper treatment (Bandeeri et al., 2004). This appreciation enhances the overall effectiveness of trauma imaging protocols, promoting an organized approach to patient care in the emergency setting.

11.2.3. Abdominal Trauma Protocols

Development of effective protocols for the management of abdominal trauma is an important priority in emergency medicine, as it will directly affect patient outcomes with timely and accurate imaging. Protocols initially start with a thorough clinical assessment, followed by the selection of imaging modalities. Initial instruments of choice are typically ultrasound, particularly the focused assessment with sonography for trauma (FAST), and computed tomography (CT), particularly for suspected intra-abdominal injury. An analysis conducted on pediatric trauma demonstrates that the implementation of an effective trauma response not only decreased the time taken between arrival in the emergency department (ED) and imaging acquisition but also increased the rate of FAST scans performed (Cross et al., 2019). Findings such as these highlight the importance of operational effectiveness and protocol optimization in the triage process for abdominal trauma cases (Figure 11.7).

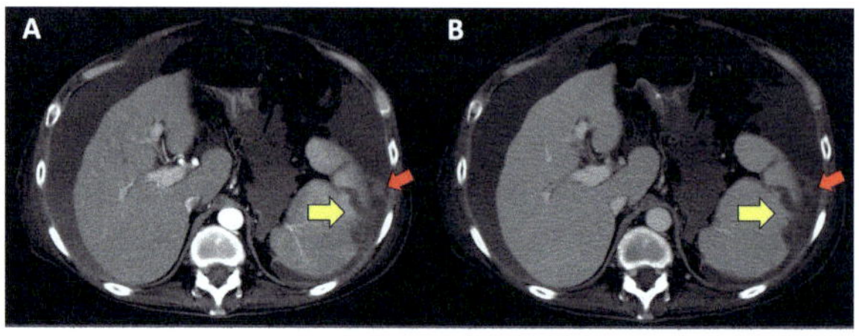

Figure 11.7. Non-traumatic splenic rupture secondary to hemorrhagic infarct in diffuse large B-cell lymphoma.

Source: https://casereports.bmj.com/content/12/1/e229052.

The imaging protocol serves more than a diagnostic purpose; it is essential in the appropriate management and decision-making regarding surgical interventions. Evidence supports that abdominal trauma protocols must use whole-body multidetector computed tomography (MDCT) in high-risk patients, balancing the detection of life-threatening injuries against potential radiation exposure (Blaz et al., 2009). In cases of trauma where the mechanism of injury is catastrophic, comprehensive imaging can reveal injuries not evident on clinical examination alone. As is indicated by the study, there were severe injuries revealed even for those patients who were found to be stable, evidence that stringent imaging protocols must be followed to avoid missed diagnoses, which can lead to severe complications or unnecessary delays in surgery. Finally, optimization of these protocols must be an ongoing process that continually adapts to new evidence and technological advancements. Imaging protocols should be continuously assessed, particularly in the decision to utilize each modality based on the status of a patient and the mechanism of injury. As mentioned in the literature, optimized triage and lower-dose imaging protocols are essential to reduce radiation risk while achieving the highest possible diagnostic yield (Blaz et al., 2009). These advancements not only improve patient safety but also streamline trauma care. Thus, as protocols in trauma are enhanced, utilization of evidence-based imaging protocols remains a cornerstone for optimal management of abdominal trauma, offering patients the best possible care in emergent conditions.

11.3. Contrast Agents in Imaging

In emergency and trauma imaging, the use of contrast agents is pivotal for enhancing the diagnostic capabilities of various modalities. These agents, which include iodine-based compounds for X-rays and CT scans, as well as gadolinium-based agents for MRI, significantly improve the visualization of anatomical structures and pathological conditions. Their ability to define vascular structures, differentiate among tissue types, and identify abnormalities accelerates clinical decision-making during emergencies. However, their selection and application require careful focus on the medical history of a patient, particularly when renal dysfunction or allergic response leads to side effects ranging from mild discomfort to lethal anaphylaxis or nephrotoxicity (N/A, 2002). The accurate use of contrast media is also emphasized in trauma imaging, where rapid but accurate assessment is required. In suspected hemorrhage or organ injury, for instance, the application of contrast can detect active bleeding or injury to intra-abdominal organs that may be overlooked on a non-contrast study. Further, imaging protocol innovation has witnessed increased utilization of optimized contrast to minimize patient exposure while maximizing diagnostic yield. The integration of real-time imaging techniques and dynamic imaging improves information derived from these physiological process events during traumatic injury in guiding interventions in real time. Despite the benefits, physicians must exercise caution regarding the timing of contrast injection and any relevant regulations to prevent risks associated with their application (Kitsiou et al., 2013). With advancing medical imaging technology, more investigation of substitute contrast agents and better delivery systems can enhance patient safety and diagnostic efficacy. Investigations into non-iodinated and non-gadolinium-based substitutes are underway to limit side effects while maintaining or improving image quality. In the trauma and emergency fields, where time is of the essence, these developments have the potential to transform patient evaluation protocols. While clinicians weigh the nuances of acute care, understanding the indications, contraindications, and latest advances in contrast agent technology remains rudimentary. Such understanding not only prescribes clinical practices but also underscores the necessity of a multidisciplinary team to deliver optimal patient outcomes under risky conditions (N/A, 2002).

11.3.1. Types of Contrast Agents Used

Among trauma and emergency imaging protocols, choosing the right contrast agents is key to improving diagnostic yield. The two major contrast agents used in medical imaging are iodinated and gadolinium-based. Iodinated contrast media are predominantly utilized during computed tomography (CT) scans (Figure 11.8).

Their high atomic number effectively increases the attenuation of X-rays, which is a critical feature to visualize vascular pathology and structures. For trauma, the rapid identification of internal hemorrhage or organ injury is of immediate concern, and therefore, the iodinated agents are part of the imaging protocols. Moreover, their wide variety of formulation possibilities allows for customized use to serve patients with varying medical histories and individualized imaging needs. On the contrary, gadolinium contrast media are used primarily in magnetic resonance imaging (MRI). While they have differing uses compared to iodinated drugs, they also enhance vascular structures and areas of ischemia or infarction. The chemical properties of gadolinium provide a better contrast, and this plays a significant role in imaging soft tissues because cases of trauma often involve damage to soft tissues.

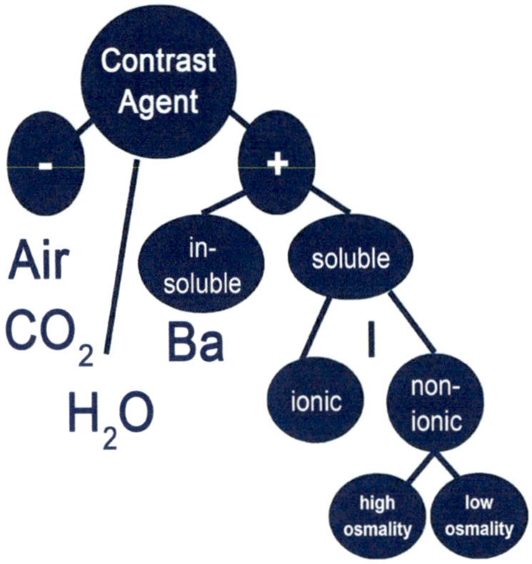

Figure 11.8. Commonly used iodinated contrast agents.

Source: https://www.google.com/url?sa=i&url=https%3A%2F%2Fhowradiologyworks.com%2Fcontrast-agents-radiographic-contrast-agents-and-iodinated-contrast-media%2F&psig=AOvVaw1oqvs4z94RUyEuqteiB_kg&ust=1750837389096000&source=images&cd=vfe&opi=89978449&ved=0CBQQjRxqFwoTCPjCqtfHiY4DFQAAAAAdAAAAABAE.

When patients have renal impairment, gadolinium preparations with lower nephrotoxicity are utilized, thereby maximizing patient safety. Such agents are judiciously used so that imaging results are correctly interpreted, and finally, they determine treatment guidance. Contrast agent is also selected based on consideration of possible adverse effects as well as contraindications, particularly in an emergency setting. Allergenic patients or those with previous sensitization to some contrast media need special care, as reactions could be mild or even lethal. Conscious of these risks, imaging protocols typically incorporate premedication to avoid untoward reactions. Also, cases involving trauma where speed is essential might limit the potential of undertaking proper pre-procedure risk assessment. Therefore, understanding the pharmacological profiles and safety concerns associated with various contrast agents is crucial for healthcare professionals performing trauma imaging. Such a comprehensive strategy to the use of contrast media assists in making imaging protocols meet both the urgency of the clinical scenario and safety of the patient.

11.3.2. Risks and Benefits of Using Contrast

The application of contrast media to emergency and trauma imaging protocols is extremely significant, primarily for the visibility of pathological conditions and anatomical structures. The contrast agents optimize the resolution of blood vessels, soft tissues, and some organs, an aspect that is extremely critical in emergencies where diagnosis is determined by rushed treatment. For instance, in cases of internal bleeding or vascular injury, the administration of iodinated contrast can be utilized to help identify hemorrhagic regions and guide surgical interventions. This application not only accelerates diagnosis but also reduces the risk of misdiagnosis, thereby improving patient outcomes. Moreover, the advances in imaging apparatus and contrast media continue to expand the scope of conditions under which contrast use is deemed helpful, making it a vital component of today's emergency diagnosis (Figure 11.9).

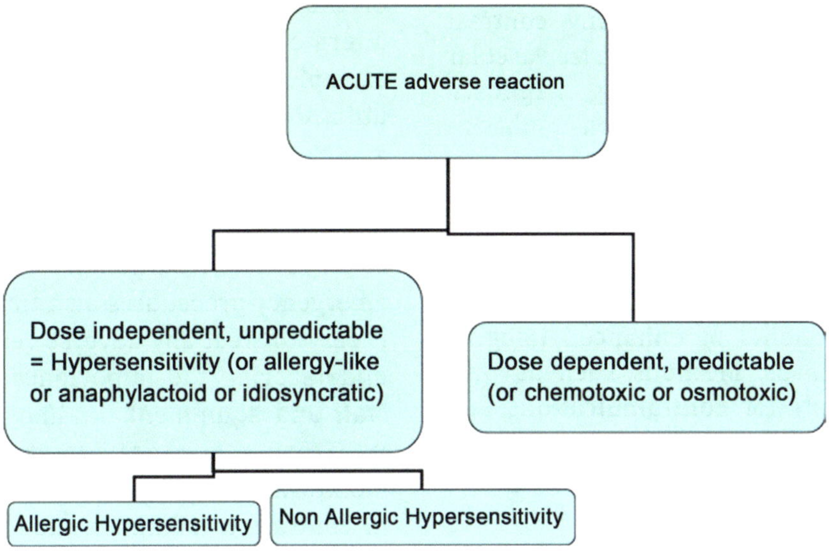

Figure 11.9. Acute adverse reactions to contrast media.

Source: https://media.springernature.com/lw685/springer-static/image/chp%3A10.1007%2F174_2013_926/MediaObjects/80608_3_En_926_Fig1_HTML.gif.

But intravenous use of contrast media is not free from risk, and this needs careful assessment before use. Contrast media-induced side effects, ranging from mild allergic to full-blown anaphylactic reactions, are a significant problem in emergency cases. On top of these, contrast-induced nephropathy (CIN) poses a significant risk, particularly to patients with intrinsic renal impairment. CIN can have further complications to make treatment in already life-critical patients even more challenging. Thus, doctors have to balance the short-term diagnostic benefit against the danger of serious side effects. Procedures need to be developed that screen the patient rigorously for possible contraindications so as to minimize these dangers, particularly in rapidly evolving trauma situations where one has to make snap judgments under pressure. In light of the above benefits and risks, appropriate usage of contrast in emergency imaging is essential. Clinicians need to weigh the potential for immediate definitive results against the risk of side effects, especially in populations who may be more susceptible, such as the elderly or patients with renal insufficiency. Implementation of evidence-based guidelines can help inform decisions about when and how contrast should be used effectively. Moreover, ongoing education on the latest advancements in contrast agents, as well as safety protocols, is crucial for healthcare professionals in emergency and trauma settings. This comprehensive information not only enhances the quality of care a patient receives but also contributes towards achieving optimal outcomes in critical settings where timely and accurate diagnosis is still the key focus.

11.3.3. Guidelines for Contrast Administration

For trauma and emergency imaging, contrast agent injection is critical to emphasize vascular pathology and structures during diagnosis. Protocols for contrast administration emphasize patient evaluation to prevent side effects, especially among high-risk patients, such as those with renal disease or allergic reactions to iodinated contrast media. Using a patient-centered approach allows medical professionals to weigh the benefits of enhanced imaging against the hazards. Methods such as pre-screening patients for contraindications and contraindicated medications are important for building a protocol that weighs safety against diagnostic integrity on a case-by-case basis. Such diligence is necessary, particularly given the increased risk in emergency settings where timely diagnosis is paramount (Figure 11.10).

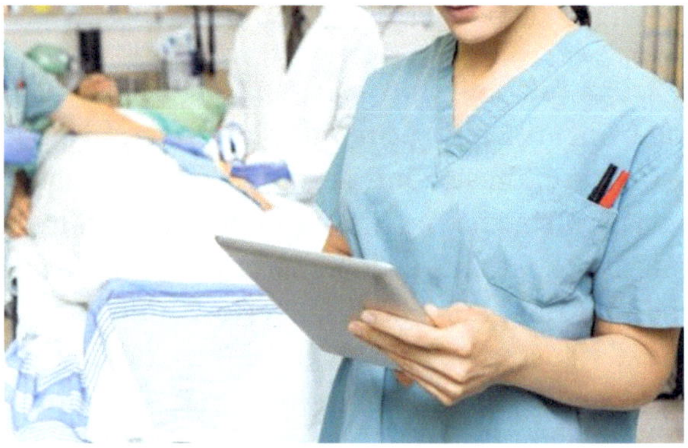

Figure 11.10. Nurse administering contrast agent via IV under radiologist supervision.

Source: https://healthimaging.com/sites/default/files/assets/articles/NurseTablet1.JPG.

A second essential factor of contrast administration in emergency care is the selection of appropriate contrast agents based on the clinical case. There are several contrast agents, for example, iodinated solutions for computed tomography (CT) and gadolinium-based substances for magnetic resonance imaging (MRI), that have varying levels of safety and performance. The selection should be made according to the particular imaging requirements of the case, considering the probability of allergic reactions and nephrotoxicity. For example, iodinated contrast has been effectively utilized in post-partum hemorrhage conditions where vascular imaging is most critical, as evidenced by studies showing its utilization in pelvic artery embolization procedures (Renzo et al., 2015). Additionally, the availability of emergency procedures on a timely basis makes it easy to treat any adverse reaction promptly, underscoring the importance of well-trained staff and equipment for imaging procedures. Instituting proper post-administration monitoring protocols is also of utmost concern in contrast to administration protocols. Post-imaging, patients must be monitored for any delayed allergy or renal complications that may occur, particularly after the administration of iodinated contrast media. Proper hydration protocols coupled with clinical monitoring minimize contrast-induced nephropathy risks—a critical concern in emergency procedures with high volume contrast (Acosta et al., 2020). In addition, institutional guidelines may have documented records of patient reactions and outcomes that may be utilized to enhance subsequent guidelines as well as improve the overall body of knowledge in terms of contrast safety. These guideline updates, aside from enhancing individual patient care, also assist in enhancing the efficiency of imaging procedures overall for emergency and trauma settings and ultimately patient outcomes via evidence-based procedural guidelines.

11.4. Challenges in Emergency Imaging

Under emergency imaging conditions, there are many barriers to providing timely and accurate diagnostics. One of the challenges is the heterogeneity of imaging protocols across various hospitals. The differences may lead to confusion among healthcare professionals, especially in contexts of high-pressure situations like trauma centers where quick action needs to be taken. Furthermore, the rapid emergence of imaging technologies makes the training and transformation of healthcare professionals a continuous process. Without education about new technology or methods, medical professionals cannot utilize these innovations effectively, ultimately compromising patient care. Ensuring all members of staff are fully updated with current and new procedures is crucial to the improvement of outcomes in emergencies, supporting the necessity of well-structured and standardized training programs in facilities (Kim et al., 2014). The integration of point-of-care ultrasound (POCUS) into emergency imaging algorithms has potential benefits but also drawbacks. Although POCUS can significantly enhance diagnostics through the provision of real-time imaging at the bedside, integration is not without challenge. Poor-resource environments are often accompanied by barriers such as the unavailability of trained personnel and equipment that is equally lacking. Also, while POCUS guidelines have been shown to be valuable in such fields as tropical infectious diseases, they are less studied in other critical fields. This paucity of research serves to underscore the need for large-scale studies that validate the application of POCUS in trauma and emergency settings. By eliminating these training and technical deficits, healthcare facilities can make the most of POCUS in emergency imaging, delivering quality care to patients regardless of their socioeconomic or geographic circumstances (Abdalla et al., 2015).

Additionally, the variability in patient characteristics has a significant impact on emergency imaging outcomes. The patients' age, size, and existing health conditions can hamper proper interpretation of the image and compliance with the protocols set. For instance, pediatric patients will react differently to certain imaging techniques than adults, necessitating specialist protocols tailored to their needs. Such complication is compounded by the occurrence of comorbid conditions, which make imaging appearances nonspecific and lead to misdiagnosis. Imaging protocols in emergencies should therefore be adaptable and based on proper knowledge of patient demographics. There must be collaborative efforts to create enhanced imaging standards applicable across a range of populations, with the main priority on continuous monitoring and optimization within emergency and trauma imaging protocols (Kim et al., 2014).

11.4.1. Time Limitations in Emergency Situations

In emergency settings, time constraints are a significant force behind the decision-making protocols that guide imaging guidelines. Emergency settings need urgent assessment and intervention due to the unpredictable course of trauma and medical emergencies. Given the need to provide timely diagnoses, health care providers typically work under tremendous pressure to expedite imaging procedures without compromising patient safety or diagnostic accuracy. Delays in the procurement of required imaging can lead to negative outcomes like higher morbidity and mortality. For instance, operations conducted under emergency conditions are strongly associated with higher operative mortality, underscoring the need for efficient imaging protocols that enable swift surgical intervention (Chu et al., 2010). Hence, it becomes crucial to develop smooth communication and workflow enhancements for the purpose of lessening imaging delays so that patients are offered timely and appropriate care in relation to the urgency of their conditions (Figure 11.11).

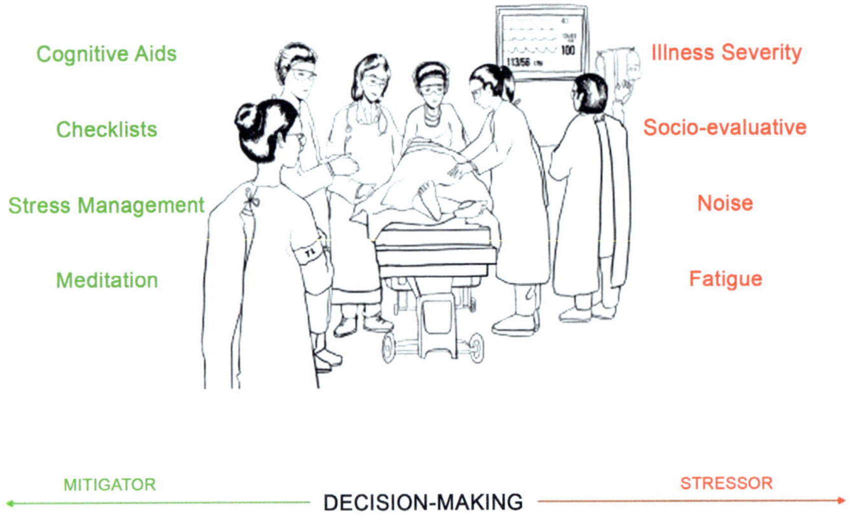

Figure 11.11. Illustrates decision-making under time pressure in trauma rooms.

Source: https://ars.els-cdn.com/content/image/1-s2.0-S0300957219306343-gr2.jpg.

Moreover, sophisticated imaging equipment can make it more problematic to manage time in the setting of emergencies. The more sophisticated the technology, the more machinery is able to generate, which may have a gigantic impact on the options of treatments. Nevertheless, the urgency of quick interpretation of sophisticated images may reinforce the pressure of time. Automated surgical tools, such as robotic platforms that rely on high-end imaging modalities, can be a blessing and a curse in relieving such time constraints. While the systems can enhance accuracy and efficiency in emergency care scenarios, careful consideration of human-robot interaction and workflow in emergency settings is needed (Das et al., 2017). Therefore, weighing the advantages of high-tech imaging against the mandates of timely patient treatment is an intrinsic concern in emergency imaging protocol design. Lastly, time factors extend beyond individual patient care and impact system-wide efficiencies of emergency medical treatment. In resource-limited environments, in which the capabilities of emergency treatment are generally strained, creating effective imaging protocols assumes greater significance. The analysis of surgical programs in developing countries using the retrospective methodology illustrates how early imaging and successful surgical interventions are correlated, particularly in emergency situations (Chu et al., 2010). This underscores the need for healthcare systems to prioritize developing protocols that address the complexity of urgent imaging across diverse settings. Through the implementation of strategic initiatives that remove bottlenecks and streamline imaging procedures, healthcare professionals are able to make a radical difference in patient outcomes, ultimately reconfiguring the direction of emergency and trauma care. That such guidelines are context-sensitive and evidence-based is essential for maximizing the delivery of urgent medical care against the relentless pressure of emergency care.

11.4.2. Patient Safety and Radiation Exposure

In the context of trauma and emergency imaging, patient safety is the utmost concern, including that of radiation exposure. The request for computed tomography (CT) scans has skyrocketed because they can quickly give essential information in emergency circumstances. Yet the hazards of radiation exposure require striking a precise balance between obtaining key diagnostic information and protecting patient well-being. Clinicians are wise to use imaging protocols that minimize radiation without sacrificing diagnostic usefulness (Figure 11.12).

Body Region Scanned	Radiation Exposure (mSv)
Head	2
C-spine	4
CTA neck	4
Facial Bones	5
Chest	7
CTA chest	15
Abdomen and Pelvis	14

Figure 11.12. Cumulative radiation dose in emergency trauma imaging procedures.

Source: https://www.jlgh.org/getattachment/Past-Issues/Volume-7---Issue-1/Radiation-Exposure-in-Trauma-Patients/wutable1.jpg.aspx?width=450&height=215.

This is particularly critical in vulnerable groups, such as children, who are most likely to be at risk of radiation-induced carcinogenesis late effects. Thus, there is a need for accurate guidelines and regulations to steer doctors toward more cautious use of imaging technologies. Current studies highlight the importance of adhering to established imaging guidelines to optimize patient protection against radiation while balancing radiation exposure. For instance, the Pediatric Emergency Care Applied Research Network (PECARN) guidelines recommend screening for head CT scans in children with minor head injury. In a retrospective analysis, it was demonstrated that while more subjects met these criteria before the publication of guidelines, there is still significant room for improvement in compliance after guideline introduction. Despite PECARN's recommendations for more selectivity, incidental findings that may lead to anxiety and additional interventions were reported to still occur frequently. This underscores the need for ongoing education and awareness among clinicians of these guidelines to enhance patient outcomes and reduce unnecessary radiation exposure (Bingham et al., 2020). In addition to the clinical guidelines that govern imaging practice, research and quality improvement activities remain important in enhancing patient safety for emergency imaging. Incidental findings are ethical dilemmas that must be handled cautiously because, although they sometimes point to a serious health problem, they can also lead to unwarranted psychological distress in patients. Health centers should thus integrate multidisciplinary approaches through the assessment of imaging methods and the incorporation of education programs aimed at radiation safety. Advanced imaging devices such as MRI and ultrasound may also provide alternative methods with low risks as they do not necessitate the use of ionizing radiation. Continued quality measure improvement will result in imaging protocols evolving in directions that make patients safer and lower radiation exposure risks in trauma and emergency care (Kitsiou et al., 2013).

11.4.3. Institutional-Level Variation in Imaging Protocols

The absence of standardization in imaging protocols across institutions remains the biggest challenge in emergency and trauma medicine. Every institution would develop its own set of imaging guidelines based on local practices, resources, and populations, resulting in variability in the quality and specificity of imaging. Such variability may result in overuse and underuse of imaging modalities, thereby affecting patient outcomes. For instance, one center might implement a highly aggressive imaging policy for certain types of trauma, while another institution might adopt a more conservative policy, potentially overlooking bad injuries. Controlling this variability is necessary to standardize care to the point that all patients receive timely and appropriate evaluation without exposing them to errors arising from these different protocols (Figure 11.13).

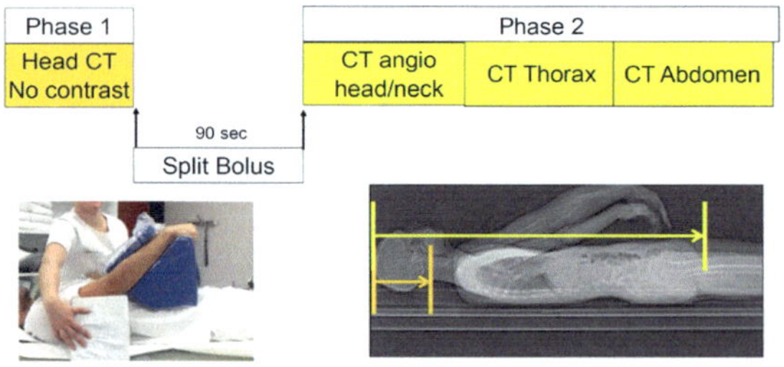

Figure 11.13. The protocol for whole-body CT scans in trauma patients.

Source: https://media.springernature.com/lw685/springer-static/image/art%3A10.1007%2Fs00068-021-01862-2/MediaObjects/68_2021_1862_Fig2_HTML.png.

In recent years, efforts to standardize imaging protocols have increased, particularly in more complex areas such as pediatric practice. The case in point is that of Pediatric Cervical Spine Injury (PCSI), which saw a study report on the variability in use of CT across institutions. Prior to the institution of an updated institutional protocol, CT scans for PCSI were improperly ordered 54% of the time. Following implementation, there was a considerable reduction in unnecessary CT orders, and rates of compliance greatly improved, providing evidence of the effectiveness of evidence-based guidelines. These projects demonstrate how harmonizing imaging protocols will improve compliance with clinical guidelines without exposure to unnecessary radiation, particularly important for high-risk populations such as children (Grether-Jones et al., 2025).

Data such as the RSNA Abdominal Traumatic Injury CT (RATIC) also provide a wide structure for inferring the effects of variation in imaging protocols. The RATIC dataset provides a wide range of adult abdominal CT scans and establishes standardized annotations created by expert radiologists. The annotations allow for better understanding of traumatic injuries and provide consistency across institutions. By using tools such as the RATIC dataset, institutions can implement more standardized procedures, reducing the room for error in diagnostic imaging for traumatic injury assessments. Besides, the collective setting of such datasets encourages sharing the best practices. It enables innovations in machine learning algorithms that can improve diagnosis ability, hence closing the gap resulting from inconsistency in protocols (Afat et al., 2024).

11.5. Advances in Imaging Technology

The advancement of imaging technology has also essentially transformed emergency and trauma imaging guidelines significantly, enhancing the speed and accuracy of diagnosis in emergency scenarios. Advances such as computed tomography (CT) and magnetic resonance imaging (MRI) have improved on the ability of medical professionals to obtain clear and accurate images of the internal parts of the body. The modalities form part of the evaluation of trauma cases, enabling quick assessments that are pivotal in the delivery of effective intervention. The introduction of high-definition imaging modalities and software technologies has reduced the time required for image acquisition, making it easier to streamline emergency department workflows. This technology helps make decisions in a timely fashion, ensuring patients are treated promptly and according to their needs. As imaging continues to advance, it becomes ever more important for emergency protocols to be improved, with better trauma management outcomes. Moreover, the utilization of established standards, for example, the Pediatric Emergency Care Applied Research Network (PECARN) criteria, depicts how imaging technology has influenced practice. PECARN standards were developed to guide clinicians in determining whether CT scans should be used in young people presenting with head trauma, a highly vulnerable population. Post-publication evidence has highlighted inconsistencies in the use of these protocols, as indicated by a study that quantified imaging trends over different periods. Findings revealed reduced usage of unnecessary CT scans upon the implementation of PECARN guidelines, which is an indication of the effectiveness of protocols in enhancing imaging use. Notably, a retrospective study supported that, while the controversies surrounding incidental findings on CTs were prevalent, clinicians prioritized evidence-based guidelines, exemplifying heightened criticality in imaging decisions to minimize risk and optimize patient care (Bingham et al., 2020).

Last but not least, further imaging modality research using artificial intelligence (AI) and machine learning algorithms can help to refine emergency imaging protocols further. These technologies will assist in radiology by automatically reviewing images, detecting patterns, and alerting to abnormalities for urgent review. With improving AI algorithms, they can also assist in reducing missed diagnoses and improving overall patient outcomes. This integration of newer technologies into emergency and trauma settings presents the future of medical imaging, where greater accuracy and speed could be the new standard. Hence, emergency departments must adapt their protocols in such a way that they incorporate these innovations to facilitate imaging practices to keep up with the latest innovations. Hence, the interaction of more sophisticated imaging technology with emergency protocol development will ultimately lead to improved trauma care and enhanced patient safety (N/A, 2002).

11.5.1. Innovations in Imaging Equipment

Technological advancements in imaging have, in turn, had a great impact on emergency and trauma imaging practice, in which correct diagnosis must be made as soon as possible. Enhanced imaging equipment, such as point-of-care ultrasound scanners and advanced computed tomography (CT) scanners, enables faster evaluation in the area of care. Such advancements enhance the skill of emergency medical responders to make sound decisions in time. For instance, point-of-care ultrasound can be used in the field to detect fluid buildup or organ injury, which is absolutely essential for trauma evaluations. Also, technologies like dual-energy CT and high-definition imaging enhance the visualization of complex injuries, significantly improving the overall diagnostic process and outcomes. As hospitals adopt these novel imaging techniques, educating personnel in their use moves to the forefront to maximize impact and reduce time to treatment, thus revolutionizing emergency care models (Kitsiou et al., 2013). Another significant development is the integration of artificial intelligence (AI) into imaging protocols, which assumes a revolutionary function in radiology image interpretation (Figure 11.14).

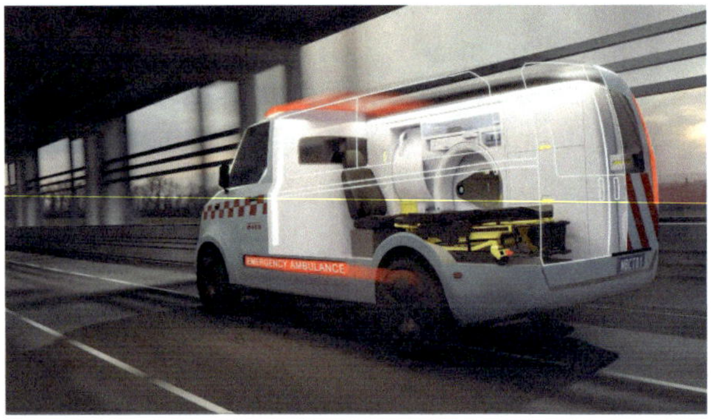

Figure 11.14. State-of-the-art mobile CT scanner deployed in an emergency vehicle.

Source: https://cdn.prod.website-files.com/6668118baa010ac66aad292b/66e7c7ed9d75b459c90faeb6_image1.jpg.

AI software can quickly analyze big amounts of imaging information in minutes, picking up on patterns and anomalies that human radiologists can overlook. AI can automatically assess case severity by examining first-in films and promptly route higher-priority cases to the most severe patients. AI use is particularly vital in emergency departments where case volume risks overwhelming radiology staff. Additionally, AI algorithms can provide timely advice and recommendations, improving the accuracy of diagnostic protocols. This technology not only enhances the role of the human element in diagnostics but also streamlines work procedures, ultimately contributing to improved patient management and treatment regimens in trauma settings (Alexandrov et al., 2023).

Additionally, improvements in imaging devices like magnetic resonance imaging (MRI) and hybrid imaging equipment, for example, PET/CT, are transforming post-trauma assessment practices. MRIs have traditionally been less convenient in emergencies due to their slower scan times and prerequisites; however, technology is reducing these obstacles, making it possible to perform rapid MRI scans for acute injuries. These technologies enable accurate soft-tissue evaluation and aid in identifying conditions that cannot be detected on standard imaging scans. Hybrid imaging also facilitates combined anatomical and functional assessment, thus allowing holistic information on patient status. With such technologies increasingly being used in emergency intervention, they can potentially maximize diagnosis and improve management strategies, so patients with trauma are treated with the best possible results (Kitsiou et al., 2013).

11.5.2. Role of Artificial Intelligence in Imaging

The use of artificial intelligence (AI) in imaging has changed the equation of emergency and trauma procedures by vastly enhancing diagnostic quality and speed. Machine learning computer software can examine vast volumes of imaging data, picking up patterns that human observers would find hard to detect. With this capability, radiologists and emergency medicine physicians can diagnose critical conditions such as internal hemorrhage or fracture sooner, enabling timely intervention. Artificial intelligence-enabled tools can triage patients through real-time interpretation of imaging findings, thus reducing wait times and patient outcomes. Moreover, AI models can improve themselves through repeated exposure to new data sets, thus establishing a convergent learning environment that evolves with new medical practice and knowledge (Figure 11.15).

With advances in imaging technology, the application of AI continues to grow, particularly in the domain of automated diagnosis. These systems utilize convolutional neural networks and other types of AI models to process images from various modalities like CT scans and MRIs. These systems have the potential to aid in detecting fine changes or abnormalities indicative of trauma that might be life-threatening, thus aiding the clinical decision process.

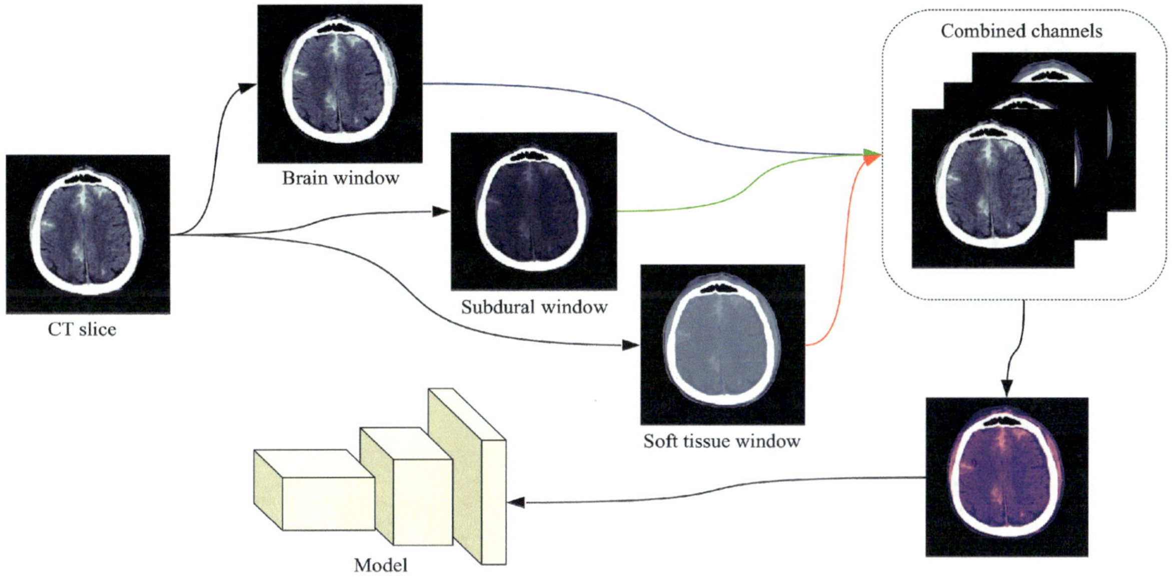

Figure 11.15. Artificial Intelligence interface highlighting automatic hemorrhage detection on CT.

Source: https://www.mdpi.com/sensors/sensors-20-05611/article_deploy/html/images/sensors-20-05611-g001.png.

The precision enabled by AI not only enhances the quality of care but also reduces the risk of human error in high-risk environments such as emergency rooms. While AI cannot fully replace the expertise of trained professionals, the application of AI to trauma imaging represents a complementary solution that can significantly enhance patient management plans within emergency departments. Still, the integration of AI into imaging has not been without problems. Ethical concerns regarding data privacy, algorithmic bias, and calls for regulatory controls take center stage. The use of AI systems introduces concerns regarding responsibility and potential overdependence on technology, potentially harming clinical judgment. To better manage these concerns, sustained collaboration between technologists and clinicians is critical to distill AI tools into alignment with the complex demands of emergency and trauma care. The development of robust protocols that incorporate AI without compromising human control will be crucial in making sure that emergency and trauma imaging protocols leverage these innovations without compromising patient safety and quality of care. Such systematic approaches will likely chart the future of emergency medicine, as evidenced by new applications of technologies that augment imaging practice and care delivery.

11.5.3. Future Trends in Emergency Imaging

New emergency imaging systems can potentially transform the speed and validity of diagnoses and treatment by medical personnel in trauma patients. New developments in machine learning and artificial intelligence have the potential to enhance image interpretation, reducing the types of diagnostic errors that occur in high-stakes settings. These systems are able to analyze vast quantities of imaging information much more rapidly than human operators, enabling quicker evaluation and triage decisions. Besides, AI can assist practitioners in identifying latent anomalies that may otherwise go unnoticed and hence improve patient outcomes. By incorporating such advanced technologies into imaging protocols, medical centers can adopt a more scientifically sound approach that is especially suited to the exigent requirements of emergency and trauma cases, which will subsequently pave the way for more future protocols that focus on efficiency as much as they do on accuracy in diagnosis (Champagne et al., 2019) (Figure 11.16).

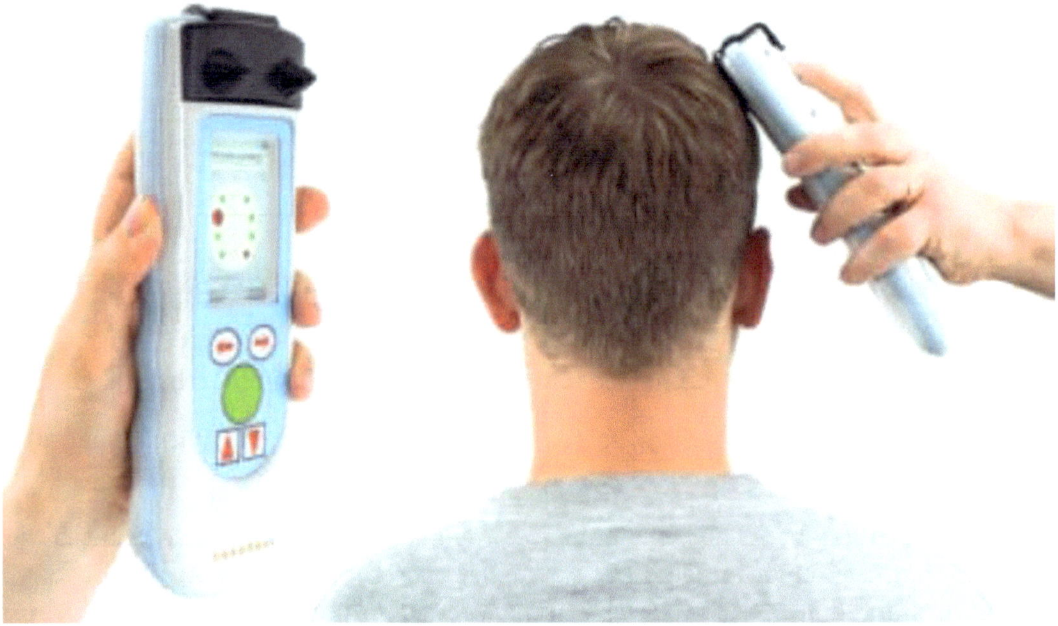

Figure 11.16. Prototype handheld ultrasound device with wireless capabilities for trauma triage.

Source: https://res.cloudinary.com/tbmg/c_scale,w_400,f_auto,q_auto/v1542239274/sites/mdb/articles/2013/features/45601-168.jpg.

Another key trend that is shaping the future of emergency imaging is the role of portable imaging technology in trauma practice. As a result of rising demand for rapid diagnostics in pre-hospital settings, there has been an increasing use of wireless imaging and handheld ultrasounds. Portable equipment allows clinicians to conduct examinations outside the imaging department, thereby facilitating faster patient assessment on site. This shift not only speeds diagnosis of life-threatening injuries, such as internal bleeding, but also supports informed decision-making before transport to healthcare facilities. The growing adoption and use of such technologies are testaments to the evolving landscape of emergency medical services, where rapid access to imaging can significantly influence treatment decisions and patient mortality rates (Eaton et al., 2025). In addition, as the healthcare system continues to embrace telemedicine, the future of emergency imaging will increasingly be about closer integration of remote interpretations into routine patient care. With tele-radiology, images captured in emergency situations are transmitted to radiologists for immediate review, no matter where they are. This integration not only takes pressure off of local radiology departments but also accesses specialized expertise that may be impossible for every institution. In addition, storage of imaging data in the cloud promises greater collaboration among medical personnel with real-time viewing of patient history and imaging findings across platforms. Taken together, these advancements point to an era in which emergency imaging protocols are no longer just about image acquisition but also about creating an integrated, seamless healthcare system that can be effectively responded to in trauma care (Champagne et al., 2019).

SUMMARY

In concluding the review of trauma and emergency imaging protocols, it can be seen that a good response mechanism plays a critical role in improving patient outcomes, particularly in cases involving trauma. Management of injuries is contingent upon obtaining imaging studies quickly, which aids in assessing the degree and type of trauma sustained. This factor is most critical in the pediatric population, where timely intervention significantly affects morbidity and mortality. As evidenced by recent data, optimized trauma response protocols have been shown to benefit patients, most notably by reducing imaging acquisition delays and accelerating decisions on definitive management. These findings underscore the necessity for optimized protocols that improve operational efficiency, thereby enabling healthcare providers to deliver timely and life-saving interventions (Cross et al., 2019). Furthermore, the application of protocol-driven imaging not only simplifies diagnosis but also facilitates a more organized approach in emergency departments. By optimising procedures for the application of imaging modalities, health professionals can more effectively deliver patient care in high-pressure situations where a rapid assessment is imperative. The advantages of fast imaging, such as quicker time to entry into the operating room, further underscore the requirement for continued advancement of protocols for trauma imaging in emergency medicine. Such advancement of protocols is part of a broader commitment to maximizing trauma care and enhancing survival and overall health outcomes of patients with acute injury (Cross et al., 2019). Lastly, the implications of these findings go beyond immediate clinical benefit; they can serve to reshape training and operational models within the setting of emergency care. Simplified imaging protocols can be included in teaching curricula, thereby positioning emerging healthcare providers to address the challenges of trauma care. Furthermore, ongoing research into the effectiveness and outcomes of new imaging techniques will continue to refine these protocols to enable even greater improvement in trauma care. These beneficial effects, such as reduced time to definitive care and increased patient flow through emergency departments, show that investments in trauma and imaging protocols pay substantial dividends in both patient health and operating efficiency.

CLOSER LOOK

EMERGENCY AND TRAUMA IMAGING PROTOCOLS

The application of emergency and trauma imaging protocols is increasingly recognized as an important factor for effective management of acute medical disease. An initial and appropriate use of imaging modalities such as computed tomography (CT) and magnetic resonance imaging (MRI) is one of the most important issues in this context. These imaging modalities, in addition to facilitating accurate diagnoses, are also useful for guiding therapeutic interventions. The need for rapid diagnosis in acute settings cannot be stressed enough, as delay can be fatal for patient outcomes. Furthermore, health systems are increasingly facilitating standardized imaging protocols as an attempt to optimize clinical workflows and minimize unnecessary radiation exposure, thus increasing patient safety and care efficiency. Healthcare provision segmentation demands realignment of imaging procedures to align with optimal practice and regulatory compliance (Anne et al., 2008). For SCI specifically, however, more recent systematic reviews underscore the use of MRI in assessing the severity of the injury and prognosis of recovery. According to research, specific MRI findings, such as the duration of intramedullary hemorrhage, may also provide valuable prognostic information regarding neurological recovery. The findings indicate that longer hemorrhages are associated with poorer outcomes, and the diameter of the spinal canal in which the lesion is located may influence the potential for recovery (Aarabi et al., 2017). This data is key to developing imaging protocols tailored to the task at hand that are not only immediately diagnostic but also consider long-term outcomes and prognosticate on recovery. The addition of evidence-based MRI assessment to imaging protocols for trauma, therefore, enhances clinical decision-making and personalizes interventions according to patient requirements. Ultimately, the development of emergency and trauma imaging protocols must be based upon continuous assessment and revision as medical evidence evolves. Ongoing research and systematic reviews are critical components of revising these protocols to ensure they address emergent clinical concerns effectively. Based on the SCI study, a robust imaging paradigm should consider both the short-term diagnostic needs and long-term considerations of injury assessments. Besides, this need for high-quality evidence also underscores the importance of prospective studies to enhance existing protocols, thereby improving functional outcomes and coordinated patient care across the healthcare continuum. Proper implementation of this can significantly enhance the efficacy of emergency services, thereby enhancing overall health outcomes (Anne et al., 2008).

The application of advanced imaging modalities in emergency medical care is now a primary driver for patient care enhancement in acute illnesses. Imaging by radiology used to be mainly limited to basic X-rays and standard CT scans; however, current practices have evolved toward multimodal imaging. Such newer modalities enable physicians to perform extensive evaluation of conditions such as acute ischemic stroke (AIS) and trauma cases. Through providing detailed views of the patients' anatomical and physiological status, these imaging techniques facilitate timely and precise intervention. This evolutionary process not only enhances real-time clinical decision-making but also substantiates the concept of personalized medicine in emergency conditions, thereby transforming emergency care (Liang et al., 2017).

Multimodal imaging, in particular, is pivotal in triage and emergency patient management. Its ability to combine disparate imaging modalities—functional imaging with conventional diagnostic imaging, for instance—offers an increasingly sophisticated perspective on patient states. For example, stroke imaging now routinely employs advanced techniques that contribute significantly to clinical assessment and treatment planning. As emergency department resources implement these advanced protocols, the imperative of continuing education and training comes into sharper focus. Emergency care practitioners must stay abreast of evolving technology and its applications in clinical practice to sustain best practices and achieve optimal patient outcomes. This ever-evolving landscape requires an integrative system wherein imaging not only serves as a diagnostic tool but also becomes the basis for effective emergency management (Liang et al., 2017). Furthermore, the evolution of imaging in emergency care reflects broader healthcare trends that emphasize safety and service quality. With more imaging technologies being used, emergency departments adopt protocols that expedite imaging in terms of waiting time and increased diagnostic sensitivity. Such projects as quality improvement and patient safety rely heavily on imaging in clinical pathways, leading to a shift towards protocols that prioritize efficiency and rapid response. With new modalities such as artificial intelligence (AI) interpretation gaining attention, the prospect of radical impact on emergency care is more and more evident. These technologies hold potential not only for improved outcomes for patients but also potential for future research and development in the realm of trauma imaging.

REFERENCES

1. Kurpad, S., Martin, A. R., Tetreault, L. A., Fischer, D. J., Skelly, A. C., Mikulis, D., Flanders, A., Aarabi, B., Mroz, T. E., Tsai, E. C., & Fehlings, M. G. (2017). Impact of baseline magnetic resonance imaging on neurologic, functional, and safety outcomes in patients with acute traumatic spinal cord injury. *Global Spine Journal, 7*(3_suppl), 151S-174S. https://doi.org/10.1177/2192568217703666Abdalla, A. B., Adler, B., Belard, R., Reddy, B. K., Bonnard, P., et al. (2015). Point-of-care ultrasound assessment of tropical infectious diseases—A review of applications and perspectives. https://core.ac.uk/download/286716207.pdf (accessed on 15th July 2025).
2. Acosta, S., Azuma, N., Bastos Gonçalves, F., Björck, M., et al. (2020). Editor's choice: European Society for Vascular Surgery (ESVS) 2020 clinical practice guidelines on the management of acute limb ischemia.
3. Afat, S., Aweidah, L., Ball, R. L., Becircić, A., et al. (2024). The RSNA Abdominal Traumatic Injury CT (RATIC) dataset. http://arxiv.org/abs/2405.19595 (accessed on 15th July 2025).
4. Alexandrov, A. W., Brandler, E. S., Chapman, S. N., Czap, A. L., et al. (2023). Prehospital stroke care Part 2: On-scene evaluation and management by emergency medical services practitioners. https://core.ac.uk/download/619410174.pdf (accessed on 15th July 2025).
5. Bandeeri, N., Henry, J. A., Meredith, C., Treacy, P. J., et al. (2004). The prevalence of cocaine-associated chest pain in a London hospital. https://core.ac.uk/download/5230488.pdf (accessed on 15th July 2025).
6. Barlas, G., Eadie, L., & Wilson, P. (2018). Tele sonography in emergency medicine: A systematic review. https://core.ac.uk/download/157674756.pdf (accessed on 15th July 2025).
7. Bingham, P., Hook, M., Shah, P., Tsao, J. W., et al. (2020). Implementation of Pediatric Emergency Care Applied Research Network (PECARN) guidelines for traumatic brain injury in a rural tertiary care center. https://core.ac.uk/download/289036100.pdf (accessed on 15th July 2025).
8. Blaz, M., Golebiowski, M., Palczewski, P., Swiatkowski, M., et al. (2009). Is whole-body trauma MDCT justified in patients in good clinical condition but with dangerous trauma mechanism? https://core.ac.uk/download/161629231.pdf (accessed on 15th July 2025).
9. Bloemers, F., Jug, M., Komadina, R., Nau, C., et al. (2024). Thoracolumbar injuries: Prehospital and emergency management, imaging, classifications and clinical implications. https://core.ac.uk/download/653304289.pdf (accessed on 15th July 2025).
10. Champagne, N., Eadie, L., Regan, L., Wilson, P., et al. (2019). The effectiveness of ultrasound in the detection of fractures in adults with suspected upper or lower limb injury: A systematic review and subgroup meta-analysis. https://core.ac.uk/download/187115971.pdf (accessed on 15th July 2025).
11. Chu, K. M., Ford, N., & Trelles, M. (2010). Operative mortality in resource-limited settings: The experience of Médecins Sans Frontières in 13 countries. https://core.ac.uk/download/pdf/9417613.pdf (accessed on 15th July 2025).
12. Copeland, L. I. B. T., James, D., Duinkerken, M. S. I., & Kelsey, J. (2018). Jefferson Digital Commons quarterly report: April–June 2019. https://core.ac.uk/download/220159103.pdf (accessed on 15th July 2025).

13. Cross, K., Fallat, M. E., Laniewicz, M., Nti, B., et al. (2019). A novel streamlined trauma response team training improves imaging efficiency for pediatric blunt abdominal trauma patients. https://core.ac.uk/download/187423820.pdf (accessed on 15th July 2025).
14. Das, N., & Yip, M. (2017). Robot autonomy for surgery. http://arxiv.org/abs/1707.03080 (accessed on 15th July 2025).
15. Dhoot, R., Dohle, C., Donnelly, J., Douglas, L., et al. (2024). Neurohospitalist core competencies. https://core.ac.uk/download/635939728.pdf (accessed on 15th July 2025).
16. Di Renzo, G. C., Epicoco, G., Fischer, M., Gerli, S., et al. (2015). Endovascular management of massive post-partum hemorrhage in abnormal placental implantation deliveries. https://core.ac.uk/download/141695765.pdf (accessed on 15th July 2025).
17. Doornberg, J. N., Duckworth, A., McQueen, M. M., Stirling, P., et al. (2021). Diagnosis of suspected scaphoid fractures. https://core.ac.uk/download/548240293.pdf (accessed on 15th July 2025).
18. Eadie, L., MacAden, A. S., Mort, A., Regan, L., et al. (2016). Remotely supported prehospital ultrasound: Real-time communication for diagnosis in remote and rural communities. https://core.ac.uk/download/80685951.pdf (accessed on 15th July 2025).
19. Eaton, C., Harris, P., Henner, A., Lança, L., et al. (2025). Tuning template for radiography in Europe. https://core.ac.uk/download/159067679.pdf (accessed on 15th July 2025).
20. Epstein, S. E., Gunther-Harrington, C. T., Li, R. H. L., Sharpe, A. N., et al. (2020). Cats with thermal burn injuries from California wildfires show echocardiographic evidence of myocardial thickening and intracardiac thrombi. https://core.ac.uk/download/323070249.pdf (accessed on 15th July 2025).
21. Gauthier, A. K., Shih, A., McCarthy, D., Davis, K., Nuzum, R., & Schoenbaum, S. C. (2008). Organizing the U.S. health care delivery system for high performance. https://core.ac.uk/download/71353608.pdf (accessed on 15th July 2025).
22. Grether-Jones, K., Kohler, J., Murphy, M., Yu, H., et al. (2025). Reducing radiation exposure in pediatric cervical spine imaging for trauma: A multi-disciplinary quality improvement initiative. https://core.ac.uk/download/640801105.pdf (accessed on 15th July 2025).
23. Kim, E., Kuppermann, N., & Tzimenatos, L. (2014). The Pediatric Emergency Care Applied Research Network: A history of multicenter collaboration in the United States. https://core.ac.uk/download/323069086.pdf (accessed on 15th July 2025).
24. Liang, J. W., Matos Diaz, I., Ostojic, L., Velickovic, T., et al. (2017). Acute stroke multimodal imaging: Present and potential applications toward advancing care. https://core.ac.uk/download/155271594.pdf (accessed on 15th July 2025).
25. Loo, J. A., Loo, R. R. O., Shen, S., Wanner, N., et al. (2014). Addressing the needs of traumatic brain injury with clinical proteomics. https://core.ac.uk/download/323079747.pdf (accessed on 15th July 2025).
26. N/A. (2008). Focal Spot, Winter 2007/2008. https://core.ac.uk/download/129069362.pdf (accessed on 15th July 2025).
27. N/A. (2025). Risk of permanent corneal injury in microgravity: Spaceflight-associated hazards, challenges to vision restoration, and role of biotechnology in long-term planetary missions. https://core.ac.uk/download/654686532.pdf (accessed on 15th July 2025).

INDEX

Symbols

A

B

C

I

J

L

M

N

O

P

R

S

T

U

V

W

X